ENDOCRINE PATHOLOGY

ENDOCRINE PATHOLOGY

VIRGINIA A. LIVOLSI, M.D.
Professor of Pathology
The University of Pennsylvania Medical Center
Philadelphia, Pennsylvania

SYLVIA L. ASA, M.D.
Chief of Pathology
The Princess Margaret Hospital
Toronto, Ontario, Canada

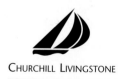

CHURCHILL LIVINGSTONE

An Imprint of Elsevier Science
New York   Edinburgh   London   Philadelphia

CHURCHILL LIVINGSTONE
An Imprint of Elsevier Science

The Curtis Center
Independence Square West
Philadelphia, Pennsylvania 19106

Library of Congress Cataloging-in-Publication Data

Endocrine pathology / [edited by] Virginia A. LiVolsi, Sylvia Asa.

   p. cm.

  ISBN 0–443–06595–0

   1. Endocrine glands—Diseases. 2. Endocrine glands—Tumors. I. Livolsi, Virginia A. II.
Asa, Sylvia L.
  [DNLM: 1. Endocrine Diseases—pathology. 2. Endocrine Glands—physiology. 3.
Endocrine Glands—physiopathology. 4. Hormones—physiology. WK 140 E5582 2002]

  RC648 .E419 2002

  616.4—dc21   00-065823

Acquisitions Editor: Marc Strauss
Senior Production Manager: Natalie Ware
Illustration Specialist: Walt Verbitski
Book Designer: Steven Stave

ENDOCRINE PATHOLOGY   ISBN 0–443–06595–0

Manufactured in China

Last digit is the print number: 9   8   7   6   5   4   3   2   1

This book is dedicated to our teachers, colleagues, and especially our patients, who have all taught us the nature and consequences of endocrine diseases.

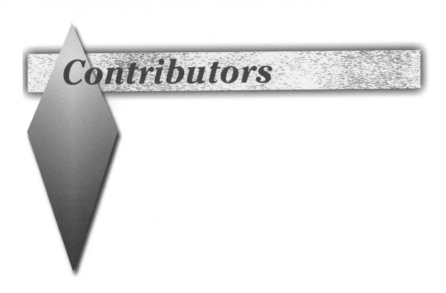

Contributors

ROBYN L. APEL, M.D.
Sullivan-Nicolaides Pathology
Ipswich, Australia
The Parathyroid Glands

SYLVIA L. ASA, M.D.
Chief of Pathology
The Princess Margaret Hospital
Toronto, Ontario, Canada
Pathology of the Pituitary Gland
The Parathyroid Glands

CONSTANTINE A. AXIOTIS, M.D.
Professor of Pathology
State University of New York Health Science Center
    at Brooklyn;
Director of Anatomic Pathology
Kings County Hospital Center
Brooklyn, New York
The Neuroendocrine Lung

ZUBAIR W. BALOCH, M.D., PH.D.
Assistant Professor of Pathology and Laboratory
    Medicine
University of Pennsylvania;
Staff Pathologist
University of Pennsylvania Medical Center
Philadelphia, Pennsylvania
Pathology of the Thyroid Gland

ANA-MARIA BAMBERGER
Department of Pathology
University of Hamburg
Hamburg, Germany
Placenta

CHRISTOPH BAMBERGER
Department of Medicine
University of Hamburg
Hamburg, Germany
Placenta

CAROL C. CHEUNG, M.D.
Department of Laboratory Medicine
Mount Sinai Hospital
Toronto, Ontario, Canada
Pathology of the Pituitary Gland

DAVID E. ELDER, M.D.
Department of Pathology
University of Pennsylvania Medical Center
Philadelphia, Pennsylvania
Merkel Cell Carcinoma

ROSALIE ELENITSAS, M.D.
Assistant Professor of Dermatology and
    Dermatopathology
University of Pennsylvania Medical Center
Philadelphia, Pennsylvania
Merkel Cell Carcinoma

C.S. FOSTER, M.D.
Department of Pathology
University of Liverpool
Liverpool, United Kingdom
Testis

EMMA E. FURTH, M.D.
Associate Professor
Department of Pathology and Laboratory Medicine
Department of Internal Medicine
University of Pennsylvania Medical Center
Philadelphia, Pennsylvania
Gastrointestinal Tract

DAVID B.P. GOODMAN, M.D., PH.D.
Professor of Pathology and Laboratory Medicine
University of Pennsylvania School of Medicine;
Director, Endocrine-Oncology Laboratory
University of Pennsylvania Health System
Philadelphia, Pennsylvania
The Contribution of Laboratory Medicine to the Diagnosis
and Management of Endocrine Tumors

PAUL KOMMINOTH, M.D.
University of Zürich
Institute of Pathology
Kantonsspital Baden
Baden, Switzerland
Paraganglia and the Adrenal Medulla

RONALD R. DE KRIJGER, M.D., PH.D.
Senior Staff
Department of Pathology
Erasmus University of Rotterdam
Rotterdam, The Netherlands
Paraganglia and the Adrenal Medulla

VIRGINIA A. LIVOLSI, M.D.
Professor of Pathology and Laboratory Medicine
University of Pennsylvania Medical Center
Philadelphia, Pennsylvania
Pathology of the Thyroid Gland

IRINA LUBENSKY, M.D.
Laboratory of Pathology
National Institutes of Health
Bethesda, Maryland
Endocrine Pancreas

ANNE MARIE MCNICOL, M.D.
Reader in Pathology
University of Glasgow;
Honorary Consultant Pathologist
North Glasgow University Hospitals NHS Trust
Glasgow, United Kingdom
The Adrenal Cortex

MARIA J. MERINO, M.D.
Chief, Surgical Pathology
Laboratory of Pathology
National Cancer Institute
National Institutes of Health
Bethesda, Maryland
Neuroendocrine Tumors of the Ovary

R. YOSHIYUKI OSAMURA, M.D.
Professor of Pathology
Tokai University School of Medicine
Boseidai Isehara-city, Kanagawa, Japan
Dispersed Neuroendocrine Cells and Their Tumors

ADRIANA REYES, M.D.
Staff Pathologist
Department of Pathology
M.D. Anderson Hospital
Houston, Texas
Neuroendocrine Tumors of the Ovary

ARTHUR S. TISCHLER, M.D., PH.D.
Professor of Pathology
Tufts University
Department of Pathology
New England Medical Center
Boston, Massachusetts
Paraganglia and the Adrenal Medulla

HONG WU, M.D.
Staff Pathologist
Fox Chase Cancer Center
Philadelphia, Pennsylvania
Merkel Cell Carcinoma

PAUL ZHANG, M.D.
Assistant Professor of Pathology and Laboratory
    Medicine
University of Pennsylvania Medical Center
Philadelphia, Pennsylvania
Merkel Cell Carcinoma

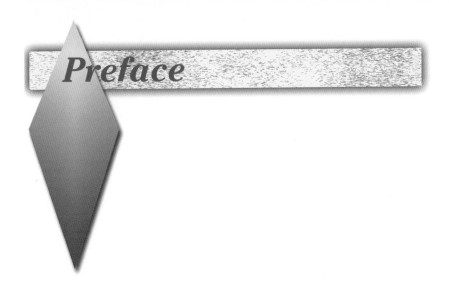

Preface

The field of endocrine pathology has progressed rapidly during the past decade. The specialties of cytopathology, genetics, and molecular biology have been applied to endocrine disorders, and new insights have been obtained. The chapters in this text include classical approaches to the diagnosis of endocrine diseases and information about modern techniques that enhance the diagnostic ability of the pathologist and service to the patient.

This book includes discussions not only of the classical endocrine organs (pituitary, thyroid, parathyroid, and adrenal) but also of those organs and tissues not normally considered "endocrine organs" that can give rise to hormonally active proliferations and tumors (e.g., skin, gastrointestinal tract, lung, and placenta). These discussions maintain the philosophy that endocrine hyperplasias and neoplasias frequently reflect systemic disorders and that the anatomical pathologist must be familiar with and utilize modern techniques to assist in the understanding of these lesions and their clinical importance and relevance.

The authors of the individual chapters are experts in their fields and have been at the forefront of application of this philosophy. We thank each of them and the editorial staff at W.B. Saunders for their efforts in making this project a reality.

Virginia A. LiVolsi, M.D.
Sylvia L. Asa, M.D., Ph.D.

Contents

CHAPTER 1
The Contribution of Laboratory Medicine to the Diagnosis and Management of Endocrine Tumors 1
DAVID B.P. GOODMAN
SENSITIVITY AND SPECIFICITY 2
COMPETITIVE-BINDING ASSAYS FOR HORMONE CONCENTRATION MEASUREMENT 3
CLINICAL APPLICATION OF LIGAND-BINDING ASSAYS 6
PEPTIDE HORMONE HETEROGENEITY 6
LIGAND-BINDING ASSAYS OF THYROID HORMONES 6
AUTOANTIBODIES AND LIGAND-BINDING ASSAYS 6
AUTOMATED LIGAND-BINDING ASSAYS 6
CIRCULATING TUMOR MARKERS 7
CA 125 7

CHAPTER 2
Dispersed Neuroendocrine Cells and Their Tumors 11
R. YOSHIYUKI OSAMURA
HISTOCHEMICAL APPROACHES TO THE DISPERSED NEUROENDOCRINE CELLS AND THEIR TUMORS 11
SURGICAL PATHOLOGY OF NEUROENDOCRINE TUMORS 11

CHAPTER 3
Pathology of the Pituitary Gland 31
CAROL C. CHEUNG AND SYLVIA L. ASA
THE NORMAL PITUITARY GLAND 31

SPECIMEN HANDLING AND DIAGNOSTIC TECHNIQUES 34
CONGENITAL AND DEVELOPMENTAL DISORDERS 34
CYSTIC LESIONS OF THE PITUITARY 35
INFLAMMATORY DISORDERS OF THE PITUITARY GLAND 36
VASCULAR DISORDERS OF THE PITUITARY 38
METABOLIC DISORDERS AFFECTING THE PITUITARY 39
HYPERPLASIA OF THE PITUITARY 39
PRIMARY TUMORS OF ADENOHYPOPHYSIAL CELLS 40
PRIMARY TUMORS OF THE NEUROHYPOPHYSIS AND HYPOTHALAMUS 50
PRIMARY TUMORS OF THE SELLA TURCICA 52
METASTATIC TUMORS TO THE HYPOPHYSIS AND SELLA TURCICA 54
MISCELLANEOUS LESIONS 54

CHAPTER 4
Pathology of the Thyroid Gland 61
ZUBAIR W. BALOCH AND VIRGINIA A. LIVOLSI
INTRODUCTION 61
THYROID DEVELOPMENT 61
NORMAL THYROID 62
GOITER 62
THYROIDITIDES 65
THYROID NEOPLASMS 67
CALCITONIN CELL LESIONS OF THYROID 81
MIXED MEDULLARY, FOLLICULAR, AND COMPOSITE TUMORS 83
THYROID PARAGANGLIOMA 83
ANAPLASTIC CARCINOMA 84
SPINDLE CELL SQUAMOUS CARCINOMA OF THYROID 84

SECONDARY (METASTATIC) TUMORS OF THE THYROID 88

CHAPTER 5

The Parathyroid Glands 103
ROBYN L. APEL AND SYLVIA L. ASA
THE NORMAL PARATHYROID GLAND 103
ADDITIONAL PATHOLOGIC EXAMINATION TECHNIQUES 108
HYPERPARATHYROIDISM: CLINICAL FEATURES 111
PATHOLOGY OF HYPERPARATHYROIDISM 118
HYPOPARATHYROIDISM: CLINICAL FEATURES 133
PATHOLOGY OF MISCELLANEOUS LESIONS OF THE PARATHYROID GLANDS 135
CONCLUSION 137

CHAPTER 6

Paraganglia and the Adrenal Medulla 149
PAUL KOMMINOTH, RONALD R. DE KRIJGER, AND ARTHUR S. TISCHLER
HISTORICAL ASPECTS AND TERMINOLOGY 149
EMBRYOLOGY 150
DISTRIBUTION 150
HISTOLOGY AND PHYSIOLOGY 151
PATHOLOGY 152
ADVANCES IN IMMUNOHISTOCHEMISTRY 152
HYPERPLASIA OF THE ADRENAL MEDULLA 153
HYPERPLASIA OF EXTRA-ADRENAL PARAGANGLIA 154
TUMORS OF THE ADRENAL MEDULLA 154
EXTRA-ADRENAL SYMPATHETIC PARAGANGLIOMAS 159
EXTRA-ADRENAL PARASYMPATHETIC PARAGANGLIOMAS 161
PROLIFERATIVE LESIONS OF NEURONAL LINEAGE 163

CHAPTER 7

The Adrenal Cortex 171
ANNE MARIE MCNICOL
NORMAL ADRENAL CORTEX 171
DEVELOPMENTAL AND CONGENITAL ABNORMALITIES 175
ADRENAL CORTICAL HYPERFUNCTION 178
ADRENAL CORTICAL TUMORS: GENERAL CONSIDERATIONS 184
PATHOGENESIS OF ADRENAL CORTICAL TUMORS 189
OTHER TUMORS 190
TUMOR-LIKE LESIONS 190

CHRONIC ADRENAL CORTICAL INSUFFICIENCY 191
ACUTE ADRENAL INSUFFICIENCY 193
INVOLVEMENT IN SYSTEMIC DISEASES 193

CHAPTER 8

Endocrine Pancreas 205
IRINA LUBENSKY
INTRODUCTION 205
NORMAL ENDOCRINE PANCREAS 205
TUMORS OF THE ENDOCRINE PANCREAS 209
PREOPERATIVE AND INTRAOPERATIVE LOCALIZATION OF PANCREATIC ENDOCRINE TUMORS 218
MORPHOLOGY OF PANCREATIC ENDOCRINE TUMORS 220
UNCOMMON TUMORS AND TUMOR-LIKE LESIONS OF THE PANCREAS 226
PATHOGENESIS AND MOLECULAR ALTERATIONS 228
TREATMENT 230

CHAPTER 9

Gastrointestinal Tract 237
EMMA E. FURTH
EMBRYOLOGY OF THE GUT AND ENTEROENDOCRINE CELLS 237
CARCINOID AND NEUROENDOCRINE TUMORS 241

CHAPTER 10

The Neuroendocrine Lung 261
CONSTANTINE A. AXIOTIS
DEVELOPMENT 261
MICROSCOPIC ANATOMY 264
PHYSIOLOGY 266
PATHOPHYSIOLOGY AND PATHOLOGY 268
CARCINOGENESIS AND MOLECULAR BIOLOGY OF NEUROENDOCRINE NEOPLASIA 272
PULMONARY NEOPLASMS WITH NEUROENDOCRINE DIFFERENTIATION 275
CLASSIFICATION 276
PATHOLOGY OF NEUROENDOCRINE NEOPLASMS 279

CHAPTER 11

Merkel Cell Carcinoma 297
HONG WU, ROSALIE ELENITSAS, PAUL ZHANG, AND DAVID E. ELDER
CLINICAL FEATURES 297
HISTOPATHOLOGY 299
TREATMENT AND PROGNOSIS 309

CHAPTER 12

*Neuroendocrine Tumors of
the Ovary* 313
ADRIANA REYES AND MARIA J. MERINO
PRIMARY CARCINOID TUMORS OF THE
OVARY 313
SMALL CELL CARCINOMA, PULMONARY TYPE ... 319
SMALL CELL CARCINOMA, HYPERCALCEMIC
TYPE 320
EPITHELIAL TUMORS WITH NEUROENDOCRINE
DIFFERENTIATION 322
SECONDARY (METASTATIC)
NEUROENDOCRINE TUMORS 324

CHAPTER 13

Testis 329
C.S. FOSTER
INTRODUCTION 329
SERTOLI'S CELL TUMORS 329
LEYDIG'S CELL TUMORS 336

SERTOLI-LEYDIG CELL TUMOR 339
GRANULOSA–STROMAL CELL
TUMORS 340
FIBROMA-THECOMA TUMORS 343
MIXED AND UNCLASSIFIED TUMORS 344
OTHER TESTIS NEOPLASMS 345
SECONDARY NEOPLASMS 348

CHAPTER 14

Placenta 351
ANA-MARIA BAMBERGER AND
CHRISTOPH BAMBERGER
MACROSCOPIC AND
MICROSCOPIC STRUCTURE
OF THE HUMAN PLACENTA 351
PLACENTAL HORMONES:
EXPRESSION, REGULATION, AND
FUNCTION 352
ENDOCRINE PATHOLOGY OF THE
HUMAN PLACENTA 354

Index 361

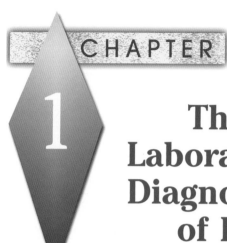

The Contribution of Laboratory Medicine to the Diagnosis and Management of Endocrine Tumors

David B. P. Goodman

The clinical pathology laboratory plays two critical roles in the diagnosis and management of endocrine tumors. First, during the preoperative evaluation of patients, measurement of circulating hormone concentrations provides evidence of loss of feedback loops that are normally operative in controlling hormone secretion. As well, assessment of hormone concentration is important in evaluating ectopic hormone production frequently observed when hormone is produced by tumors outside endocrine glands. Second, measurement of hormone concentration is important postoperatively as a tumor marker to monitor the completeness of initial surgical therapy and the return of disease either at the primary site or as a distant metastasis.

Originally, hormones were categorized into three classes based on their chemical structure: peptide and protein hormones, steroid hormones, and amino acid–related hormones. As new hormones are discovered, this simple categorization does not remain valid: e.g., prostaglandins are produced from fatty acids. Hormones are chemical messengers that send a signal from one point to another in a physiologic system. There are four hormonal communication systems, each with distinct anatomic relationships.

Systematic. In this classic endocrine system, hormone is synthesized and stored in specific cells in a defined endocrine gland. Hormone is released on receipt of an appropriate physiologic signal, a change in some component in the blood (e.g., glucose $[K^+][Ca^{2+}]$), or receipt of a neural signal. Once secreted into the blood stream, the hormone can then travel to a distant cellular target. Frequently, the hormone, particularly if it is a hydrophobic molecule like a steroid hormone, is carried in the blood stream complexed to a specific transport protein (e.g., transcortin for cortisol, vitamin D–binding protein for $1,25(OH)_2D3$). The target cell for a specific hormone is determined by the presence of specific high-affinity receptors for that hormone at the target cell. As a consequence of the presence of hormone at the target cell, a signal transduction process follows, and a specific set of biologic responses is generated. Frequently, some aspects of the biologic response result in a change in the concentration of some blood component such that a feedback signal is sent to the originating endocrine gland to decrease the biosynthesis and secretion of the hormone. In the pancreas, beta cells secrete insulin in response to elevated glucose. Insulin then acts on liver, muscle, and adipose tissue to decrease blood glucose concentration, and the decreased blood glucose feeds back to the pancreatic beta cells to diminish insulin secretion.

Paracrine. In the paracrine system, the distance from the secretion site to the target cell is greatly reduced. Secreted hormone diffuses from the secreting cell to immediately adjacent target cells. For example, testosterone is secreted by the Leydig cells in the testes and diffuses to adjacent seminiferous tubules.

Autocrine. A variation of the system is when the hormone-secreting cell and the target cell are the same. Examples of autocrine hormones are the prostaglandins, thromboxanes, leukotrienes, and lipoxins.

Neurotransmitters. It is now generally accepted that neurotransmitters are hormones, chemical messengers. Thus, a neuron normally innervates a single cell. The electric signal may travel a long distance over the axon. This electric signal is then transformed into a chemical mediator, the neurotransmitter, which is secreted by the axon. The neurotransmitter diffuses locally across the synapse to the adjacent receptor. Thus, neurotransmitters such as acetylcholine and norepinephrine may be considered paracrine hormones.

An understanding of the utility of determining hormone concentration in blood is essential in the management of endocrine tumors. The analytic test procedures are assessed for precision (reproducibility) and accuracy (closeness to correct or true value). A test may be referred to as sensitive (capable of measuring small quantities) and/or specific (free of interference by other substances). These terms are used in quite a different way when describing the clinical utility of a test (see below).

The distinction between a test result being a true positive (TP) or true negative (TN) is determined with reference to a selective normal range based on 95% confidence limits. Because some normal people fall outside this range (*false positive* [FP]) and some with disease fall within it (*false negative* [FN]), the term reference range (RR) is preferred. For any particular disease, attention is focused at either the upper or lower limit of this range, so we are really considering a reference value (RV). A major problem is to define for each analyte the RV that provides the greatest usefulness in the process of coming to a decision. This is called the decision threshold or decision point.

SENSITIVITY AND SPECIFICITY

To properly utilize hormone concentration analysis, several statistical constructs must be understood.[1, 2] These laboratory test statistics are best illustrated as a 2×2 decision matrix (Fig. 1–1). The *sensitivity* of a test is a measure of its positivity, the percentage of patients with the disease that fall beyond the RV (Fig. 1–2). This is 100% at point A.

$$\text{Sens} = \frac{\text{TP}}{\text{TP} + \text{FN}} \times 100$$

$$= \% \text{ of disease cases that give} \\ \text{a positive result with the RV chosen}$$

The *specificity* of a test is a measure of its negativity, the percentage of patients without the disease that fall within the RR. It is 100% at point C in Figure 1–2.

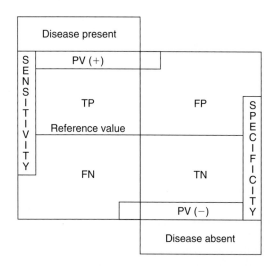

Figure 1–1. A 2×2 decision. The matrix illustrates the meanings of sensitivity, specificity, and predictive value (PV) of a clinical laboratory assay.

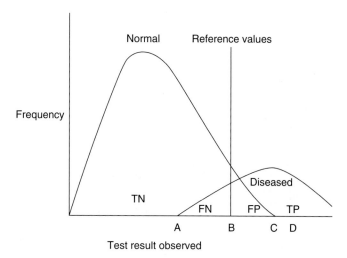

Figure 1–2. Distribution of results for a biochemical analyte in normal and diseased populations. *A, B, C,* and *D* are decision points referred to in the text.

$$\text{SPEC} = \frac{\text{TN}}{\text{TN} + \text{FP}} \times 100$$

$$= \% \text{ of nondisease cases that give a} \\ \text{negative result with the RV selected}$$

Moving the RV toward the normal range increases sensitivity for ruling disease out. Moving the RV toward the disease range increases specificity for ruling disease in. The particular clinical situation will give the optimal choice of RV. Very few laboratory analyses have such high sensitivity and specificity that they are pathognomonic for a particular disease. Tests currently employed utilizing molecular diagnostic techniques to determine DNA polymorphisms may eventually hold this position.

The essential characteristic of any test is its predictive value (PV). PV depends not only on sensitivity and specificity but also on disease prevalence. The PV is also affected by RV and the TP or TN rates. The PV indicates the information that can be gained by performing the test.

The predictive value of a positive test:

$$\text{PV} (+) = \frac{\text{TP}}{\text{TP} + \text{FP}} \times 100$$

The predictive value of a negative test:

$$\text{PV} (-) = \frac{\text{TN}}{\text{TN} + \text{FN}} \times 100$$

Laboratory data are most useful ruling out rather than ruling in a diagnosis. A test with a high PV$^+$ works best in a high-prevalence population. In a low-prevalence population, tests with high PV are more useful. As the prevalence increases, the PV of a positive test increases, and the PV of a negative test decreases. As the diagnosis becomes less likely, the PV of a negative test increases, and the PV of a positive test decreases. Note that 100−PV is the probability that a patient has a particular disease in spite of a negative test result.

The efficiency of a laboratory test is the percentage of all results that are true results, whether TP or TN. Efficiency is expressed as follows:

$$\frac{TP + TN}{Total\ tests} \times 100$$

This is the same as $\dfrac{sens + spec}{2}$

The efficiency of flipping a coin is 50%. A perfect test would have 100% efficiency. Generally, a laboratory test is not worthwhile unless its efficiency is greater than 80%.

A receiver operating characteristic (ROC) curve is useful both in assessing the clinical value of different tests and in selecting the best RV for the test chosen. The ROC curve is based on the relation of the true positive to the false positive rate. It is obtained by plotting the TP ratio [TP (TP + FN) = SENS] versus the FP ratio [FP/(FP + TN) = 100−SPEC] for a series of reference values. One can also calculate a *likelihood ratio,* which is the ratio of these two conditional probabilities. The ratio of TP to FP for detecting disease and the ratio of FN to TN for excluding diseases are as follows:

For a positive test $\dfrac{\%\ TP}{\%\ FP} = \dfrac{SENS}{100 - SPEC}$

For a negative test $\dfrac{\%\ FN}{\%\ TN} = \dfrac{100 - SENS}{SPEC}$

COMPETITIVE-BINDING ASSAYS FOR HORMONE CONCENTRATION MEASUREMENT

Berson and Yalow's[3] observations in the 1950s on the behavior of insulin-binding antibodies gave rise to the technique known as competitive assay. Ligand assay has proliferated because it permits sensitive and accurate quantitation of a variety of compounds (peptides, steroids, vitamins, thyroid hormones, drugs) of biologic importance over a wide range of concentrations.[4] Before development of ligand assay technology, many hormones were measured by crude chemical or in vivo assays using various laboratory animals.

Ligand competition-binding assays have several principles in common. They depend on similar behavior of the standard to be measured and that of the unknown. They depend on the laws of mass action to partition the compound to be measured between the free state and the state of being bound to a binding reagent with a specific but limited capacity to bind the compound. They depend on a means

of distinguishing bound compound from free compound. Many different specific binding agents have been used in ligand-binding assays, including antibiotics, naturally occurring proteins, hormone receptors, and enzymes. All of these binding reagents have advantages and disadvantages. The most important differences in the binding agents relate to their affinity (how avidly they bind the compound to be measured) and specificity (how specifically they bind only the compound being measured). The association constant (Ka) of a binding reagent is obtained by measuring how strongly a compound is bound to a binding reagent. Generally, the greater the Ka of a binding reagent, the more stable the association of the binding reagent and specifically bound compound.[5]

Radioimmunoassay

Radioimmunoassay (RIA) is based on the interaction between a radioisotopically-labeled compound and an antibody directed against it that can be inhibited by an unlabeled compound (Fig. 1–3). RIA is commonly used because antibodies can be prepared to a wide variety of compounds including proteins, peptides, steroids, and medications.

Potential drawbacks to RIA include cross-reactivity of antibody with compounds other than the one to be measured; difficulty inducing antibody to the same compounds; multiple antibodies formed to the antigen in each individual immunized animal and the resultant difference in characteristics or immunologic properties of different antibodies in one animal for a specific compound; and antibodies induced to the same specific antigen in different animals of the same species will vary in their properties, making it necessary to characterize the individual antibodies from different animals to the same antigen. Finally, in an RIA immunologic reactivity rather than biologic activity is being measured.

When an animal is immunized with an antigen, that animal may produce more than one antibody to the antigen. Currently, cell lines are more usually developed that produce antibody to a single antigen determinant. These monoclonal, antibody-forming cell lines—hybridomas—are produced by fusing an antibody-forming mouse spleen cell with myeloma cells. These hybridomas are capable of producing large quantities of monoclonal homogeneous antibody.

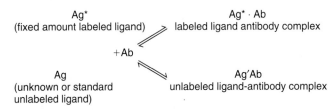

Figure 1–3. Representation of the principle of competitive radioimmunoassay.

This can be contrasted with heterogeneous or poly-clonal antibodies that recognize different antigen determinants of the same compound that are formed when an animal is immunized.[6]

Radioassay

Binding proteins that occur in nature may be used as specific binding reagents. Compared with RIA, these binding proteins have a lower binding affinity and are less specific.[7] Serum ordinarily contains proteins that bind cortisol thyroid hormone, testosterone, and vitamin B_{12}. When these proteins are used in an assay, similar serum-binding proteins must be destroyed by either heating the sample or precipitation of interfering binding activity prior to radioassay analysis. The advantage of radioassay using naturally occurring binding proteins relates to their availability and relative inexpensiveness, ease of preparation, storage stability, and consistency from one preparation to another. The disadvantage of these naturally occurring binding proteins is that they have lower affinity (sensitivity) and specificity than RIA. Binding proteins are also available for a limited number of compounds.[4]

Receptor Assays

Receptors for various compounds have been localized on cellular membranes and in both the cytoplasm and the nuclei of cells. These receptors are generally directed toward the biologically active portion of a molecule, which need not be the most immunologically active portion. Disadvantages of receptor assays are that they tend to be unstable; they must be prepared from a source where they are present in small amounts, then concentrated; the techniques used to separate receptors often decrease the number of intact receptors isolated and may adversely alter the binding characteristics of those receptors; receptors may be altered to recognize small changes in compounds produced by radioisotope labeling, making the labeled compound a less than optimal tracer for a particular assay; receptor assays are generally less sensitive than RIAs; and receptors may be occupied by nonspecific binding agents. Advantages of receptor assays include uniformity of characteristics from preparation to preparation and assessment of biologic activity as opposed to immunologic activity.

Ligand Labels for Competitive Binding Assays

Labels in competitive binding assays have included radioactive isotope–labeled molecules, enzyme activity, fluorescence, and chemiluminescence. The labeled molecule need not behave exactly as the unlabeled compound, but the two compounds must display similar behavior in the assay system.[5, 8]

Immunoassays can be divided into two types: homogeneous, in which free label can be distinguished from bound label without physical separation of the two, and heterogeneous, in which free and bound label must be separated physically before the assay is completed. It is desirable for the labeled and unlabeled compounds to have similar affinities for the binder. If the affinity of the labeled compound is less than that of the unlabeled compound, the sensitivity of the assay will be decreased. Additionally, if the labeled compound interacts with the binder differently than does the unlabeled compound or has biochemical properties different from those of the unlabeled compound, assay results may not be predictable.[4, 5, 8]

Radioactive Labels

Radiolabels have been used in immunochemical assays because they offer great flexibility and allow for extremely sensitive assays. Two principal types of label are employed: beta emitters such as tritium (^{3}H) and gamma emitters such as iodine 125 (^{125}I). Each isotope group has different properties, which form the basis for their being employed in specific assays. ^{3}H has a long half-life (12.3 years) when compared with ^{125}I (60.2 days), and ^{3}H is easily incorporated into organic compounds. However, ^{3}H has several disadvantages: the specific activity of ^{3}H is much less than for ^{125}I-labeled compounds, and ^{3}H, a beta emitter, can be assayed using only a liquid scintillation counting system. Gamma-emitting radioisotopes have several advantages over beta-emitting radioisotopes when used in immunoassays. Gamma detection is possible directly from the assay tube. Because of its high specific activity, less gamma-emitting radioisotope is required for reliable determination of the quantity of isotope in a sample, and counting time is reduced.[9]

Labeled Binders— Immunoradiometric Assays

Immunoradiometric assays (IRMAs) differ from RIAs and radioassays in that the compound to be measured binds to a labeled antibody present in the assay in excess. Free and bound antibodies are separated, often by exposing the reaction mixture to antigen coupled to a solid phase. The radioactive-labeled antibody that is not bound to the solid phase–attached antigen reflects the concentration of antigen in the sample (Fig. 1–4). In some IRMAs, two antibodies are reacted to the antigen being measured. One of the antibodies is coupled to a solid phase and the other, which is radiolabeled, is added to the assay after incubation with the solid phase–bound antigen-specific unlabeled antibody. This type of assay is called a two-site IRMA or sandwich IRMA. In a two-site IRMA, the amount of radiolabeled antibody attached to the solid phase reflects the concentration of antigen present.[10]

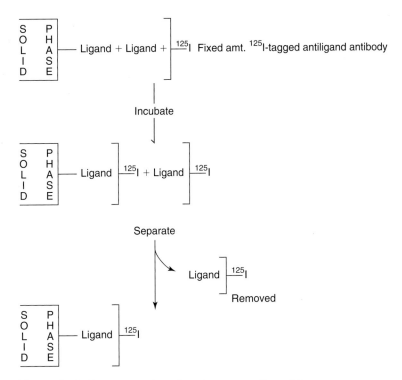

Figure 1–4. Representation of an immunoradiometric assay.

Enzyme Labels, Enzyme-Linked Immunosorbent Assays

Enzymes may be employed in place of radioisotope to label antigens or antibodies. In this approach, analogous to that of RIA, the enzyme is coupled to the antigen to be studied. Enzymatic activity is then determined in either bound or free antigen after separation of the two moieties. Enzymes are convenient to use because they are stable. Urease, peroxidase, and alkaline phosphatase are frequently employed. Enzymes may be bound to antigen-specific antibodies and used in a method analogous to that of an IRMA sandwich assay. In enzyme-labeled systems, in which the antigen is covalently linked to the enzyme, binding of the antigen to antibody may decrease enzyme activity. Thus, by determining enzymatic activity, the amount of antibody-bound and free enzyme–labeled antigen in the sample can be determined. This particular enzyme-linked immunosorbent assay is homogeneous because it is not necessary to separate bound and free antigen before assessing enzyme activity. It is called an enzyme multiplied immunoassay technique. The inhibition of enzyme activity in antibody-bound enzyme-labeled antigen results from either conformational changes occurring in the enzyme as a result of antibody binding to the antigen-enzyme complex or as a result of antibody preventing conformational changes necessary for the enzyme activity. Disadvantages of enzyme-linked immunosorbent assay arise due to enzyme labels hindering antigen-antibody binding, resulting in diminished assay sensitivity. Additionally, enzymatic labeling of antigens and antibodies may be difficult, and naturally occurring substances may inhibit or interfere with quantitation of enzyme activity.[11]

Fluorescent Labels

The advantages of fluorescent labels include their low cost, stability, relative inexpensiveness of instrumentation used to measure fluorescence, and the speed of assay performance. Fluorescent label immunoassays are inherently less sensitive than RIAs. Additionally, the sensitivity of these assays is diminished by background fluorescence. Time-resolved fluorometry minimizes background fluorescence by using a pulse of light to excite the fluorescent label. Fluorescence is then measured during a specific time after excitation. Some fluorescent immunoassays do not require separation of bound and free label to quantitate the analyte being measured. This technology includes the fluorescence polarization method of immunoassay and homogeneous assays using nonfluorescent precursors as enzyme substrate. In fluorescent polarization immunoassay, polarized light excites a fluorescent label. As this label is bound, the degree of polarization of the fluorescent emission from the label increases. The disadvantage of this method is a nonlinear relationship between the concentration of the test compound and the polarization of the fluorescent emission. This type of assay also has a limited concentration range over which the compound being assayed can be accurately measured.[12]

CLINICAL APPLICATION OF LIGAND-BINDING ASSAYS

Discrepancies in Hormone Ligand-Binding Assays

Hormone ligand assays have greatly increased understanding of endocrine physiology and pathophysiology. However, data obtained from ligand-binding assays must be evaluated critically.[13] Examples of discrepancies when clinical observations and bioassay data are compared with results obtained in ligand-binding assays are numerous. Confounding factors may include immunologic or binder-active hormone with diminished biologic activity[14]; biologically active hormones that are immunologically or binder nonreactive in a given assay[15]; immunologically related hormones with different biologic functions[16]; hormone fragments that are immunologically active but biologically inactive[14, 17]; the influence of drugs or other substances that interfere with an assay, such as native antibody, against the ligand being assayed or against the binding agent[18]; and the influence of disease or an unusual circumstances on hormone clearance.[19]

PEPTIDE HORMONE HETEROGENEITY

When a serum sample is treated by various separation techniques and then assayed for ligand binding activity, many polypeptide hormones are found to exist in multiple or heterogeneous forms.[20] Adrenocorticotropic hormone (ACTH) and gastrin-producing tumors are good examples. Neoplasms often produce a very large polypeptide called big ACTH.[21] This molecule has only about 5% of the biologic activity of native ACTH, and it often causes Cushing's syndrome. If native ACTH is assayed following serum fractionation in such cases, the concentration of biologically active ACTH might be underestimated. Conversely, when such a serum is assayed without fractionation, high levels of ACTH might be observed in the absence of clinical illness. This would be due to the presence of an increased concentration of immunologically reactive but biologically inactive big ACTH. In the case of gastrin, normal gastrin (a 34-amino-acid peptide) as well as a 17-amino-acid peptide is produced in response to feeding. Both peptides are biologically active, but the 17-amino-acid peptide is cleared considerably faster. Consequently, a clinical condition such as a gastrinoma could theoretically arise in which the 17-amino-acid peptide was produced and immunologic reactivity for gastrin might be normal in the presence of hypersecretion of gastrin and gastric acid (Zollinger-Ellison syndrome).[20]

LIGAND-BINDING ASSAYS OF THYROID HORMONES

Ligand-binding assay is one of the prime tools employed in assessing thyroid functions. As with steroid hormones, a plasma-binding protein for thyroid hormone was the basis for some early thyroid hormone ligand-binding assays, as is true for cortisol-binding globulin and sex hormone–binding globulin. Therefore, thyroid hormone levels increase in pregnancy, estrogen therapy, and chronic liver disease. However, the fraction of free thyroxine would remain normal. As is the case with other hormones where plasma-binding proteins are present, absolute certainty about hormone status requires measurement of the free fraction of hormone. In assessing thyroid status, currently utilized thyroid-stimulating hormone assays have sufficient sensitivity to accurately assess thyroid status over the entire clinical spectrum.[22]

AUTOANTIBODIES AND LIGAND-BINDING ASSAYS

Assay problems and pathophysiologic states can arise as a result of antibody production to an antigen (hormone or ligand), the immunoglobulin used to assay an antigen, or the antigen's receptor site. The use of monoclonal antibody in immunoassay and the increasing clinical application of mouse monoclonal antibody for targeted imaging and immunotherapy have created a new problem. Treated patients produce heterophilic antibodies against murine antibodies, which interfere with immunoassays. In most cases, the cross-linking of divalent heterophilic antibody to both the primary monoclonal antibody and the enzyme-conjugated secondary monoclonal antibody mimics an antigen, resulting in a falsely elevated value. However, interference with antigen binding by the heterophilic antibodies can decrease the results of an immunoassay.[23] It is known that 15%–40% of individuals may have one or more heterophilic antibodies. Heterophilic antibody interference can be reduced by addition of mouse serum or nonspecific mouse immunoglobulin to the immunoassay, which will complex the heterophilic antibody and make it unavailable for binding to the murine monoclonal employed in the assay.

AUTOMATED LIGAND-BINDING ASSAYS

The pressure to contain costs has necessitated the development of less expensive hormone assay techniques. This cost saving, along with vastly improved assay turnaround times, has been realized recently with the development of automated assays systems for ligand-binding assays. These automated systems vary considerably and generally include automated pipetting, separation steps, assay calculation, and reporting assay data in an appropriate format. The fact that assay pipetting, washing, and quantitation are automated leads to reduced inter- and intra-assay variability.

CIRCULATING TUMOR MARKERS

It is recognized that if metastases are not present at the time the primary tumor is diagnosed, the chances of curing the patient are excellent. Unfortunately, metastasis has already occurred in most patients by the time their tumor is diagnosed.[24] Therefore, early diagnosis or screening before the appearance of symptoms and before metastasis has occurred is highly desirable. Circulating tumor markers have been shown to be elevated several months before the appearance of symptoms. It is therefore conceivable that the measurement of circulating tumor markers could be useful for the early detection of disease or for providing prognostic information. In addition, most assays for serum tumor markers are quantitative, noninvasive, less expensive, and capable of handling a large number of specimens.

Prostate-Specific Antigen and Free Prostate-Specific Antigen

Because of its tissue specificity, prostate-specific antigen (PSA) was the first tumor marker recommended for screening prostate cancer in men older than 50 years. To improve both the sensitivity and specificity of prostate cancer detection, measurement of serum PSA was also recommended in combination with a digital rectal examination.[25] The attempt was to detect prostate cancer at an early, curable stage when the tumor is still confined inside the gland and when the serum PSA concentration is 4.0–10.0 ng/mL.[26] Two new procedures have also been proposed in support of screening: measurement of (1) the rate of increase in PSA concentration over time and (2) the density obtained by dividing the PSA concentration by the volume of the prostate gland determined by transrectal ultrasound.[27] A mildly elevated PSA associated with a small gland may be indicative of cancer, whereas the same PSA value in a patient with a large gland may be indicative of benign prostatic hyperplasia (BPH). An age-adjusted PSA reference range was also found useful in improving PSA screening.[28]

PSA is present in serum in two major forms: free PSA and PSA complexed to α_1-antichymotrypsin. The majority of PSA in serum from a patient with prostate cancer is complexed, and only less than 5% is free. On the other hand, 5%–50% of free PSA may be found in patients with BPH and prostatitis. These patients are responsible for the false positive rates of PSA detected during screening. Measuring the percentage of free PSA or the ratio of free PSA to α_1-antichymotrypsin may help in differentiating BPH from prostate cancer and eliminate unnecessary biopsies.[26]

CA 125

The feasibility of screening women for ovarian cancer by measuring CA 125 is still being evaluated. In most cases, at the time of detection the tumor will have advanced to a stage in which the possibility of cure is low. The diagnosis of ovarian cancer has usually relied on surgery. Although CA 125 is not specific for ovarian cancer, it has the advantage of being elevated at the early stages (stage 1) of cancer development.[29]

Monitoring Therapy

One of the two most useful applications of tumor markers is in monitoring the course of disease, particularly during therapy. The levels of tumor marker indicate whether the patient is experiencing relapse or remission. During the course of chemotherapy, the level of tumor marker may indicate when there is a need for a redesign of medication because some tumor cells have developed drug resistance. It is critical to determine whether any changes in the level of tumor marker are due to changes in tumor activity and not to problems revolving around the precision of the test. Specificity of a tumor marker does not play as important a role in monitoring as it does in diagnosis. However, one must be aware of other benign episodes during treatment that may cause a change in the level of tumor marker because of its poor specificity.

Detection of Recurrence

Monitoring tumor markers for the detection of recurrence following surgical removal of tumor is the second most useful application of tumor markers. Because cancers have been identified in patients being monitored, the specificity of the tumor marker used is less critical than its sensitivity. While monitoring for recurrence, the rate of change of a serial tumor marker is more important than it is while monitoring treatment. The rate of increase of tumor marker concentration becomes a major factor: both the frequency of testing and the therapeutic strategy are largely determined by the rate of change of tumor marker observed. Because the levels of most tumor markers in benign and malignant disease overlap, it is usually too late when unambiguous elevations are recognized. It is, therefore, critical to watch for changes in tumor marker concentration, even though it may still be below the normal cutoff point. PSA is the only tumor marker that, because of its tissue specificity, will indicate the recurrence when it becomes detectable following prostatectomy. Tumor markers are excellent for monitoring recurrences because the appearance of most circulating tumor markers has a "lead time" of several months (3–6 months) before arriving at a stage at which many of the physical procedures could be used for detection.[30] The ease of drawing blood and the sensitivity of the tumor marker assay also make the noninvasive monitoring process appealing.

Individual Tumor Markers

Following is a description of several tumor markers whose utility has been shown in the management of endocrine tumors.

α-Fetoprotein

α-Fetoprotein (AFP) is elevated in more than 70% patients with nonseminomatous cancer. However, AFP is also elevated transiently in pregnancy and in many benign liver diseases, such as hepatitis and cirrhosis.[31, 32] Analysis of AFP and human chorionic gonadotropin (hCG) can help in reducing the clinical staging errors in patients with testicular tumors and aid in the differential diagnosis of various germ cell tumors. AFP is not elevated in seminomas; increased levels rule out the presence of a pure seminoma. The use of AFP combined with hCG is highly predictive for the recurrence of testicular cancer.

CA 125

CA 125 was first defined using a murine monoclonal antibody CA 125 raised against a serous ovarian carcinoma cell line. This epitope is associated with a high-molecular-weight mucin-like glycoprotein expressed in coelomic epithelium during embryonic development and human ovarian carcinoma cells.[33, 34] Elevated CA 125 levels are found in more than 80% of nonmucinous epithelial ovarian carcinomas, such as the serous cystadenocarcinoma of the ovary, but less frequently in endometrial or clear cell carcinomas. It is essentially undetectable in mucinous cystadenocarcinomas.[35] CA 125 is not specific; elevated levels can be observed in pelvic inflammatory disease, pregnancy, and in breast, pulmonary, and gastrointestinal disease. However, the appearance of elevated CA 125 has been found to occur 1–4 months before the diagnosis of recurrent disease.[36] CA 125 is most useful for detecting epithelial tumors, which account for 90% of ovarian cancers, at an early stage and for monitoring without surgical restaging.

Calcitonin

Elevated serum calcitonin is found in medullary carcinoma of the thyroid, particularly after stimulation with pentagastrin. Elevated levels are also detectable in bronchogenic carcinomas; small cell lung cancer; breast, liver, and renal cancers; and carcinoid tumors.[37]

Chromogranin A

Chromogranin A is a major soluble protein of the chromaffin granule, which is a catecholamine storage vesicle.[38] Chromogranin A is a useful marker of exocytotic sympathoadrenal activity in patients with pheochromocytoma.[39] Plasma chromogranin A is also elevated in patients with peptide-producing tumors. Elevated levels are found in endocrine pancreatic tumors, carcinoid tumors, pheochromocytomas, and small cell lung carcinomas.[40, 41]

Human Chorionic Gonadotropin

Human chorionic gonadotropin (hCG) is elevated in serum during pregnancy but present only in trace amounts (<0.3 IU/L) in normal serum. Elevated hCG can be found in trophoblastic tumors, choriocarcinoma, and germ cell tumors of the testes and ovary. More than 60%–70% of patients with nonseminomas and occasionally those with seminomas have elevated free β-hCG.[42] Ectopic β-hCG is also occasionally elevated in ovarian cancer. Increased sensitivity in monitoring recurrence in nonseminomatous testicular cancer can be achieved by using both β-hCG and AFP. Analysis of serum hCG may be particularly helpful in treating patients with seminomatous cancer because no other tumor marker has been found to be elevated in these patients. Seminomatous testicular cancer contains both intact hCG and free β- or free α-hCG subunits in equal amounts. Therefore, only one assay is necessary to monitor these patients. On the other hand, only hCG or β-hCG subunits may be found in patients with nonseminomatous cancers. Measurement of both free subunits and intact hCG will increase the sensitivity for these patients with nonseminomatous cancers.[43, 44]

Parathyroid Hormone-Related Peptide

The circulating forms of parathyroid hormone-related peptide (PTH-RP) include both a large N-terminal peptide and a C-terminal peptide with close sequence homology to parathyroid hormone. PTH-RP induces hypercalcemia by binding to and activating parathyroid hormone receptors. PTH-RP is secreted by tumors associated with hypercalcemia. Elevated levels of PTH-RP can be found in a majority of patients with cancer-associated hypercalcemia. Determining PTH-RP may be useful in differentiating hyperparathyroidism, sarcoidosis, vitamin D toxicity, and various malignancies, including squamous cell, renal, bladder, and ovarian carcinoma. Patients with impaired renal function but without hypercalcemia or cancer may have elevated PTH-RP levels.[43]

Urinary Gonadotropin Peptide

In addition to intact hormone and free β subunit of hCG, a small urinary gonadotropin fragment (UGF) or a 10-kd urinary gonadotropin peptide (UGP), called the core fragment or beta-core, can be detected in urine and serum of patients with gynecologic malignancies. UGF is composed of segments of the β-hCG chain attached by 4 disulfide linkages. UGF may be a product of trophoblast tissue or may originate from peripheral degradation of circulating hormones by the kidney. UGP is immunologically distinct from hCG and β-hCG.

Unlike CA 125, which is associated with serous ovarian cancer, UGP can be detected in serous and in mucinous, endometrioid, and other types of non-serous ovarian cancer. UGP may be superior to CA 125 at detecting ovarian cancers at an early stage. Conceivably, combined use of UGP and CA 125 would improve sensitivity for detection of ovarian cancers.[46, 47]

References

1. Galen RS, Gambino SR: Beyond Normality: The Predictive Value and Efficiency of Medical Diagnosis. John Wiley and Sons, New York, 1975.
2. Galen RS: The normal range. Arch Pathol Lab Med 1977; 101:561.
3. Yalow RS, Berson RS: Assay of plasma insulin in human subjects by immunological methods. Nature 1959; 184:1648.
4. Henry JB, Alexander DR, Eng DC: Evaluation of endocrine function. In Henry JB, ed.: Clinical Diagnosis and Management by Laboratory Methods, 19th ed. WB Saunders, Philadelphia, 1996, p 322.
5. Thompson SG: Principles of competitive binding assays. In Kaplan LA, Pescer AJ, eds.: Clinical Chemistry. Mosby–Year Book, St. Louis, 1996, p 250.
6. Campbell AM: Production and purification of antibodies. In Diamandis EP, Christopoulos TK, eds.: Immunoassay. Academic Press, San Diego, 1996, p 96.
7. Brien TG: Free cortisol in human plasma. Horm Metab Res 1980; 12:643.
8. Hunter WM: Preparation and assessment of radioactive tracers. Br Med Bull 1974; 30:18.
9. Segel IH: Isotopes in Biochemistry in Biochemical Calculations. John Wiley, New York, 1976, p 354.
10. Baker TS: Immunoradiometric assays. In Collins WP, ed.: Alternative Immunoassays. John Wiley, New York, 1985, p 59.
11. Gosling JP: Enzyme immunoassay. In Diamandis EP, Christopher TK, eds.: Immunoassay. Academic Press, San Diego, 1996, p 287.
12. Christopoulos TK, Diamandis EP: Fluorescence immunoassay. In Diamandis EP, Christopoulos TK, eds.: Immunoassay. Academic Press, San Diego, 1996, p 309.
13. Odell WD, Ross GT: Correlation of bioassay and immunoassay potencies for FSH, LH, TSH, and hCG. In Odell WD, Daughady WH, eds.: Principles of Competitive Binding Assays. Lippincott, Philadelphia, 1971, p 401.
14. Faglia G, Beck-Peccoz P, Ballabio M, et al.: Excess of beta subunit of thyrotropin (TSH) in patients with idiopathic central hypothyroidism due to secretion of TSH with reduced biological activity. J Clin Endocr Metab 1983; 56:908.
15. Zapf J, Rinderknecht E, Humbel RE: Nonsuppressible insulin-like activity (NSILA) from human serum: Recent accomplishments and their physiologic implications. Metabolism 1978; 27:1803.
16. Greenwood FC, Hunter WM, Klopper A: Assay of human growth hormone in pregnancy at parturition and in lactation: Detection of a growth hormone–like substance from the placenta. Br Med J 1964; 1:22.
17. CR Kahn: Ectopic production of chorionic gonadotropin and its subunits by islet cell tumor. N Engl J Med 1977; 297:565.
18. Morrow LB: Interference in endocrine testing. In Streck WF, Lockwood DH, eds.: Endocrine Diagnosis: Clinical and Laboratory Approach. Little, Brown, Boston, 1983, p 297.
19. Cohen KL: Metabolic, endocrine and drug interference with pituitary function tests: A review. Metabolism 1977; 28:1165.
20. Yalow RS: Heterogeneity of peptide hormones: Its relevance in clinical medicine. Adv Clin Chem 1978; 20:1.
21. Gewirtz G, Yalow RG: Ectopic ACTH production in carcinoma of the lung. J Clin Invest 1974; 53:1022.
22. Klee GG, Hay ID: Biochemical testing of thyroid function. Endocr Metab Clin North Am 1997; 26:763.
23. Kricka LJ, Schmorfeld-Pruss D, Senior M, et al.: Interference by human antimouse antibody in two-site immunoassays. Clin Chem 1998; 36:892.
24. Berlin NT: Early diagnosis of cancer. Prev Med 1974; 3:185.
25. Catalona WJ, Smith DS, Ratliff T, et al.: Measurement of prostate-specific antigen in serum as a screening test for prostate cancer. New Engl J Med 1991; 324:1156.
26. Cutalona WJ, Smith DS, Wolfert RL, et al.: Evaluation of percentage of free serum prostate–specific antigen to improve specificity of prostate cancer screening. JAMA 1995; 274:1214.
27. Benson MC, Whang IS, Olsson LA, et al.: The use of prostate-specific antigen density to enhance the predictive value of intermediate levels of serum prostate–specific antigen. J Urol 1992; 147:817.
28. Oesterling JE: Prostate-specific antigen: A critical assessment of the most useful tumor marker for adenocarcinoma of the prostate. J Urol 1991; 145:907.
29. Frische HA, Bast RC: CA 125 in ovarian cancer: Advances and controversy. Clin Chem 1998; 44:1379.
30. Chan DW, Beveridge RA, Muss H, et al.: Use of Truquant BR radioimmunoassay for early detection of breast cancer recurrence in patients with stage II and stage III disease. J Clin Oncol 1997; 15:2322.
31. Vessella RL, Lange PH: Utility of tumor markers in testicular tumors and prostate cancer. Lab Med 1985; 16:298.
32. Vogelgang NJ, Lange PH: Acute changes of AFP and hCG during induction chemotherapy of germ tumors. Cancer Res 1982; 42:4855.
33. Bast RC Jr, Freenay M, Lazarus H, et al.: Reactivity of a monoclonal antibody with human ovarian carcinoma. J Clin Invest 1981; 68:1331.
34. Davis HM, Zurawski VR Jr, Bast C, et al.: Characterization of CA 125 antigen associated with human epithelial ovarian carcinoma. Cancer Res 1986; 46:6143.
35. Jacobs I, Bast RC Jr: The CA 125 tumor-associated antigen: A review of the literature. Human Reprod 1989; 41:12.
36. Zurawski VR, Orjaseter H, Andersen A, et al.: Elevated serum CA 125 levels prior to diagnosis of ovarian neoplasm: Relevance for early detection of ovarian cancer. Int J Cancer 1988; 42:677.
37. Austin LA, Heath H III: Calcitonin physiology and pathophysiology. New Engl J Med 1981; 304:269.
38. Aschez-Colbrie R, Hagn C, Schober M: Chromogranin A, B, and C: Widespread constituents of secretory vesicle. N Y Acad Sci 1987; 493:120.
39. O'Connor DT, Bernstein KN: Radioimmunoassay of chromogranin A in plasma as a measure of exocytotic sympathoadrenal activity in normal subjects and patients with pheochromocytoma. New Engl J Med 1984; 311:764.
40. Said JW, Vimadalal S, Nash G: Immunoreactive neuron-specific enolase, bombesin, and chromogranin as markers for neuroendocrine lung tumors. Hum Pathol 1985; 16:236.
41. Eriksson B, Arnberg H, Oberg K, et al.: Chromogranins: New sensitive markers for neuroendocrine tumors. Acta Oncol 1988; 25:325.
42. Saller B, Clara R, Spottl G, et al.: Testicular cancer secretes intact human choriogonadotropin (hCG) and its free beta subunits: Evidence that hCG (+hCGB) assays are the most reliable in diagnosis and follow-up. Clin Chem 1990; 362:264.
43. Ruther U, Luthgens M, Baker H, et al.: Human chorionic gonadotropin in patients with pure seminoma. J Tumor Marker Oncol 1989; 477:88.
44. Tes RK, Lea CL, Oliver RT, et al.: Composition of intact hormone and free subunits in the human chorionic gonadotropin–like material found in serum and urine of patients with carcinoma of the bladder. Clin Endocrinol 1990; 33:355.
45. Bartis W, Brady TF, Orloff JJ, et al.: Immunochemical characterization of circulatory parathyroid hormone–related protein in patients with humoral hypercalcemia of cancer. New Engl J Med 1990; 322:1106.
46. Hussa RO, Fein HG, Pattillo RA, et al.: A distinctive form of human chorionic gonadotropin beta-subunit-like material produced by cervical carcinoma cells. Cancer Res 1986; 46:1948.
47. Cole LA, Nam JH, Chambers JT, et al.: Urinary gonadotropin fragment: A new tumor marker. II: Differentiating a benign from malignant pelvic mass. Gynecol Oncol 1990; 36:391.

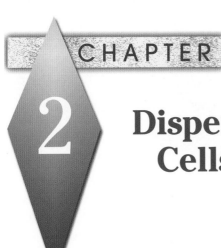

CHAPTER

2

Dispersed Neuroendocrine Cells and Their Tumors

R. Yoshiyuki Osamura

The peptide hormones are secreted not only from the endocrine organs, including the pituitary glands, pancreatic islets, and adrenal medulla, but also from the more widely distributed neuroendocrine cells such as thyroid C cells and gastrointestinal and bronchopulmonary neuroendocrine cells. The latter system is called "dispersed neuroendocrine cells."[1, 2, 2a] Moreover, neuroendocrine tumors occur in nonendocrine organs such as the liver, biliary system, kidney, testis, ovary, skin, auditory canal, soft tissue, and so on. The pathogenetic possibility is that these tumors may be derived from the dispersed neuroendocrine cells. Multiple endocrine neoplasia (MEN) is another phenomenon in human endocrine oncology that has drawn attention from the aspect of genetics and histogenesis. This chapter provides a discussion of the neuroendocrine tumors that derive from the dispersed neuroendocrine cells as well as the authentic endocrine tumors.

HISTOCHEMICAL APPROACHES TO THE DISPERSED NEUROENDOCRINE CELLS AND THEIR TUMORS[3-5]

Tinctorial Histochemistry, Immunohistochemistry, and In Situ Hybridization

Neuroendocrine cells are histochemically detected on the basis of (1) general neuroendocrine characteristics and (2) the presence of specific peptide hormones. For the former, classic staining for argyrophilic (Grimelius' staining) and argentaffin (Fontana-Masson staining) reaction have been used widely and extensively. Currently, immunohistochemical staining for secretory granule–related proteins is frequently used.[1-3]

These markers include chromogranins (A, B, C), secretogranin, and endocrine granule constituent. Prohormone convertases (PCs) also reside in the secretory granules and could be used to detect the endocrine nature of the cells. Other markers include neural cell adhesion molecule and SNAP-25, which are proteins associated with the cell membrane. Neuron-specific enolase is also frequently used as a most primitive neuroendocrine marker, although it is not specific to neuroendocrine cells (Figs. 2–1 to 2–7).

Recent application of nonradioisotopic in situ hybridization has been also used to detect messenger RNA (mRNA) of chromogranins and other neuroendocrine markers.[4, 5]

Electron microscopic identification of dense-cored neurosecretory granules is another tool for diagnostic characterization of neuroendocrine cells and tumors.

Identification of Specific Hormones

The identification of specific hormones relies completely on either immunohistochemistry or in situ hybridization. Immunohistochemistry is now more widely used. Many peptide hormones can be detected using commercially available polyclonal or monoclonal antibodies. In situ hybridizations can be performed using nonradioisotopic techniques with synthetic oligonucleotides. New amplification techniques such as tyramide (catalyzed) signal amplification have been applied to detect minute amount of hormones and hormone mRNA. Reverse transcriptase-polymerase-chain reaction (RT-PCR) and in situ reverse-transcriptase polymerase-chain reaction (in situ RT-PCR) are sensitive tools to detect minute amounts of mRNA. These specific methods are sometimes mandatory for the diagnosis of dispersed endocrine cells and their tumors.[4, 5]

SURGICAL PATHOLOGY OF NEUROENDOCRINE TUMORS

In our practice of diagnostic surgical pathology, we occasionally encounter neuroendocrine tumors,

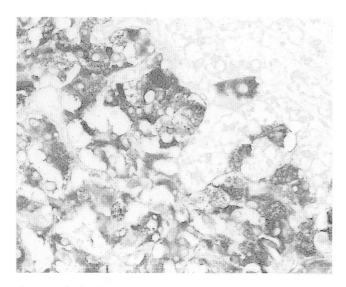

Figure 2-1. Chromogranin A in the human adrenal medulla. Localization in the cytoplasm.

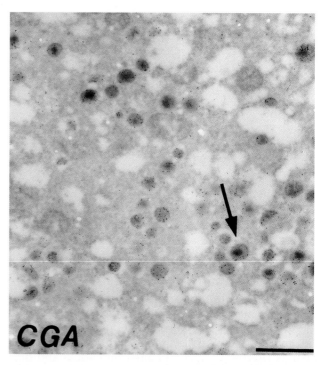

Figure 2-2. Localization of chromogranin A (CGA) in secretory granules of adrenal medulla. Localization at the periphery of the secretory granule (immunoelectron microscopy postembedding method).

which produce peptide hormones and their precursors. These tumors occur in the endocrine organs with eutopic or ectopic hormone production and in nonendocrine organs with ectopic hormone production. The tumor cells usually contain dense, cored neurosecretory granules in their cytoplasm. Diagnosing neuroendocrine tumors in surgical pathology is important in order to detect the source of bioactive substances and predict biologic behavior of the tumor cells.

A. Surgical pathology of the neuroendocrine tumors.[6]
   1. Neuroendocrine tumors arising from endocrine organs can usually be diagnosed on the basis of typical histologic appearance (i.e., medullary carcinoma of the thyroid [MCT], pheochromocytoma, pancreatic islet cell tumors).
   2. Neuroendocrine tumors in nonendocrine organs:
      a. Tumors are diagnosed as carcinoid on the basis of hematoxylin and eosin–stained sections.
      b. Small cell carcinoma should be diagnosed as neuroendocrine carcinoma.

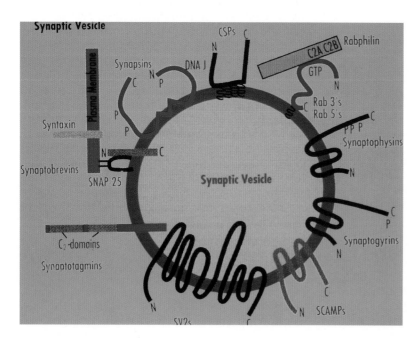

Figure 2-3. Scheme of the synaptic vesicle– (or secretory granule–) related proteins.

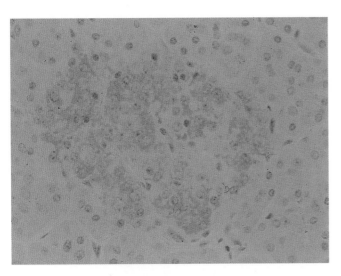

Figure 2-4. Synaptophysin in the human pancreatic islet. Localization in the cytoplasm.

c. Ordinary adenocarcinomas with endocrine cells are identified by special staining. For neuroendocrine tumors arising from endocrine organs and those in nonendocrine organs that are diagnosed as carcinoid, special staining and electron microscopy results are mostly supportive of the hematoxylin and eosin–stain diagnosis. For small cell carcinoma, which should be diagnosed as neuroendocrine carcinoma, and ordinary adenocarcinomas with endocrine cells, special staining, such as Grimelius' argyrophil method and immunohistochemical detection of neuroendocrine markers, and/or electron microscopy are mandatory for correct diagnosis.

B. Neuroendocrine tumors in the endocrine organs: thyroid, pancreas, and adrenal medulla.

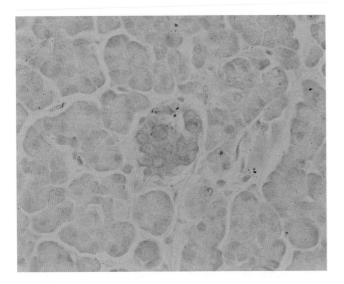

Figure 2-5. SNAP-25 in the human pancreatic islet. Localization in cell membrane.

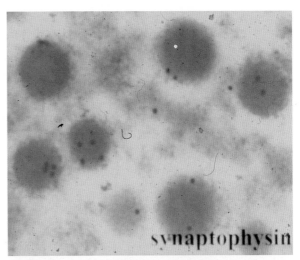

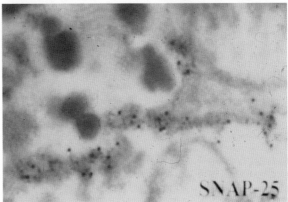

Figure 2-6. Intracellular localization of synaptophysin in the secretory granules and SNAP-25 in cell membrane (immunoelectron microscopy postembedding method).

1. MCT is derived from C cells and produces calcitonin (CT), and carcinoembryonic antigen (CEA) (Figs. 2–8 to 2–11). The tumor is composed of spindle cells and frequently demonstrates amyloid deposition in the stroma. Other peptides produced by MCT include pro-opiomelanocortin (POMC), serotonin, and somatostatin, among others. MCT can occur in combination with pheochromocytomas as a member of MEN-IIa and IIb. In these situations it is important to analyze mutation of the tumor suppressor gene *RET*.
2. Pheochromocytomas are characterized by granular pleomorphic cells with an organoid pattern and sometimes by clear cells. The tumors are well-known multihormonal tumors producing met-enkephalin, somatostatin, CT, and, less frequently, other peptides (Figs. 2–12 to 2–15). The tumors also produce noradrenaline and adrenaline. Met-enkephalin is detected in most pheochromocytomas and has been claimed to be one of the tumor markers. Some tumor cells show colocalization of met-enkephalin and somatostatin. The tumor cells are usually positive for chromogranin A in the cytoplasm and contain dense-cored neurosecretory granules. The

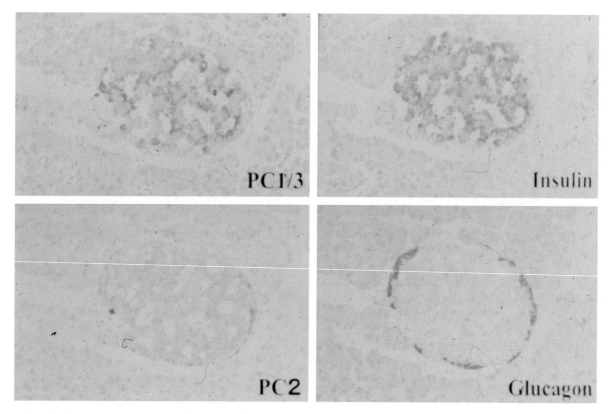

Figure 2-7. Prohormone convertase (PC)1/3 and PC2 in the pancreatic islet. Localization of PC1/3 and PC2 in insulin (B) cells and PC2 in glucagon (A) cells.

pheochromocytomas are also known as "10% tumors," because 10% occur extra-adrenally, 10% are bilateral in the adrenal medulla, and 10% metastasize. The tumor can occur as a component of MEN-IIa and IIb, as mentioned. The paraganglioma can occur in nonendocrine tissues, such as the urinary bladder.

3. Pancreatic islet cell tumors contain various biologically important factors; they are frequently functional and multihormonal. Malignant behavior is usually related to the type of hormone produced. These tumors occur in patients with MEN-I. Neuroendocrine tumors of the pancreas can occur as functioning tumors or as nonfunctioning tumors. Functioning tumors show eutopic hormone production, including insulin (insulinoma), glucagon (glucagonoma), somatostatin (somatostatima), or pancreatic polypeptide. Ectopic hormone production includes gastrin (gastrinoma), vasoactive intestinal peptide, or growth hormone–releasing hormone. Of particular interest in this group of tumors is that the biologic behavior of the pancreatic neuroendocrine tumors is related to the hormones they mainly produce (i.e., most insulinomas are benign; in contrast, most glucagonomas, somatostatinomas, and gastrinomas are malignant, exhibiting metastases). The pertinent clinical and pathologic findings for each type of pancreatic neuroendocrine tumors are discussed as follows

a. Insulinomas are the most frequent pancreatic endocrine tumors and comprise about 70% to 75% of all pancreatic endocrine tumors. The incidence of these tumors is equal in both sexes, and it generally occurs in individuals between the ages of 30 and 60 years. Infants with nesidioblastosis sometimes acquire endocrine tumors in the pancreas. All patients with insulinomas are symptomatic and hypoglycemic. Almost all insulinomas are localized in the pancreas and are usually (90%) solitary, thus making surgical excision a possible treatment. The tumor may be associated with MEN-I. Insulinomas are mostly benign; 4% to 16% are malignant, exhibiting metastasis. Histologically, the tumor shows solid and trabecular patterns and ultrastructural dense-cored neurosecretory granules with characteristic crystalline cores (Figs. 2–16 to 2–18). The tumor is frequently multihormonal, and pancreatic polypeptide is one of the concomitantly produced hormones.

b. Glucagonomas are rare among pancreatic endocrine tumors. This tumor type causes diabetes mellitus and necrolytic migratory erythema. It primarily affects individuals 40 to 70 years of age and slightly more women than men. More than 60% of symptomatic glucagonomas are malignant. Frequently, the tumor is multihormonal and produces

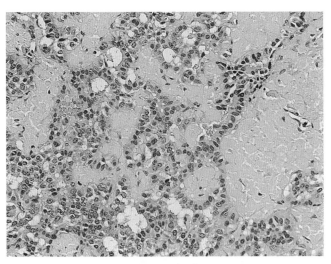

Figure 2-8

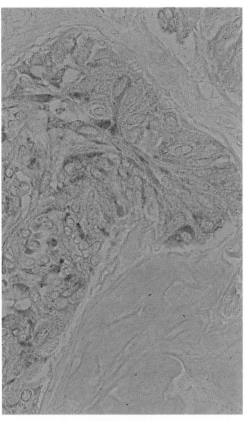

Figure 2-9

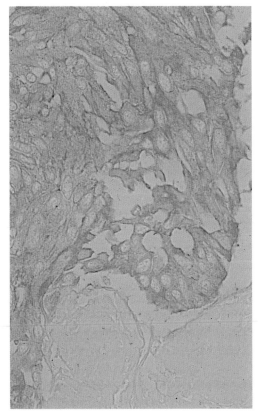

Figure 2-10

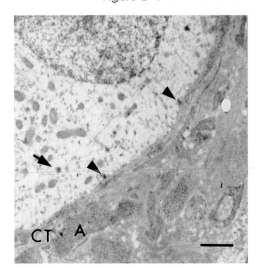

Figure 2-11

Figures 2-8 to 2-11. Medullary carcinoma of the thyroid (MCT). H&E staining shows neuroendocrine cells and amyloid deposition (Fig. 2–8). The tumor cells are positive for calcitonin (Fig. 2–9) and carcinoembryonic antigen (CEA) (Fig. 2–10). Immunoelectron microscopy (postembedding method) shows calcitonin (CT) in the secretory granules and amyloid (Fig. 2–11).

pancreatic polypeptide, insulin, and somatostatin in addition to glucagon. It is sometimes associated with MEN-I.

c. Gastrinomas are relatively rare among pancreatic neuroendocrine tumors, comprising about 20% to 25%. Patient age generally ranges from 30 to 50 years, but individuals between the ages of 20 and 92 years have been affected. This tumor causes intractable ulcers in the stomach, duodenum, and jejunum with bleeding. Gastric acid secretion is greatly increased. The calcium-stimulated gastrin secretion is useful for the differential diagnosis of gastrinomas. Frequent association

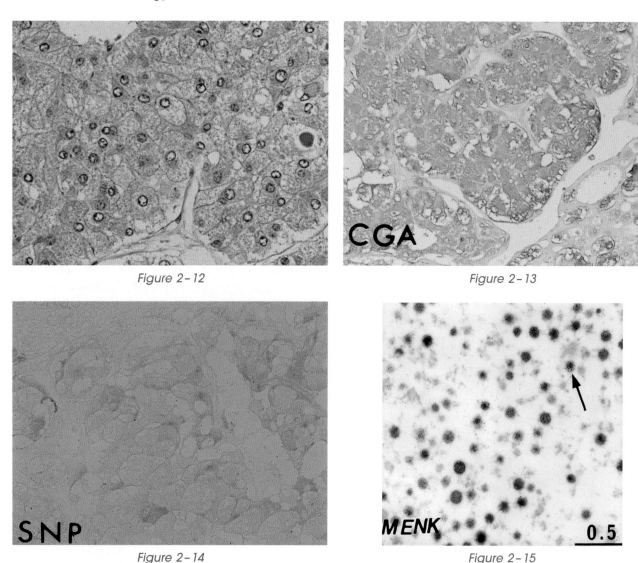

Figure 2-12

Figure 2-13

Figure 2-14

Figure 2-15

Figures 2–12 to 2–15. Pheochromocytoma of the adrenal medulla. H&E staining shows basophilic cytoplasm in the cytoplasm of the tumor cells (Fig. 2–12). They are positive for chromogranin A (CGA) (Fig. 2–13) and synaptophysin (SNP) (Fig. 2–14). Immunoelectron microscopy (postembedding method) shows met-enkephalin (MENK) in the secretory granules of the tumor cells (Fig. 2–15).

with parathyroid tumors indicates the diagnosis of MEN-I. All patients with gastrinomas should have their parathyroid hormone and calcium levels monitored. Eighty percent of gastrinomas occur in the pancreas, and approximately 60% (ranges 70% to 90%) of gastrinomas metastasize, frequently to the liver. Ultrastructurally, the tumor cells contain dense-cored neurosecretory granules, with an average diameter of about 240 nm. The tumor is frequently multihormonal, with the additional production of pancreatic peptide.

d. Patients with somatostatinomas demonstrate diabetes mellitus, steatorrhea, and hypochlorhydria. Some patients experience gallstones. The tumor is mostly solitary and is localized in the pancreas. It is sometimes associated with neurofibromas and pheochro-

mocytomas. The tumor is frequently malignant. Ultrastructurally, the tumor cells contain dense-cored neurosecretory granules. The tumor is sometimes multihormonal and produces pancreatic polypeptide as an additional hormone (Figs. 2–19 to 2–23).

e. Tumors producing vasoactive intestinal peptide (VIP) and the diarrheogenic syndrome comprise about 3% to 5% of all pancreatic neuroendocrine tumors. Patients present with watery diarrhea, hypokalemia, and hypo- or achlorhydria. Two-thirds of patients experience abdominal colic and intermittent high fecal fat output. About 50% to 75% of tumors are malignant. Histologically, the tumor shows islet cell arrangements or ganglioneuromas. The tumors are frequently multihormonal and produce pancreatic polypeptide as an additional hormone.

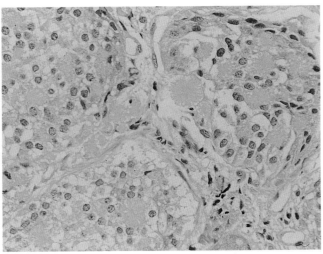

Figure 2-16

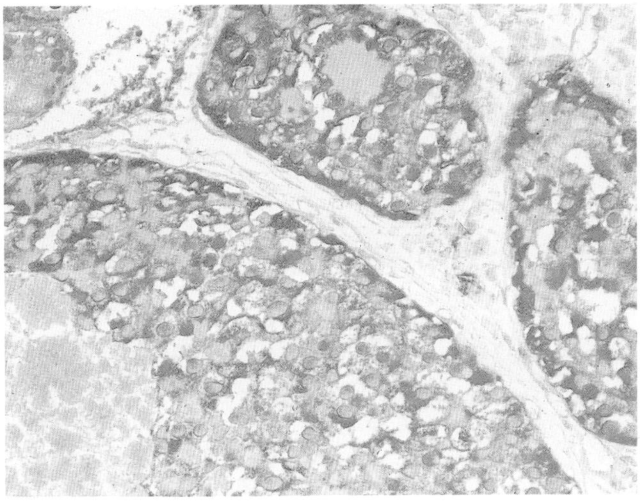

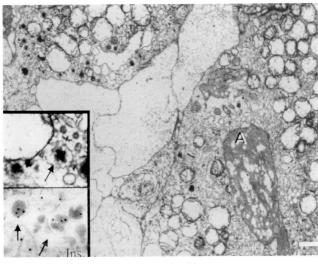

Figure 2-17

Figure 2-18

Figures 2-16 to 2-18. Insulinoma of the pancreas. H&E staining shows neuroendocrine cells and scanty amyloid deposition (Fig. 2–16). The tumor cells are positive for insulin. Amyloid is weakly positive for insulin (Fig. 2–17). Electron microscopy shows the presence of secretory granules, some of which exhibit crystalloid appearance (inset). The secretory granules contain insulin by immunoelectron microscopy (postembedding method) (Fig. 2–18).

f. Some pancreatic islet cell tumors are frequently nonfunctioning clinically. However, at the cellular levels, the tumor cells contain various peptide hormones by immunohistochemistry.

C. Neuroendocrine tumors in dispersed endocrine cells of lung, gastrointestinal tract, and other nonendocrine tissues.

1. Neuroendocrine cells with neuroendocrine markers, hormone production, and electron microscopic demonstration of secretory granules are also identified in systemic organs, including lung, gastrointestinal tract, and biliary tract. In the human fetal lung, clusters of neuroendocrine cells appear in the bronchi as neuroepithelial bodies, which physiologically disappear in adults. Neuroendocrine tumors may occur in the so-called nonendocrine organs. This type of tumor includes the carcinoids occurring in the kidneys and liver, Merkel cell tumors of the skin, and neuroendocrine carcinomas of the breast and prostate.

a. Carcinoids are tumors of neuroendocrine nature and were first reported by Oberdorfer in 1900. This tumor consists of characteristic trabecular and organoid structures with "ribbon-like" patterns. The tumors occur in systemic organs and represent tumors of the dispersed neuroendocrine cells. They are usually classified on the basis of the tissue origins (i.e., foregut, midgut, and hindgut). The carcinoids of each tissue origin are summarized in Table 2–1. Of particular interest, each group

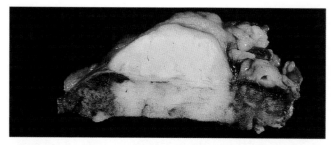

Figure 2-19

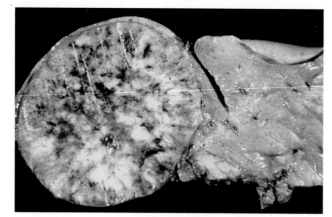

Figure 2-20

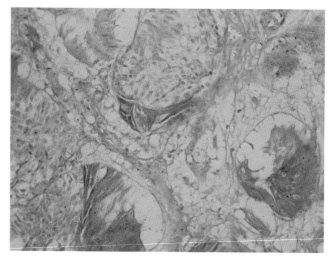

Figure 2-22

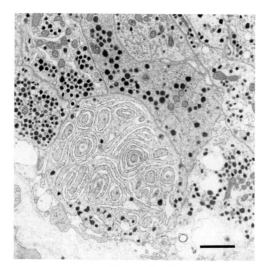

Figure 2-23

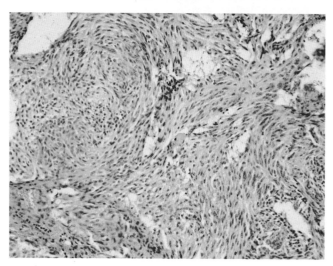

Figure 2-21

Figures 2-19 to 2-23. Somatostatinoma of the pancreas with liver metastasis. Fig. 2-19 shows the primary tumor in the pancreas. Fig. 2-20 shows metastatic tumor in the liver. The tumor is composed of many clusters of mildly atypical spindle neuroendocrine cells (H&E staining, Fig. 2-21). The tumor cells are focally positive for somatostatin (Fig. 2-22). Electron microscopy shows well-developed endoplasmic reticula and a few secretory granules (Fig. 2-23).

of carcinoids has some tendency to exhibit characteristic functional differentiation, such as peptide hormone production (see Table 2-1). The carcinoids are usually multihormonal, especially bronchial carcinoids. The carcinoids can occur in other organs such as the breast, prostate, and middle ear. Occasionally, in patients with type A gastritis, there are diffuse and multinodular proliferations of

neuroendocrine cells designated as "diffuse carcinoids" (Figs. 2-24 to 2-28).

b. Neuroendocrine carcinomas are poorly differentiated tumors of neuroendocrine nature with apparent malignant biologic nature. Morphologically, the tumors frequently exhibit small anaplastic cells with marked nuclear atypia. These tumors occur in the esophagus, lung, prostate, and other tissues and usually contain

Table 2-1. Clinicopathologic Comparison of TBC, ABC, SCCL, and LCNCL

Carcinoid Type	Cytologic/Histologic Features	Hormone Production and NE Markers	5-Year, 10-Year Survival
TBC	Nests and cords of regular cells with infrequent mitoses	CT, GRP, ACTH, α-SU	87%, 87%
ABC	Increased mitoses and cellularity, nuclear pleomorphism, increased chromatin and N/C ratio, distorted, architecture and necrosis	Similar to above	56%, 35%
SCCL	Small anaplastic cells with marked nuclear atypia and markedly high N/C ratio	NSE, CT, GRP, ACTH	9%, 5%
LCNCL	Organoid, trabecular, palisading, or rosette-like formation; marked nuclear atypia; frequent mitoses and necrosis	CGA, α-SU, NCAM, CT, GRP, SS, PP, 5-HT, ACTH	27%, 9%
			Worse prognosis than non-SCCL, even in early stages

TBC, typical bronchial carcinoid; ABC, atypical bronchial carcinoid; SCCL, small cell carcinoma of the lung; LCNCL, large cell neuroendocrine carcinoma of the lung; NE, neuroendocrine; N/C, nuclear-cytoplasmic; CT, calcitonin; GRP, gastrin-releasing peptide; ACTH, adrenocorticotropic hormone; α-SU, α-subunit; NSE, neuron-specific enolase; CGA, chromogranin; SS, somatostatin; PP, pancreatic polypeptide; 5-HT, serotonin.

a few secretory granules in the cytoplasm. In the stomach and, less frequently, in other organs, adenocarcinoma of signet-ring type can occasionally exhibit neuroendocrine features and is included in this category of the tumors.

c. Adenocarcinomas of various organs sometimes gain a neuroendocrine nature without altering morphology. This type of tumor includes gastric tubular adenocarcinoma with histochemical neuroendocrine characteristics, determined by argyrophilic staining, and positivity for chromogranins and synaptophysin.

2. Neuroendocrine tumors of the lung.
   a. Bronchial neuroendocrine tumors include tumorlets, carcinoids, and small cell carcinomas. Large cell neuroendocrine carcinomas of

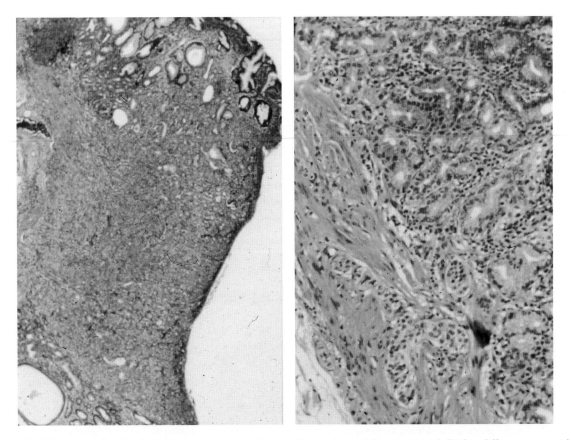

Figure 2-24. Diffuse carcinoid of the stomach in type A gastritis. Left: nodular carcinoid. Right: diffuse carcinoid.

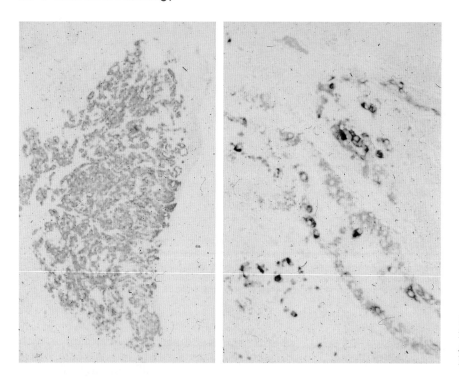

Figure 2-25. Chromogranin A in diffuse carcinoid of the stomach in type A gastritis. Left: nodular carcinoid. Right: diffuse carcinoid.

the lung (LCNCL) are included in this category also (see Table 2–1). Tumorlets are proliferative lesions of neuroendocrine cells associated with bronchiectasis. Functionally, these lesions are immunohistochemically positive for calcitonin (CT), gastrin-releasing peptide (GRP), and adrenocorticotropic hormone (ACTH). These cells are considered to be a reactive proliferation of neuroendocrine cells in inflammatory lesions.

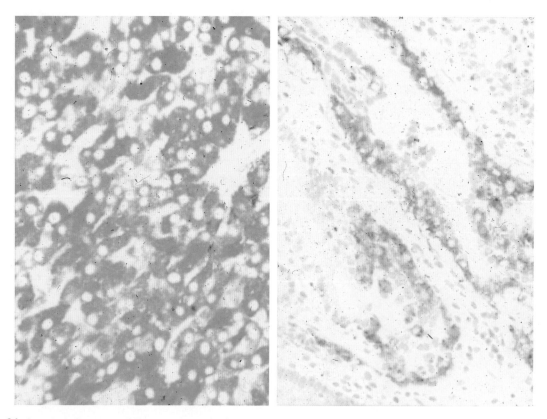

Figure 2-26. Synaptophysin in diffuse carcinoid of the stomach in type A gastritis. Left: nodular carcinoid. Right: diffuse carcinoid.

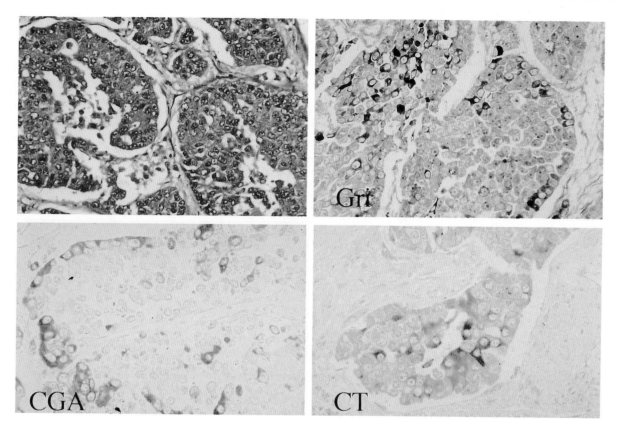

Figure 2-27. Large cell neuroendocrine carcinoma of the lung. Left upper: H&E staining. Right upper: Argyrophilia in the tumor cells (Grimelius' staining) (Gri). Left lower: Chromogranin A (CGA) in the tumor cells. Right lower: Calcitonin (CT) in the tumor cells.

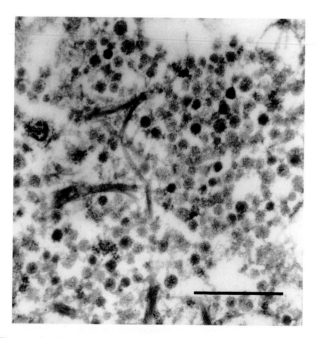

Figure 2-28. Electron microscopy shows many small secretory granules (from formalin-fixed tissue).

(1) Bronchial carcinoids occur mostly in individuals younger than 40 years, with an equal incidence in both sexes. Bronchial carcinoids are neoplastic lesions of bronchial neuroendocrine cells (frequently designated as Kulchitsky cells) and are immunohistochemically multihormonal, including CT, GRP, ACTH, and α-subunit. Occasionally, bronchial carcinoids occur in patients with MEN. The carcinoids are usually found in the main bronchus as polypoid tumors. Microscopically, these tumors are composed of nests and cords of regular cells with infrequent mitoses. Clinically, the bronchial carcinoids give rise to symptoms such as cough caused by intramural polypoid growths. Forty percent of carcinoids show to metastasis to the regional lymph nodes, and 5% to 10% show metastasis to the liver, causing hepatomegaly. The ability[7] to elaborate serotonin occasionally causes carcinoid syndrome.

(2) Atypical bronchial carcinoid is characterized by increased mitoses, nuclear pleomorphism, increased chromatin, increased nuclear-cytoplasmic ratio, increased cellularity and distorted architecture, and

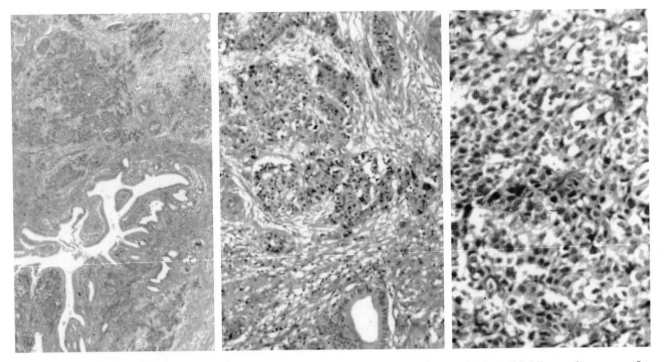

Figure 2-29. Carcinoid of the gallbladder. Left: low magnification view near the cystic duct. Middle: medium magnification. Right: high magnification.

necrosis in comparison to bronchial carcinoids. Seventy percent of these tumors metastasize to the regional lymph nodes. This tumor is now considered to be classified between classic bronchial carcinoids and small cell carcinomas.

(3) Large-cell neuroendocrine carcinoma of the lung (LCNCL)[8-11] (see Table 2–1). LCNCLs, as defined by Travis,[8] are characterized by a neuroendocrine appearance on light microscopy, including an organoid, trabecular, palisading, or

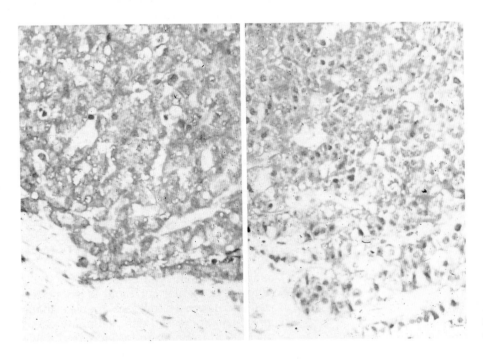

Figure 2-30. Synaptophysin (left) and chromogranin A (right) in carcinoid of the gallbladder.

rosette-like growth pattern, large tumor cells with a low nuclear-cytoplasmic ratio, polygonal shape, finely granular eosinophilic cytoplasm, coarse chromatin, and frequent nucleoli, high mitotic rate (greater than 10 per 10 high-power fields), frequent tumor necrosis, and neuroendocrine features on immunohistochemistry or electron microscopy or both. Jiang and colleagues[11] reported on 22 patients (2.87% of 766) (see Figs. 2–27 and 2–28) who underwent surgical resection for lung cancer, having had a worse prognosis than those with non–small cell lung carcinoma (NSCLC). In their series, chromogranin A, glycoprotein α-subunit, and NCAM had a positivity of 54.5%, 54.5%, and 72.7%, respectively, by immunohistochemistry. Prohormones of GRP (pro-GRP), CT, human chorionic gonadotropin α-subunit, serotonin (5-HT), somatostatin, pancreatic polypeptide, ACTH, and calcitonin gene-related peptide (CGRP) were positive, with rates of 22.7%, 45.5%, 36.4%, 18.2%, 40.9%, 4.5%, 22.7%, and 18.2%, respectively. LCNCL can be easily diagnosed when the tumor exhibits an organoid pattern, but it should be distinguished from poorly differentiated adenocarcinoma and poorly differentiated squamous cell carcinoma.[11] In Jiang's series, LCNCLs had a poorer prognosis than NSCLCs. Dresler et al[10] pointed out that LCNLs identified on histologic examination have a remarkably poor prognosis, even in the very early stage. Adjuvant therapy did not improve survival. Pro-GRP and ACTH/ POMC have been emphasized as tumor markers for small cell neuroendocrine carcinoma, because the tumors lack the prohormone-converting enzymes (PCs 1/3 and 2).

(4) Small cell carcinomas are composed of small anaplastic cells of neuroendocrine nature, generally associated with a poor prognosis. The tumor cells are frequently positive for neuron-specific enolase, but the positivities for the other neuroendocrine markers (e.g., argyrophilia, and immunoreactivity for chromogranins and/ or synaptophysin) vary. Occasionally, the tumor cells produce CT, GRP, or ACTH, and patients are symptomatic, such as in Cushing's syndrome. The peptide hormones are generally produced as prohormones, which are subject to proteolytic fragmentation, designated as "processing," by specific enzymes in the cells. These enzymes are composed of PC3 and PC2. The tumorlets and carcinoids are equipped with PCs as well as peptide production. The small cell carcinomas are usually negative for peptide production and lack PCs. This is the basic mechanism for release of prohormones such as POMC in small cell neuroendocrine carcinomas.

b. Gastrointestinal (GI) carcinoids can occur anywhere in the gastrointestinal tract.[12] This group of tumors has three tissue origins: foregut, midgut, and hindgut. Carcinoids of the stomach[13–16] and gallbladder[17] (Figs. 2–29 to 2–30) are derived from the foregut, those of the ileum and right side of the colon from the midgut, and tumors of the rectum and left side of the colon from the hindgut. Sixty to eighty percent occur in the midgut (appendix and terminal ileum), and 10% to 20% occur in the hindgut (primarily in the rectum). With the advent of rectal endoscopy, rectal carcinoids are frequently removed by biopsy. Because of the biologic behavior of GI carcinoids, all carcinoids are considered to be potentially malignant. Aggressive behavior correlates with site of origin and depth of local penetration as well as the size of the tumors. Appendiceal[18] (Figs. 2–31 to 2–35) and rectal carcinoids are seldom malignant and very rarely show extensive metastasis. In contrast, ileal, gastric, and colonic carcinoids are frequently malignant. A large proportion have already metastasized by the time they are detected. Deep invasion more than halfway through the wall in extra-appendiceal carcinoids correlates with a high prevalence (90%) of nodal and distant metastases. Sixty percent of tumors larger

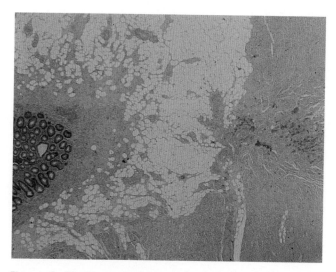

Figure 2–31. Carcinoid of the appendix. Carcinoid is present at the tip of the appendix.

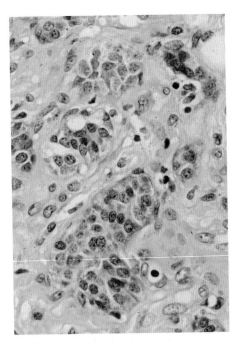

Figure 2-32. Higher magnification of carcinoid of the appendix. Many clusters of carcinoid cells.

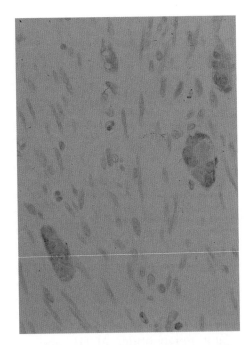

Figure 2-33. Serotonin (5-HT) in the appendiceal carcinoid cells.

than 2 cm show metastases at first detection. In contrast, tumors smaller than 1 cm in diameter rarely (less than 5%) metastasize. The functional characteristics generally are the same as those of tumors with tissue origins: gastric carcinoids (foregut) are frequently positive for gastrin and α-subunit; ileal carcinoids (midgut) are positive for serotonin; and rectal carcinoids (hindgut) are positive for glicentin, neuropeptide Y, and peptide YY. Ileal (midgut) carcinoids are characterized by serotonin production and often multihormonal production. Metastatic carcinoids in the liver cause carcinoid syndrome, which is characterized by a paroxysmal flushing, asthma-like wheezing,

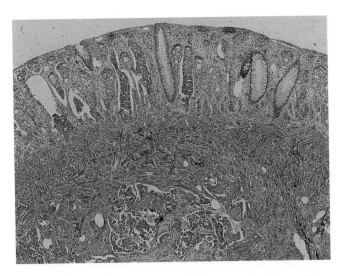

Figure 2-34. The carcinoid cells are present in submucosa and in the mucosa.

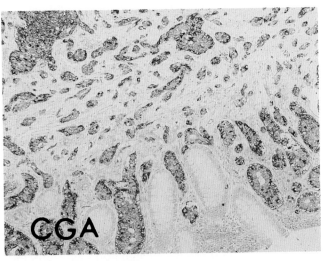

Figure 2-35. Chromogranin A (CGA) in the rectal carcinoid. The carcinoid cells are strongly positive for chromogranin A.

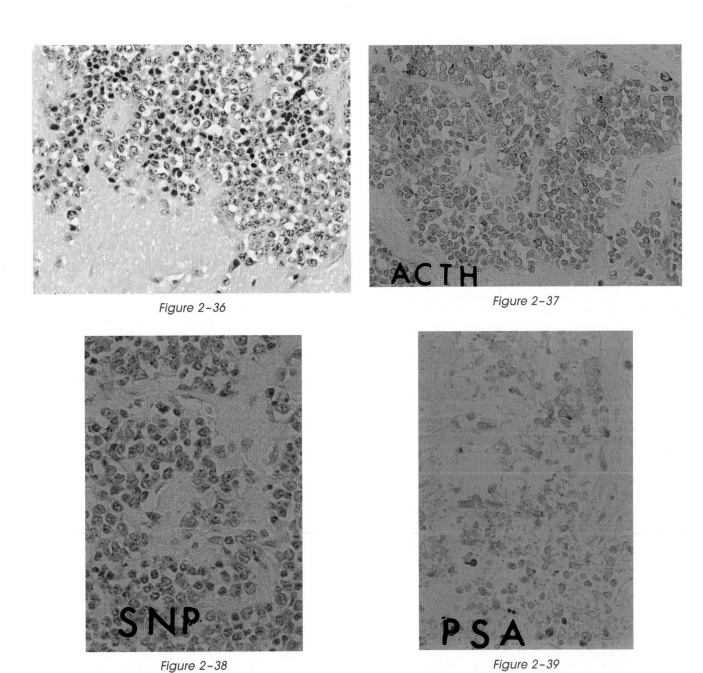

Figure 2-36

Figure 2-37

Figure 2-38

Figure 2-39

Figures 2-36 to 2-39. Neuroendocrine carcinoma of the prostate with ectopic ACTH production. H&E staining (Fig. 2-39) shows small anaplastic tumor cells. They are positive for ACTH (Fig. 2-37), synaptophysin (SNP) (Fig. 2-38), and prostate-specific antigen (PSA) (Fig. 2-39).

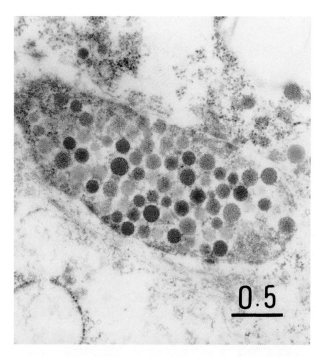

Figure 2-40. Electron micrograph of neuroendocrine carcinoma of the prostate with ectopic ACTH production. The cytoplasmic processes are filled with secretory granules.

right-sided heart failure, explosive and watery diarrhea, abdominal pain, and pellagra-like lesions of the skin and mucosa. Most often carcinoid syndrome is caused by ileal carcinoids, but it can occur with other carcinoids. It usually is seen only in the presence of hepatic metastasis.

D. Nonendocrine tissues, such as breast, prostate, kidney, liver, testis, and uterine cervix,[19] sometimes exhibit neuroendocrine tumors, most frequently carcinoids in the kidney and ovary.[20] In the prostate,[21, 22] the neuroendocrine tumors are most frequently of the small cell carcinoma type (Figs. 2–36 to 2–40). Carcinoids of the kidney[23–25] are rare and are frequently argyrophilic. The renal carcinoids can occasionally metastasize; the most frequent metastatic sites are the liver and the retroperitoneal lymph nodes. Very rarely are these tumors symptomatic, e.g., presenting with Cushing's syndrome. Carcinoids of the ovary occur in combination with struma ovarii, and occasionally these tumors lack struma. Carcinoids of the ovary are similar in hormonal expression to rectal carcinoids (i.e., glicentin, neuropeptide Y, and peptide YY). Neuroendocrine tumors in the breast[26] can be classified as neuroendocrine carcinomas or carcinomas with neuroendocrine differentiation (Figs. 2–41 to 2–44). These tumors are argyrophilic, and carcinoids of the breast are occasionally symptomatic, such as when they cause Cushing's syndrome by producing ACTH. Infrequently, ductal carcinomas of the breast are argyrophilic and positive for chromogranin A. Neuroendocrine tumors of the prostate are usually poorly differentiated carcinomas with argyrophilia and positive neuroendocrine markers. They are focally positive for prostate-specific antigen, indicating the actual prostatic origin of this tumor. Neuroendocrine carcinomas of the prostate are occasionally symptomatic, and we have seen a patient with neuroendocrine carcinoma of the prostate with Cushing's syndrome.[21, 22]

1. Carcinoids of the liver[27] are rare and must be distinguished from hepatocellular carcinoma with neuroendocrine differentiation because of the better prognosis in the former group. The latter tumor can be identified by α-fetoprotein positivity in the tumor cells. In one of our patients, the tumor had two components: one with strong positivity for chromogranin and synaptophysin and the other with strong positivity for SNAP-25, keratin, and α-subunit (Figs. 2–45 to 2–47). These findings may indicate two neuroendocrine patterns in a single tumor.

2. The thymus is an organ that gives rise to carcinoids, occasionally symptomatic tumors that cause Cushing's syndrome. Morphologically, the tumor is similar to those in other organs. Thymic carcinoids should be differentiated from germinomas and pulmonary peripheral carcinoids. The dem-onstration of thymic tissue in or adjacent to the tumor is important in establishing the diagnosis.

3. Primitive carcinomas of the skin of a neuroendocrine nature are designated as Merkel cell carcinomas.[28, 29] These tumors are immunohistochemically positive for neuroendocrine markers such as synaptophysin and chromogranin A as well as for keratin and, sometimes, for neurofilaments (Figs. 2–48 to 2–52). These intermediate filaments are characteristically present as cytoplasmic globules. Occasionally, the tumors are symptomatic, such as in Cushing's syndrome.

4. Very occasionally, the middle ear exhibits the histogenesis of carcinoids,[30, 31] the cellular origin of which is not clear. Morphologically, carcinoids of the middle ear demonstrate morphology similar to that of carcinoids of other organs.

5. Whether peripheral neuroepithelial tumors fall in the category of neuroendocrine tumors is subject to controversy.[32, 33] These tumors occur in the soft tissue and are composed of many small anaplastic cells arranged in solid clusters. Immunohistochemically, the tumors are positive for neuron-specific enolase and CD99 (MIC-1). On electron microscopic examination, the tumor cells contain very occasional small secretory granules, which is one of the diagnostic findings.

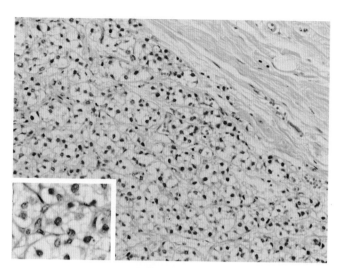

Figure 2-41

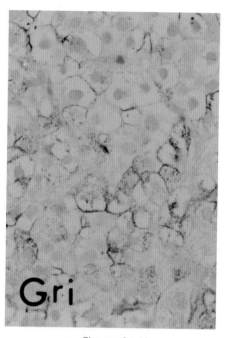

Figure 2-42

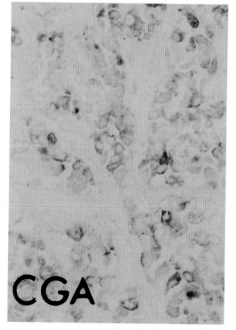

Figure 2-43

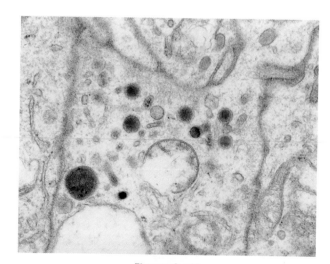

Figure 2-44

Figures 2-41 to 2-44. Neuroendocrine carcinoma of the breast. H&E staining shows many clear tumor cells in the well-demarcated nodule. Higher magnification shows clear cytoplasm (inset) (Fig. 2-41). The tumor cells are argyrophilic (Grimelius' staining), (Fig. 2-42) (Gri) and chromogranin A (CGA) (Fig. 2-43). Electron microscopy shows a few secretory granules in the cytoplasm (Fig. 2-44).

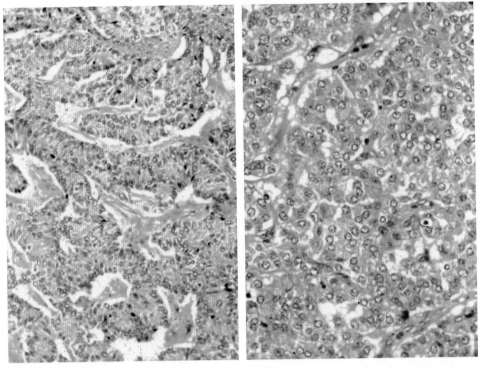

Figure 2–45

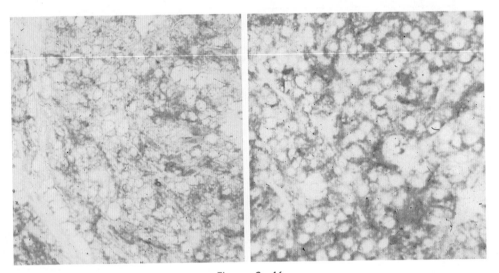

Figure 2–46

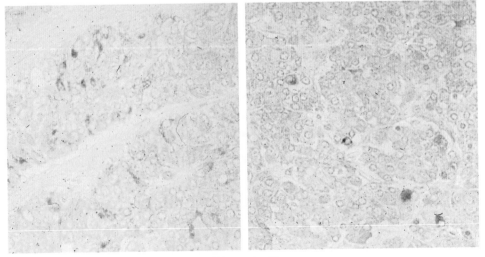

Figure 2–47

Figures 2–45 to 2–47. Carcinoid of the liver. Figure 2–45 shows trabecular (left) or organoid (right) pattern of the tumor. Figure 2–46 shows strongly positive synaptophysin in both trabecular (left) and organoid (right) pattern. Trabecular pattern (left) is more frequently positive for chromogranin A than organoid pattern (right) (Fig. 2–47).

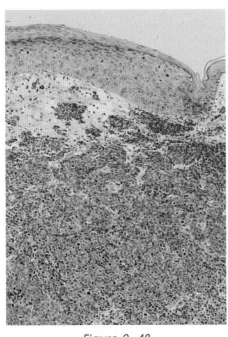

Figure 2–48

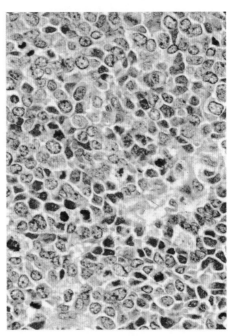

Figure 2–49

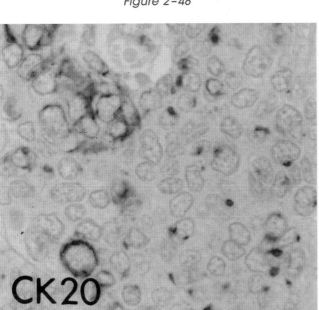

Figure 2–50

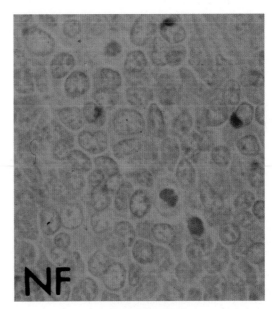

Figure 2–51

Figures 2–48 to 2–51. Merkel's cell carcinoma of the skin. H&E staining (Fig. 2–48) shows many small anaplastic tumor cells in the dermis. The overlying epidermis shows the features of Bowen's disease. The higher magnification shows many anaplastic tumor cells (Fig. 2–49). The tumor cells are positive for keratin 20 (CK20) (Fig. 2–50) and neurofilaments (NF) (Fig. 2–51).

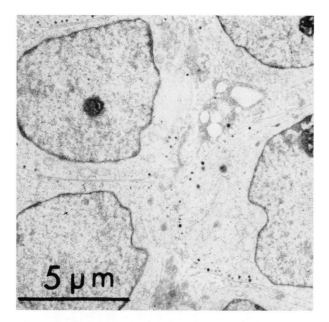

Figure 2-52. Electron micrograph of Merkel's cell carcinoma of the skin. The tumor cells show a few small secretory granules in the cytoplasm.

References

1. DeLellis RA, Dayal Y: Neuroendocrine system. In Sternberg SS, ed.: Histology for Pathologists, 2nd ed. Lippincott-Raven, Philadelphia, 1997, p. 1133.
2. DeLellis RA, Tischler AS: The dispersed neuroendocrine cell system. In Kovacs K, Asa SL, eds.: Functional Endocrine Pathology, 2nd ed. Blackwell Science; Malden, MA, 1998, p 529.
2a. DeLellis RA, Tischler AS, Wolfe HJ: Multidirectional differentiation in neuroendocrine neoplasms. J Histochem Cytochem 1984; 32:899.
3. Langley K: The neuroendocrine concept today. Ann N Y Acad Sci 1994; 733:1.
4. Lloyd RV: Use of molecular probes in the study of endocrine disease. Hum Pathol 1987; 18:1192.
5. Lloyd RV: Introduction to molecular endocrine pathology. Endoc Pathol 1993; 4:64.
6. Capella C, Heitz, Pu, Höfler H, et al: Revised classification of neuroendocrine tumors of the lung, pancreas and gut. Virchows Archiv 1995; 425:547.
7. Arrigoni MG, Woolner LB, Bernatz PE: Atypical carcinoid tumors of the lung. Thorac Cardiovasc Surg 1972; 64:413.
8. Travis WD, Linnoila RI, Tsokos MG, et al: Neuroendocrine tumors of the lung with proposed criteria for large cell neuroendocrine carcinoma. Am J Surg Pathol 1991; 15:529.
9. Travis WD, Gal AA, Colby TV, et al: Reproducibility of neuroendocrine lung tumor classification. Hum Pathol 1998; 29:272.
10. Dresler CM, Ritter JH, Patterson GA, et al: Clinicopathologic analysis of 40 patients with large cell neuroendocrine carcinoma of the lung. Ann Thorac Surg 1997; 63:180.
11. Jiang S-X, Kameya T, Shoji M, et al: Large cell neuroendocrine carcinoma of the lung: A histologic and immunohistochemical study of 22 cases. Am J Surg Pathol 1998; 22:526.
12. Kloppel G, Heitz PU, Capella C, et al: Pathology and nomenclature of human gastrointestinal neuroendocrine (carcinoid) tumors and related lesions. World Surg 1996; 20:132.
13. Reinecke P, Borchard F: Pattern of gastric endocrine cells in microcarcinoidosis—An immunohistochemical study of 14 gastric biopsies (see comments). Virchows Arch 1996; 428:237.
14. Ahlman H, Kolby L, Lundell L, et al: Clinical management of gastric carcinoid tumors. Digestion 1994; 55:77.
15. Waldum HL, Aase S, Kvetnoi I, et al: Neuroendocrine differentiation in human gastric carcinoma. Cancer 1998; 83:435.
16. Bordi C: Gastric carcinoid: An immunohistochemical and clinicopathologic study of 104 patients. Cancer 1995; 75:129.
17. Yamamoto M, Nakajo S, Miyoshi N, et al: Endocrine cell carcinoma (carcinoid) of the gallbladder. Am J Surg Pathol 1989; 13:292.
18. Burke AP, Sobin LH, Federspiel BH, et al: Goblet cell carcinoids and related tumors of the vermiform appendix. Am J Clin Pathol 1990; 94:27.
19. Falchetti M, Berenzi A, Benetti A, et al: Neuroendocrine tumors of the uterine cervix: Cytomorphologic, histochemical and immunohistochemical aspects. Arch Anat Cytol Pathol 1989; 37:88.
20. Wolpert HR, Fuller AF, Bell DA, et al.: Primary mucinous carcinoid tumor of the ovary: A case report. Int J Gynecol Pathol 1989; 8:156.
21. di Sant' Agnes P: Neuroendocrine cells of the prostate and neuroendocrine differentiation in prostatic carcinoma: A review of morphologic aspects. Urology 1998; 51:121.
22. Ro JY, Tetu B, Ayala AG, et al: Small cell carcinoma of prostate gland: Immunohistochemical and electron microscopic studies of 18 cases. Cancer 1987; 59:977.
23. Unger PD, Russell A, Thung SN, et al: Primary renal carcinoid. Arch Pathol Lab Med 1990; 114:68.
24. Goldblum JR, Lloyd RV: Primary renal carcinoid: Case report and literature review. Arch Pathol Lab med 1993; 117:855.
25. Federspiel BH, Burke AP, Sobin LH, et al: Rectal and colonic carcinoids: A clinicopathologic study of 84 cases. Cancer 1990; 65:135.
26. Maluf HM, Koerner FC: Carcinoma of the breast with endocrine differentiation: A review. Virchows Arch 1994; 425:449.
27. Norgaard T, Bardram L: Endocrine liver tumor differential diagnosis from hepatocellular carcinoma. Histopathology 1985; 9:777.
28. Chan JKC, Suster S, Wenig BM, et al: Cytokeratin 20 immunoreactivity distinguishes Merkel cell (primary cutaneous neuroendocrine) carcinomas and salivary gland small cell carcinoma from small cell carcinomas of various sites. Am J Surg Pathol 1997; 21:226.
29. Drijkoningen M, De Wolf-Peeters C, Van Limbergen E, et al: Merkel cell tumor of the skin: An immunohistochemical study. Hum Pathol 1986; 17:301.
30. Riddell DA, LeBoldus GM, Joseph MG, et al: Carcinoid tumor of the middle ear: Case report and review of the literature. J Otolaryngol 1994; 23:276.
31. Ruck P, Pfisterer EM, Kaiserling E, et al: Carcinoid tumor of the middle ear: A morphological and immunohistochemical study with comments on histogenesis and differential diagnosis. Pathol Res Pract 1989; 185:496.
32. Hibshoosh H, Lattes R: Immunohistochemical and molecular genetic approaches to soft tissue tumor diagnosis: A primer. Semin Oncol 1997; 24:515.
33. Fletcher CD: Soft tissue tumors: The impact of cytogenetics and molecular genetics. Verh Dtsch Ges Pathol 1997; 81:318.

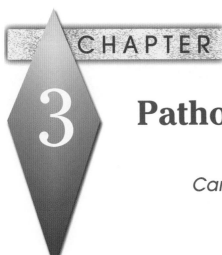

CHAPTER 3

Pathology of the Pituitary Gland

Carol C. Cheung and Sylvia L. Asa

THE NORMAL PITUITARY GLAND

The human pituitary gland is the master endocrine organ that drives metabolism and maintains homeostasis. It regulates the activity of many target organs including the thyroid, the adrenals, the liver, the mammary glands, and the reproductive organs. It is located at the base of the brain in the midline, enclosed inferiorly and laterally by the bony sella turcica and superiorly by the diaphragma sella, which represents a reflectio n of the dura mater surrounding the entire gland[1, 2] (Fig. 3–1). Lateral to the sella are the cavernous sinuses; anteroinferior is the sphenoid sinus; anterosuperior is the optic chiasm; superior to it is the hypothalamus. On average, the bean-shaped gland (Fig. 3–2) measures 0.6 cm superior-inferior × 0.9 cm anterior-posterior × 1.3 cm medial-lateral; and has an average weight of 0.6 g. Females tend to have larger glands, especially during or after pregnancy; this reflects hyperplasia of prolactin-producing cells and can result in an increase in weight of up to 1 g.[3, 4]

The pituitary is composed of two anatomically and functionally distinct parts: the neurohypophysis and the adenohypophysis (Fig. 3–3).

The adenohypophysis is embryologically derived from Rathke's pouch.[5] It is composed of the pars distalis, the pars intermedia, and the pars tuberalis. Adenohypophysial development and cytodifferentiation are regulated by various transcription factors.[6, 7] Many of these are implicated in early pituitary organogenesis, including the bicoid-related pituitary homeobox factor Ptx1[8]; pituitary homeobox factor 2 (Ptx2), structurally related to Ptx1[9]; two members of the *Lhx* gene family, a group of LIM homeobox genes, *Lhx3* and *Lhx4*[10]; and P-LIM, another LIM homeobox protein transcription factor that is selectively expressed in the pituitary with highest levels at the early stages of Rathke's pouch development.[11] Another early determinant of pituitary differentiation is the Rathke's pouch homeobox *(Rpx)* protein, which is identified in the pituitary primordium before the onset of known pituitary hormone production.[12]

The prophet of Pit-1 is a paired-like homeodomain protein that is expressed early in pituitary development. It induces Pit-1 expression and plays a role in downregulation of *Rpx*.[13, 14] Inactivating mutations of the prophet of Pit-1 have been identified as the cause of Pit-1 deficiency in Ames' dwarf mice[13] and in humans with combined pituitary hormone deficiency.[15, 16]

Id, a member of the helix-loop-helix family of transcription factors, is also found early in development and in some pituitary tumor cell lines but is decreased or absent in differentiated cells.[17] Its role in pituitary cytodifferentiation remains unclear.

The molecular factors that determine hormone production have now been identified as transcription factors that target specific hormone genes. These factors have clarified three main pathways of cell differentiation.[6, 7] Corticotropin upstream transcription-binding element drives corticotroph differentiation; the factors implicated in this activity are not entirely clear but include neuroD1/beta 2.[18, 19] Expression of steroidogenic factor-1 (SF-1) is required for gonadotroph differentiation.[20] Somatotrophs, lactotrophs, mammosomatotrophs, and thyrotrophs all derive from growth hormone (GH)-producing precursors that express the transcription factor Pit-1[21–24] with the additional expression of estrogen receptor (ER)α,[25] which enhances prolactin (PRL) secretion, or thyrotroph embryonic factor, which stimulates thyrotrophin (TSH)-beta production.[26]

The *pars distalis* is composed of acini (Fig. 3–4) that contain the specialized cell types, all of which have their own unique hormonal function and characteristics.[1]

GH-producing *somatotrophs* are located in the lateral wings of the anterior pituitary and account for approximately 50% of the cell population. On light microscopy, they appear strongly acidophilic with central, round nuclei. Ultrastructurally, somatotrophs are round or oval with centrally located nuclei. Rough endoplasmic reticulum and Golgi's complexes vary, depending on the secretory activity of the cell. Secretory granules ranging in size from 150 to 800 nm are scattered throughout the cytoplasm.

31

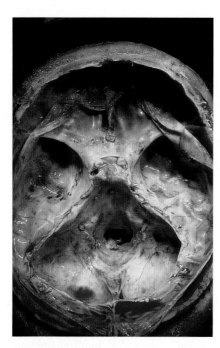

Figure 3–1. Gross anatomy of the pituitary. This view of the base of skull with brain removed shows the sella turcica with the exposed pituitary stalk and an intact diaphragma sella.

PRL-secreting *lactotrophs* are scattered randomly throughout the adenohypophysis; however, they can most often be found in the posterolateral aspects of the gland. In males and nulliparous females, they constitute approximately 9% of the cell population; in multiparous females, they can represent up to 31% of the adenohypophysial cells. With hematoxylin and eosin (H&E) staining, they are usually sparsely granulated and chromophobic; however,

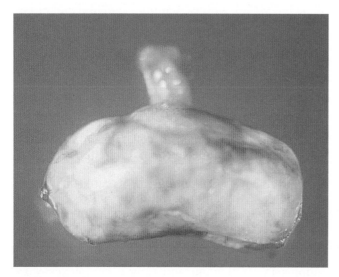

Figure 3–2. Gross photograph; coronal view of pituitary. The pituitary stalk inserts posteriorly. The adenohypophysis has a yellow color and lobulated glandular consistency.

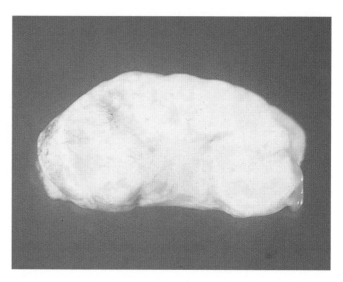

Figure 3–3. Gross photograph; horizontal view of pituitary. The yellow adenohypophysis comprises the bulk of the pituitary mass. The neurohypophysis is white and is located posteriorly.

some may be densely granulated and acidophilic. Ultrastructurally, densely granulated lactotrophs with numerous secretory granules are more commonly seen in children. Adult pituitaries more often contain sparsely granulated lactotrophs. These are elongated or polygonal cells with processes that often encircle gonadotrophs. The rough endoplasmic reticulum is arranged in parallel arrays that occasionally form concentric structures known as Nebenkern formations. Golgi's complexes are prominent. Secretory granules are sparse and range in size from 150 to 250 nm. A diagnostic feature of PRL-secreting cells is the extrusion of granules at the lateral cell border, a phenomenon known as misplaced exocytosis.

Mammosomatotrophs, which produce both GH and PRL, resemble somatotrophs on routine histology. Both GH and PRL can be localized in the cytoplasm

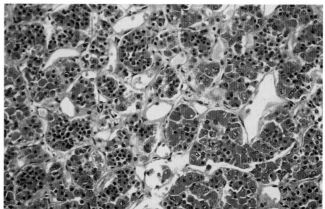

Figure 3–4. Histology of normal pituitary. The adenohypophysis is composed of acini of cells with acidophilic, basophilic, or chromophobic cytoplasm (H&E stain).

by immunohistochemistry. Ultrastructurally, these cells resemble densely granulated somatotrophs; however, the secretory granules are more pleomorphic, ranging from small, ovoid granules measuring up to 400 nm, to large, irregular, elongated granules measuring up to 2000 nm. In addition, they exhibit the hallmark of PRL secretion: misplaced exocytosis.

Thyrotrophs, which produce TSH, represent approximately 5% of adenohypophysial cells and are most commonly found in the anteromedial aspect of the gland. They are angular chromophobic cells with long cytoplasmic processes that abut basement membranes. They exhibit cytoplasmic immunoreactivity for α-subunit and β-TSH. Ultrastructural examination confirms the long processes and the angularity of the cells. The nuclei are usually round and eccentric. The rough endoplasmic reticulum contains dilated cisternae; the Golgi complexes are globular. Secretory granules are located just inside the plasma membrane and range in size from 100 to 200 nm.

Corticotrophs, which produce pro-opiomelanocortin (POMC) and its derivatives including adrenocorticotropin (ACTH), melanotropin, and lipotropin, represent approximately 15%–20% percent of adenohypophysial cells. They are concentrated in the central mucoid wedge but can also be found in the lateral wings, the intermediate lobe, and even in the posterior lobe (see below). These medium-sized cells are basophilic and have strong cytoplasmic positivity with the periodic acid–Schiff (PAS) stain (Fig. 3–5). They have characteristic "enigmatic bodies," which are large, unstained, perinuclear vacuoles representing dilated lysosomes. Ultrastructurally, corticotrophs are oval with oval nuclei and prominent, round nucleoli usually attached to the inner surface of the nuclear membrane. The cytoplasm contains moderately developed rough endoplasmic reticulum with abundant free ribosomes. The enigmatic body is a large membrane-bound structure with an electron-dense periphery, which often displaces the Golgi

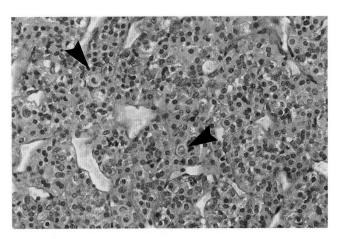

Figure 3–6. Crooke's hyaline change. In situations of glucocorticoid excess, corticotrophs *(arrows)* exhibit accumulation of cytoplasmic hyaline filaments that displace PAS-positive material to the cell periphery and juxtanuclear areas (PAS-diastase stain).

apparatus. Small bundles of intermediate filaments may be scattered throughout the cytoplasm. The secretory granules exhibit a characteristic pleomorphism with respect to both size and shape. When corticotrophs are exposed to excess glucocorticoids, they undergo a reversible morphologic modification known as *Crooke's hyaline change.* Crooke's cells exhibit perinuclear accumulation of intermediate filaments that peripherally displace the PAS-positive, ACTH-immunoreactive secretory granules (Fig. 3–6). On light microscopy, the accumulated filaments have a pale, homogenous, glassy appearance, and they stain for low-molecular-weight cytokeratins.

Gonadotrophs, which produce the two gonadotropins, follicle-stimulating hormone (FSH) and luteinizing hormone (LH), account for 10% of adenohypophysial cells. They are scattered throughout the pars distalis and pars tuberalis. With increasing age, these cells tend to undergo squamous metaplasia. Ultrastructurally, gonadotrophs are oval with eccentric spherical nuclei. The cytoplasm contains prominent dilated, rough, endoplasmic reticulum containing flocculent electron-dense material. The Golgi apparatus is prominent and globular. Secretory granules, which are scattered throughout the cytoplasm, range in size from 250 nm in males to up to 600 nm in females.

The adenohypophysis includes other cells that are not hormonally active. *Follicular cells* are found around small follicles; they are thought to derive from hormone-secreting cells in response to trauma, compression, or degeneration. *Folliculostellate cells* are stromal sustentacular cells that surround acini of the normal gland; they are immunoreactive for S-100 protein or glial fibrillary acidic protein (Fig. 3–7). Scattered cells in the gland that have features of adenohypophysial hormone-secreting cells cannot be classified and are called *null cells*, and the normal gland also contains occasional *oncocytes*.

The *pars intermedia* represents the vestigial remnant of Rathke's pouch. In the adult human, it is

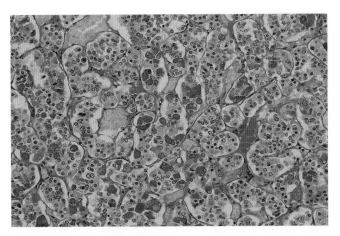

Figure 3–5. Corticotrophs in normal pituitary. Corticotrophs in the nontumorous adenohypophysis have diffuse cytoplasmic PAS-positivity that is diastase resistant (PAS-diastase stain).

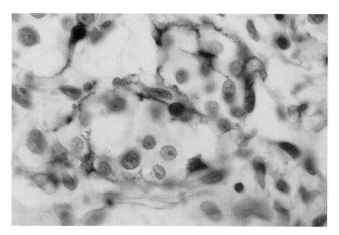

Figure 3–7. Folliculostellate cells. Pituitary acini are surrounded by sustentacular cells with elongated cell processes that stain for S-100 protein (immunohistochemical stain for S-100 protein).

composed of cystic spaces lined by the various hormone-containing cell types, predominantly corticotrophs. With aging, these corticotrophs proliferate into the posterior lobe in a phenomenon known as basophil invasion. Basophils are structurally similar to corticotrophs of the pars distalis; however, they have   functional differences and are thought to cleave POMC differently from the ACTH-producing cells of the pars distalis, and in situations of glucocorticoid excess, they do not undergo Crooke's hyaline change.

The *pars tuberalis* is the superior portion of the adenohypophysis that wraps itself around the neural stalk. It is composed primarily of gonadotrophs that, with age, undergo squamous metaplasia.[27]

The *neurohypophysis* is composed of the infundibulum, the pituitary stalk, and the pars nervosa of the pituitary. The cell types of the neurohypophysis include pituicytes, which are modified glial cells, and the axonal processes of neurons whose cell bodies are located in the hypothalamus. The neurohypophysis stores and releases the hypothalamic hormones oxytocin and vasopressin.

The superior, middle, and inferior hypophysial arteries, all of which originate from the internal carotid arteries, supply the pituitary gland.[28–30] The superior hypophysial arteries supply the infundibulum of the neurohypophysis and eventually form the portal vessels that transport regulatory hormones from the hypothalamus to the pituitary gland. In addition, this capillary network also provides up to 30% of the adenohypophysial arterial supply. The middle hypophysial arteries supply blood directly to the adenohypophysis, and the inferior hypophysial arteries supply the pars nervosa. Venous blood from the pituitary gland drains mainly into the internal jugular veins; however, there is evidence that reversal of flow in the short portal vessels can allow these to serve as efferent channels that permit adenohypophysial secretion to affect neurohypophysial and hypothalamic function.[31, 32]

SPECIMEN HANDLING AND DIAGNOSTIC TECHNIQUES

Intraoperative consultation is not usually indicated for patients with the most common form of pituitary disorder, pituitary adenomas. However, it may be indicated in some situations in which the distinction of an inflammatory lesion, metastatic tumor, or other unusual primary tumor may alter surgical management. Two common approaches are used for intraoperative diagnosis: the cytologic smear and the traditional frozen section. Each has advantages and drawbacks.[1] The amount of tissue required for smears is less than for frozen sections, allowing maximal use of small biopsy samples, and there is no freezing artefact induced by this method, but the interpretation requires experience.

Because surgical resection specimens tend to be small, appropriate handling is essential. Tissue should be processed for histologic and immunohistochemical evaluation. A small piece should be submitted for electron microscopy; although most specimens do not require ultrastructural examination, occasional rare lesions are diagnosed based on specific ultrastructural features—which lesion will fall into this category cannot be predicted. In some centers, tissue is frozen for molecular analysis or placed in culture media for in vitro studies, but these are, at present, predominantly research techniques.

For histologic and immunohistochemical analysis, tissue is usually fixed in 10% neutral buffered formalin. Routine histochemical stains should include H&E, the Gordon-Sweet silver stain for reticulin, PAS, and occasionally Congo red staining for amyloid. Immunohistochemical analysis should include stains for the various pituitary hormones and transcription factors as well as for low-molecular-weight cytokeratins that identify subtypes of pituitary adenomas.

For electron microscopy, small pieces of tissue should be initially fixed in 2.5% glutaraldehyde, post-fixed with osmium, and embedded in epoxy resin.

CONGENITAL AND DEVELOPMENTAL DISORDERS

Ectopic Adenohypophysis

The path followed by Rathke's pouch during fetal development may contain deposits of fully functional adenohypophysial tissue.[33–35] The sphenoid sinus is the most common site to find ectopic pituitary tissue. Up to 20% of the population harbors ectopic adenohypophysial tissue in suprasellar locations.[36, 37] These ectopic foci may be incidental findings, or they can undergo hyperplastic or neoplastic change.

Pituitary Aplasia/Hypoplasia

These disorders are usually associated with severe congenital malformations such as those seen in the Cornelia de Lange syndrome[38] or Arnold-Chiari malformation.[39] They result in hypopituitarism with subsequent thyroid and adrenal hypoplasia or aplasia.[40-44] At least one form of this disorder associated with septo-optic dysplasia has been attributed to a mutation of the *Rpx-1* gene (also known as *Hesx-1*).[45]

Partial hypopituitarism with pituitary dwarfism and hypothyroidism has been attributed to Pit-1 deficiency due to mutations in the *pit-1* gene.[46-48] In animal models of this disorder, there is hypoplasia of somatotrophs, lactotrophs, and thyrotrophs.[49]

Pituitary Duplication or Dystopia

These lesions are also usually associated with other congenital malformations.[50, 51]

Empty Sella Syndrome

This condition results from a defective or absent diaphragma sella.[52] Increased cerebrospinal fluid pressure causes sellar enlargement and flattens the pituitary against the floor of the sella turcica (Fig. 3–8). Pituitary function is usually unaffected.[53] However, up to 5% of patients have hyperprolactinemia, which is most likely secondary to distortion of the pituitary stalk[54]; it may rarely be associated with a prolactin-secreting adenoma.

CYSTIC LESIONS OF THE PITUITARY

Rathke's Cleft Cysts

Remnants of Rathke's pouch commonly form small cysts (<5 mm) in the vestigial pars intermedia. These small cysts occasionally enlarge into true Rathke's cleft cysts that are symptomatic. Although this condition may occasionally be seen in children, it is most common in adults.

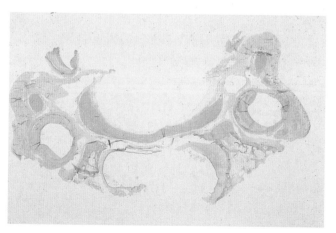

Figure 3-8. Empty sella syndrome. A coronal whole-mount of the sella turcica shows the adenohypophysis compressed at the base of the sella turcica (H&E stain).

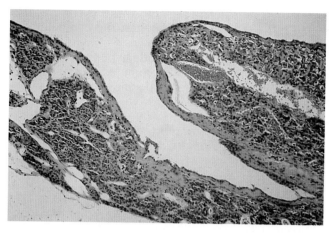

Figure 3-9. Rathke's cleft cyst. A cyst lined by flattened epithelium with surrounding fibrosis is identified within adenohypophysis (H&E stain).

These cysts are nonfunctional but may cause hypopituitarism or diabetes insipidus by compression of surrounding structures.[55] Suprasellar extension may give rise to mass effects such as visual field defects and headaches. Severe cases can lead to hydrocephalus, aseptic meningitis and, rarely, abscess formation.[56] Computed tomography (CT) scans usually reveal low-density cystic areas with peripheral enhancement; magnetic resonance imaging (MRI) findings tend to be more variable.[57]

Treatment by drainage, with or without surgical excision, usually results in resolution of mass effects; however, hypopituitarism and diabetes insipidus may persist, requiring permanent hormone replacement. Recurrence rates are low.

Microscopic examination reveals a cystic lesion lined by ciliated cuboidal or columnar epithelium (Fig. 3–9) with occasional goblet cells and areas of squamous metaplasia.

Arachnoid Cysts

Arachnoid cysts originate in the arachnoid of the sellar and parasellar areas; they may be congenital or acquired.

Clinically, they can present with mass effects from suprasellar extension or hypopituitarism and/or diabetes insipidus due to pituitary compression.[55] Radiologically, they appear cystic on CT and MRI.

Treatment involves drainage of cyst contents and partial surgical excision.

Grossly, cystic structure filled with clear fluid is seen. Microscopically, the cyst wall consists of arachnoid laminar connective tissue lined by a layer of simple flattened epithelium.

Dermoid and Epidermoid Cysts

Dermoid and epidermoid cysts (also known as cholesteatomas) originate from ectopic or traumatically implanted epithelial cells. In addition to the sellar and suprasellar regions, these cysts are also found intracranially, most often at the cerebellopontine angle.[58]

Clinical manifestations include hypopituitarism, hyperprolactinemia due to stalk compression, visual field defects, and a variety of nonspecific neurologic symptoms. Radiologic evaluation revealsa cystic lesion.

Surgical resection is usually curative. Complications include either the rupture of the cyst with subsequent meningitis or the development of squamous cell carcinoma.[59, 60]

As in other areas of the body, epidermoid cysts have a lining composed of keratinizing squamous epithelium. The lining of dermoid cysts contains skin appendages such as hair follicles and sweat glands.

INFLAMMATORY DISORDERS OF THE PITUITARY GLAND

Inflammatory conditions can cause mass effects and/or hypothalamic-hypophysial dysfunction. Primary or idiopathic inflammatory conditions include lymphocytic hypophysitis, granulomatous hypophysitis, and xanthomatous hypophysitis.[61] Secondary inflammatory conditions affecting the pituitary gland include infections and various systemic diseases.

Lymphocytic Hypophysitis

This chronic inflammatory condition of the pituitary gland is seen most commonly in young postpartum or pregnant females.[62] The disorder is much less common in males; the female-to-male ratio is 8.5:1. The mean ages of presentation are 34.5 years in females and 44.7 years in males. An autoimmune cause has been proposed as the basis for lymphocytic hypophysitis because of its association with a number of other autoimmune endocrine disorders, such as thyroiditis, adrenalitis, atrophic gastritis, and lymphocytic parathyroiditis. There is evidence for pituitary antibodies in patients with this disease.[63]

Clinical Features

Clinically, the symptoms and signs of lymphocytic hypophysitis tend to be nonspecific; therefore, the diagnosis is usually established at histologic examination. The most common manifestation is mild-to-moderate hyperprolactinemia; isolated hormone deficiencies are rare. In addition, it can present with mass effects such as headache and visual field deficits. Rarely, patients present with isolated diabetes insipidus, and the inflammatory process is restricted to the posterior lobe and stalk, which can exhibit localized enlargement; this disorder has been named infundibular neurohypophysitis.[64-66]

Radiologic findings can mimic features of an adenoma; the gland is enlarged and may even exhibit suprasellar extension. Careful MRI examination with contrast enhancement documents no discrete delineation between a tumor and the usually enhancing normal gland.

The natural history of untreated lymphocytic hypophysitis is variable; it may result in permanent hypopituitarism due to extensive destruction of adenohypophysial cells, or it may run a self-limited course followed by a full recovery. Treatment for this condition is supportive with appropriate hormone replacement. Corticosteroids have been proposed to decrease inflammation, but the efficacy of this treatment has yet to be determined. Transsphenoidal surgery should be considered if the patient suffers progressive mass effects or deterioration as evidenced by radiologic or neurologic changes. However, surgery has resulted in deleterious effects in occasional case reports.

Pathology

The usual gross appearance of the gland is that of an inflamed, enlarged, and soft mass. The gland may appear atrophic and fibrotic if the disease course is prolonged.

Microscopic examination reveals a diffuse mixed inflammatory infiltrate composed mainly of lymphocytes and plasma cells forming occasional lymphoid follicles; this is accompanied by variable numbers of neutrophils, eosinophils, and macrophages. There is destruction of the adenohypophysial tissue; the remaining islands of normal parenchyma exhibit variable oncocytic change (Fig. 3–10). The amount of fibrosis varies with the duration of the disease.

The lymphocytic infiltrate is immunoreactive for leukocyte common antigen and B-cell and T-cell markers. Residual adenohypophysial cells contain the various pituitary hormones. Rarely, there seems to be preferential destruction of one hormone-containing cell type.

On electron microscopy, the adenohypophysial cells exhibit degenerative changes, including crinophagy and oncocytosis. Numerous lymphocytes and plasma cells can be easily identified.

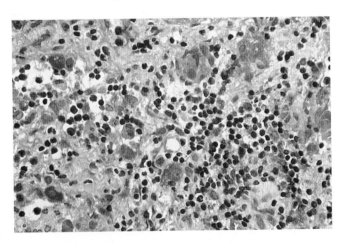

Figure 3–10. Lymphocytic hypophysitis. The adenohypophysis is infiltrated by chronic inflammatory cells. Residual parenchymal cells exhibit oncocytic change (PAS stain).

Granulomatous Hypophysitis

Idiopathic granulomatous hypophysitis is a rare chronic inflammatory disorder of unknown pathogenesis that was first described in 1917.[67-70] It represents 1% of all pituitary disorders, with an annual incidence of 1 in 10 million. As of 1991, only 31 cases were described in publications, 21 from autopsy material. Unlike lymphocytic hypophysitis, there is no gender predilection. The mean age of presentation in females is 21.5 years; in males, it is 50 years.

Clinical Features

Clinically, patients may present with visual field deficits, cranial nerve palsies, or headaches, which may be accompanied by nausea and vomiting; this is in contrast to headaches caused by adenomas that are not associated with nausea and vomiting.[71, 72] Other clinical manifestations include variable degrees of adenohypophysial failure,[73] hyperprolactinemia,[74] diabetes insipidus, and meningitis with cerebrospinal fluid leukocytosis.[75]

Radiologic evaluation usually reveals an intrasellar mass with or without suprasellar extension.[72] Sometimes, a tongue-like extension along the basal hypothalamus can be seen.

Treatment is somewhat controversial; transsphenoidal biopsy/resection and subsequent administration of corticosteroids have been proposed.[61, 76]

Pathology

Microscopically, this condition is characterized by collections of histiocytes with scattered lymphocytes and plasma cells; multinucleated giant cells may be present (Fig. 3–11). Because it is a primary condition of the pituitary gland, a diagnosis of granulomatous hypophysitis cannot be made unless causes of secondary hypophysitis can be ruled out (see below).

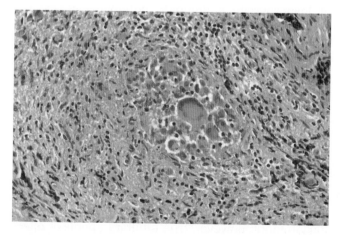

Figure 3–11. Granulomatous hypophysitis. The pituitary contains well-formed granulomas with foreign body–type giant cells (H&E stain).

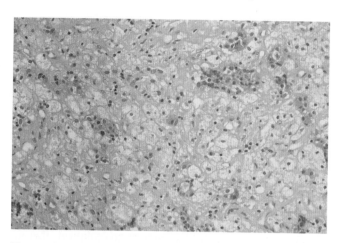

Figure 3–12. Xanthomatous hypophysitis. Nests of residual adenohypophyseal cells are seen within a sea of foamy histiocytes (H&E stain).

Xanthomatous Hypophysitis

This relatively new clinicopathologic entity described by Folkerth et al.[77] is characterized by a chronic inflammatory infiltrate composed mainly of foamy histiocytes with scattered lymphocytes and plasma cells. The patients reported have been young females. Clinical presentation included headache, nausea, menstrual irregularity, and diabetes insipidus. One patient had elevated prolactin levels. In most patients, a preoperative diagnosis of pituitary adenoma was suspected based on the presence of a localized lesion in the pituitary.[61, 77] Histologically, the condition is characterized by infiltration of the adenohypophysis by foamy histiocytes (Fig. 3–12) with areas of granulation tissue. The histiocytes are immunoreactive with antibodies to CD68; they are nonimmunoreactive for S-100 and CD1a. The presence of lipid within the infiltrating histiocytes has been confirmed by electron microscopy. This disorder may represent a reactive process[61]; however, it remains idiopathic. A diagnosis of xanthomatous hypophysitis can be made only after causes of secondary hypophysitis are ruled out.

Secondary Hypophysitis

These are inflammatory lesions of the pituitary gland; they have a definite cause[78] or occur as part of a systemic process. A number of infectious agents can involve the pituitary gland, including fungi, mycobacteria, brucellosis, and syphilis.[79] They can result in acute or chronic hypophysitis with occasional abscess formation. Other causes of secondary hypophysitis include sarcoidosis,[80] vasculitides such as Takayasu's disease[81] and Wegener's granulomatosis,[82] Crohn's disease,[83] Whipple's disease, ruptured Rathke's cleft cyst,[84, 85] necrotizing adenoma,[78] and meningitis.[75]

AIDS may involve the pituitary gland.[86] The involvement is usually infectious in nature and results in acute or chronic inflammation with necrosis. The pathogens are generally opportunistic organisms including *Pneumocystis carinii*, *Toxoplasma gondii*, and *cytomegalovirus*.

VASCULAR DISORDERS OF THE PITUITARY

Pituitary Infarction

Ischemic necrosis of the pituitary can result from a number of insults, including head injury, hemorrhagic shock, disseminated intravascular coagulation, thrombocytopenia, and stroke.[87-90] Two particular conditions resulting in pituitary infarction, Sheehan's syndrome and pituitary apoplexy, are discussed here.

Sheehan's Syndrome

Sheehan's syndrome refers to postpartum necrosis of the pituitary gland; it is usually related to hypotension secondary to postpartum hemorrhage.[91] The necrosis, which usually involves the adenohypophysis, may be focal or may involve virtually the entire gland. Most commonly, there is central necrosis with a rim of viable cells at the periphery of the gland (Fig. 3–13). Subsequent fibrosis may lead to further damage of functional cells. Clinical manifestations appear only with significant tissue destruction. The neurohypophysis, with its independent blood supply, is usually spared.

Pituitary Apoplexy

This condition constitutes a true endocrine emergency in which acute hemorrhagic infarction of a sellar tumor (usually an adenoma) results in rapid

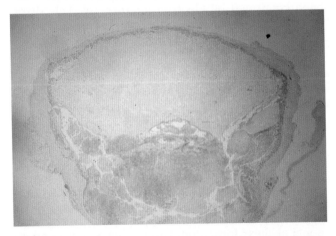

Figure 3–13. Sheehan's syndrome. In this autopsy pituitary, the adenohypophysis has been replaced by fibrous tissue. A thin rim of viable pituitary cells is identified at the periphery of the gland (hematoxylin-phloxine-saffron stain). (Photograph courtesy of Dr. K. Kovacs, Toronto, Canada.)

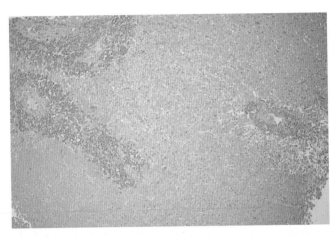

Figure 3–14. Pituitary apoplexy. A pituitary adenoma is almost entirely infarcted; viable cells are seen only around vascular channels (H&E stain).

expansion of the tumor, leading to symptoms and signs of elevated intracranial pressure.[92]

Clinical Features

Clinical manifestations include acute onset headache, visual impairment, cranial nerve palsies (especially diplopia due to compression of the oculomotor and abducens cranial nerves as they traverse the cavernous sinus), altered level of consciousness, weakness, meningeal irritation, diabetes insipidus, acute hypopituitarism, and even sudden death. There is usually no previous history of pituitary adenoma. Factors predisposing to pituitary apoplexy include carotid angiography, radiation therapy, trauma, coagulopathy, temporal arteritis, diabetes mellitus, and atherosclerosis.

Appropriate treatment involves immediate administration of glucocorticoids. Fluid and electrolyte status must be carefully monitored for neurohypophysial dysfunction such as diabetes insipidus or syndrome of inappropriate antidiuretic hormone. Surgical decompression is required if the patient exhibits altered mental function or severe visual impairment; early decompression is the most important determinant to visual recovery. The clinical course of this condition is variable and unpredictable; rarely does spontaneous recovery occur. Long-term hormonal replacement therapy is a common outcome.

Pathology

Histologic examination reveals infarction and hemorrhage (Fig. 3–14). These features are commonly found focally on morphologic examination of pituitary tumors; however, true pituitary apoplexy refers to those extreme cases where hemorrhagic infarction of the pituitary is accompanied by the appropriate clinical features.

METABOLIC DISORDERS AFFECTING THE PITUITARY

Hypophysial Amyloidosis

Amyloid deposition involving the pituitary gland usually occurs as part of a systemic disorder, such as multiple myeloma, or in association with a pituitary adenoma,[93–97] most commonly prolactinoma. The amyloid is seen either in vessel walls or in the interstitium. Histologically, it appears as an extracellular, amorphous, eosinophilic substance that stains with Congo red and exhibits characteristic apple-green birefringence under polarized light.

Hypophysial Hemosiderosis

Deposition of iron occurs in the pituitary gland of patients with hemochromatosis; preferential deposition in gonadotrophs is common.[98, 99] The accumulation of iron may result in fibrosis with subsequent pituitary dysfunction.

HYPERPLASIA OF THE PITUITARY

Hyperplasia is an increase in the number of cells of a particular organ or tissue in response to a stimulus; this process may be physiologic or pathologic. Hyperplasia must be distinguished from neoplasia, which implies independent cell proliferation. Any cell population within the pituitary gland can undergo hyperplastic changes.[1, 100, 101] *Somatotroph hyperplasia* most often results from ectopic production of GH-releasing hormone by pheochromocytomas, endocrine tumors of lung, pancreas, or other elements of the dispersed endocrine system.[102–104] Rarely, hyperplasia may be associated with a gangliocytoma of the hypothalamus.[105] *Mammosomatotroph hyperplasia* may also be due to ectopic GH-releasing production. It is the characteristic pituitary lesion in McCune-Albright syndrome[106, 107]; rarely, it may be idiopathic.[108] *Lactotroph hyperplasia* is physiologic during pregnancy or other conditions of estrogen excess, but pathologic idiopathic lactotroph hyperplasia is a rare cause of hyperprolactinemia.[109, 110] *Corticotroph hyperplasia* can be associated with Cushing's disease, either alone or in conjunction with an adenoma.[111–113] In some patients, it is attributed to ectopic or eutopic excess of corticotropin-releasing hormone. It is a physiologic response to glucocorticoid insufficiency in patients with untreated Addison's disease. *Thyrotroph hyperplasia* develops in patients with prolonged primary hypothyroidism.[114–116] *Gonadotroph hyperplasia* can be seen in patients with prolonged primary hypogonadism.[117, 118]

Clinical Features

Excessive hormone secretion from hyperplastic cells results in distinctive clinical syndromes that can mimic those of functional adenomas. Radiologic evaluation may reveal no identifiable abnormality, but usually there is diffuse sellar enlargement. Only when pituitary enlargement is dramatic with suprasellar extension can pituitary hyperplasia result in mass effects such as headache, nausea, vomiting, visual field deficits, and cranial nerve palsies.

Hyperplasia is usually reversible if the underlying condition is treated appropriately. However, in patients with idiopathic lactotroph or corticotroph hyperplasia, the underlying stimulus to adenohypophysial cell proliferation/hypersecretion is not identifiable. Patients with lactotroph hyperplasia can be treated with dopaminergic agonists. Those with Cushing's syndrome may require total hypophysectomy to achieve clinical control.

Pathology

Although they may have similar clinical presentations, a reticulin stain can reliably distinguish adenohypophysial hyperplasia from adenohypophysial adenoma. A hyperplastic lesion will exhibit expanded acini within an intact reticulin framework (Fig. 3–15), whereas an adenoma will show breakdown of the reticulin fiber network (Fig. 3–16). Immunohistochemistry shows predominance of the hyperplastic cell type with other hormone-containing cells interspersed throughout the gland. Ultrastructural examination is not a reliable method for distinguishing hyperplasia from adenoma. However, it has defined the basis of cell enlargement that defines thyroidectomy cells in patients with primary hypothyroidism and gonadectomy cells in patients with primary hypogonadism; in both situations, the target cells develop ample, vacuolated cytoplasm that is occupied almost entirely by dilated, rough, endoplasmic reticulum with flocculent material.

Hyperplastic changes may be diffuse or focal. In some cases, an adenoma can coexist with hyperplasia.[104, 111–113, 117, 118]

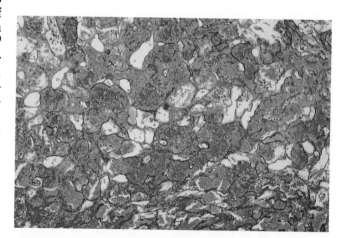

Figure 3–15. Pituitary hyperplasia. In the patient with primary hypothyroidism, pituitary enlargement is due to thyrotroph hyperplasia. The reticulin stain documents intact acinar architecture (Gordon-Sweet silver stain).

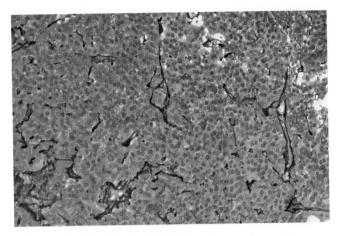

Figure 3-16. Pituitary adenoma. In pituitary adenoma, there is total breakdown of the reticulin fiber network (Gordon-Sweet silver stain).

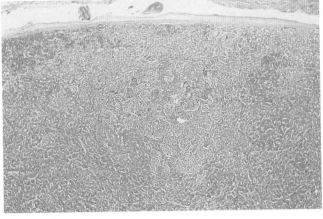

Figure 3-17. Pituitary microadenoma. This autopsy pituitary contains an incidental chromophobic microadenoma (hematoxylin-phloxine-saffron stain).

PRIMARY TUMORS OF ADENOHYPOPHYSIAL CELLS

Primary tumors of the adenohypophysis include pituitary adenomas and the rare malignant pituitary carcinoma.

Pituitary Adenomas

Pituitary adenomas are benign neoplasms that arise from adenohypophysial cells and represent up to 25% of all intracranial tumors.[1] They are present in approximately 20% of the general population.[1] Their prevalence increases with advancing age; both sexes are equally affected.

Multiple endocrine neoplasia (MEN) syndromes are familial disorders in which several endocrine glands develop neoplasms or hyperplasias.[119] Pituitary adenomas are most commonly associated with MEN-1 (Wermer's syndrome), an autosomal-dominant disorder with incomplete penetrance.[120] This syndrome is characterized by the development of parathyroid hyperplasia or adenoma, pancreatic endocrine cell hyperplasia, dysplasia and tumor, and pituitary adenoma. The various tumors develop metachronously rather than synchronously in individual patients and in no specific order. Approximately two-thirds of affected patients develop a pituitary adenoma, most often producing prolactin and/or GH.[121] This disease results from a germline mutation of the *MEN-1* gene on chromosome 11q13 that encodes the tumor suppressor protein "menin."[122] Loss of heterozygosity of the intact allele is responsible for subsequent tumor formation.[123]

The cause of the more common sporadic pituitary adenoma is not yet known. A number of etiologic factors have been implicated, including genetic events, hormonal stimulation, and growth factors[6]; it is likely that all of these interact to initiate transformation and promote tumor cell proliferation.

Classification of Pituitary Adenomas

There are several classification schemes for pituitary adenomas: functional, anatomic/radiologic, histologic, immunohistochemical, ultrastructural, and clinicopathologic.[1]

The *functional classification* is used clinically. It groups adenomas according to the hormonal syndromes with which they are associated. This includes the various functioning adenomas and the clinically "silent" or nonfunctioning adenomas.

The *anatomic/radiologic classification* categorizes pituitary adenomas based on size and degree of invasion.[124] Four grades are recognized: grade I adenomas have a diameter less than 1 cm (Fig. 3–17); grade II adenomas are intrasellar tumors larger than 1 cm (Fig. 3–18); grade III adenomas are associated with localized erosion of the sella turcica; grade IV adenomas are large, expansive lesions with extensive extrasellar involvement, including invasion of the hypothalamus, cavernous sinus, bone, and even

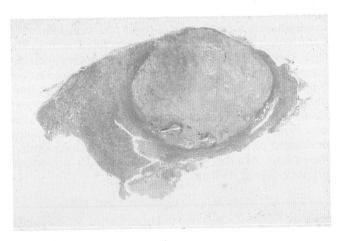

Figure 3-18. Pituitary macroadenoma. This 1-cm pituitary adenoma replaces one lateral lobe of the gland (hematoxylin-phloxine-saffron stain).

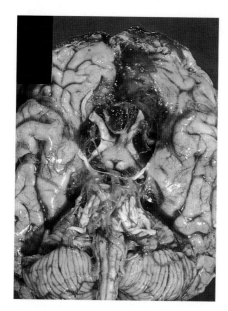

Figure 3–19. Invasive pituitary adenoma. This very large pituitary tumor has destroyed the sella turcica and has invaded laterally as well as anteriorly into the frontal lobe.

brain parenchyma (Figs. 3–19 and 3–20). Each grade is subclassified based on the degree of suprasellar extension, identified as small (A), moderate (B), or large (C).

Ectopic pituitary adenomas can arise in embryonic remnants of Rathke's cleft that are found in extrasellar locations, including the sphenoid sinus, parapharyngeal area, suprasellar regions, middle nasal meatus, petrous temporal bone, clivus, hypothalamus, and third ventricle.[125–133] Epidemiologically, these tumors resemble their intrasellar counterparts. Compared with intrasellar pituitary adenomas, higher proportions of ectopic adenomas are functional, with the most common clinical presentation being Cushing's disease. Silent ectopic adenomas usually

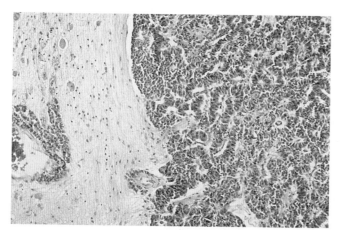

Figure 3–20. Invasive pituitary adenoma. Microscopically, this pituitary tumor has invaded brain parenchyma (H&E stain).

present with mass effects, and their diagnosis depends on careful examination of resected tissue specimens.

The *histologic classification*, based on histochemical stains, divides adenomas into acidophilic, basophilic, and chromophobic. This classification is of limited value and has largely been abandoned.

The *immunohistochemical classification* categorizes pituitary adenomas based primarily on hormone content, with additional information provided by immunoreactivity for transcription factors and keratins[1] (Table 3–1).

Although electron microscopy can be extremely valuable in the diagnosis of certain tumors, the *ultrastructural classification* of adenomas is less commonly used.[134]

The *clinicopathologic classification* represents the most effective classification scheme.[1] It categorizes adenomas using both morphologic and clinical features as shown in Table 3–2.

Functioning Somatotroph Adenomas

Somatotroph adenomas arise from GH-producing cells and represent 10%–15% of pituitary adenomas.

Clinical Features

GH excess in adults manifests as acromegaly, which is characterized by acral enlargement, prognathism, and soft-tissue thickening involving the face and lips.[135] Gigantism results from excessive GH before epiphyseal plate closure. These changes are associated with reduced life expectancy due to diabetes mellitus, cardiovascular abnormalities, and an increased incidence of malignancies, primarily colon and breast carcinoma. Because the onset of acromegaly is somewhat insidious, the problem is often not recognized until the patient presents with mass effects or features of hypopituitarism.

Biochemically, the diagnosis of acromegaly or gigantism is based on detection of elevated serum levels of GH and somatomedin C, also known as insulin-like growth factor-1. Failure to suppress GH following oral glucose administration is a reliable indicator of acromegaly. Some acromegalic patients exhibit a paradoxical stimulation of GH by thyrotropin-releasing hormone. Hyperprolactinemia can be prominent in some patients; this may be the result of stalk compression in macroadenomas or the elaboration of PRL in addition to GH by the tumor.

Sellar enlargement can be demonstrated in most patients with CT scan, but MRI is the imaging technique of choice to identify a pituitary adenoma and delineate residual normal tissue, which enhances with contrast more readily than does tumor tissue.

Somatotroph adenomas are difficult to cure. Surgical resection, medical treatment with somatostatin analogues, and radiation have been used with varying success.[136]

Table 3-1. Immunohistochemical Classification of Pituitary Adenomas

GH-PRL-TSH Family	Pit-1
GH-containing somatotroph adenomas	Pit-1, GH
Densely granulated somatotroph adenomas	Pit-1, GH, ± α-subunit
Sparsely granulated somatotroph adenomas	Pit-1, GH, keratin whorls
GH- and PRL-containing mammosomatotroph adenomas	Pit-1, GH, PRL, ER ± α-subunit
PRL-containing lactotroph adenomas	Pit-1, PRL, ER
Sparsely granulated lactotroph adenomas	Pit-1, PRL, ER
Densely granulated lactotroph adenomas	Pit-1, PRL, ER
PRL-cell adenomas with GH content (acidophil stem cell)	Pit-1, PRL, ER, GH, keratin whorls
TSH-containing thyrotroph adenomas	Pit-1, β-TSH, α-subunit
GH-, PRL-, and TSH-containing adenomas	Pit-1, GH, PRL, ER, α-subunit, β-TSH
ACTH Family	**?**
ACTH-containing corticotroph adenomas	ACTH, keratins
Densely granulated corticotroph adenomas	ACTH, keratins
Sparsely granulated corticotroph adenomas	ACTH, keratins
Gonadotropin Family	**SF-1, ER**
FSH/LH-containing gonadotroph adenomas	SF-1, ER, β-FSH, β-LH, α-subunit
Unclassified Adenomas	
Unusual plurihormonal adenomas	Multiple markers
Immunonegative adenomas	No immunohistochemical markers

Pathology

Grossly, these tumors are usually well demarcated and are located in the lateral wing of the adenohypophysis. Microscopically, there are several subtypes of somatotroph adenomas.

Densely Granulated Somatotroph Adenoma. This is composed of acidophilic cells arranged in a trabecular, sinusoidal, or diffuse architecture (Fig. 3–21). The tumor cells show strong, diffuse cytoplasmic immunoreactivity for GH (Fig. 3–22) and strong nuclear immunoreactivity for Pit-1.[1] Tumor cells exhibit moderate perinuclear positivity with antibodies to low-molecular-weight cytokeratins. There is variable cytoplasmic immunoreactivity for α-subunit of glycoprotein hormones. On electron microscopy,[134] the tumor cells resemble nontumorous somatotrophs; they have spherical nuclei with prominent nucleoli.

Table 3-2. Clinicopathological Classification of Pituitary Adenomas

Functioning Adenomas	Nonfunctioning Adenomas
GH-PRL-TSH Family	
Adenomas causing GH-excess	
Densely granulated somatotroph adenomas	
Sparsely granulated somatotroph adenomas	Silent lactotroph adenomas
Mammosomatotroph adenomas	
Adenomas causing hyperprolactinemia	
Lactotroph adenomas	Silent lactotroph adenomas
Acidophil stem cell adenomas	
Adenomas causing TSH excess	
Thyrotroph adenomas	Silent thyrotroph adenomas
ACTH Family	
Adenomas causing ACTH excess	
Densely granulated corticotroph adenomas	Silent corticotroph adenomas
Sparsely granulated corticotroph adenomas	
Gonadotroph Family	
Adenomas causing gonadotropin excess	
Gonadotroph adenomas	Silent gonadotroph adenomas (null cell adenomas, oncocytomas)
Unclassified Adenomas	
Unusual plurihormonal adenomas	Immunonegative adenomas

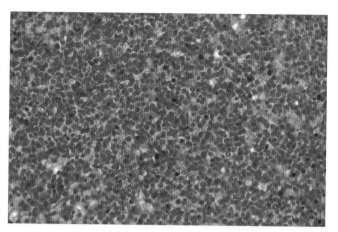

Figure 3-21. Densely granulated somatotroph adenoma. This tumor is composed of cells with abundant, strongly acidophilic cytoplasm and minimal nuclear pleomorphism (H&E stain).

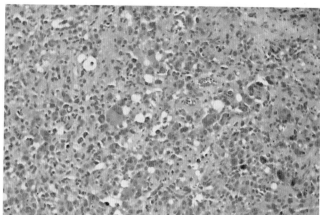

Figure 3-23. Sparsely granulated somatotroph adenoma. This tumor is characterized by highly pleomorphic cells with chromophobic cytoplasm and irregular nuclei. Occasional binucleate cells are seen; in some cells there is a pale juxtanuclear cytoplasmic vacuole that corresponds to the fibrous body (H&E stain).

Parallel arrays of rough endoplasmic reticulum are found, and Golgi's complexes are well formed. The numerous secretory granules are homogeneous, dense, and spherical, with diameters ranging from 150 to 600 nm.

Sparsely Granulated Somatotroph Adenoma. This is composed of solid sheets of chromophobic cells with striking nuclear pleomorphism and prominent nucleoli (Fig. 3–23). Immunohistochemical stains for low-molecular-weight cytokeratins reveal the characteristic feature of this tumor type, the fibrous body (Fig. 3–24), which manifests as juxtanuclear globular reactivity.[1] There is focal, weak, cytoplasmic immunoreactivity for GH and occasionally for α-subunit. Nuclear immunoreactivity for Pit-1 is usually present. Ultrastructurally,[134] the tumor cells are irregularly shaped with eccentric, pleomorphic, and often multilobulated nuclei. The rough endoplasmic reticulum can be either poorly or well developed. The characteristic fibrous body is a juxtanuclear, spherical mass composed of intermediate filaments. Secretory granules are sparse, ranging in size from 100 to 250 nm.

Mammosomatotroph Adenoma. This produces both GH and PRL. It is associated with acromegaly and is the most frequent finding in patients with gigantism and in young patients with acromegaly. Microscopically, the tumor is composed mainly of acidophilic cells arranged in a diffuse or solid pattern. Chromophobic cells may be scattered throughout. Immunohistochemically, the tumor cells are strongly immunoreactive for GH and variably immunoreactive for α-subunit and PRL.[1] Staining for low-molecular-weight cytokeratins yields a perinuclear pattern of staining similar to that of normal somatotrophs and the cells of densely granulated somatotroph

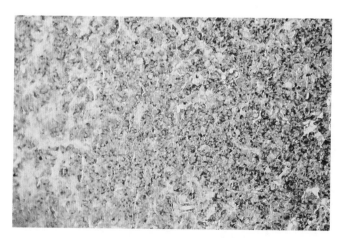

Figure 3-22. Densely granulated somatotroph adenoma. Immunohistochemistry for GH documents intense cytoplasmic reactivity throughout the cytoplasm of tumor cell (immunohistochemical stain for growth hormone).

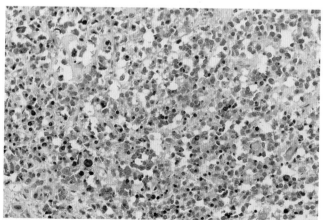

Figure 3-24. Sparsely granulated somatotroph adenoma. Immunohistochemistry for low-molecular-weight cytokeratins identifies juxtanuclear whorls of positivity that represent fibrous bodies, the hallmark of this tumor type.

adenomas. There is strong nuclear immunoreactivity for Pit-1 and occasionally for ER. Very rarely, β-TSH can be demonstrated in the cytoplasm. Ultrastructurally, the tumor cells resemble densely granulated somatotrophs[134]; however, secretory granules have mottled cores, are variably pleomorphic, and can measure up to 1000 nm. In addition, the cells exhibit misplaced exocytosis, which is the classic feature of PRL secretion.

Drug Effects

These tumors rarely show a response to dopaminergic agents. Treatment with somatostatin analogues often results in inhibition of GH excess,[137] most successfully in patients with densely granulated as compared with sparsely granulated tumors.[138] There is, however, no consistent tumor size reduction or morphologic alteration attributable to this therapy.[139]

Functioning Lactotroph Adenomas

Tumors arising from PRL-secreting adenohypophysial cells are the most common type of pituitary adenoma.[140, 141] Although almost half of adenomas found incidentally at autopsy are of this type,[142] the incidence is much lower in surgical series, probably because these tumors are often treated medically. This tumor is more common in females, who tend to present at a younger age with hormonal disturbances. Males tend to present at a later age with mass effects.[143] There are three variants of PRL-secreting pituitary adenomas: sparsely granulated and densely granulated lactotroph adenomas and the rare but aggressive acidophil stem cell tumor.

Clinical Features

In women, hyperprolactinemia most commonly manifests as galactorrhea and ovulatory disturbances, including amenorrhea and infertility. In men, hyperprolactinemia leads to decreased libido, erectile dysfunction, and only occasionally galactorrhea. In contrast to women, men tend to present later, with larger tumors that more often result in mass effects and hypopituitarism secondary to adenohypophysial destruction.[143] Large, invasive tumors may erode into sinuses and present as nasal masses. Death may result from tumor destruction of the hypothalamus or from tumor obstruction of the third ventricle. Patients with the unusual and aggressive acidophil stem cell adenoma may present with subtle features of acromegaly in addition to hyperprolactinemia.[144]

An elevated serum PRL level greater than 250 ng/mL is virtually diagnostic of a prolactin-secreting adenoma. Values less than 250 ng/mL must be interpreted with more caution because a number of physiologic, pharmacologic, and pathologic conditions may cause elevated serum PRL levels. Lactotroph adenomas tend to have a good correlation between tumor size and PRL level.

Radiologic evaluations generally reveal microadenomas in women and macroadenomas with suprasellar extension in men.

Medical treatment with bromocriptine results in a rapid fall in serum PRL levels and tumor shrinkage[140, 141]; these effects depend on the continued administration of the drug. Those tumors that show only a partial response to bromocriptine, usually macroadenomas, generally require surgical resection.

The acidophil stem cell adenoma is resistant to treatment with bromocriptine.[145] Surgical resection is necessary for these aggressive tumors; careful postoperative monitoring is required, as recurrence is common. Radiation therapy may play a role in the management of recurrent acidophil stem cell tumors.

Pathology

Microadenomas are most commonly located in the posterolateral portions of the gland. Macroadenomas may invade into dura mater, nasal sinuses, and bone. They can be soft and red, or gray and firm. Occasionally, the presence of psammoma bodies results in a gritty consistency.

Sparsely Granulated Lactotroph Adenoma. This is the more common variant. The chromophobic tumor cells are arranged in papillae, trabeculae (Fig. 3–25), or solid sheets (Fig. 3–26); tumor cells may form pseudorosettes around vascular spaces.[1] Calcification with the formation of frank psammoma bodies is occasionally present. Amyloid deposition is a rare feature. The tumor cells show strong immunoreactivity for PRL in a juxtanuclear globular pattern that corresponds to the Golgi region (Fig. 3–27). Nuclear staining for Pit-1 is usually present, and estrogen receptor positivity may be found by immunohistochemistry. Ultrastructurally,[134] the cells have large nuclei with prominent nucleoli. The rough

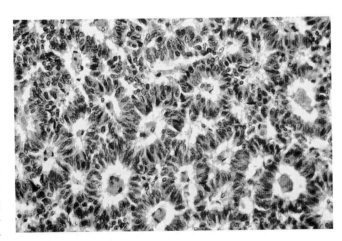

Figure 3–25. Sparsely granulated lactotroph adenoma, trabecular type. This tumor is composed of chromophobic cells arranged in trabeculae that surround vascular channels (H&E stain).

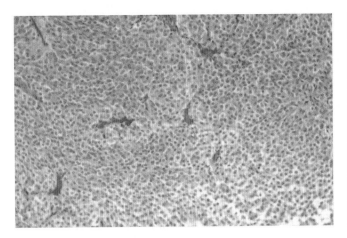

Figure 3-26. Sparsely granulated lactotroph adenoma, solid type. These tumors are usually composed of sheets of bland epithelial cells with abundant chromophobic cytoplasm (H&E stain).

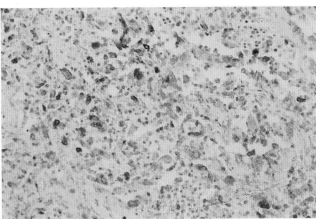

Figure 3-28. Densely granulated lactotroph adenoma. In contrast to the more common sparsely granulated variant, this rare tumor exhibits diffuse cytoplasmic positivity for PRL.

endoplasmic reticulum is prominent and arranged in distinctive parallel arrays; when arranged in concentric whorls, they are called Nebenkern formations. The large, well-developed Golgi complexes harbor immature pleomorphic granules. Secretory granules are spherical and sparse and range in size from 150 to 300 nm. Misplaced exocytosis is a diagnostic feature of PRL-producing tumors.

Densely Granulated Lactotroph Adenoma. This is much less common than the sparsely granulated variant. This tumor is composed of acidophilic cells that exhibit diffuse cytoplasmic positivity for PRL (Fig. 3–28), unlike the juxtanuclear Golgi pattern seen in the sparsely granulated adenoma. Ultrastructurally, densely granulated cells have abundant rough endoplasmic reticulum; secretory granules are numerous and can measure up to 700 nm. Misplaced exocytosis is again a diagnostic feature.

Acidophil Stem Cell Adenoma. This is usually composed of solid sheets of large cells that are slightly acidophilic due to the accumulation of mitochondria (Fig. 3–29). Large cytoplasmic vacuoles corresponding to giant mitochondria can be easily appreciated on light microscopy.[1] The classic immunohistochemical profile shows strong diffuse immunoreactivity for PRL and scant immunoreactivity for GH. Some tumors may lack detectable immunoreactivity for GH. Staining with low-molecular-weight cytokeratins usually allows the detection of scattered fibrous bodies.[1] Electron microscopy may be necessary to render a definitive diagnosis of this tumor.[134] Ultrastructurally, the cells are elongated with oval or irregular nuclei. The cytoplasm is occupied by numerous enlarged mitochondria; distinctive giant mitochondria containing electron-dense tubules are frequently seen. Fibrous bodies, or juxtanuclear bundles of cytokeratin

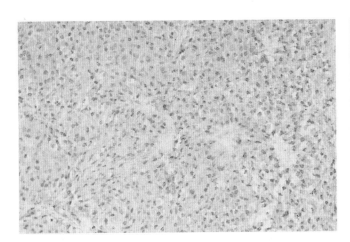

Figure 3-27. Sparsely granulated lactotroph adenoma. The immunohistochemical hallmark of this tumor is the globular juxtanuclear pattern of immunoreactivity for PRL that corresponds to the Golgi complex.

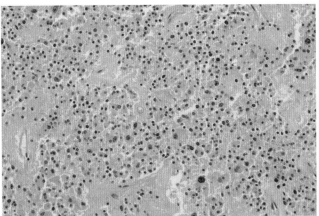

Figure 3-29. Acidophil stem cell adenoma. This oncocytic PRL-producing tumor has significant nuclear pleomorphism. Occasional tumor cells have cytoplasmic vacuoles that represent dilated mitochondria (H&E stain).

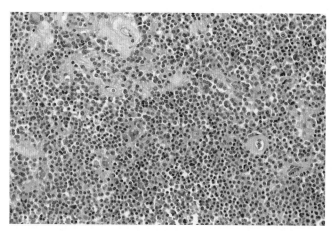

Figure 3-30. Dopamine agonist effects on lactotroph adenoma. Following treatment with dopamine agonists, sparsely granulate lactotroph adenomas shrink because of involution of tumor cell cytoplasm. These cellular tumors can be confused with lymphoma (H&E stain).

intermediate filaments, identical to those seen in sparsely granulated somatotroph adenomas, are scattered throughout the tumor. Secretory granules are scant and range in size from 150 to 200 nm. Misplaced exocytosis can be seen.

Drug Effects

Administration of dopamine agonists such as bromocriptine results in a dramatic clinical response in patients with prolactinomas. The rapid fall in serum PRL is accompanied by an almost equally rapid reduction in tumor size that is due to tumor cell shrinkage.[146] In the absence of relevant history, the changes may be a source of diagnostic confusion. The cytoplasm of the tumor cells shrinks, resulting in a marked increase in cellularity (Fig. 3–30). The resulting picture can histologically resemble a lymphoma. These changes are reversible on discontinuation of therapy; however, the alterations may be permanent in a small population of tumor cells. After chronic therapy, there is occasionally interstitial and perivascular fibrosis along with hemorrhage and hemosiderin deposition.

Functioning Thyrotroph Adenomas

Thyrotroph adenomas account for less than 1% of all pituitary neoplasms.

Clinical Features

Patients with pituitary-dependent TSH excess may exhibit features of hyperthyroidism or hypothyroidism, or they may be euthyroid.[147] Because most thyrotroph tumors are invasive macroadenomas, mass effects with visual field disturbances are common. In patients with elevated levels of serum TSH, thyroid function must be carefully evaluated to exclude primary thyroid failure, and radiologic evaluation with an MRI scan is essential for identifying the presence of a discrete sellar tumor rather than diffuse hyperplasia. Diffuse thyrotroph hyperplasia can mimic this disorder; it requires medical rather than surgical therapy.

Thyrotroph adenomas tend to be invasive and aggressive.[1] Treatment consists of surgery, radiation, or both. Medical therapy with bromocriptine and octreotide has had minimal success.

Pathology

Grossly, thyrotroph adenomas tumors tend to be invasive and fibrotic macroadenomas at the time of diagnosis.

On light microscopy, these tumors are composed of chromophobic cells with indistinct cell borders and varying degrees of nuclear pleomorphism (Fig. 3–31). Architecturally, the tumors most commonly exhibit a solid or sinusoidal pattern. Stromal fibrosis is relatively common, and occasional psammoma bodies may be present. The tumor cells show variable immunoreactivity for α-subunit and THS-beta. Immunohistochemistry highlights the polygonal structure of the tumor cells that usually have elongated processes.[1] Ultrastructurally, thyrotroph adenoma cells resemble normal thyrotrophs.[134] The polygonal cells have euchromatic nuclei and long interdigitating cytoplasmic processes that contain abundant rough endoplasmic reticulum with prominent and spherical Golgi's bodies. Secretory granules, which are spherical and range in size from 150 to 250 nm, tend to accumulate along the cell membrane. Some densely granulated tumors occasionally have larger granules measuring up to 350 nm.

Functioning Corticotroph Adenomas

Tumors composed of ACTH-secreting corticotrophs represent 10% to 15% of all pituitary adenomas. There

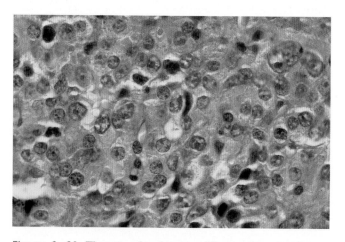

Figure 3-31. Thyrotroph adenoma. These tumors are composed of spindle-shaped cells with elongated processes and highly pleomorphic nuclei. There is focal PAS-positivity in the cytoplasm (PAS stain).

are three recognized variants: densely granulated corticotroph adenoma, sparsely granulated corticotroph adenoma, and Crooke's cell adenoma.

Clinical Features

Cushing's disease, defined as pituitary-dependent hypercortisolism, has a number of clinical manifestations, including central obesity, plethoric moon-shaped facies, hypertension, acne, hirsutism, proximal muscle weakness, menstrual irregularities, mental disturbances, osteopenia, easy bruising, buffalo hump, hyperpigmentation, and increased susceptibility to infection.[148] Cushing's disease can be fatal if not recognized and treated promptly. Laboratory investigations reveal elevated urinary-free cortisol levels with loss of diurnal plasma cortisol variation. There is failure to suppress cortisol with low-dose (1 mg) dexamethasone suppression testing, but high-dose (8 mg) testing generally yields a response. Plasma ACTH is usually elevated but to a lesser degree than in patients with ectopic ACTH secretion.

Treatment of Cushing's disease is aimed at reduction of ACTH plasma levels, with subsequent normalization of cortisol secretion. In patients with microadenomas, lateralization of the tumor with MRI, and/or inferior petrosal sinus sampling,[149, 150] followed by transsphenoidal resection of the adenoma can be curative. Large or invasive adenomas are rarely cured by surgery alone. Radiation therapy is employed in cases of unsuccessful surgical treatment but can have significant side effects in patients with glucocorticoid excess. Some studies have demonstrated success of medical therapy with anti-serotoninergic agents, such as cyproheptadine, reserpine, or metergoline, but more often, therapy for persistent Cushing's disease is directed at inhibition of cortisol synthesis. This is accomplished surgically by adrenalectomy and medically by administration of ketoconazole, aminoglutethimide, metyrapone, or low-dose mitotane. These drugs are given as a last resort because of their severe side effects. Bilateral adrenalectomy may result in Nelson's syndrome[151] and is therefore not a routine procedure, but it is often used after failure of pituitary surgery.

Pathology

The most common cause of Cushing's disease is a basophilic microadenoma.[1] This small tumor may be centrally located, as corticotrophs are most abundant in the median wedge of the anterior pituitary, but it usually exhibits lateralization of blood supply, justifying inferior petrosal sinus sampling. The macroadenoma is associated with Nelson's syndrome and represents chromophobic or sparsely granulated adenomas in patients with less florid hormone excess.

Densely granulated corticotroph adenoma. This is the most common type of corticotroph adenoma. On light microscopy, this tumor is composed

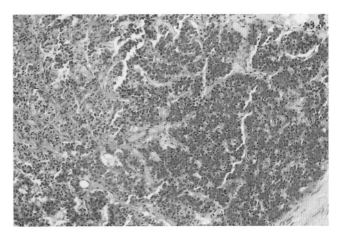

Figure 3-32. Densely granulated corticotroph adenoma. Cushing's disease is usually due to a basophilic microadenoma that can be difficult to identify on MRI (H&E stain).

of basophilic cells arranged in a sinusoidal architecture (Fig. 3-32). The tumor cells exhibit cytoplasmic PAS positivity. They are immunoreactive for ACTH, β-endorphin, and other POMC-derived peptides. Positivity for low-molecular-weight cytokeratins is seen in patients with Cushing's disease; in patients with Nelson's syndrome, the tumor cells do not accumulate keratin filaments. Ultrastructurally,[134] corticotroph cells are large and polygonal with ovoid or irregular nuclei that harbor nucleoli in contact with the inner nuclear membrane. The cytoplasm contains prominent rough endoplasmic reticulum with abundant free ribosomes, spherical Golgi's complexes, and perinuclear intermediate filaments composed of cytokeratins that are prominent in patients with Cushing's syndrome but are not conspicuous in Nelson's syndrome. The secretory granules range in size from 150 to 450 nm in diameter and are distinctive because of their marked variability in shape and electron density.

Sparsely Granulated Corticotroph Adenoma. This is less common than the densely granulated variant. By light microscopy, the tumor cells are chromophobic (Fig. 3-33) and are negative or only focally positive with the PAS stain. They exhibit strong immunoreactivity for cytokeratins and weak immunoreactivity for ACTH and other POMC-derived peptides.[1] Ultrastructurally,[134] the cells contain less well-developed organelles and scant secretory granules, but the characteristic variability of size, shape, and density of the granules characterizes them as corticotrophs.

Crooke's Cell Adenoma. This is a rare tumor that exhibits Crooke's hyaline change.[152, 153] Usually, Crooke's hyalinization is restricted to nontumorous corticotrophs; this marker of feedback suppression by glucocorticoids is rarely seen in adenomas. These tumors can be associated with Cushing's disease, but it is generally an unusual form of the disease, such as cyclical Cushing's disease. The tumor cells can exhibit marked cytologic and nuclear

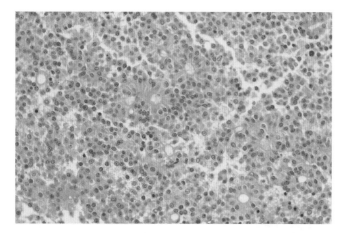

Figure 3–33. Sparsely granulated corticotroph adenoma. Patients with Cushing's disease and large adenomas usually have chromophobic tumors that are sparsely granulated, and ACTH immunoreactivity may be weak or focal (H&E stain).

atypia (Fig. 3–34). The perinuclear ring of pale hyaline material represents the accumulation of low-molecular-weight cytokeratin filaments that are intermediate filaments on electron microscopy.[154] The cells exhibit a rim of peripheral positivity when stained with PAS, and this is due to immunohistochemically detectable ACTH in secretory granules located either at the periphery of the cell or in the perinuclear region.

Functioning Gonadotroph Adenomas

These tumors are mainly diagnosed in middle-aged men with no prior history of gonadal dysfunction.[155] Although they occur in women, the clinical diagnosis is more often missed because elevation of

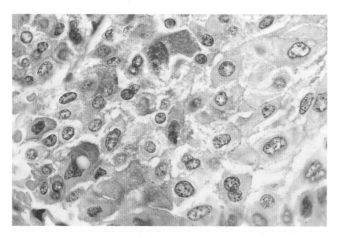

Figure 3–34. Crooke's cell adenoma. Rarely, corticotroph adenomas undergo Crooke's hyaline change. The tumor cells have pleomorphic nuclei and hyaline cytoplasm with basophilic granules limited to the cell periphery. Scattered basophilic cells can be seen (H&E stain).

gonadotropins is considered to be physiologic in postmenopausal women, and the tumors are considered to be nonfunctional.[156]

Clinical Features

Although symptoms and signs of gonadal dysfunction may occur, these tumors usually present with mass effects including headache, visual field impairment, and cranial nerve deficits. Gonadal dysfunction is rare and ironically manifests as hypogonadism[155]; rare cases of gonadal hyperfunction have been reported.[157, 158] In premenopausal young women, these tumors may mimic primary ovarian failure; the effects are generally reversible after successful surgical resection.

Elevated levels of serum FSH or LH or both are required to secure a diagnosis of gonadotroph adenoma. In most cases, levels of FSH alone are elevated; some cases have elevation of both FSH and LH; elevation of serum LH alone is rare. Gonadotrophin secretion may respond to stimulation by gonadotropin-releasing hormone and, paradoxically, to thyrotropin-releasing hormone.

Radiologic evaluation with CT and MRI usually reveals macroadenomas with suprasellar extension.

Surgery is the treatment of choice, with the transsphenoidal route being the preferred approach. The transfrontal approach is indicated only in cases in which the majority of the tumor is suprasellar. Adjuvant radiation therapy is reserved for large invasive tumors that fail surgical therapy and recur rapidly. Medical therapy with gonadotropin-releasing hormone analogues, bromocriptine, or octreotide have had minimal success; there is no conclusive evidence to support the efficacy of these drugs in the treatment of gonadotroph adenomas.

Pathology

Grossly, the tumors are soft and well-vascularized and occasionally have foci of hemorrhage or necrosis.

Microscopically, they are characterized by chromophobic cells arranged in a trabecular, papillary, or sinusoidal pattern.[159] There is usually prominent pseudorosette formation around vascular spaces (Fig. 3–35). Focal oncocytic change is quite common. Scant PAS positivity may be demonstrated in some tumor cells. The tumor cells exhibit variable intensity of immunoreactivity for α-subunit, β-FSH, and β-LH. As well, there is strong nuclear staining with steroidogenic factor-1.[1] It is common for gonadotroph adenomas to exhibit ultrastructural diversity.[134, 160] Well-differentiated tumor cells are elongated, with the nucleus occupying one pole and secretory granules accumulating at the opposite pole. Poorly differentiated cells are generally ovoid or polygonal and lack polarity. Rough endoplasmic reticulum is usually composed of short dilated profiles that contain flocculent material. Golgi's bodies are perinuclear, large,

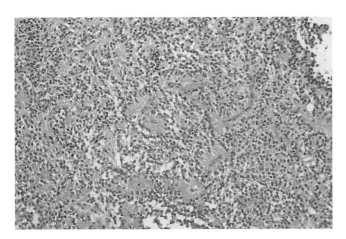

Figure 3–35. Gonadotroph adenoma. These tumors are composed of sheets and trabeculae of cells with chromophobic cytoplasm. They exhibit characteristic perivascular pseudorosettes (H&E stain).

and globular. Secretory granules are generally small (250 nm), variable in number, and located close to the cell membrane. Cells exhibiting oncocytic change have abundant mitochondria.

Clinically Nonfunctioning Pituitary Adenomas

These tumors account for approximately one-third of all pituitary adenomas. Because of their lack of clinically detectable hormonal activity, they tend to present with mass effects such as headache, visual field deficits, cranial nerve defects or, rarely, cavernous sinus syndrome.[1] If there is extensive tissue destruction, hypopituitarism results in clinical symptoms.

Less commonly, pituitary apoplexy with hemorrhage into the tumor causes a medical emergency.

Biochemically, patients may have varying degrees of hypopituitarism depending on the amount of adenohypophysial tissue destruction. There is no evidence of hormone excess; however, stalk compression without significant adenohypophysial destruction can result in mild hyperprolactinemia.

Radiologically, these tumors present as large sellar masses, usually with extensive suprasellar or parasellar extension.

Transsphenoidal surgical resection or debulking is the treatment of choice. Local recurrence is common, and adjuvant radiation therapy may be required for rapidly growing lesions. No effective medical therapy is available.

Pathology

The diagnosis of silent pituitary adenomas is based solely on morphologic features of the tumor.[1] *Silent somatotroph adenomas* have morphologic features similar to those of sparsely granulated somatotroph adenomas. *Silent lactotroph adenomas* and *silent thyrotroph adenomas* exhibit morphologic features corresponding to those of their functioning counterparts. *Silent corticotroph adenomas* are usually associated with hyperprolactinemia, even in cases without obvious stalk involvement. There are two morphologic variants. *Type I silent corticotroph adenomas* correspond morphologically to the functioning densely granulated corticotroph adenoma. *Type II silent corticotroph adenomas* are similar to the sparsely granulated functioning corticotroph adenomas. The clinical inactivity of some corticotroph adenomas may be due to aberrant cleavage of the POMC molecule. *Silent gonadotroph adenomas* are morphologically identical to the functioning gonadotroph adenomas and represent the largest group of clinically nonfunctioning adenomas. Most tumors classified as *null cell adenomas* are silent gonadotroph adenomas composed of poorly differentiated cells with scattered foci exhibiting histologic features consistent with gonadotroph differentiation; these tumors generally exhibit SF-1 staining despite lack of detectable gonadotropin content. *Oncocytomas* represent silent gonadotroph adenomas with extensive oncocytic change (Fig. 3–36). The tumor cells are usually arranged in sheets or nests and contain abundant granular eosinophilic cytoplasm, which corresponds ultrastructurally to mitochondrial accumulation in the cytoplasm. These tumors also generally exhibit SF-1 nuclear reactivity.[1]

Despite advances in morphologic classification of adenohypophysial cells, because of improved tissue fixation, more specific and sensitive antibodies, and transcription factors that identify cell differentiation, there remain pituitary adenomas that defy definitive classification based on histologic, immunohistochemical, and ultrastructural examination. *Poorly differentiated adenomas* are negative for all hormones and transcription factors and exhibit no ultrastructural markers of the known adenohypophysial cell types.[1]

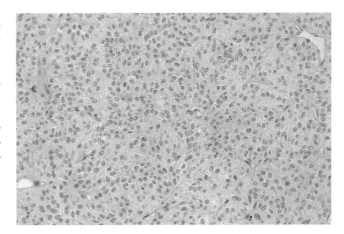

Figure 3–36. Oncocytoma. These tumors have extensive oncocytic change but usually exhibit nuclear reactivity for SF-1 and often have scattered cytoplasmic positivity for gonadotropin subunits (H&E stain).

The tumor identified as *female type gonadotroph adenoma*[161] is usually clinically silent and immunohistochemically plurihormonal and is characterized by a distinctive ultrastructural feature of dilated, saccular Golgi's bodies known as honeycomb Golgi. The cytogenesis of this lesion is not known.

Plurihormonal Pituitary Adenomas

Occasionally, pituitary adenomas elaborate multiple hormones. Most often, this is due to known regulatory factors; products of different hormone families are rarely produced. These adenomas may be fully functioning, partially functioning (in which only one component is clinically apparent), or silent.

The most common combination is excessive production of GH and PRL, or of GH, PRL, and TSH, resulting in acromegaly/gigantism accompanied by hyperprolactinemia and even hyperthyroidism. This pattern of plurihormonality is accounted for by the expression of Pit-1, which regulates the expression of these various hormones by related cells. Other combinations of unrelated hormones have been reported.[1] The interpretation of the individual combinations must be evaluated with caution and may in some cases be artefacts of antibody cross-reactivity. Due to the relative uniqueness of each case, biochemical and radiologic profiles often do not contribute to the diagnosis.

Treatment is determined on an individual basis and can include surgical resection or medical therapy. There is no conclusive evidence indicating that plurihormonal adenomas have a different prognosis when compared with their monohormonal counterparts. However, the silent subtype III adenoma is considered more aggressive, and local recurrence is not uncommon.[162] There may be a role for radiotherapy for this relatively radiosensitive lesion.

Pathology

Monomorphous plurihormonal adenomas are composed of one cell type that can produce multiple hormones; this is supported by cytoplasmic immunoreactivity for two or more hormones within the same cell. *Plurimorphous plurihormonal adenomas* are composed of at least two cell types, each of which exhibits a characteristic immunohistochemical and ultrastructural profile. These may represent "collision" tumors.[163, 164] *Silent subtype III adenomas* are rare and aggressive plurihormonal tumors that are identified by unique ultrastructural features.[162] The large tumor cells have nuclei that are located at one pole and may contain spheridia. There is abundant well-developed rough endoplasmic reticulum with prominent, tortuous Golgi's complexes and abundant groups of mitochondria. Small secretory granules are localized to attenuated, interdigitating cell processes.

Pituitary Carcinoma

Malignant tumors of adenohypophysial origin are defined by the ability to metastasize.[1, 165] Although many pituitary adenomas are widely invasive, destructive of adjacent tissues, and lethal, they are not classified as malignancies. The pathogenesis of the very rare pituitary carcinoma is not known. H-*ras* point mutations have been reported in some metastatic foci but not in the corresponding primary tumor.[166, 167] Immunoreactivity for p53 has been reported, but p53 mutations are not found in these lesions, and there is insufficient evidence to draw any conclusions regarding the mechanism of the apparent accumulation of p53 protein.[168]

Clinical Features

Pituitary carcinomas generally present initially as pituitary adenoma. They may cause a variety of hormonal abnormalities[169–174] or be clinically nonfunctioning.[175, 176] Only the subsequent development of metastases identifies the lesion as malignant.

Radiologic investigation may reveal spread to various sites, including the subarachnoid space, cervical lymph nodes, bone, liver, and lungs. Local radiology usually reveals an invasive tumor with extension beyond the confines of the sella turcica.

The prognosis is poor. Because of the limited number of reported cases, no conclusions can be drawn regarding the effectiveness of various therapeutic approaches.

Pathology

The definition of pituitary carcinoma is based on the presence of metastatic disease. The most common sites include the subarachnoid space, brain parenchyma (not including areas of direct invasion), cervical lymph nodes, bone, liver, and lungs. Examination of the primary tumor usually reveals nonspecific morphologic features such as hypercellularity, hemorrhage, necrosis, mitoses, nuclear pleomorphism, and invasion; none of these features, either individually or in combination, are reliable indicators of malignancy. Immunohistochemistry and electron microscopy are used mainly to characterize the tumor based on the classification scheme applied to the more common adenomas.[177]

PRIMARY TUMORS OF THE NEUROHYPOPHYSIS AND HYPOTHALAMUS

Neuronal Tumors

These tumors are also known as "gangliocytomas" or "ganglioneuromas."[1] They are neoplasms composed of mature neurons, most likely derived from the ganglion cells of the hypothalamus. Clinically, they can present with mass effects, hypothalamic dysregulation, hypopituitarism, and hyperprolactinemia.[178] Because these tumors have the ability to synthesize hypothalamic peptides, they may sometimes be associated with other hormonal syndromes including acromegaly, precocious puberty, or Cushing's disease.[178] Treatment involves surgical resection. Grossly, they vary in size and appearance. Microscopically, they are composed of mature ganglion cells with abundant cytoplasm that contains Nissl's substance and of large nuclei with prominent nucleoli. Binucleate or even multinucleated cells are not uncommon. The tumor cells are distributed within a variable stroma composed of neuroglia—fibrous tissue with small-vessel proliferation. These tumors are immunoreactive for synaptophysin and neurofilament. Ultrastructurally, the tumor cells resemble mature neurons, with abundant endoplasmic reticulum, mitochondria, and neurofilaments. Secretory granules are concentrated in neuronal processes. The neuronal lesions associated with acromegaly have often been composite tumors with a pituitary adenoma component, usually a sparsely granulated somatotroph adenoma.

Gliomas

These are neoplasms of neuroglia and include astrocytomas, oligodendrogliomas, and ependymomas.[1] The pilocytic astrocytoma, which is most common in young patients, is the most common glial tumor of the sellar region.[179] These lesions can be sporadic, associated with inherited conditions, or may follow cranial irradiation.[180, 181] Clinically, they usually present with mass effects, hypothalamic hypopituitarism, and hyperprolactinemia from decreased dopaminergic inhibition of prolactin. Radiologic characteristics vary with each tumor type. Low-grade gliomas that occur in children have a good prognosis. Postirradiation gliomas and those affecting the optic nerve are aggressive and rapidly lethal.

Meningiomas

Meningiomas are neoplasms of the meninges and are most commonly of arachnoid origin. They occur more frequently in females. Meningiomas of the sellar region account for up to 20% of all meningiomas. They can present with neurologic deficits, visual field defects, hypopituitarism, and hyperprolactinemia due to stalk compression.[182] Completely intrasellar meningiomas are rare.[183] They have been reported following radiotherapy for pituitary adenoma.[184-186] Treatment consists of complete surgical resection.

Granular Cell Tumors

Granular cell tumors are benign neoplasms of uncertain histogenesis found in the neurohypophysis or distal pituitary stalk.[187, 188] They resemble granular cell tumors in other sites. Most of these tumors are small and are incidental autopsy findings. Occasionally, they present with visual field deficits. Diabetes insipidus is rare. Clinically apparent tumors generally undergo surgical resection. Grossly, the tumors are tan, firm, and well demarcated from the surrounding tissue. Microscopically, the tumors are unencapsulated and composed of cells with abundant, granular, eosinophilic cytoplasm. The granules are PAS-positive and diastase-resistant. The tumor cells exhibit variable immunoreactivity for the histiocytic markers α_1-antitrypsin, α_1-antichymotrypsin, and cathepsin B. They are usually nonimmunoreactive for glial fibrillary acidic protein and S-100 protein.[189] Ultrastructurally, the granular cells have phagolysosomes containing debris and electron-dense material.

Chordomas

Chordomas are rare midline tumors derived from notochord remnants. They are most common in the sacral region but can occur in other sites, including the vertebrae, the clivus, and the sella turcica.[190] They usually occur in patients older than 30 years. These tumors are slow-growing but locally aggressive. Clinically, patients with parasellar chordomas can present with hypopituitarism. Radiologically, the tumors are lobulated, osteolytic lesions with foci of calcification. Elevation of the periosteum is a characteristic feature. The treatment of choice is surgical excision. Tumors that are incompletely resected can be irradiated. Mean survival from time of diagnosis is approximately 5 years. Grossly, chordomas are gelatinous, lobulated, and calcified. Microscopically, the tumors are composed of large polygonal cells called physaliphorous cells because of their bubbly cytoplasmic vacuoles containing glycogen and neutral mucins. The cells are arranged in solid sheets or trabeculae within a stroma of acidic mucin. The tumor cells are immunoreactive for low-molecular-weight cytokeratins, epithelial membrane antigen, S-100 protein, and sometimes carcinoembryonic antigen. Ultrastructurally, desmosomes and microvilli are present. The rough endoplasmic reticulum forms concentric rings around mitochondria.

Schwannomas

These tumors are also known as neurolemmomas. Schwannomas of this region are derived from the Schwann cells surrounding cranial nerves. They are rare tumors that can present as a sellar mass with or without hypopituitarism or hyperprolactinemia.[191-193] These tumors are usually benign. Surgical resection is the treatment of choice. Histologically, these tumors are identical to schwannomas elsewhere in the body. They are usually encapsulated lesions composed of spindle-shaped cells arranged into the classic Antoni A and Antoni B areas. Verocay's bodies result from palisading of tumor cells in Antoni A areas. The tumor cells are immunoreactive for S-100 protein. Ultrastructural examination reveals basal lamina and pathognomonic long-spacing collagen.

PRIMARY TUMORS OF THE SELLA TURCICA

These are primary, nonhypophysial tumors that arise in the region of the sella turcica. They include craniopharyngiomas, germ cell tumors, lymphomas, leukemias, Langerhans' cell histiocytosis, and tumors of mesenchymal origin.

Craniopharyngioma

This benign but locally invasive tumor, which originates from the remnants of Rathke's pouch, represents 2%–4% of all intracranial neoplasms.[194] It is the most common sellar tumor in children and accounts for 10% of all childhood central nervous system tumors. Craniopharyngiomas can occur at all ages; the peak incidence occurs from 5 to 20 years old, with a second smaller peak occurring in the sixth decade. Some series show a male predominance.

Clinical Features

Three-quarters of patients have mass effects with headaches and visual field disturbances.[55] Patients may have psychiatric disturbances, nausea, vomiting, and somnolence. Hypopituitarism is identified in the majority but is not often the presenting complaint. In contrast to patients with large pituitary adenomas, hyperprolactinemia is found in less than half of patients,[195, 196] and about 25% of patients have diabetes insipidus. Children may present with dwarfism.

Radiologic evaluation reveals a variably cystic lesion; only 10% of craniopharyngiomas are entirely solid with no cystic component. An enlarged or eroded sella turcica is encountered in 50% of cases; suprasellar calcification is present in more than 50% of cases. MRI is the preferred technique for determining the extent of the lesion; there is often a strong T1 signal in the absence of contrast because of high lipid content.

The natural history of these lesions is extensive infiltration with significant tissue damage. Infiltration may involve the hypothalamus or extend to as high as the third ventricle. Complete surgical resection is curative.[197] However, the highly infiltrative nature of this lesion often results in incomplete resection with a subsequent high recurrence rate of 10% to 62%; this is especially true in younger patients. Postoperative radiation has been advocated to reduce recurrence. Hormone replacement may be necessary for persistent hypopituitarism.

Complications of untreated disease include hydrocephalus, if there is extension and obstruction of the third ventricle, and rupture with abscess formation. A single case of malignant transformation in a craniopharyngioma has been reported.[198]

Pathology

Craniopharyngiomas are entirely suprasellar in 85% of cases; an intrasellar component is present in only 15%. Most of these tumors are larger than 1 cm at the time of diagnosis. They are well circumscribed but not necessarily encapsulated and usually contain a thick oil-like fluid resembling black sludge. Other features recognized grossly include cholesterol and calcification.

On light microscopy, the tumor is characterized by islands of epithelial cells and cysts within a loose fibrous stroma (Fig. 3–37). Cholesterol clefts are commonly present. There is often keratinous debris, which forms the nidus for foci of calcification. Occasionally, there is a mixed chronic inflammatory infiltrate composed of lymphocytes, plasma cells, and macrophages. Although well delineated grossly, microscopically these tumors frequently have infiltrative borders with associated gliosis of the adjacent brain. Two histologic types are identified: the adamantinomatous variant and the papillary variant. The *adamantinomatous variant* has a prominent stellate component and resembles the dental ameloblastic organ and other adamantinomas. The less common *papillary variant* is more frequently found in adults. This tumor is characterized by pseudopapillary squamous epithelium in a solid or cystic pattern; palisading, fibrosis, and cholesterol accumulation are usually absent. This variant has a somewhat better prognosis than the adamantinomatous variant.

By immunohistochemistry, the presence of cytokeratin reactivity confirms the epithelial nature of these tumors. Ultrastructural examination reveals tonofilaments, intercellular junctions, and the absence of secretory granules.

Germ Cell Tumors

These are midline tumors that arise from residual germ cells. They include germinomas, embryonal carcinomas, teratomas, endodermal sinus tumors, and

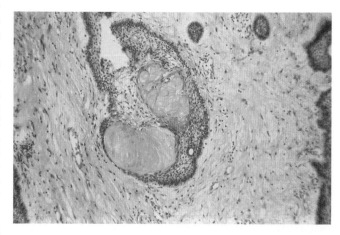

Figure 3–37. Craniopharyngioma. Epithelial-lined cysts are suspended within a loose stroma. Keratin debris is present within the islands of epithelium (hematoxylin-phloxine-saffron stain).

choriocarcinomas. These tumors represent less than 1% of intracranial tumors in adults.[199] In children, however, germ cell tumors account for approximately 6.5% of all intracranial neoplasms.[200] They are relatively rare after age 20, with males more frequently affected than females. The most common site of intracranial involvement is the pineal gland, followed by the suprasellar region.[201] Within the sellar region, pure germinomas and pure teratomas are the predominant subtypes. Mixed germ cell tumors are also common; they usually contain a germinoma in combination with some other component.[202, 203]

Clinical Features

Clinical manifestations include hypopituitarism, diabetes insipidus, and visual field defects. If sufficiently large, they may cause raised intracranial pressure, hydrocephalus, psychosis, and dementia. Involvement of the hypothalamus can lead to anorexia or bulimia. Tumors that produce β-hCG may result in precocious puberty. Germ cell tumors do not have diagnostic radiologic findings.[201, 204]

Germ cell tumors can be difficult to treat. The exception to this is the germinoma, which is radiosensitive, with long-term cure in 70% of patients. Despite combined treatment with surgery, radiation, and chemotherapy, the other germ cell tumors tend to recur and metastasize.[205–207]

Pathology

Intracranial germ cell tumors are histologically identical to germ cell tumors arising in other sites. Germinomas are immunoreactive for placental alkaline phosphatase. Embryonal carcinomas are immunoreactive for α-fetoprotein, pregnancy glycoprotein SP1, and the β-subunit of human chorionic gonadotropin (hCG). Endodermal sinus tumors produce α-fetoprotein. Choriocarcinomas contain β-hCG, placental lactogen, and SP1.[203, 208]

Hematologic Tumors

Neoplastic proliferations of myeloid, lymphoid, or plasmacytoid cells within the hypophysis and hypothalamus usually occur as part of a systemic disorder. However, very rarely, the hypophysis and/or hypothalamus may be the primary site of involvement.[209–211]

Clinical Features

Involvement of the hypophysial-hypothalamic region most commonly manifests as diabetes insipidus; less commonly, it can result in the syndrome of inappropriate antidiuretic hormone, hypopituitarism, and mass effects.

On MRI, the lesions are isodense on T1-weighted images, are hyperintense on T2-weighted images, and enhance with contrast.

Management of primary sellar hematologic neoplasms is the same as that for other primary hematologic tumors of the central nervous system.[212–214]

Pathology

Grossly, the lesions are often subcapsular; rarely, they may be intraparenchymal. Histologically, these neoplasms are similar to their extracranial counterparts. They are most commonly non-Hodgkin's lymphomas composed of B cells.[215]

Langerhans' Cell Histiocytosis

Langerhans' cell histiocytosis is characterized by proliferation of the Langerhans' cell, which is a special type of histiocyte with dendritic processes and antigen-presenting capabilities. This disease can be unifocal, multifocal, or disseminated. It is separated into three clinicopathologic entities: Letterer-Siwe disease, eosinophilic granuloma, and Hand-Schüller-Christian disease.[1]

Clinical Features

Langerhans' cell histiocytosis may involve the neurohypophysis and hypothalamus, resulting in diabetes insipidus and, less commonly, hypopituitarism with associated hyperprolactinemia. Involvement of the adenohypophysis is rare.[216–218]

On CT and MRI scans, the lesions are usually multifocal, ill-defined, hypodense, contrast-enhancing masses. Involvement of the pituitary stalk is common.[219, 220]

Treatment depends on the distribution of the disease and can include surgery and irradiation. The prognosis is variable.[217, 218]

Pathology

By light microscopy, Langerhans' cells have abundant pink cytoplasm with characteristic indented or kidney bean–shaped nuclei. They are usually accompanied by a mixed inflammatory infiltrate including lymphocytes, plasma cells, and eosinophils. Langerhans' cells are immunoreactive for CD1a and S-100 protein. Ultrastructurally, the presence of Birbeck's granules within the cytoplasm is diagnostic.[215, 221]

Mesenchymal Tumors

Tumors arising from mesenchyme can be derived from vessels, fat, bone, cartilage, or fibrous tissue. They can be benign or malignant and can involve any site in the body, including the sellar region.[222] Involvement of the sellar turcica by such neoplasms is uncommon; they usually manifest with mass effects and variable hypofunction of anterior or posterior pituitary function. Various examples of such tumors have been reported in the sellar region, including hemangioma,[223, 224] glomangioma,[225] hemangioblastoma,[226] lipoma,[1] enchondroma,[227] chondroma,[228, 229] chondrosarcoma,[230] chondromyxoid fibroma,[231] giant cell tumor,[232] alveolar soft-part sarcoma,[233] osteosarcoma,[234] and fibrosarcoma.[235]

The tumors that involve the sellar turcica can be sporadic or can occur as part of a clinical syndrome such as von Hippel–Lindau disease.[226] However, most commonly, sarcomas of the sellar region develop as a result of previous irradiation for lesions such as pituitary adenoma or craniopharyngioma.[236]

METASTATIC TUMORS TO THE HYPOPHYSIS AND SELLA TURCICA

The pituitary gland, being a highly vascular organ, can be the target of bloodborne metastases from many malignancies. Metastatic tumors to the pituitary gland are not an uncommon event; the prevalence has been reported to be as high as 26.7%. Involvement of the neurohypophysis is more common than that of the adenohypophysis. The most common sites of origin are lung, breast, and gastrointestinal tract.[237–240]

Clinical Features

Metastatic tumors to the pituitary gland are usually not among the most prominent clinical complaints of patients with disseminated malignancy; they are usually discovered at autopsy. They may occasionally present as a sellar tumor in a patient with an occult primary. Clinically, they are distinguished from primary pituitary adenomas by the prominence of diabetes insipidus and mass effects such as headaches, visual field defects, ptosis, and ophthalmoplegia; hypopituitarism is less evident and occurs when adenohypophysial involvement is extensive. In rare cases, metastatic involvement of a pituitary adenoma may result in rapid increase in tumor size and/or sudden worsening symptoms.[241–244]

Because of the disseminated nature of malignancies that involve the pituitary, treatment is usually palliative; surgery with or without radiation may result in symptomatic relief.[245]

Pathology

The morphologic features of the metastatic tumor usually conform to those of the primary malignancy. The major differential diagnosis for metastatic tumors to the hypophysis is a pituitary adenoma. Problems may arise because nuclear pleomorphism

and mitotic activity can be prominent features in some adenomas; this is especially true for the sparsely granulated somatotroph adenoma.[1]

MISCELLANEOUS LESIONS

Other rare and unusual lesions of the pituitary region include inflammatory pseudotumors,[246] aneurysm,[247] meningoencephalocele,[248] hamartomas and choristomas,[249, 250] and brown tumor of bone.[132] The details of the clinical and pathologic features of these entities are reported individually.

References

1. Asa SL: Tumors of the Pituitary Gland. In Atlas of Tumor Pathology, Third Series. Armed Forces Institute of Pathology, Washington, D.C., 1998.
2. Asa SL, Kovacs K, Melmed S: The hypothalamic-pituitary axis. In Melmed S, ed.: The Pituitary. Blackwell Scientific Publications, Boston, 1995, p. 3.
3. Asa SL, Penz G, Kovacs K, et al.: Prolactin cells in the human pituitary: A quantitative immunocytochemical analysis. Arch Pathol Lab Med 1982; 106:360.
4. Elster AD, Sanders TG, Vines FS: Size and shape of the pituitary gland during pregnancy and postpartum: Measurement with MR imaging. Radiology 1991; 181:531.
5. Asa SL, Kovacs K: Functional morphology of the human fetal pituitary. Pathol Annu 1984; 1:275.
6. Asa SL, Ezzat S: The cytogenesis and pathogenesis of pituitary adenomas. Endocr Rev 1998; 19:798.
7. Asa SL, Ezzat S: Molecular determinants of pituitary cytodifferentiation. Pituitary 1999; 1:159.
8. Tremblay JJ, Lanctot C, Drouin J: The pan-pituitary activator of transcription, Ptx1 (pituitary homeobox 1) acts in synergy with SF-1 and Pit-1 and is an upstream regulator of the Lim-homeodomain gene Lim3/Lhx3. Mol Endocrinol 1998; 12:428.
9. Gage PJ, Camper SA: Pituitary homeobox 2, a novel member of the bicoid-related family of homeobox genes, is a potential regulator of anterior structure formation. Hum Mol Genet 1997; 6:457.
10. Sheng HZ, Moriyama K, Yamashita T, et al.: Multistep control of pituitary organogenesis. Science 1997; 278:1809.
11. Bach I, Rhodes SJ, Pearse RV, et al.: P-Lim, a LIM homeodomain factor, is expressed during pituitary organ and cell commitment and synergizes with Pit-1. Proc Natl Acad Sci U S A 1995; 92:2720.
12. Hermesz E, Machem S, Mahon KA: Rpx: A novel anterior-restricted homeobox gene progressively activated in the prechordal plate, anterior neural plate and Rathke's pouch of the mouse embryo. Development 1996; 122:41.
13. Sornson MW, Wu W, Dasen JS, et al.: Pituitary lineage determination by the prophet of Pit-1 homeodomain factor defective in Ames dwarfism. Nature 1996; 384:327.
14. Gage PJ, Brinkmeier MLSLM, Knapp LT, et al.: The Ames dwarf gene, df, is required early in pituitary ontogeny for the extinction of Rpx transcription and initiation of lineage-specific cell proliferation. Mol Endocrinol 1996; 10:1570.
15. Wu W, Cogan JD, Pfäffle RW, et al.: Mutations in *prop-1* cause familial combined pituitary hormone deficiency. Nat Genet 1998; 18:147.
16. Fofanova O, Takmura N, Kinoshita E, et al.: Compound heterozygous deletion of the *prop-1* gene in children with combined pituitary hormone deficiency. J Clin Endocrinol Metab 1998; 83:2601.
17. Jackson SM, Barnhart KM, Mellon P, et al.: Helix-loop proteins are present and differentially expressed in different cell lines from the anterior pituitary. Mol Cell Endocrinol 1993; 96:167.

18. Therrien M, Drouin J: Cell-specific helix-loop-helix factor required for pituitary expression of the pro-opiomelanocortin gene. Mol Cell Biol 1993; 13:2342.

19. Poulin G, Turgeon B, Drouin J: NeuroD1/beta2 contributes to cell-specific transcription of the proopiomelanocortin gene. Mol Cell Biol 1997; 17:6673.

20. Ingraham HA, Lala DS, Ikeda Y, et al.: The nuclear receptor steroidogenic factor 1 acts at multiple levels of the reproductive axis. Genes Dev 1994; 8:2302.

21. Rosenfeld MG: POU-domain transcription factors: Pou-er-ful developmental regulators. Genes Dev 1991; 5:897.

22. Asa SL, Puy LA, Lew AM, et al.: Cell type–specific expression of the pituitary transcription activator Pit-1 in the human pituitary and pituitary adenomas. J Clin Endocrinol Metab 1993; 77:1275.

23. Friend KE, Chiou Y-K, Laws ER Jr, et al.: Pit-1 messenger ribonucleic acid is differentially expressed in human pituitary adenomas. J Clin Endocrinol Metab 1993; 77:1281.

24. Pellegrini I, Barlier A, Gunz G, et al.: Pit-1 gene expression in the human pituitary and pituitary adenomas. J Clin Endocrinol Metab 1994; 79:189.

25. Day RN, Koike S, Sakai M, et al.: Both Pit-1 and the estrogen receptor are required for estrogen responsiveness of the rat prolactin gene. Mol Endocrinol 1990; 4:1964.

26. Drolet DW, Scully KM, Simmons DM, et al.: TEF, a transcription factor expressed specifically in the anterior pituitary during embryogenesis, defines a new class of leucine zipper proteins. Genes Dev 1991; 5:1739.

27. Asa SL, Kovacs K, Bilbao JM: The pars tuberalis of the human pituitary: A histologic, immunohistochemical, ultrastructural and immunoelectron microscopic analysis. Virchows Arch [A] 1983; 399:49.

28. Stanfield JP: The blood supply of the human pituitary gland. J Anat 1960; 94:257.

29. Daniel PM, Prichard MML: Observations on the vascular anatomy of the pituitary gland and its importance in pituitary function. Am Heart J 1966; 72:147.

30. Gorczyca W, Hardy J: Arterial supply of the human anterior pituitary gland. Neurosurgery 1987; 20:369.

31. Bergland RM, Page RB: Can the pituitary secrete directly to the brain?: Affirmative anatomical evidence. Endocrinology 1978; 102:1325.

32. Bergland RM, Page RB: Pituitary-brain vascular relations: A new paradigm. Science 1979; 204:18.

33. Melchionna RH, Moore RA: The pharyngeal pituitary gland. Am J Pathol 1938; 14:763.

34. Boyd JD: Observations of the human pharyngeal hypophysis. J Endocrinol 1956; 14:66.

35. Ciocca DR, Puy LA, Stati AO: Identification of seven hormone-producing cell types in the human pharyngeal hypophysis. J Clin Endocrinol Metab 1985; 60:212.

36. Hori A: Suprasellar peri-infundibular ectopic adenohypophysis in fetal and adult brains. J Neurosurg 1985; 62:113.

37. Colohan ART, Grady MS, Bonnin JM, et al.: Ectopic pituitary gland simulating a suprasellar tumor. Neurosurgery 1987; 20:43.

38. Björklöf K, Brundelet PJ: Typus degenerativus amstelodamensis (Cornelia de Lange first syndrome): Congenital hypopituitarism due to a cyst of Rathke's cleft? Acta Pediatr Scand 1965; 54:275.

39. Fujita K, Matsuo N, Mori O, et al.: The association of hypopituitarism with small pituitary, invisible stalk, type 1 Arnold-Chiari malformation, and syringomyelia in several patients born in breech position: A further proof of birth injury theory on the pathogenesis of "idiopathic hypopituitarism." Eur J Pediatr 1992; 151:266.

40. Ehrlich RM: Ectopic and hypoplastic pituitary with adrenal hypoplasia. J Pediatr 1957; 51:377.

41. Moncrieff MW, Hill DS, Archer J, et al.: Congenital absence of pituitary gland and adrenal hypoplasia. Arch Dis Child 1972; 47:136.

42. Kauschansky A, Genel M, Walker Smith GJ: Congenital hypopituitarism in female infants: Its association with hypoglycemia and hypothyroidism. Am J Dis Child 1979; 133:165.

43. Kosaki K, Matsuo N, Tamai S, et al.: Isolated aplasia of the anterior pituitary as a cause of congenital panhypopituitarism. Horm Res 1991; 35:226.

44. Pholsena M, Young J, Couzinet B, et al.: Primary adrenal and thyroid insufficiencies associated with hypopituitarism: A diagnostic challenge. Clin Endocrinol (Oxf) 1994; 40:693.

45. Dattani MT, Martinez-Barbera JP, Thomas PQ, et al.: Mutations in the homeobox gene HESX1/Hesx1 associated with septo-optic dysplasia in human and mouse. Nature Genet 1998; 19:125.

46. Tatsumi K, Miyai K, Notomi T, et al.: Cretinism with combined hormone deficiency caused by a mutation in the Pit-1 gene. Nature Genet 1992; 1:56.

47. Pfäffle RW, DiMattia GE, Parks JS, et al.: Mutation of the POU-specific domain of Pit-1 and hypopituitarism without pituitary hypoplasia. Science 1992; 257:1118.

48. Radovick S, Nations M, Du Y, et al.: A mutation in the POU-homeodomain of Pit-1 responsible for combined pituitary hormone deficiency. Science 1992; 257:1115.

49. Li S, Crenshaw EB III, Rawson EJ, et al.: Dwarf locus mutants lacking three pituitary cell types result from mutations in the POU-domain gene pit-1. Nature 1990; 347:528.

50. Roessmann U: Duplication of the pituitary gland and spinal cord. Arch Pathol Lab Med 1985; 109:518.

51. Priesel A: Über die dystopie der neurohyophyse. Virchows Arch Pathol Anat Physiol Klin Med 1927; 266:407.

52. Jordan RM, Kendall JW, Kerber CW: The primary empty sella syndrome: Analysis of the clinical characteristics, radiographic features, pituitary function and cerebrospinal fluid adenohypophysial hormone concentrations. Am J Med 1977; 62:569.

53. Bergeron C, Kovacs K, Bilbao JM: Primary empty sella: A histologic and immunocytologic study. Arch Intern Med 1979; 139:248.

54. Gharib H, Frey HM, Laws ER Jr, et al.: Coexistent primary empty sella syndrome and hyperprolactinemia: Report of 11 cases. Arch Intern Med 1983; 143:1383.

55. Shin JL, Asa SL, Woodhouse LJ, et al.: Cystic lesions of the pituitary: Clinicopathological features distinguishing craniopharyngioma, Rathke's cleft cyst, and arachnoid cyst. J Clin Endocrinol Metab 1999; 84:3972.

56. Obenchain TG, Becker DP: Abscess formation in a Rathke's cleft cyst: Case report. J Neurosurg 1972; 36:359.

57. Kucharczyk W, Peck WW, Kelly WM, et al.: Rathke's cleft cysts: CT, MR imaging, and pathologic features. Radiology 1987; 165:491.

58. Yamakawa K, Shitara N, Genka S, et al.: Clinical course and surgical prognosis of 33 cases of intracranial epidermoid tumors. Neurosurgery 1989; 24:568.

59. Abramson RC, Morawetz RB, Schlitt M: Multiple complications from an intracranial epidermoid cyst: Case report and literature review. Neurosurgery 1989; 24:574.

60. Lewis AJ, Cooper PW, Kassel EE, et al.: Squamous cell carcinoma arising in a suprasellar epidermoid cyst: Case report. J Neurosurg 1983; 59:538.

61. Cheung CC, Ezzat S, Smyth HS, et al.: The spectrum and significance of primary hypophysitis. J Clin Endocrinol Metab 2000.

62. Thodou E, Asa SL, Kontogeorgos G, et al.: Lymphocytic hypophysitis: Clinicopathological findings. J Clin Endocrinol Metab 1995; 80:2302.

63. Crock PA: Cytosolic autoantigens in lymphocytic hypophysitis. J Clin Endocrinol Metab 1998; 83:609.

64. Imura H, Nakao K, Shimatsu A, et al.: Lymphocytic infundibuloneurohypophysitis as a cause of central diabetes insipidus. N Engl J Med 1993; 329:683.

65. Hasimoto K, Takao T, Makino S: Lymphocytic andenohypophysitis and lymphocytic infundibuloneurohypophysitis. Endocr J 1997; 44:1.

66. Kamel N, Dagci Illgin S, Corapicioglu D, et al.: Lymphocytic infundibuloneurohypophysitis presenting as diabetes insipidus in a man. J Endocrinol Invest 1998; 21:537.

67. Del Pozo JM, Roda JE, Montoya JG, et al.: Intrasellar granuloma: Case report. J Neurosurg 1980; 53:717.

68. Oeckler RCT, Bise K: Non-specific granulomas of the pituitary: Report of six cases treated surgically. Neurosurg Rev 1991; 14:185.

69. Rickards AD, Harvey PW: Giant-cell granuloma and the other pituitary granulomata. Q J Med 1989; 23:425.

70. Scanarini M, d'Ercole AJ, Rotilio A, et al.: Giant-cell granulomatous hypophysitis: A distinct clinicopathological entity. J Neurosurg 1989; 71:681.

71. Inoue T, Kaneko Y, Mannoji H, et al.: Giant cell granulomatous hypophysitis manifesting as an intrasellar mass with unilateral ophthalmoplegia. Neurol Med Chir (Tokyo) 1997; 37:766.

72. Vasile M, Marsot-Dupuch K, Kujas M, et al.: Idiopathic granulomatous hypophysitis: Clinical and imaging features. Neuroradiol 1997; 39:7.

73. Hassoun P, Anayssi E, Salti I: A case of granulomatous hypophysitis with hypopituitarism and minimal pituitary enlargement. J Neurol Neurosurg Psychiatr 1985; 48:949.

74. Holck S, Laursen H: Prolactinoma coexistent with granulomatous hypophysitis. Acta Neuropathol (Berl) 1983; 61:253.

75. Yoshioka M, Yamakawa N, Sarro H, et al.: Granulomatous hypophysitis with meningitis and hypopituitarism. Intern Med 1992; 31:1147.

76. Rossi GP, Pavan E, Chiesura-Corona M, et al.: Bronchocentric granulomatosis and central diabetes insipidus successfully treated with corticosteroids. Eur Respir J 1994; 7:1893.

77. Folkerth RD, Price DL, Schwartz M, et al.: Xanthomatous hypophysitis. Am J Surg Pathol 1998; 22:736.

78. Glauber HS, Brown BM: Pituitary macroadenoma associated with intrasellar abscess: A case report and review. Endocrinologist 1992; 2:169.

79. Berger SA, Edberg SC, David G: Infectious disease in the sella turcica. Rev Infect Dis 1986; 5:747.

80. Veseley DL, Maldonodo A, Levey GS: Partial hypopituitarism and possible hypothalamic involvement in sarcoidosis: Report of a case and review of the literature. Am J Med 1977; 62:425.

81. Toth M, Szabo P, Racz K, et al.: Granulomatous hypophysitis associated with Takayasu's disease. Clin Endocrinol 1996; 45:499.

82. Lohr KM, Ryan LM, Toohill RJ, et al.: Anterior pituitary involvement in Wegener's granulomatosis. J Rheumatol 1988; 15:855.

83. De Bruin WI, van't Verlaat JW, Graamans K, et al.: Sellar granulomatous mass in a pregnant woman with active Crohn's disease. Neth J Med 1991; 39:136.

84. Albini CH, MacGillvray MHFJE, Woorhess ML, et al.: Triad of hypopituitarism, granulomatous hypophysitis, and ruptured Rathke's cleft cyst. Neurosurg 1988; 22:133.

85. Cannavo S, Romaon C, Calbucci F, et al.: Granulomatous sarcoidotic lesion of hypothalamic-pituitary region associated with Rathke's cleft cyst. J Endocrinol Invest 1997; 20:77.

86. Sano T, Kovacs K, Scheithauer BW, et al.: Pituitary pathology in acquired immunodeficiency syndrome. Arch Pathol Lab Med 1989; 113:1066.

87. Sheehan HL, Davis JC: Pituitary necrosis. Br Med Bull 1968; 24:59.

88. Kovacs K: Necrosis of anterior pituitary in humans. Neuroendocrinology 1969; 4:179.

89. Kovacs K: Adenohypophysial necrosis in routine autopsies. Endokrinologie 1972; 60:309.

90. Kovacs K, Bilbao JM: Adenohypophysial necrosis in respirator-maintained patients. Pathol Microbiol 1974; 41:275.

91. Sheehan HL: Post-partum necrosis of the anterior pituitary. J Pathol Bacteriol 1937; 45:189.

92. Cardoso ER, Peterson EW: Pituitary apoplexy: A review. Neurosurgery 1984; 14:363.

93. Voigt C, Saeger W, Gerigk CH, et al.: Amyloid in pituitary adenomas. Pathol Res Pract 1988; 183:555.

94. Landolt AM, Kleihues, P, Heitz PhU: Amyloid deposits in pituitary adenomas: Differentiation of two types. Arch Pathol Lab Med 1987; 111:453.

95. Bilbao JM, Horvath E, Hudson AR, et al.: Pituitary adenoma producing amyloid-like substance. Arch Pathol Lab Med 1975; 99:411.

96. Bilbao JM, Kovacs K, Horvath E, et al.: Pituitary melanocorticotrophinoma with amyloid deposition. J Can Sci Neurol 1975; 2:199.

97. Mori H, Mori S, Saitoh Y, et al.: Growth hormone–producing pituitary adenoma with crystal-like amyloid immunohistochemically positive for growth hormone. Cancer 1985; 55:96.

98. Livadas DP, Sofroniadou K, Souvatzoglou A, et al.: Pituitary and thyroid insufficiency in thalassaemic haemosiderosis. Clin Endocrinol 1979; 20:435.

99. Kletzky OA, Costin G, Marrs RP, et al.: Gonadotropin insufficiency in patients with thalassemia major. J Clin Endocrinol Metab 1979; 48:901.

100. Horvath E: Pituitary hyperplasia. Pathol Res Pract 1988; 183:623.

101. Saeger W, Lüdecke DK: Pituitary hyperplasia: Definition, light and electron microscopical structures and significance in surgical specimens. Virchows Arch [A] 1983; 399:277.

102. Sano T, Asa SL, Kovacs K: Growth hormone–releasing hormone-producing tumors: Clinical, biochemical, and morphological manifestations. Endocr Rev 1988; 9:357.

103. Ezzat S, Asa SL, Stefaneanu L, et al.: Somatotroph hyperplasia without pituitary adenoma associated with a long-standing growth hormone–releasing hormone-producing bronchial carcinoid. J Clin Endocrinol Metab 1994; 78:555.

104. Zimmerman D, Young WF Jr, Ebersold MJ, et al.: Congenital gigantism due to growth hormone–releasing hormone excess and pituitary hyperplasia with adenomatous transformation. J Clin Endocrinol Metab 1993; 76:216.

105. Asa SL, Scheithauer BW, Bilbao JM, et al.: A case for hypothalamic acromegaly: A clinicopathological study of six patients with hypothalamic gangliocytomas producing growth hormone–releasing factor. J Clin Endocrinol Metab 1984; 58:796.

106. Kovacs K, Horvath E, Thorner MO, et al.: Mammosomatotroph hyperplasia associated with acromegaly and hyperprolactinemia in a patient with the McCune-Albright syndrome. Virchows Arch [A] 1984; 403:77.

107. Weinstein LS, Shenker A, Gejman PV, et al.: Activating mutations of the stimulatory G protein in the McCune-Albright syndrome. N Engl J Med 1991; 325:1688.

108. Moran A, Asa SL, Kovacs K, et al.: Gigantism due to pituitary mammosomatotroph hyperplasia. N Engl J Med 1990; 323:322.

109. Peillon F, Dupuy M, Li JY, et al.: Pituitary enlargement with suprasellar extension in functional hyperprolactinemia due to lactotroph hyperplasia: A pseudotumoral disease. J Clin Endocrinol Metab 1991; 73:1008.

110. Jay V, Kovacs K, Horvath E, et al.: Idiopathic prolactin cell hyperplasia of the pituitary mimicking prolactin cell adenoma: A morphological study including immunocytochemistry, electron microscopy, and in situ hybridization. Acta Neuropathol (Berl) 1991; 82:147.

111. Kubota T, Hayashi M, Kabuto M, et al.: Corticotroph cell hyperplasia in a patient with Addison disease: Case report. Surg Neurol 1992; 37:441.

112. McKeever PE, Koppelman MCS, Metcalf D, et al.: Refractory Cushing's disease caused by multinodular ACTH-cell hyperplasia. J Neuropathol Exp Neurol 1982; 41:490.

113. McNicol AM: Patterns of corticotropic cells in the adult human pituitary in Cushing's disease. Diagn Histopathol 1981; 4:335.

114. Khalil A, Kovacs K, Sima AAF, et al.: Pituitary thyrotroph hyperplasia mimicking prolactin-secreting adenoma. J Endocrinol Invest 1984; 7:399.

115. Chan AW, MacFarlane IA, Foy PM, et al.: Pituitary enlargement and hyperprolactinaemia due to primary hypothyroidism: Errors and delays in diagnosis. Br J Neurosurg 1990; 4:107.

116. Grubb MR, Chakeres D, Malarkey WB: Patients with primary hypothyroidism presenting as prolactinomas. Am J Med 1987; 83:765.

117. Kovacs K, Horvath E, Rewcastle NB, et al.: Gonadotroph cell adenoma of the pituitary in a woman with long-standing hypogonadism. Arch Gynecol 1980; 229:57.

118. Nicolis G, Shimshi M, Allen C, et al.: Gonadotropin-producing pituitary adenoma in a man with long-standing primary hypogonadism. J Clin Endocrinol Metab 1988; 66:237.

119. Ezzat S, Asa SL: Syndromes of multiple endocrine neoplasia and hyperplasia. In Kovacs K, Asa SL, eds.: Functional Endocrine Pathology. Blackwell Scientific Publications, Boston, 1996, p. 2.

120. Wermer P: Genetic aspects of adenomatosis of endocrine glands. Am J Med 1954; 16:363.
121. Scheithauer BW, Laws ER Jr, Kovacs K, et al.: Pituitary adenomas of the multiple endocrine neoplasia type I syndrome. Semin Diagn Pathol 1987; 4:205.
122. Chandrasekharappa SC, Guru SC, Manickam P, et al.: Positional cloning of the gene for multiple endocrine neoplasia-type 1. Science 1997; 276:404.
123. Dong Q, Debelenko LV, Chandrasekharappa SC, et al.: Loss of heterozygosity at 11p13: Analysis of pituitary tumors, lung carcinoids, lipomas, and other uncommon tumors in subjects with familial multiple endocrine neoplasia type 1. J Clin Endocrinol Metab 1997; 82:1416.
124. Hardy J: Transsphenoidal microsurgery of the normal and pathological pituitary. In Clinical Neurosurgery, Proceedings of the Congress of Neurological Surgeons, 1968. Williams & Wilkins, Baltimore, 1969, p. 185.
125. Rasmussen P, Lindholm J: Ectopic pituitary adenomas. Clin Endocrinol (Oxf) 1979; 11:69.
126. Dyer EH, Civit T, Abecassis J-P, et al.: Functioning ectopic supradiaphragmatic pituitary adenomas. Neurosurgery 1994; 43:529.
127. Anand NK, Osborne CM, Harkey HLI: Infiltrative clival pituitary adenoma of ectopic origin. Head Neck Surg 1993; 108:178.
128. Coire CI, Horvath E, Kovacs K, et al.: Cushing's syndrome from an ectopic pituitary adenoma with peliosis: A histological, immunohistochemical and ultrastructural study and review of the literature. Endocr Pathol 1997; 8:65.
129. Kleinschmidt–De Masters BK, Winston KR, Rubinstein D, et al.: Ectopic pituitary adenomas of the third ventricle: Case report. J Neurosurg 1990; 72:139.
130. Lloyd RV, Chandler WF, Kovacs K, et al.: Ectopic pituitary adenomas with normal anterior pituitary glands. Am J Surg Pathol 1986; 108:546.
131. Matsumura A, Meguro K, Doi M, et al.: Suprasellar ectopic pituitary adenoma: Case report and review of the literature. Neurosurgery 1990; 26:681.
132. Shenker Y, Lloyd RV, Weatherbee L, et al.: Ectopic prolactinoma in a patient with hyperparathyroidism and abnormal sellar radiography. J Clin Endocrinol Metab 1986; 62:1065.
133. Slonim SM, Haykal HA, Cushing GW, et al.: MRI appearances of an ectopic pituitary adenoma: Case report and review of the literature. Neuroradiol 1993; 35:546.
134. Kovacs K, Horvath E: Tumors of the pituitary gland. In Atlas of Tumor Pathology, Second Series, Fascicle 21. Armed Forces Institute of Pathology, Washington, D.C., 1986.
135. Ezzat S, Forster MJ, Berchtold P, et al.: Acromegaly: Clinical and biochemical features in 500 patients. Medicine 1994; 73:233.
136. Frohman LA: Therapeutic options in acromegaly. J Clin Endocrinol Metab 1991; 72:1175.
137. Ezzat S, Snyder PJ, Young WF, et al.: Octreotide treatment of acromegaly: A randomized, multicenter study. Ann Intern Med 1992; 117:711.
138. Moriyama E, Tsuchida S, Beck H, et al: Lymphocytic adenohypophysitis: Case report. Neurol Med Chir 1986; 26:339.
139. Ezzat S, Horvath E, Harris AG, et al.: Morphological effects of octreotide on growth hormone–producing pituitary adenomas. J Clin Endocrinol Metab 1994; 79:113.
140. Blackwell RE: Diagnosis and management of prolactinomas. Fertil Steril 1985; 43:5.
141. Grossman A, Besser GM: Prolactinomas. Br Med J 1985; 290:182.
142. Burrow GN, Wortzman G, Rewcastle NB, et al.: Microadenomas of the pituitary and abnormal sellar tomograms in an unselected autopsy series. N Engl J Med 1981; 304:156.
143. Grisoli F, Vincentelli F, Jaquet P, et al.: Prolactin secreting adenoma in 22 men. Surg Neurol 1980; 13:241.
144. Horvath E, Kovacs K, Singer W, et al.: Acidophil stem cell adenoma of the human pituitary: Clinicopathologic analysis of 15 cases. Cancer 1981; 47:761.
145. Asa SL, Kovacs K, Horvath E, et al.: Hormone secretion in vitro by plurihormonal pituitary adenomas of the acidophil cell line. J Clin Endocrinol Metab 1992; 75:68.
146. Tindall GT, Kovacs K, Horvath E, et al.: Human prolactin-producing adenomas and bromocriptine: A histological, immunocytochemical, ultrastructural and morphometric study. J Clin Endocrinol Metab 1982; 55:1178.
147. Beck-Peccoz P, Brucker-Davis F, Persani L, et al.: Thyrotropin-secreting pituitary tumors. Endocr Rev 1996; 17:610.
148. Aron DC, Findling JW, Tyrrell JB: Cushing's disease. Endocrinol Metab Clin North Am 1987; 16:705.
149. Oldfield EH, Doppman JL, Nieman LK, et al.: Petrosal sinus sampling with and without corticotropin-releasing hormone for the differential diagnosis of Cushing's syndrome. N Engl J Med 1991; 325:897.
150. Booth GL, Redelmeier DA, Grosman H, et al.: Improved diagnostic accuracy of inferior petrosal sinus sampling over imaging for localizing pituitary pathology in patients with Cushing's disease. J Clin Endocrinol Metab 1998; 83:2291.
151. Nelson DH, Meakin JW, Thorn GW: ACTH-producing pituitary tumors following adrenalectomy for Cushing's syndrome. Ann Intern Med 1960; 52:560.
152. Felix IA, Horvath E, Kovacs K: Massive Crooke's hyalinization in corticotroph cell adenomas of the human pituitary: A histological, immunocytological and electron microscopic study of three cases. Acta Neurochir 1981; 58:235.
153. Franscella S, Favod-Coune C-A, Pizzolato G, et al.: Pituitary corticotroph adenoma with Crooke's hyalinization. Endocr Pathol 1991; 2:111.
154. Neumann PE, Horoupian DS, Goldman JE, et al.: Cytoplasmic filaments of Crooke's hyaline change belong to the cytokeratin class: An immunocytochemical and ultrastructural study. Am J Pathol 1984; 116:214.
155. Snyder PJ: Gonadotroph cell adenomas of the pituitary. Endocr Rev 1985; 6:552.
156. Daneshdoost L, Gennarelli TA, Bashey HM, et al.: Recognition of gonadotroph adenomas in women. N Engl J Med 1991; 324:589.
157. Djerassi A, Coutifaris C, West VA, et al.: Gonadotroph adenoma in a premenopausal woman secreting FSH and causing ovarian hyperstimulation. J Clin Endocrinol Metab 1995; 80:591.
158. Välimäki MJ, Tiitinen A, Alfthan H, et al.: Ovarian hyperstimulation caused by gonadotroph adenoma secreting follicle-stimulating hormone in 28-year-old woman. J Clin Endocrinol Metab 1999; 84:4204.
159. Asa SL, Gerrie BM, Kovacs K, et al.: Structure-function correlations of human pituitary gonadotroph adenomas in vitro. Lab Invest 1988; 58:403.
160. Asa SL, Gerrie BM, Singer W, et al.: Gonadotropin secretion in vitro by human pituitary null cell adenomas and oncocytomas. J Clin Endocrinol Metab 1986; 62:1011.
161. Horvath E, Kovacs K: Gonadotroph adenomas of the human pituitary: Sex-related fine-structural dichotomy: A histologic, immunocytochemical, and electron-microscopic study of 30 tumors. Am J Pathol 1984; 117:429.
162. Horvath E, Kovacs K, Smyth HS, et al.: A novel type of pituitary adenoma: Morphological feature and clinical correlations. J Clin Endocrinol Metab 1988; 66:1111.
163. Apel RL, Wilson RJ, Asa SL: A composite somatotroph-corticotroph pituitary adenoma. Endocr Pathol 1994; 5:240.
164. Syro LV, Horvath E, Kovacs K: Double adenoma of the pituitary: A somatotroph adenoma colliding with a gonadotroph adenoma. J Endocrinol Invest 2000; 23:37.
165. Saeger W, Lübke D: Pituitary carcinomas. Endocr Pathol 1996; 7:21.
166. Cai WY, Alexander JM, Hedley-Whyte ET, et al.: Ras mutations in human prolactinomas and pituitary carcinomas. J Clin Endocrinol Metab 1994; 78:89.
167. Pei L, Melmed S, Scheithauer B, et al.: H-ras mutations in human pituitary carcinoma metastases. J Clin Endocrinol Metab 1994; 78:842.
168. Thapar K, Scheithauer BW, Kovacs K, et al.: p53 Expression in pituitary adenomas and carcinomas: Correlation with invasiveness and tumor growth fractions. Neurosurgery 1996; 38:765.
169. Frost AR, Tenner S, Tenner M, et al.: ACTH-producing pituitary carcinoma presenting as the cauda equina syndrome. Arch Pathol Lab Med 1995; 119:93.

170. Kouhara H, Tatekawa T, Koga M, et al.: Intracranial and intraspinal dissemination of an ACTH-secreting pituitary tumor. Endocrinol Jpn 1992; 39:177.

171. Mixson AJ, Friedman TC, Katz DA, et al.: Thyrotropin-secreting pituitary carcinoma. J Clin Endocrinol Metab 1993; 76:529.

172. Petterson T, MacFarlane IA, MacKenzie JM, et al.: Prolactin secreting pituitary carcinoma. J Neurol Neurosurg Psychiatry 1992; 55:1205.

173. Stewart PM, Carey MP, Graham CT, et al.: Growth hormone–secreting pituitary carcinoma: A case report and literature review. Clin Endocrinol (Oxf) 1992; 37:189.

174. Walker JD, Grossman A, Anderson JV, et al.: Malignant prolactinoma with extracranial metastases: A report of three cases. Clin Endocrinol (Oxf) 1993; 38:411.

175. Luzi P, Miracco C, Lio R, et al.: Endocrine inactive pituitary carcinoma metastasizing to cervical lymph nodes: A case report. Hum Pathol 1987; 18:90.

176. Beauchesne P, Trouillas J, Barral F, et al.: Gonadotropic pituitary carcinoma: Case report. Neurosurg 1995; 37:810.

177. Zahedi A, Booth GL, Smyth HS, et al.: Distinct clonal composition of primary and metastatic adrenocorticotrophic hormone-producing pituitary carcinoma. Clin Endocrinol 2001 (in press).

178. Puchner MJA, Lüdecke DK, Saeger W, et al.: Gangliocytomas of the sellar region: A review. Exp Clin Endocrinol 1995; 103:129.

179. Rossi ML, Bevan JS, Esiri MM, et al.: Pituicytoma (pilocytic astrocytoma). J Neurosurg 1987; 67:768.

180. Kitanaka C, Shitara N, Nakagomi T, et al.: Postradiation astrocytoma: Report of two cases. J Neurosurg 1989; 70:469.

181. Zampieri P, Zorat PL, Mingrino S, et al.: Radiation-associated cerebral gliomas: A report of two cases and review of the literature. J Neurosurg Sci 1989; 33:271.

182. Grisoli F, Vincentelli F, Raybaud C, et al.: Intrasellar meningioma. Surg Neurol 1983; 20:36.

183. Slavin MJ, Weintraub J: Suprasellar meningioma with intrasellar extension simulating pituitary adenoma. Arch Ophthalmol 1987; 105:1488.

184. Spallone A: Meningioma as a sequel of radiotherapy for pituitary adenoma. Neurochirurgia 1982; 25:68.

185. Sridhar K, Ramamurthi B: Intracranial meningioma subsequent to radiation for a pituitary tumor: Case report. Neurosurgery 1989; 25:643.

186. Kasantikul V, Shuangshoti S, Phonprasert C: Intrasellar meningioma after radiotherapy for prolactinoma. J Med Assoc Thai 1988; 71:524.

187. Buley ID, Gatter KC, Kelly PMA, et al.: Granular cell tumours revisited: An immunohistological and ultrastructural study. Histopathology 1988; 12:263.

188. Cone L, Srinivasan M, Romanul FCA: Granular cell tumor (choristoma) of the neurohypophysis: Two cases and a review of the literature. Am J Neuroradiol 1990; 11:403.

189. Nishioka H, Ii K, Llena JF, et al.: Immunohistochemical study of granular cell tumors of the neurohypophysis. Virchows Arch [B] 1991; 60:413.

190. Mathews W, Wilson CB: Ectopic intrasellar chordoma. J Neurosurg 1974; 39:260.

191. Ishige N, Ito C, Saeki N, et al.: Neurinoma with intrasellar extension: A case report. Neurol Surg 1985; 13:79.

192. Perone TP, Robinson B, Holmes SM: Intrasellar schwannoma: Case report. Neurosurgery 1984; 14:71.

193. Wilberger JE Jr: Primary intrasellar schwannoma: Case report. Surg Neurol 1989; 32:156.

194. Banna M: Craniopharyngioma: Based on 160 cases. Br J Radiol 1976; 49:206.

195. Cusimano MD, Kovacs K, Bilbao JM, et al.: Suprasellar craniopharyngioma associated with hyperprolactinemia, pituitary lactotroph hyperplasia, and microprolactinoma: Case report. J Neurosurg 1988; 69:620.

196. Wheatley T, Clark JDA, Stewart S: Craniopharyngioma with hyperprolactinaemia due to a prolactinoma. J Neurol Neurosurg Psychiatry 1986; 49:1305.

197. Laws ER Jr: Craniopharyngioma: Diagnosis and treatment. Endocrinologist 1992; 2:184.

198. Scheithauer BW: The hypothalamus and neurohypophysis. In Kovacs K, Asa SL, eds.: Functional Endocrine Pathology. Blackwell Scientific Publications, Boston, 1991, p. 170.

199. Kleihues P, Burger PC, Scheithauer BW: Histological Typing of Tumours of the Central Nervous System: World Health Organization International Histological Classification of Tumours. Springer-Verlag, Berlin, 1993.

200. Rueda-Pedraza ME, Heifetz SA, Sesterhenn IA, et al.: Primary intracranial germ cell tumors in the first two decades of life: A clinical, light-microscopic, and immunohistochemical analysis of 54 cases. Perspect Pediatr Pathol 1987; 10:160.

201. Jennings MT, Gelman R, Hochberg F: Intracranial germ-cell tumors: Natural history and pathogenesis. J Neurosurg 1985; 63:155.

202. Furukawa F, Haebara H, Hamashima Y: Primary intracranial choriocarcinoma arising from the pituitary fossa: Report of an autopsy case with literature review. Acta Pathol Jpn 1986; 36:773.

203. Kageyama N, Kobayashi T, Kida Y, et al.: Intracranial germinal tumors. Prog Exp Tumor Res 1987; 30:255.

204. Chang T, Teng MMH, Guo W-Y, et al.: CT of pineal tumors and intracranial germ-cell tumors. Am J Neuroradiol 1989; 10:1039.

205. Allen JC, Kim JH, Packer RJ: Neoadjuvant chemotherapy for newly diagnosed germ-cell tumors of the central nervous system. J Neurosurg 1987; 67:65.

206. Baskin DS, Wilson CB: Transsphenoidal surgery of intrasellar germinomas: Report of two cases. J Neurosurg 1983; 59:1063.

207. Sakai N, Yamada H, Andoh T, et al.: Primary intracranial germ-cell tumors: A retrospective analysis with special reference to long-term results of treatment and the behavior of rare types of tumors. Acta Oncol 1988; 27:43.

208. Nakagawa Y, Perentes E, Ross GW, et al.: Immunohistochemical differences between intracranial germinomas and their gonadal equivalents: An immunoperoxidase study of germ cell tumours with epithelial membrane antigen, cytokeratin and vimentin. J Pathol 1988; 156:67.

209. Sheehan T, Cuthbert RJG, Parker AC: Central nervous system involvement in haematological malignancies. Clin Lab Haematol 1989; 11:331.

210. Singh VP, Mahapatra AK, Dinde AK: Sellar-suprasellar primary malignant lymphoma: Case report. Indian J Cancer 1993; 30:88.

211. Samaratunga H, Perry-Keene D, Apel RL: Primary lymphoma of the pituitary gland: A neoplasm of acquired MALT? Endocr Pathol 1997; 8:335.

212. Masse SR, Wolk RW, Conklin RH: Peripituitary gland involvement in acute leukemia in adults. Arch Pathol 1973; 96:141.

213. Fine HA, Mayer RJ: Primary central nervous system lymphoma. Ann Intern Med 1993; 119:1093.

214. Hochberg FH, Miller DC: Primary central nervous system lymphoma. J Neurosurg 1988; 68:835.

215. Warnke R, Dorfman R, Weiss L, et al.: Tumors of the lymphoid system. In Atlas of Tumor Pathology, Third Series. Armed Forces Institute of Pathology, Washington, D.C., 1995.

216. Vadakekalem J, Stamos T, Shenker Y: Sometimes the hooves do belong to zebras! An unusual case of hypopituitarism. J Clin Endocrinol Metab 1995; 80:17.

217. Nisho S, Mizuno J, Barrow DL, et al.: Isolated histocytosis X of the pituitary gland: Case report. Neurosurgery 1987; 21:718.

218. Ober KP, Alexander E Jr, Challa VR, et al.: Histiocytosis X of the hypothalamus. Neurosurgery 1989; 24:93.

219. Schmitt S, Wichmann W, Martin E, et al.: Primary stalk thickening with diabetes insipidus preceding typical manifestations of Langerhans cell histiocytosis in children. Eur J Pediatr 1993; 152:399.

220. Tien RD, Newton TH, McDermott MW, et al.: Thickened pituitary stalk on MR images in patients with diabetes insipidus and Langerhans cell histiocytosis. Am J Neuroradiol 1990; 11:703.

221. Ornvold K, Ralfkiaer E, Carstensen H: Immunohistochemical study of the abnormal cells in Langerhans cell histiocytosis (histiocytosis X). Virchows Arch [A] 1990; 416:403.

222. Fechner RE, Mills SE: Tumors of the bones and joints. In Atlas of Tumor Pathology, Third Series, Fascicle 8. Armed Forces Institute of Pathology, Washington, D.C., 1993.
223. Chang WH, Khosla VK, Radotra BD, et al.: Large cavernous hemangioma of the pituitary fossa: A case report. Br J Neurosurg 1991; 5:627.
224. Sansone ME, Liwnicz BH, Mandybur TI: Giant pituitary cavernous hemangioma: Case report. J Neurosurg 1980; 53:124.
225. Asa SL, Kovacs K, Horvath E, et al.: Sellar glomangioma. Ultrastruct Pathol 1984; 7:49.
226. Dan NG, Smith DE: Pituitary hemangioblastoma in a patient with von Hippel–Lindau disease. J Neurosurg 1975; 42:232.
227. Miki K, Kawamoto K, Kawamura Y, et al.: A rare case of Maffucci's syndrome combined with tuberculum sellae enchondroma, pituitary adenoma and thyroid adenoma. Acta Neurochir 1987; 87:79.
228. Dutton J: Intracranial solitary chondroma: Case report. J Neurosurg 1978; 49:460.
229. Angiari P, Torcia E, Botticelli RA, et al.: Ossifying parasellar chondroma: Case report. J Neurosurg Sci 1987; 31:59.
230. Sindou M, Daher A, Vighetto A, et al.: Chondrosarcome parasellaire: Rapport d'un cas opéré par voie ptériono-temporale et revue de la littérature. Neurochirurgie 1989; 35:186.
231. Viswanathan R, Jegathraman AR, Ganapathy K, et al.: Parasellar chondromyxofibroma with ipsilateral total internal carotid artery occlusion. Surg Neurol 1987; 28:141.
232. Wolfe JTI, Scheithauer BW, Dahlin DC: Giant-cell tumor of the sphenoid bone. Review of 10 cases. J Neurosurg 1983; 59:322.
233. Bots GTAM, Tijssen CC, Wijnalda D, et al.: Alveolar soft-part sarcoma of the pituitary gland with secondary involvement of the right cerebral ventricle. Br J Neurosurg 1988; 2:101.
234. Amine ARC, Sugar O: Suprasellar osteogenic sarcoma following radiation for pituitary adenoma: Case report. J Neurosurg 1976; 44:88.
235. Ahmad K, Fayos JV: Pituitary fibrosarcoma secondary to radiation therapy. Cancer 1978; 42:107.
236. Piatt JH, Blue JM, Schold SC, et al.: Glioblastoma multiforme after radiotherapy for acromegaly. Neurosurgery 1983; 13:85.
237. McCormick PC, Post KD, Kandji AD, et al.: Metastatic carcinoma to the pituitary gland. Br J Neurosurg 1989; 3:71.
238. Roessmann U, Kaufman B, Friede RL: Metastatic lesions in the sella turcica and pituitary gland. Cancer 1970; 25:478.
239. van Seters AP, Bots GTAM, Van Dulken H, et al.: Metastasis of an occult gastric carcinoma suggesting growth of a prolactinoma during bromocriptine therapy: A case report with a review of the literature. Neurosurgery 1985; 16:813.
240. de la Monte SM, Hutchins GM, Moore GW: Endocrine organ metastases from breast carcinoma. Am J Pathol 1984; 114:131.
241. Max MB, Deck MDF, Rottenberg DA: Pituitary metastasis: Incidence in cancer patients and clinical differentiation from pituitary adenoma. Neurology 1981; 31:998.
242. Molinatti PA, Scheithauer BW, Randall RV, et al.: Metastasis to pituitary adenoma. Arch Pathol Lab Med 1985; 109:287.
243. Post KD, McCormick PC, Hays AP, et al.: Metastatic carcinoma to pituitary adenoma: Report of two cases. Surg Neurol 1988; 30:286.
244. Ramsay JA, Kovacs K, Scheithauer BW, et al.: Metastatic carcinoma to pituitary adenomas: A report of two cases. Exper Clin Endocrinol 1988; 92:69.
245. Branch CL Jr, Laws ER Jr: Metastatic tumors of the sella turcica masquerading as primary pituitary tumors. J Clin Endocrinol Metab 1987; 65:469.
246. Gartman JJ Jr, Powers SK, Fortune M: Pseudotumor of the sellar and parasellar areas. Neurosurgery 1989; 24:896.
247. Dussault J, Plamondon C, Volpe R: Aneurysms of the internal carotid artery simulating pituitary tumours. Can Med Assoc J 1969; 101:51.
248. Durham LH, Mackenzie IJ, Miles JB: Transsphenoidal meningohydroencephalocoele. Br J Neurosurg 1988; 2:407.
249. Schochet SS Jr, McCormick WF, Halmi NS: Salivary gland rests in the human pituitary: Light and electron microscopical study. Arch Pathol 1974; 98:193.
250. Kato T, Aida T, Abe H, et al.: Ectopic salivary gland within the pituitary gland: Case report. Neurol Med Chir 1988; 28:930.

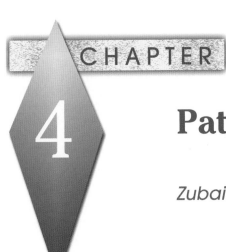

Pathology of Thyroid Gland

Zubair W. Baloch and Virginia A. LiVolsi

INTRODUCTION

The first description of the thyroid gland is ascribed to Galen (120–200 A.D.). Thomas Wharton (1641–1673) first coined the term "thyroid" because of the organ's proximity to the thyroid cartilage. The word thyroid is derived from the Greek "thyros," meaning "shield," because it was originally considered to protect the larynx.[1-2]

The term "goiter" is derived from the Latin word "gutter," meaning throat. The ancient Chinese, who treated it with seaweed and burnt sponge (although it is unlikely they recognized the role of iodine in this therapy), apparently recognized goiter.[1-2]

King first described the endocrine function of the thyroid in 1836. Parry first recognized the association of hyperthyroidism with goiter in 1786; Graves followed in 1836; Von Basedow in 1840 noted the association of goiter, exophthalmos, and palpitations. The latter two have their names associated with the disease of autoimmune hyperthyroidism: Graves in England and North America and Basedow in continental Europe.[1-4]

THYROID DEVELOPMENT

The thyroid gland develops from the fusion of three structures: one median anlage and two lateral anlagen. The median anlage forms the greater portion of the gland and develops from the base of the tongue in the foramen cecum.[5-6] It can be identified in human embryos near the end of the first month of gestation. The median anlage develops into a diverticulum, expands laterally, becomes bilobed, and descends from the tongue to its final position in the anterior neck. During this descent, it maintains its contact with the foregut by the thyroglossal duct. Usually, the duct atrophies; however, its caudal portions may persist in many embryos and leads to pyramidal lobe in about 75% of mature human thyroids.[2, 5] The entire length of the thyroglossal duct can also remain in some subjects, may become

cystic and inflamed, and even infected. In rare cases, it can serve as a site for papillary carcinoma arising in the thyroid tissue present in its wall.[2, 5] The two lateral anlagen develop as ultimobranchial bodies from the endoderm of the fourth and fifth branchial pouches. In fish, amphibians, and birds, the ultimobranchial bodies remain as separate entities, whereas in most mammals and humans they fuse to the lateral aspect of the median anlage. The ultimobranchial body gives rise to parafollicular or calcitonin cells (C cells) and solid cell nests in the thyroid.[6-9]

The functional capacity of the thyroid gland is evident by 11 to 12 weeks of gestation. Both thyroxine and thyroid-stimulating hormone (TSH) are detectable in fetal circulation after 12 weeks, and their concentration increases progressively during gestation.[10]

Developmental Anomalies

The most common developmental anomalies of the thyroid gland, which lead to congenital hypothyroidism, are aplasia and hypoplasia.[11] These defects are encountered in about 1 in 3000 to 4000 live births in North America.[11] Abnormal descent of the thyroid can cause ectopic or aberrant thyroid along the thyroglossal duct; the ectopias are named according to the level at which they are found. These include lingual, sublingual, suprahyoid, and infrahyoid.[12-19] In addition, because of the close association of the gland with development of other tissues, thyroid tissue can be found in the esophagus, larynx, trachea, soft tissues of the neck, heart and great vessels.[16-19] Lingual thyroid represents one of the common aberrant locations; rarely, this may produce a mass at the base of tongue and can lead to dysphagia, dyspnea, or severe hemorrhage in young children.[12-14, 19] An important clinical consideration is that the lingual thyroid may represent the only thyroid present in the patient.[12-14]

Similarly, because of developmental effects, other derivatives of branchial or pharyngeal pouches can

61

be found within the thyroid gland; that is, the intrathyroidal parathyroid, salivary gland remnants, and thymus.[20, 21] Some authors have suggested that these intrathyroidal rests can serve as origin for some rare tumors of thyroid such as mucoepidermoid carcinoma, squamous carcinoma, and carcinoma showing thymus-like differentiation.[21] The normal thyroid gland can occasionally show the presence of fat, cartilage, and/or muscle; similarly, deposits of thyroid tissue can be seen embedded within muscle and fat close to the thyroid.[22, 23] One should be aware of this developmental aberration because it can be mistaken for an infiltrative neoplasm.[23]

Is it normal to see benign-appearing thyroid tissue in cervical lymph nodes? This question still faces an unresolved debate. Some thyroid experts believe that thyroid tissue found within lymph nodes medial to the jugular vein represents benign inclusions, whereas similar occurrences in lymph nodes lateral to jugular vein, even lacking all described malignant nuclear features, are true metastases from papillary carcinoma.[2, 24-26] On the other hand, studies have shown that such deposits can be seen in cervical nodes when the thyroid gland failed to reveal any tumor on serial sectioning.[26-29] It is theoretically possible that small fibrous "scars" seen in the thyroid devoid of any obvious cancer may represent totally involuted papillary cancers.[2, 23] It has been suggested that presence of thyroid tissue within lymph nodes might also represent entrapment of thyroid tissue within jugular lymph sacs during development,[2] whereas others believe that these thyroid inclusions are due to transport of normal thyroid tissue by normal lymphatics.[25, 26] Klinck[27] suggested that the benign ectopic thyroid tissue is usually wedge-shaped, whereas the true metastases are rounder. This observation was found not to be useful by Meyer and Steinberg,[28] and they emphasized the need to rely more on cytologic features. In their study, they documented benign thyroid inclusions in 5 out of 106 autopsy cases; only 1 case showed a primary tumor, in the contralateral thyroid lobe.[28] Thus, according to these studies, it is not entirely impossible that, rarely, thyroid tissue deposits within cervical lymph nodes may represent developmental rests. However, in some instances the lymph node metastases from a documented thyroid papillary carcinoma may appear cytologically benign; therefore, one cannot completely rely on the cytologic details to differentiate between benign thyroid inclusions and true metastasis.[23]

NORMAL THYROID

The normal thyroid gland consists of two lateral lobes joined by an isthmus and enveloped by a thin capsule. The capsule harbors sizable venous channels and is continuous with the pretracheal fascia, which anchors it to the cricoid cartilage; these anatomic features are responsible for the thyroid's movement during swallowing. The reported figures for the normal weight of the thyroid are largely dependent on the geographic region of study. In nongoitrous areas, the normal weight of the thyroid gland ranges from 15 to 35 g; in the United States, the normal thyroid glands weigh 10 to 20 g.[2, 27, 29]

The parenchyma of the thyroid gland is subdivided by delicate fibrous septa into lobules. A lobule consists of 20 to 40 functional units of thyroid, termed follicles, and is supplied with blood by a lobular artery. The lobular artery gives rise to a rich capillary network that, along with lymphatics, surrounds individual follicles. Each follicle is lined by low-cuboidal or low-columnar epithelium and is filled with thyroglobulin-containing colloid. A basal lamina envelops the entire follicle.[2, 23, 27, 29] Calcium oxalate crystals can be found in colloid in both normal and diseased thyroids; these increase with increasing age.[2, 23, 30, 31]

The C cells are usually found within the same basement membrane as follicular cells separated from colloid by follicular cells. They are difficult to identify in routine histologic preparations; however, performing immunostains for calcitonin can recognize them.[2, 23, 29, 32-34] On electron microscopy, the follicular cells show a basal nucleus with homogenous chromatin. There is well-formed rough endoplasmic reticulum, Golgi's apparatus, small mitochondria, and apical secretory vesicles. The C cells show numerous membrane-bound neurosecretory granules containing calcitonin.[35, 36]

GOITER

The term goiter denotes both nodular and diffuse enlargement of thyroid and is usually used for a benign and hyperplastic process or a process of unknown cause.[2, 23] The affected patient may be hypothyroid, euthyroid, or hyperthyroid. Clinically, goiter is divided by the functional activity of the gland into toxic and nontoxic variants.[2, 23, 37-39]

Goiter is the compensatory hyperplasia of the thyroid because of low output of the thyroid hormone. The basic mechanism involves increased production of TSH because of low levels of thyroid hormone leading to increased thyroid mass to overcome the deficient state.[2, 23, 40] Worldwide, the most common cause of thyroid hormone deficiency is insufficient dietary iodine leading to iodine-deficiency goiter.[41-42] The goiter is termed endemic when more than 10% of a given population is affected; this is more common in geographic regions where nutritional deficiency of iodine is prevalent.[40-42]

Sporadic goiter is extremely common in areas that are not known to suffer from iodine-deficient diet.[2, 23, 40] The specific cause for this condition is unknown; decreased intake of iodine, external goitrogens, and undetectable impairment in thyroid hormone synthesis including mild cases of dyshormonogenesis have been implicated.[2, 23, 43-49]

Increased production of TSH, despite normal levels of thyroid hormones, can be seen in pituitary thyrotroph adenoma leading to hyperplasia and thyrotoxicosis.[49-51] In diffuse toxic goiter (Graves' disease), circulating immunoglobulins mimic the effects of TSH causing thyroid growth and excess hormone production.[46, 52, 53] Rarely, germline mutations of TSH receptor can also lead to hereditary or sporadic diffuse toxic goiter (non-Graves' type).[2, 52]

Pathology

The morphologic changes in both endemic and sporadic goiter are similar; they represent a spectrum of changes and include hyperplasia, colloid accumulation, and nodule formation.[2, 23, 42, 54] The hyperplastic stage is characterized by diffuse enlargement of the gland; microscopically, the follicles are collapsed, contain small quantities of colloid, and are lined by tall columnar epithelium.[42, 54] In some cases, the cellular atypia and crowding of the nuclei are prominent and can be mistaken for a neoplastic process. One may encounter foci of papillary growth in some follicles[23] (Fig. 4–1).

A process called involution, in which the follicles become distended with colloid and are lined by small cuboidal and/or flat epithelium, follows the

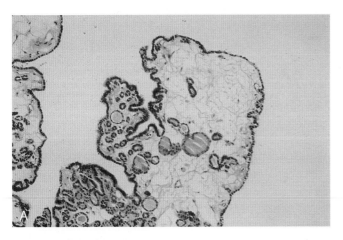

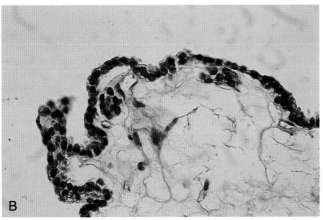

Figure 4–1. Papillary hyperplasia in nodular goiter *(A);* high-power view showing nonvascular edematous stalk lined by flattened follicular epithelium *(B).*

initial stage of hyperplasia. Grossly, when removed at this stage, the gland shows a glistening and mucoid cut surface because of excess colloid. Microscopically, the gland reveals areas of hyperplasia intermixed with atrophic changes. As the goiter persists, the gland goes through multiple cycles of hyperplasia and involution resulting in nodular goiter, which is characterized by poorly circumscribed or partially encapsulated areas of hyperplasia and intervening distended colloid-filled follicles lined by flattened epithelium. There may also be areas of degenerative changes as a result of distortion and compromise of blood supply; these include fibrosis, granulation tissue formation, old hemorrhage, and dystrophic calcification.[2, 23, 54]

Some hyperplastic nodules are circumscribed and encapsulated and may be mistaken for adenoma.[2, 23, 29] This especially holds true for larger nodules that show a distinct growth pattern different from that of the surrounding thyroid. It can be difficult to distinguish these cases from true adenomas.[23, 29] Consequently, some pathologists prefer to classify such lesions as adenomatoid nodules or adenomatoid goiter. Several investigators have explored the pathogenesis of thyroid nodules by studying the clonal composition of such lesions.[55-58] These studies have shown that up to 70% of dominant nodules in nodular goiter are clonal proliferations.[56-57] Kopp et al[58] found both monoclonal and polyclonal nodules within the same gland and suggested that this represents separate pathogenetic mechanisms or that polyclonal nodules may reflect a step involved in the formation of monoclonal lesions, thus representing an event in the hyperplasia-neoplasia sequence.

It has been estimated that thyroid nodules affect 4% to 7% (approximately 15 million) of the population in the United States and that only 4%–10% of these harbor malignancies.[2, 23, 59] Today, fine-needle aspiration (FNA) has proved to be an effective procedure for selecting patients requiring thyroid surgery. The technique of FNA is rapid, safe, and well tolerated by patients, and it can be performed on an outpatient basis either manually by palpation or under radiologic guidance by a pathologist, clinician, or radiologist.[59-68]

Cytology of Nodular Goiter

The cytologic specimen smeared on a clean glass slide and stained with Diff-Quik stain, in our opinion, shows the best morphologic depiction of nodular goiter.[64] This is characterized by abundant watery colloid, which usually stains blue-pink and sometimes shows a "chicken wire" artifact because of drying. The follicular cells appear small and dark, arranged in monolayer sheets, and grouped with follicle formation or as single cells.[62-64] Hürthle's cell metaplasia is also a common finding.[62] Macrophages, usually filled with hemosiderin granules, are also noted; however, their number depends on the presence or absence of degenerative changes or a cystic component. The hyperplastic nodules show a cellular specimen with a prominent Hürthle's cell change, and the follicular cells are usually arranged in sheets with abundant cytoplasm and may assume oval to spindle shapes (tissue culture pattern).[62, 68]

Diffuse Toxic Goiter (Graves' Disease)

Caleb H. Parry (1755–1822), Robert James Graves (1796–1853), and Carl Adolph Basedow (1799–1854) were not the first ones to recognize the combination of goiter, exophthalmos, and palpitations; ancient Greeks described it as early as 5th century B.C. Both Parry and Graves thought that the clinical findings in this disorder constituted a syndrome. Graves first published an account of this condition in 1843 and, since then, it has been commonly known as Graves' disease (GD).[1–4, 69, 70]

GD is an autoimmune thyroid disorder characterized by hyperthyroidism, diffuse thyroid enlargement, exophthalmos and, less commonly, pretibial myxedema.[71–75] The patient's serum contains autoantibodies, which stimulate the thyrotropin receptor and have been designated as thyroid-stimulating immunoglobulins (TSI).[76–79] It is generally believed that patients with GD are genetically susceptible to this disorder; clustering of GD within families, prevalence in monozygotic twins, and expression of specific HLA (HLA-B8, -DR3) haplotypes suggest this.[80–83] However, despite multiple studies, no specific susceptibility genes have been identified.[82]

In GD the thyroid gland shows symmetric and diffuse enlargement with smooth capsule. The cut surfaces are fleshy, red-brown, and lack the normal glistening because of paucity of colloid storage.[2, 23, 74] On light microscopy, the gland shows hypertrophy and hyperplasia. The follicles are of different sizes and shapes with minimal or absent colloid and are lined by tall columnar cells. The follicular cells are usually piled up and form papillary projection into the lumina of follicles (Fig. 4–2A) In some instances the follicular cells may show nuclear clearing; together with the papillary architecture, they can be mistaken for papillary carcinoma.[2, 23, 29] However, in GD these changes are diffusely distributed throughout, the cells are round, basely placed, and lack other nuclear features of papillary carcinoma.[2, 23, 74] A concomitant lymphocytic infiltrate is seen interspersed between follicles and/or in the interstitial tissue (see Fig. 4–2B). This lymphocytic infiltrate can be sparse or extensive. Cytotoxic-suppressor T cells predominate between the epithelial cells, whereas the lymphocytes seen in interstitial tissues mainly consist of helper-inducer cells.[2, 71, 84]

If treated surgically, almost all patients with GD undergo preoperative therapy, which leads to alterations in the classic histologic picture.[85–86] Some cases show larger follicles filled with colloid, residual foci of papillary hyperplasia, oxyphilic metaplasia, and sclerosis, whereas other cases may reveal a diffuse lymphocytic thyroiditis and follicular

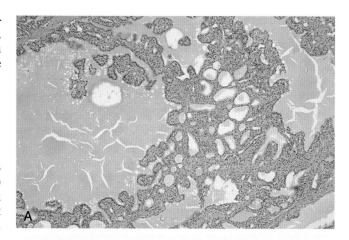

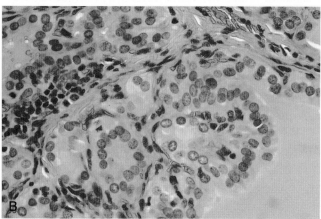

Figure 4–2. Diffuse papillary hyperplasia in Graves' disease *(A);* high-power view showing papillary projection lined by hyperplasia epithelium and an interstitial lymphocytic infiltrate *(B).*

atrophy with Hürthle's cell metaplasia, resembling Hashimoto's thyroiditis.[2, 23, 85, 86]

Cytology of GD

The patients with GD usually do not undergo FNA; only patients with solitary nodules, which are found to be cold on radioiodine scan, are selected for FNA.[2, 68, 87] The cytologic smears are cellular and show a hyperplastic appearance. One may also observe lymphocytes, epithelioid cells, and granulomata. In our experience, cases of GD can show enlarged follicular cells in loosely cohesive groups with prominent nucleoli and ample eosinophilic cytoplasm. Occasionally, the cells may display focal nuclear chromatin clearing; however, other diagnostic nuclear features of papillary carcinoma are absent.[2, 23, 87–89]

Dyshormonogenetic Goiter

This rare condition is caused by inborn errors of thyroid metabolism. These errors can involve any step in the pathway of thyroid hormone synthesis and are usually inherited in an autosomal-recessive fashion. The severity of the disease depends on the completeness of the biochemical defect; some cases may show only goiter without hypothyroidism, whereas others with severe defect lead to neonatal hypothyroidism (cretinism).[90-96]

The decrease in thyroid hormone production causes sustained elevation of TSH and compensatory hyperplasia of the gland.[94-96] On light microscopy, the changes are similar to those of nodular goiter. The hyperplastic nodules are extremely cellular and are divided by broad fibrous septa. The growth pattern is commonly trabecular or microfollicular with minimal or absent colloid; some areas may also show papillary hyperplasia. The follicular cells commonly show marked atypia, characterized by nuclear enlargement, hyperchromasia, and multinucleation.[90-93] This cytologic atypia can be mistaken for a malignancy.[2, 90-93] Malignant tumors arising in the background of dyshormonogenetic goiter are extremely rare; the diagnosis of malignancy depends on unequivocal demonstration of vascular invasion and/or metastasis.[97-99]

THYROIDITIDES

Thyroiditis is usually classified into acute, subacute, and chronic, according to the clinical mode of presentation. Almost all thyroiditides present as diffuse enlargement of the thyroid with and without pain, compressive symptoms, and alterations in thyroid function.[2, 23, 100]

Acute Thyroiditis (Acute Suppurative Thyroiditis)

This condition is rare and most commonly represents an infectious process; however, it occasionally can be seen in initial phases of exposure of the thyroid gland to radiation.[101-108] The initial description of this phenomenon by Bauchet[109] in 1857 documented this condition in five patients; later, Hazard reviewed the literature describing acute thyroiditis in 1955.[110]

Acute thyroiditis is most commonly seen in malnourished children and immunocompromised patients or following major trauma to the neck in healthy individuals. In the majority of cases the infectious elements reach the thyroid via lymphatics, but a vascular route has also been documented.[101, 110] There is often a preceding or concomitant history of upper respiratory or pharyngeal infection.[2, 23, 101] The list of causative organisms includes pyogenic organisms, fungi, and the less common agents such as *Actinomyces,* mycobacteria, syphilis, and *Pneumocystis carinii.*[102-108] The last of these has been reported in HIV syndrome.[107] On microscopic examination, the thyroid shows acute inflammation and microabscess formation. In longstanding cases the abscess may extend into the mediastinum or even rupture through the anterior neck skin or into the esophagus and trachea.[2, 23, 101]

Subacute Thyroiditis (de Quervain's Disease)

Synonyms for this condition include acute simple thyroiditis, noninfectious thyroiditis, granulomatous thyroiditis, and de Quervain's disease.[100, 111, 112] De Quervain described this condition in 1904 and later in 1936.[113, 114] It is now thought that the disease is most likely caused by a viral agent and (in classic cases) leads to painful, asymmetric enlargement of a previously normal gland.[115-117] It commonly affects middle-aged women and is associated with the HLA-B35 haplotype. Subacute thyroiditis may persist from several weeks to months and usually disappears spontaneously without any permanent damage to the gland. Antithyroid antibody titers maybe mildly elevated with mild thyrotoxicosis, but these are believed to be the aftermath of thyroid follicle destruction caused by the inflammatory process.[115-119]

Grossly, the gland is slightly enlarged and may be adherent to the surrounding tissues. On light microscopy, the morphologic patterns may vary with the stage of the disease. The early stages are characterized by single follicle destruction, with a concomitant infiltrate of macrophages and giant cells leading to focal granuloma formation; the surrounding thyroid may also show interstitial infiltrates of lymphocytes, eosinophils, and plasma cells. This picture usually progresses to a more florid granulomatous process, which is followed by the healing process characterized by fibrosis and regeneration of the follicular epithelium.[118-121] Often, large areas of the gland are involved.[2, 23]

It is important pathologically to distinguish this condition from palpation thyroiditis.[2, 23] The latter is caused by repeated manipulations of the gland during physical examinations, which leads to rupture of follicles, extrusions of luminal contents, macrophage infiltration, and foreign body giant cell reaction. This "lesion" involves one to five follicles, and its focality distinguishes it from subacute thyroiditis.[2, 23, 122]

Chronic Thyroiditis

This category includes Hashimoto's disease, nonspecific chronic thyroiditis, and Reidel's disease.[2, 23] Reidel's disease, although classified as a chronic thyroiditis, is a distinct histopathologic entity and usually does not share any similarities with other chronic inflammatory lesions of the thyroid.[2, 123, 125-127] There is a small number of cases reported that show simultaneous involvement of thyroid by both Hashimoto's thyroiditis and Reidel's disease.[124-127] This most likely represents incidental co-occurrence of these two entities; however, a common underlying mechanism cannot be excluded entirely.[125, 127]

Autoimmune Thyroiditis (Hashimoto's Thyroiditis)

This entity is also known as chronic lymphocytic thyroiditis, struma lymphomatosa, and lymphadenoid goiter.[128-130]

Hashimoto first reported this condition in 1912 in a case series of four patients.[128] All patients were women; the thyroid showed lymphocytic infiltration, follicular atrophy, fibrosis, and eosinophilic metaplasia of the follicular cells.[128] This disease is more common in women, with a female-to-male ratio of approximately 10:1.[128-133] The autoimmune bases for this condition comes from the fact that there are circulating antibodies to the thyroglobulin, thyroid peroxidase (microsomal antigen), colloid antigen, and thyroid hormones.[130-134] In addition, there is increased prevalence of HLA-DR5 and a strong family history of autoimmune disorders, especially Graves' disease.[83]

The enlargement of the thyroid is gradual over a span of months to years. The initial stages of the disease may show transient hyperthyroidism because of destruction of the thyroid follicles; however, eventually the majority of cases develop clinical or subclinical hypothyroidism.[129-133]

Grossly, the gland is symmetrically enlarged and is not fixed to the surrounding structures. The cut surface is usually lobulated, smooth, and pale pink.[2, 23, 130] The microscopic picture is characterized by diffuse infiltration of the thyroid parenchyma by lymphoplasmacytic infiltrates, formation of lymphoid follicles, follicular atrophy, Hürthle's cell metaplasia, decreased or absent colloid, and varying amounts of fibrosis.[23, 129-133] The lymphocytes consist of a polymorphous population of both B and T cells. The T and B ratio is 50:50 in the gland; however, it is normal (80:20) in the blood. Both plasma cells and B cells exhibit IgG, IgM, IgA heavy chains and kappa and lambda light chains. Most of the T cells between thyroid follicles and follicular cells are CD4+, whereas, scattered CD8+ cells are found throughout the gland.[135-137]

Hürthle's cell (oncocytic, eosinophilic) metaplasia can be focal or extensive and may give rise to partially encapsulated nodules or small cellular aggregates.[2, 23, 129, 130] In the majority of cases, the Hürthle cells may show focal atypia characterized by enlarged nuclei, prominent nucleoli, and mitoses and can be mistaken for malignancy.[23, 29] Similarly, the follicular cells embedded within lymphocytic infiltrate may show prominent nuclear clearing and nuclear grooves and can be misdiagnosed as papillary carcinoma[23, 29, 138] (Fig. 4–3). Therefore, it is prudent that one should follow strict criteria for diagnosing malignancy in the background of chronic lymphocytic thyroiditis. In addition, the glands affected by lymphocytic thyroiditis may show hyperplasia of the ultimobranchial body/solid cell nests, which may show follicular arrangement with nuclear elongation and chromatin clearing and can be mistaken for foci of papillary carcinoma.[2, 23] Ultimobranchial body nests usually show squamous differentiation, cyto-

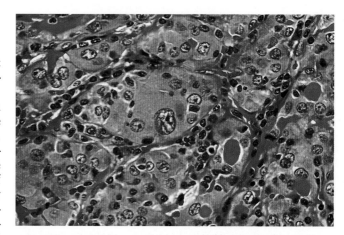

Figure 4–3. Nuclear atypia in a case of lymphocytic thyroiditis that can be mistaken for papillary cancer nuclei.

plasmic vacuolation, nuclear inclusions, and associated fibrosis; they lack the infiltrative growth pattern observed in foci of papillary carcinoma.[2, 8, 23]

In some cases of lymphocytic thyroiditis, the lymphocytic infiltrate can be extensive and may be mistaken for lymphoma. Although primary thyroid lymphomas usually arise in the background of chronic lymphocytic thyroiditis, thyroid lymphomas usually show a monomorphic infiltrate, which will replace and infiltrate the thyroid follicles and follicular cells.[139, 140] In addition, immunohistochemical stains for T and B cells, demonstration of light chain restriction by immunostains or flow cytometry, and molecular studies are always helpful for demonstrating clonality in these lesions.[2, 139, 140]

Cytology of Hashimoto's Thyroiditis

Usually patients with known lymphocytic thyroiditis who develop nodules or cold areas on scan are selected for FNA. The specimens from such cases usually show scant colloid, Hürthle's cells, follicular cells, lymphocytes, and few plasma cells. The lymphocytes are usually seen in the background, percolating between cell groups, and in some cases one may see an intact lymphoid follicle.[2, 63, 141] The Hürthle cells may display nuclear atypia and, similarly, follicular cells may show some chromatin clearing and margination; however, one should refrain from interpreting these changes as malignant.[2, 63, 142, 143] Papillary carcinoma arising in the background of thyroiditis is seen as a separate population, devoid of lymphocytic infiltrate and with appropriate nuclear features.[142, 143]

Fibrous Variant of Hashimoto's Thyroiditis

This variant is characterized by extreme fibrosis leading to effacement of a major portion of thyroid parenchyma.[144, 145] This has been reported in 10% to

13% of cases diagnosed as Hashimoto's thyroiditis. This variant can be distinguished from Reidel's disease by diffuse involvement of the entire gland, maintenance of lobular architecture and, most importantly, by lack of extension of fibrotic process beyond the thyroid capsule. [124-127, 144, 145]

Reidel's Disease

This is a rare fibroinflammatory disorder of thyroid[2, 23, 123, 146-150] Bernhard Reidel[146] first reported two cases of this in 1896, followed by an additional case in 1897. The cause of Reidel's disease remains unknown. The early literature proposed that it may represent end-stage Hashimoto's thyroiditis; currently, however, it is agreed that Hashimoto's thyroiditis and Reidel's disease are two distinct entities, distinguishable on the basis of their clinicopathologic features.[2, 23, 146-149]

Clinically, Reidel's disease presents as a painless enlargement of thyroid with pressure symptoms because of tracheal and esophageal involvement. Hypothyroidism and hypoparathyroidism may ensue, depending on the extent of destruction and replacement of the thyroid and parathyroid by a fibrosclerotic process.[147, 148]

Grossly, the gland is woody and hard and presents as a mass with fixation to the adjacent structures of the neck. The cut surface is yellow-white and lacks lobulation and vascularity. On light microscopy, the histologic picture features total loss of follicular parenchyma of thyroid and replacement by hyalinized collagenous bands. In addition, there is phlebitis and luminal obliteration of the small and large veins within and outside of the thyroid; perineural involvement by inflammatory cells can also be found.[2, 23, 146-149]

The clinicopathologic features that distinguish Reidel's disease from fibrosing Hashimoto's thyroiditis include extension of fibroinflammatory process beyond the confines of the thyroid capsule, preservation of the thyroid gland not involved by the process, lack of Hürthle's cell metaplasia, and phlebitis.[124-127, 146, 147] The plasma cells in Reidel's disease express lambda chains and IgA whereas, in Hashimoto's thyroiditis, there is dominance of kappa chains and IgG. Antithyroid antibodies are absent (or, rarely, present in small amounts) in Reidel's disease.[125-127]

Rarely, Reidel's disease is associated with similar fibroinflammatory processes involving the retroperitoneum, orbit, mediastinum, bile ducts, parotid, pituitary, and testis; hence, this condition can be part of idiopathic fibrosis.[124, 150]

Combined Reidel's Disease and Fibrosing Hashimoto's Thyroiditis

To date, a handful of cases has been documented in the literature, which shows simultaneous involvement of the thyroid by Reidel's disease and fibrosing Hashimoto's thyroiditis.[124-127] The patients usually present with thyroid enlargement and serologic profile of Hashimoto's thyroiditis. However, the microscopic picture is that of Reidel's disease. In some cases, the immunohistochemical profile of inflammatory infiltrate is also consistent with Hashimoto's thyroiditis.[124-127] We believe that these processes still represent distinct clinicopathologic entities and that this simultaneous occurrence is just coincidental.

THYROID NEOPLASMS

Tumors of the thyroid gland can be classified as primary (epithelial and nonepithelial) neoplasms and secondary tumors.[2, 23, 29, 151] The primary epithelial neoplasms originate from either follicular or C cells. The tumors originating from follicular cells display a wide variety of morphologic appearances and biologic behavior. Even though thyroid tumors are rare, this variability in clinical behavior has evoked a great interest in thyroid tumors by clinicians and pathologists.[2, 23, 29] Thyroid cancer accounts for 1.3% of all malignancies and 0.4% percent of cancer deaths in the United States.[152] These low mortality rates are because of the indolent behavior of papillary carcinoma, which represents the majority of thyroid cancers.[152, 153] Other thyroid tumors, such as anaplastic carcinomas, present as aggressive tumors leading to death within 1 year of their diagnosis. This heterogeneity in the clinical behavior of malignant thyroid tumors emphasizes the need of correct histologic diagnosis and classification of thyroid tumors.[2, 23, 29, 153, 154]

The majority of primary epithelial tumors of the thyroid are of follicular origin and include follicular adenoma and carcinoma (Hürthle's and non-Hürthle's) and papillary carcinoma and its variants as well as insular and so-called poorly differentiated carcinoma and anaplastic carcinoma. Other primary epithelial tumors include the C cell–derived tumor medullary carcinoma, tumor originating from both follicular and C cells, the mixed medullary and follicular carcinomas, and the least common squamous carcinoma and related tumors. The nonepithelial tumors are very rare; the most common in this category include malignant lymphoma and other miscellaneous tumors arising from the mesenchymal components. Finally, secondary/metastatic tumors on the thyroid can mimic primary thyroid neoplasms.[2, 23, 29, 151]

Benign Tumors

Follicular Adenoma (Hürthle's and Non-Hürthle's)

To date, controversy exists among pathologists about what defines a follicular adenoma. A majority of endocrine pathologists believe that follicular adenoma is an encapsulated neoplasm that is different from the surrounding parenchyma by both growth pattern and cytologic features arising as a solitary nodule in an otherwise histologically normal gland.[29, 37-39, 54] However, this definition, which is supported by others is, in our view, too restrictive.[2, 23] The reasons are (1) in some instances, it is difficult to clearly separate hyperplastic/adenomatous nodules arising in the background of goiter or thyroiditis from adenomas[37-39, 54] and (2) up to 70% of the adenomatous nodules are clonal, thus representing neoplastic proliferations.[55-58] Therefore, we believe that diagnosis of an adenoma should include a follicular-derived completely encapsulated nodule with a distinct growth pattern confined within the boundaries of its capsule that is different from the surrounding thyroid parenchyma. These proliferations can be rarely multiple and are seen in the background of normal thyroid or in the setting of nodular goiter, toxic goiter, and thyroiditis.[2, 23, 29, 54]

On gross examination, the follicular adenoma presents as a circumscribed and rarely as a dumbbell-shaped encapsulated proliferation.[2, 23, 29, 153] The surrounding parenchyma is usually compressed around the lesion and can sometimes give rise to a secondary plane of separation. The cut surface can show signs of excess colloid or cystification and hemorrhage (usually because of previous FNA) and fibrosis. The adenomas can range in size from a few millimeters to several centimeters.[2, 29]

On light microscopy, the adenomas can be purely Hürthle's cells, non-Hürthle's cells or, rarely, a mixture of both cell types. Adenomas can be further classified according to various growth patterns and cell types. These include simple or normofollicular, macrofollicular, microfollicular, trabecular, and solid.[2, 23, 29] (The other rare varieties such as atypical, signet-ring cell, and hyalinizing trabecular adenoma are discussed separately.)

The adenomas with follicular growth pattern usually show follicles of varying sizes and shape; however, one growth pattern that is macrofollicular or microfollicular is prominent. As expected from the designation, the macrofollicular adenomas show abundant luminal colloid, whereas the microfollicular lesions show small follicles tightly packed together with scant colloid.[2, 23, 29] Tightly packed cells arranged in solid cord or trabeculae with rare follicles and prominent vascularity characterize the trabecular/solid growth patterns. The cells of non-Hürthle's follicular adenoma are usually small and round with even chromatin pattern and small nucleoli. The cells from Hürthle's cell adenoma show abundant granular eosinophilic cytoplasm, round vesicular nuclei, and prominent cherry red nucleoli.[23]

The mesenchymal components of an adenoma vary from case to case. Some adenomas can show prominent hyalinization, and others may show prominent vasculature. Dystrophic calcification can be seen in both the tumor stroma and the capsule. In addition, some cases may show areas of squamous metaplasia, often near areas of hemorrhage. Because a majority of thyroid nodules undergo FNA, some cases, especially of Hürthle's cell type, may show prominent post-FNA alterations, which may include such varieties as focal areas of hemorrhage, fibrosis, endothelial proliferation, pseudovascular and capsular invasion, and even partial or total infarction.[2, 23]

Immunohistochemically, all adenomas stain for thyroglobulin and show a cytokeratin profile similar to that of normal thyroid parenchyma.[2, 23, 29, 155-162] It has been shown that the follicular adenomas usually do not stain for CK-19, a marker more commonly expressed in papillary carcinoma.[155-162]

Multiple studies have been published regarding the capability of different markers helpful in differentiating between follicular adenoma and carcinoma.[163-168] Follicular adenomas usually lack expression of p53 and CA 19-9 and show lower levels of Ki-67 and *bcl-2* as compared with follicular carcinoma.[163-168] Some investigators have also investigated HBME-1 and CD-15 antibodies in this regard, which have shown decreased expression in adenomas.[167, 168] *Ret*-oncogene rearrangements have been reported in 45% of adenomas in patients with radiation exposure, as compared with 84% in radiation-induced papillary cancers.[169] These studies do point out some differences between adenomas and carcinomas, however; until a specific marker is discovered, one should rely on morphologic criteria alone to differentiate between follicular adenoma and carcinoma.

Rare Variants of Follicular Adenoma

Atypical Follicular Adenoma

Hazard and Kenyon[170] first proposed this term in 1954. These lesions are follicular tumors that show some alarming features, including spontaneous necrosis, infarction, and numerous mitoses or excess cellularity and lack invasive growth.[2, 23, 29, 170] Almost all behave in a benign fashion.[2, 23, 29] Bronner and LiVolsi[171] designated a group of Hürthle's cell adenomas as atypical on the basis of nuclear pleomorphism, mitoses, necrosis, and infarction in the absence of previous FNA and capsular herniation and trapping. None of the tumors in this series behaved in a malignant fashion.

Hyalinizing Trabecular Adenoma/ Paraganglioma-Like Adenoma of the Thyroid

This rare neoplasm of thyroid was first described by Carney et al[172]; it was defined as a benign encapsulated follicular-derived neoplasm composed of elongated cells arranged around capillaries in a background of hyaline and occasionally calcified extracellular matrix[172-174] (Fig. 4–4). The individual tumor cells may show nuclear grooves, inclusions, and psammoma bodies, which can be mistaken for papil-

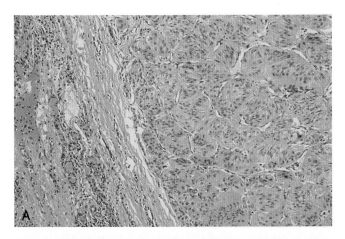

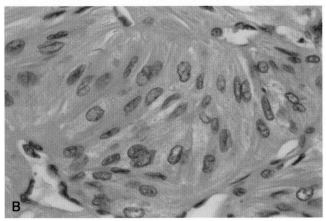

Figure 4–4. Low-power view of hyalinizing trabecular adenoma showing an encapsulated tumor with trabecular growth pattern *(A)*; high-power view showing oval- to spindle-shaped tumor cells arranged with cleared chromatin arranged in nests *(B)*.

lary carcinoma, especially in FNA specimens.[175, 176]. In 1999,[177] yellow cytoplasmic inclusions containing glycosaminoglycan, proteoglycan, and lipid in the cytoplasm of the tumor cells of this lesion were described. Ultrastructurally, these inclusions were consistent with giant lysosomes. Although this feature was found to be universal in hyalinizing trabecular adenomas, other benign tumors such as follicular adenomas may also show this feature.[177]

Bronner et al[178] suggested the term paraganglioma-like adenoma of thyroid (PLAT) because of the peculiar arrangement of tumor cells around vessels. In addition, these authors and others have described this pattern in other follicular tumors and in adenomatoid nodules in nodular goiter.[178, 179] A majority of authors believe that HTA is benign because most of these cases behave in a benign fashion.[172–174] However, a few reports have documented cases of malignant hyalinizing trabecular neoplasms that showed capsular and vascular invasion.[180, 181] These reports and others have argued against the categorization of HTA as a distinct tumor of thyroid; Li et al[180] classified the thyroid lesion that showed both hyalinization and trabecular architecture into

four groups: HTA in normal thyroid; HTA-like changes associated with nodular hyperplasia or lymphocytic thyroiditis; hyalinizing trabecular carcinoma with capsular and/or vascular invasion, and focal HTA-like changes associated with papillary carcinoma.

Some authors believe that HTA/PLAT is closely related to papillary carcinoma; this assumption is based on the similar cytologic characteristics, frequent coexistence, and similar immunoprofile.[181, 182] Fonseca et al[182] suggested that HTA may represent a encapsulated variant of papillary carcinoma; they based this inference on the observation that there were no differences in the expression of stratified epithelial-type cytokeratins in HTA and papillary carcinoma.

Signet-Ring Cell Follicular Adenoma

This represents a distinctive morphologic form of follicular adenoma.[183–188] It is characterized by the presence of large vacuoles in the cytoplasm of the follicular cells that leads to lateral displacement of the nucleus, giving rise to signet-ring cell formation (hyperplastic nodules in goiter can sometimes show this change).[185, 186] Rarely, the entire lesion will show this formation; usually, the signet-ring cells make up the majority and are intermixed with groups of follicular cells of normal cytologic features.[184–188]

It has been shown that the cytoplasmic vacuoles contain thyroglobulin and that by ultrastructural studies these vacuoles represent either intracellular lumina or dilated vesicles.[189, 190] Some authors have suggested that the signet-ring cell transformation of the follicular cell may represent an arrest of folliculogenesis.[190] In rare instances, the cytoplasm may also show mucin positivity; such lesions have been termed mucin-producing or signet-ring cell mucinous adenoma of thyroid.[183, 185, 187–189] It is suggested that mucin staining may be because of protein-polysaccharide complexes derived from the degradation of thyroglobulin.[185, 188]

The major differential diagnosis of signet-ring cell or clear cell tumors of the thyroid includes metastatic signet-ring cell carcinoma from the gastrointestinal tract and clear cell carcinoma of the kidney. These entities can be excluded by performing immunostains for thyroglobulin.[23, 29, 184]

Malignant Tumors

Clinically detectable thyroid carcinomas constitute less than 1% of all human cancers and are a rare cause of death.[2, 23, 29, 153, 154, 191] The annual incidence of thyroid cancer in different parts of the world ranges from 0.5 to 10 cases per 100,000 population.[153, 154] Females are more commonly affected (three times more often) than males; however, this holds true mostly in the adult age group; the female preponderance is not marked in older age. It has been shown that thyroid nodules in older males more commonly harbor malignancy than similar lesions in females.[2, 23, 29, 191]

The well-differentiated tumors comprise a major portion of thyroid tumors.[151] They are more common in young adults, whereas, the less differentiated and anaplastic tumors of the thyroid are prevalent at extremes of age.[2, 23, 29, 151, 191] The well-differentiated thyroid tumors are known for their indolent biologic behavior and excellent prognosis; the reported 5-year survival rates are 90% for males and 94% for females.[191] Tubiana et al[192] monitored 546 patients with differentiated thyroid cancers for 8–40 years. According to this study, age at tumor diagnosis appeared to be the most important prognostic factor. Tumors diagnosed in patients younger than 45 years had fewer relapses and higher total survival. The other prognostic factor included tumor histology, sex, and lymph node status.

Anaplastic cancer of the thyroid is a rapidly growing fatal tumor, which commonly presents in older individuals. Even with the most aggressive therapeutic measures, only less than 5% of the patients survive for 1 year.[2, 23, 29, 193]

Despite the available and proposed classification schemes, there is still a group of thyroid tumors that needs to be further defined and properly classified. The tumors included in this category are the so-called poorly differentiated tumors of thyroid. A majority of tumors placed in this category show follicular derivation and lack specific morphologic patterns; their clinical behavior falls between those of well-differentiated and anaplastic carcinoma.[194]

Papillary Thyroid Carcinoma and Variants

Papillary thyroid carcinoma (PTC) is the most common form of thyroid malignancy; it comprises at least 80% of all malignant thyroid tumors diagnosed in nonendemic goiter regions.[23, 29, 191, 195–200] It usually presents before the age of 40 years and is three to four times more frequent in women than in men.[195–197] In addition, most thyroid cancers in the pediatric population can be classified as papillary cancer.[2, 23] Rare forms of papillary cancer have also been diagnosed as congenital tumors. Familial occurrence of PTC is being more frequently recognized.[201–204] PTC behaves in an indolent fashion, with a prolonged disease-free survival and high probability of cure.[23, 195–197, 205] However, some histologic variants of PTC follow an aggressive clinical course with distant metastasis and even prove fatal in some cases.[2, 23, 29, 205] In general, these tumors metastasize via lymphatics; vascular invasion can also be seen, especially in cases of the follicular variant and tall cell variant.[2, 23, 29, 205]

Pathology

PTC can present in various sizes and forms.[195–200] The size of this tumor can range from less than a centimeter, defined as microcarcinoma, to a large tumor mass with extension beyond the confines of thyroid.[195, 199, 206] The larger tumors tend to be more common in females than in males.[198, 199] Among the gross appearances of these tumors, the most common ones are irregular area of scar formation because of excessive intratumoral fibrosis, solid nodule, solid and cystic tumors, and totally cystic tumor with minor solid and/or papillary component. Gross deposits of calcium may be noted.[2, 23, 29, 199, 200]

On light microscopy, PTC displays three types of growth patterns: pure papillary pattern characterized by a central fibrovascular core lined by tumor cells; pure follicular pattern, which can be microfollicular, macrofollicular, or a mixture of both; and a mixed papillary and follicular growth pattern.[195–200, 206] According to the World Health Organization, the histologic diagnosis of PTC is solely defined by its "characteristic nuclear features"; thus, a tumor of thyroid with the distinctive cytologic features of papillary carcinoma, regardless of its growth pattern, should be classified as PTC.[151]

The PTC tumor cell is oval or elongated because of change in the shape of the nucleus. The nuclei show chromatin clearing and margination along the nuclear membrane, which imparts a cleared-out appearance (the "orphan Annie" nuclei) to the nucleus[207] (Fig. 4–5A). It has been shown by immuno-electron microscopy studies that the nuclei of the papillary cancer demonstrate changes in the distribution of chromatin and ribonucleoproteins along with perinuclear deposition of vimentin and desmin.[208, 209] It has been suggested that the chromatin changes within the nucleus alone or in combination with perinuclear changes may be responsible for the characteristic ground-glass nucleus.[2, 23, 29, 207–209] The other nuclear features include nuclear grooves, usually seen parallel to the long axis of the nucleus, and intranuclear inclusions that appear as circumscribed punched-out holes in the nucleus with sharp borders.[210–212] Kaneko et al[213] performed scanning and transmission electron microscopy on cytologic specimens of PTC; the specimens showed that intranuclear grooves and inclusions are formed by nuclear membranes and are essentially the same structure.

Concentric, lamellated, calcific structures known as psammoma bodies are usually present in these tumors, especially in cases with papillary growth pattern.[195–200] It is suggested that presence of psammoma bodies is virtually pathognomonic of PTC; however, one may see these in other benign follicular tumors and certain benign conditions.[2, 23, 29] Psammoma bodies are formed by deposition of calcium onto the infarcted cells present at the tips of papillae; thus, concentric lamellation is the result of repeated cycles of tumor cell death followed by calcium deposition.[2, 23, 29, 198] It has been shown that the macrophage-type cells surrounding the psammoma bodies express osteopontin-mRNA, which may play a role in the development of these structures.[214]

The other feature of PTC includes infiltrative growth pattern, which is usually seen at the periphery of

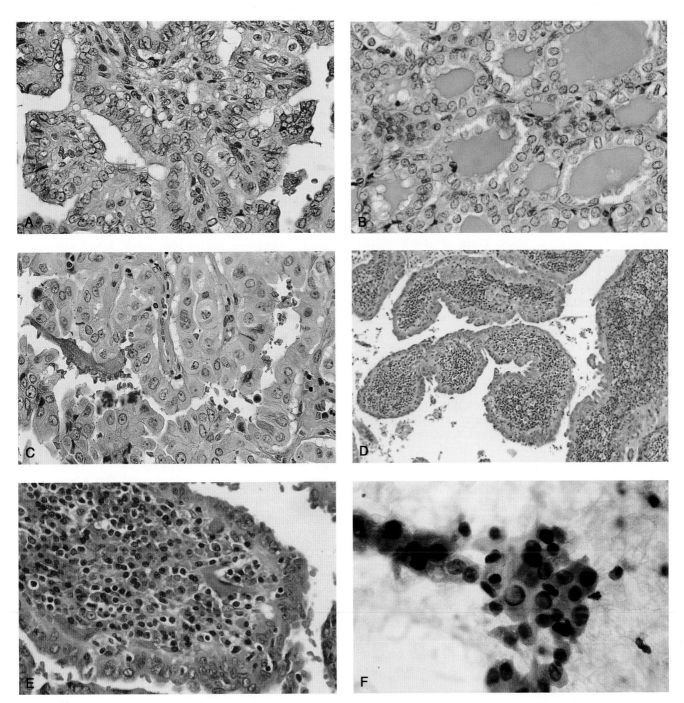

Figure 4–5. Classic variant of papillary thyroid carcinoma showing papillary fronds lined by cells with nuclear features of papillary carcinoma *(A);* follicular variant of papillary carcinoma, follicles with thick eosinophilic colloid lined by cells with papillary cancer nuclei *(B);* tall cell variant of papillary carcinoma, lined by tall eosinophilic cells *(C);* Warthin's-like papillary carcinoma, low-power view showing papillae lined by oncocytic tumor cells and a lymphocytic infiltrate in the stalk *(D)* and high-power view showing tumor cells with nuclear features of papillary carcinoma *(E);* Papanicolaou's stained FNA of thyroid, demonstrating tumor cells with elongated nuclei, nuclear chromatin clearing, and intranuclear inclusion *(F).*

main tumor mass and is associated with fibrosis. The fibrosis may be seen also within the main tumor mass.[2, 23, 29, 198]

Squamous differentiation can be seen in up to 45% of PTC.[2, 23, 29, 198] A concomitant lymphocytic infiltrate (usually sparse) can be seen at the invasive edge of the tumor; rarely, these infiltrates may be extensive.

It has been suggested that such inflammatory infiltrates most likely represent a host response to the tumor as seen in other tumors throughout the body.[2, 23, 29, 215]

PTC usually disseminates via lymphatics within and outside the thyroid gland.[2, 23, 29, 191, 215–217] Many pathologists agree that intraglandular metastasis of

PTC is responsible for its frequent presentation as multicentric tumors[2, 23]; however, some authors believe that these multiple foci of tumor represent separate clones of tumor.[29] Fialkow et al[56] and Hicks et al,[218] by using enzyme technology and molecular biology techniques, respectively, have shown that the papillary tumors are monoclonal. A similar study by Apel et al[57] showed that two separate PTCs from the same patient exhibited preferential inactivation of the same X chromosome allele. In a study, Sugg et al[219] found that the majority of multifocal thyroid carcinomas have different profiles of *RET/PTC*, suggesting independent origin. Only a few cases in this study demonstrated identical *RET/PTC* profiles, suggesting intrathyroidal spread or separate tumors with similar profiles. Thus, none of these studies have clearly excluded the idea that the multifocality in papillary cancer is due either to intrathyroidal spread of the same tumor or to separate primaries. Because of multicentric presentation of papillary cancer, many surgeons and endocrinologists prefer total thyroidectomy as the treatment of choice over partial thyroidectomy in patients with papillary cancer.[220–222]

Regional lymph node metastasis from papillary cancer can be found in 42% to 90% of patients[205, 223, 224]; however, this phenomenon does not apparently affect the prognosis.[205, 209] Vascular invasion can be identified in up to 7% and distant metastasis to bone and lungs occurs in 5% to 7% of cases.[2, 23, 29, 225, 226]

Ultrastructure

On electron microscopy, the nucleus of the PTC cell shows scant compact chromatin arranged in small masses, highly infolded nuclear membrane, paucity of nuclear pores, and cytoplasmic intranuclear inclusions. The cytoplasm may display abundant mitochondria and cytoplasmic filaments.[208, 209, 213]

Immunohistochemistry

Almost all papillary cancers express thyroglobulin.[156] Several studies have shown that papillary cancers show a different profile of cytokeratin expression than the normal thyroid parenchyma and other follicular-derived lesions.[155, 157–162, 227] As shown by us and by other investigators, cytokeratin-19 may be helpful in differentiating between PTC and other follicular-derived lesions such as papillary hyperplasia, follicular adenoma, and carcinoma.[155, 159, 162] However, one should be aware that cytokeratin-19 also stains foci of squamous metaplasia and degenerating cells found within benign nodules and Hashimoto's thyroiditis.[155] The other antigens studied in papillary cancers include S-100, neuroendocrine markers, estrogen receptors, cell-adhesion molecules alpha and beta integrins, CD44, CD57, CA125, HBME-1, and α1-antitrypsin.[168, 169, 228–234] These represent only part of the list of markers used in the immunohistochemical analysis of PTC. Despite detailed studies, no single marker has been identified as specific for papillary cancer; the morphologic diagnosis still remains the best available tool for the diagnosis of this tumor.

Prognostic Indicators in PTC

Although PTC generally behaves in a indolent fashion, the death rate can range from 4.8% to 17%.[2, 23, 191, 205] The poor prognostic factors in PTC include older age at the time of tumor diagnosis, male sex, large tumor size (>5 cm), extrathyroidal extent of local disease, and presence of distant metastasis.[205, 215, 225, 226] Tumor grading in PTC is of no value because more than 95% are classified as grade 1.[23, 29, 215] It has been shown that certain pathologic subtypes of PTC may also act as prognostic indicators; this is discussed, along with a description of each variant, later in this chapter.[205–208]

It has been suggested that ploidy analysis may be helpful in predicting long-term prognosis of PTC. Some authors have shown that diploid tumors rarely follow an aggressive clinical course, as compared with aneuploid tumors. Despite these studies, the role of ploidy analysis as an independent prognostic indicator is still questionable.[235, 236]

Several authors have explored the role of various biologic markers as predictors of aggressive behavior in PTC. These include p53, Ki-67, cell cycle proteins, proliferating cell nuclear antigen, and *bcl-2* as markers of proliferation and apoptosis, and cathepsin D, metalloproteinases, and laminin as markers for invasiveness and metastasis.[163–167, 237–240] PTC rarely or focally expresses p53 and Ki-67; *bcl-2* is expressed in the majority of PTC, indicating a low apoptotic rate.[163, 164]

Oncogenes and Well-Differentiated Thyroid Cancer

To define the role of oncogenes in the tumorigenesis of well-differentiated thyroid cancer, various oncogenes have been studied.

The *RET/PTC* oncogene is specific to the PTC. It was first described in 1987, when it was found that a mutated form of this proto-oncogene isolated from a metastatic papillary cancer could transform NIH 3t3 cells.[241] Its role in thyroid tumorigenesis has been proved in a transgenic mouse model in which thyroid-targeted *RET/PTC* expression leads to development of thyroid carcinoma with papillary morphologic features.[242–244] Similarly, tissue culture studies have shown that introduction of *RET/PTC* retroviral constructs into thyroid epithelial cells led to development of nuclear forms typical of PTC as compared with those of nonexpressing cells or cells infected with the *H-ras* gene.[245]

The *RET* proto-oncogene encodes two isoforms of a transmembrane tyrosine kinase receptor, which is involved in the development of the neural crest and the kidney.[219, 241] Somatic rearrangements of *RET*, known as *RET/PTC*, have been detected in PTC.[169, 219, 241–252] These rearrangements result in tyrosine kinase activation and translocation of the fusion protein to the cytoplasm.[241–246] To date, a family of five fusion proteins RET/ PTC1-5 have been described; each of them led to transposition of a cellular gene adjacent to the tyrosine kinase domain of RET (RET TK).[242, 253–256] Paracentric inversion of chromosome 10 causes juxtaposition of the *H4* gene (RET/PTC-1) or the *ele-1* gene (RET/PTC-3, -4) adjacent to RET TK.[253, 254] RET/PTC-2 is formed by rearrangements within chromosome 17 because of transposition of Riα subunit of cAMP-dependent protein kinase A adjacent to the RET TK.[219] RET PTC-5 has been described in PTC of two patients who were exposed to radiation in the Chernobyl accident.[256] All members of the *RET/PTC* family have been implicated in the early stages of PTC.[219, 242, 243]

In addition, some of these distinct germ-line mutations have also been found in multiple endocrine neoplasia MEN2A and 2B, familial medullary thyroid carcinoma, congenital megacolon disease, and Hirschsprung's disease.[246, 257, 258]

In sporadic papillary cancer, RET/PTC-1 is more commonly expressed, followed by RET/PTC-3, RET/-PTC-2, and RET/PTC-4.[219, 250] RET/PTC-3 is more commonly found than others in solid papillary tumors (up to 79%) than is PTC-1 or PTC-2 and usually predominates (up to 80%) in radiation-induced PTC, especially in children affected in the Chernobyl reactor accident. Similarly RET/PTC-5 has also been implicated in radiation-induced PTC.[169, 253, 255, 256, 259, 260]

So does *RET/PTC* play a critical role in papillary thyroid carcinogenesis? Several studies have strongly suggested that *RET/PTC* plays a role in the development of this tumor.[243–245, 248] In their study of multifocal papillary thyroid neoplasia, Sugg et al[219] showed that *RET/PTC* was more frequently expressed in papillary microcarcinomas than in clinically evident tumors. Other groups have reported similar findings.[248] In addition, patients with Hashimoto's thyroiditis show high expression (95%) of RET/PTC-1 and RET/PTC-3 without histopathologic evidence of papillary thyroid cancer, suggesting a possible risk of PTC in these glands or that the tumors are very small and are obscured by thyroiditis.[251] These studies suggest that rearrangement of *RET/PTC* is an early event in the development of PTC; however, its role in the progression of PTC and clinically evident tumors still needs to be defined.

Mutations in *ras* oncogene are found in follicular adenomas and carcinomas but not in PTC.[260–262] Activating mutations of the thyrotropin receptor and a subunit of the stimulatory *G (Gs)* protein gene have been reported in some functioning follicular adenomas and follicular carcinomas.[263] Inactivating point mutations of the p53 are rarely observed in differentiated thyroid cancer and are more commonly present in poorly differentiated and anaplastic carcinomas.[163–165]

Several authors have explored the role of *erbB-2* proto-oncogene in thyroid carcinomas; *erbB-2* is a member of the EGF receptor family of tyrosine kinase receptors. Some studies have shown elevated *erbB-2* RNA and protein expression in thyroid tumors.[264–267] Haugen et al[266] showed a correlation between cytoplasmic *erbB-2* expression and increased survival in female patients with thyroid carcinomas. Sugg et al found no evidence of *erbB-2* gene amplification in a large group of thyroid tumors. They found increase in the *erbB-2* RNA levels in PTC, which did not correlate with the clinical behavior of the tumor studied.[267] However, confirming the findings of Haugen et al, Sugg et al found that the cytoplasmic *erbB-2* staining was associated with a good prognosis.

Treatment Options for PTC

The treatment of PTC is still controversial among endocrinologists and surgeons.[220–222, 268–270] Usually, a clinically evident PTC, that is, one measuring more than 1.0 cm, is treated by total thyroidectomy and sampling of the palpable lymph nodes followed by radioactive iodine ablation.[205, 220, 221, 268, 270] The arguments in favor of this mode of treatment are lower recurrence rate as compared with that for partial thyroidectomy and easier ablation with radioactive iodine.[220–221, 269] However, some clinicians argue against this radical treatment because there is increased risk of surgical complications such as recurrent laryngeal nerve paralysis and hypoparathyroidism.[222, 268, 271, 272] Long-term follow-up (more than 40 years) studies have shown that intrathyroidal papillary cancer can be successfully treated by conservative surgery.[271]

Postoperatively, iodine-131 is usually given for destroying the remaining thyroid tissue, destruction of any occult foci of carcinoma, and facilitation of postablative scanning to rule out any persistent disease. It is generally not used in low-risk groups because the surgery alone provides excellent results.[220, 268–270]

Variants of PTC

The sole diagnostic feature of PTC is the typical nuclear cytology.[195–197, 207, 210, 211, 215] Histologic variants of PTC have been described on the basis of architecture, cell type, size and shape, and tumor stroma. Some of these variants are associated with indolent behavior (encapsulated subtype, cystic variant, and microcarcinoma), whereas others have been shown to follow an aggressive clinical course (tall cell, columnar cell, and trabecular variants).[2, 23, 29, 151, 153, 191, 273] The clinical behavior of other variants of PTC, such as solid, diffuse sclerosing, follicular, and oncocytic variants, is still controversial because of conflicting data and lack of large clinical series.[29, 191, 273]

Follicular Variant of PTC (FVPTC)

The follicular variant of PTC (FVPTC) is the most common histologic variant of PTC following the classic variant.[2, 23, 29, 198–200, 206] Lindsay[274] first described it; later, Chen and Rosai[275] described additional cases and named it follicular variant. FVPTC clinically behaves similar to conventional PTC; however, some authors have described more frequent distant metastases in FVPTC than in conventional PTC.[191, 198–200, 274, 275] Histologically, FVPTC is characterized by formation of follicles lined by cells with nuclear features of PTC[2, 23, 29, 274, 275] (see Fig. 5B). The growth pattern can be exclusively microfollicles, macrofollicles, or an uneven mixture of both.[275] Some tumors may show complete encapsulation by a thick capsule with dystrophic calcification, and others may show distinct areas of growth with partial encapsulation to total lack of a capsule.[2, 23, 29, 191, 275]

Some FVPTC fails to show diffuse distribution of nuclear features of papillary cancer[29]; in our experience, such cases are characterized by multifocal distribution of nuclear features of papillary cancer, and the diagnostic areas are more commonly observed underneath the tumor capsule. In our practice, we have seen that an encapsulated follicular-patterned lesion with multifocal distribution of nuclear features of papillary cancer has a greater chance of being misdiagnosed either as a follicular adenoma or follicular carcinoma than does an encapsulated lesion that displays diffusely nuclear features of papillary cancer.[276] We have seen similar cases that were misdiagnosed as follicular adenoma and that many years later developed bone metastases. It has been suggested that FVPTC can be distinguished from follicular adenoma and carcinoma by performing a panel of low- and high-molecular-weight cytokeratins.[155, 159, 162]

Three distinct variants of FVPTC have been described. The diffuse variant is characterized by replacement of the entire thyroid by tumor; lymph node and distant metastases are common in these patients.[2, 23, 29, 191] The encapsulated variant is characterized by a FVPTC, which is completely encircled by a fibrous capsule; such tumors usually behave in indolent fashion.[29] Some pathologists prefer to diagnose such tumors as neoplasms of uncertain malignant potential.

Finally, Albores-Saavedra et al[277] described 13 cases of FVPTC, which predominantly showed a macrofollicular growth pattern and on low-power microscopy resembled adenomatous/hyperplastic nodules. This particular variant is characterized by lack of diffuse distribution of features of PTC. The follicles with diagnostic nuclear features of PTC are randomly distributed in the tumor nodule and are intermixed with follicles without features of PTC. The macrofollicular variant of PTC can be easily confused with macrofollicular adenoma and/or hyperplastic/adenomatous goiter.[277]

These tumors are usually large; however, despite their size, these tumors rarely show lymph node metastases or extrathyroidal extension. The nodal metastases also show a macrofollicular growth pattern.[277]

In a separate publication, Albores-Saavedra et al[278] described five cases of the macrofollicular variant of PTC, which showed a minor (less than 5%) component of insular growth pattern. Two cases from this series showed nodal and distant (lungs and bone) metastasis. All patients were alive at follow-up (6 months to 5 years). Thus, the authors believed that the insular component did not worsen the prognosis in this series. However, a 40% prevalence of distant metastasis would be highly unusual in classic papillary cancer.

Tall Cell Variant

Hawk and Hazard first described this variant of PTC in 1976.[279] These tumors usually present in an older age group with a strong male predilection; often the lesions are large (over 5 cm). On light microscopy, these tumors show papillary formations lined by elongated tumor cells, (the height of individual cells being twice the width), eosinophilic cytoplasm, and nuclear features of PTC[23, 29, 279–282] (see Fig. 4–5C). Ultrastructural examination demonstrates increased mitochondria; however, these are not as abundant nor as morphologically abnormal as seen in Hürthle's cells.[23, 29, 280]

The antigenic profile of the tall cell variant is similar to that of classic PTC: positive for thyroglobulin and cytokeratins, especially for cytokeratin-19, and negative for calcitonin. However, tall cells have been reported to stain more strongly with CD15 (LeuM-1) and EMA than those of conventional PTC.[281] Ruter et al[283] demonstrated an increased frequency of p53 mutations in the tall cell variant compared with classic PTC (61% versus 11%). Roque et al[284] found clonal changes of chromosome 2—I[2] (q10) and trisomy 2—in the tall cell variant; these authors suggested that a gain of 2q was specific and may be important in the development of this histologic variant. There are no significant differences in the DNA content by flow cytometry between tall cell variant and classic PTC.[191]

The tall cell variant behaves more aggressively than conventional PTC: larger size at diagnosis, greater propensity toward extrathyroidal tumor extensions, vascular invasion, recurrences, shorter disease-free survival, distant metastasis, and about 25% rate of fatal outcome.[2, 23, 29, 280, 281] Whether the clinical behavior of the tall cell variant is related to its occurrence in older patients and its large size at diagnosis or to different intrinsic properties (p53 and chromosome 2 changes) remains unclear.[283, 284]

Oncocytic Papillary Neoplasms of the Thyroid

These tumors represent rare morphologic variants of thyroid tumors.[285–289] There is controversy regarding which tumors qualify for this category.[286, 287] Two types of tumors have been described under this heading: oncocytic variant of PTC and papillary Hürthle's cell neoplasms.[285–289] Oncocytic PTC represents a form of cancer in which the tumor cells display prominent cytoplasmic eosinophilia with nuclear features of PTC.[285-287] Most of these tumors show papillary architecture and minimal or no invasive growth characteristics and behave in a fashion similar to that of classic PTC.[2, 29, 285-287] In our experience, such tumors are very rare.

Papillary Hürthle's cell tumors show a papillary growth pattern but lack nuclear features of PTC.[290, 291] Hürthle's cell lesions tend to be stroma-poor. Thus, surgical manipulation and pathologic sectioning may cause separation of tumor cords and "artifactual" papillary growth pattern.[23] If a Hürthle cell lesion is encapsulated, shows no invasion, and lacks papillary cancer nuclei, the tumor should be diagnosed as benign.[2, 23, 29] Hence, papillary change only should not be equated with a malignant diagnosis. The diagnosis of malignancy depends on demonstration of capsular and/or vascular invasion.[2, 23, 29]

The diagnosis of these lesions mandates application of strict diagnostic criteria because the prognosis and clinical management of Hürthle's cell carcinoma differs significantly from that of PTC. Thus, the characteristic nuclear form is of much more importance than the tumor growth pattern.[2, 23, 29, 191]

Warthin's-Like Tumor of the Thyroid

This variant of PTC histologically resembles Warthin's tumor of the salivary gland.[292] Apel et al[292] first described this entity; additional reports subsequently appeared.[293, 294] Warthin's-like carcinoma of the thyroid is usually associated with lymphocytic thyroiditis; it is characterized by circumscribed growth, papillary architecture, central cyst formation, tumor cells with eosinophilic granular cytoplasm, nuclear features of PTC, and brisk lymphoplasmacytic infiltrate in the papillary stalks (see Fig. 4–5D and E). Clinically, these tumors behave like conventional PTC.[292-294]

PTC with Nodular Fasciitis-Like Stroma

Tumor sclerosis is a frequent finding in PTC.[2, 23, 29, 198-200] It is usually observed in the middle of or at the invasive edge of the tumor; in some cases this sclerosis can be extensive and may replace a major portion of tumor mass.[198-200]

Chan et al[295] reported an unusual histologic variant of PTC that is characterized by a unique fasciitis-like stromal component. On low power, these tumors resemble fibroadenoma or phyllodes tumor of the breast. The tumor cells are usually arranged in anastomosing cords, tubules, and papillae with nuclear features of PTC and can show varying degrees of squamous metaplasia. The stromal component is similar to that seen in cases of nodular fasciitis and consists of spindle cells arranged in irregular fascicles in a background of vascularized fibromyxoid stroma.[295-297]

Clinically these tumors behave similarly to classic PTC; the lymph node metastases from these tumors show only the carcinomatous element without the stroma. This reactive fibroblastic response is confined to the thyroid, which raises the possibility of this being a peculiar host response to tumor.[295-297]

This PTC variant should be distinguished from benign fibroproliferative lesions of the thyroid, such as fibrosing Hashimoto's thyroiditis and Reidel's disease as well as from anaplastic carcinoma.[295] Fibrosing Hashimoto's thyroiditis usually shows diffuse involvement of the thyroid with lymphoid follicle formation, fibrosis, and Hürthle's cell metaplasia.[144, 145] The follicular cells in thyroiditis can show reactive nuclear chromatin clearing, which can be mistaken for PTC.[138] However, this nuclear change is only limited to the follicular cells surrounded or infiltrated by lymphoplasmacytic infiltrate.[23, 29, 138] The true foci of papillary cancers arising in the background of thyroiditis are usually associated with fibrosis, may show invasive growth at the edges, and are devoid of or have a sparse lymphoplasmacytic infiltrate.[23] Keloidal fibrosis, chronic inflammation, phlebitis, and extension of the fibroinflammatory process beyond the thyroid capsule characterize Reidel's disease.[123]

The stromal cells in PTC with nodular fasciitis-like stroma stain negative with cytokeratin and positive with vimentin, smooth-muscle actin, and desmin. These results indicate the myofibroblastic nature of the stromal component and help in distinguishing it from the spindle-shaped tumor cells seen in cases of anaplastic carcinoma, which often stain for cytokeratin.[295-297]

Cribriform PTC

This rare, distinct variant of PTC has been described in about 1% to 2% of patients with familial adenomatous polyposis (FAP).[201-203, 298-309] The tumors, almost all occurring in females, are characterized by "multifocality" and a cribriform solid and/or spindle cell growth pattern.[202, 203, 306, 308] However, the tumors are grouped as papillary cancer based on nuclear morphologic features and thyroglobulin immunoreactivty.[201, 203, 306, 308] About 10% of reported cases have shown metastases outside the neck.[202, 303, 308] All patients show typical APC (adenomatous polyposic coli) germ-line mutations; some of the thyroid tumors studied in this group have shown *RET/PTC* activation.[309] It has been suggested that loss of function of *apc* coexists with *RET* activation in some thyroid tumors.[309] However, the molecular genetic relationships between these tumors and the known genetic mutations in FAP remain to be elucidated. Similar tumors with this unusual form may occur sporadically unassociated with colonic polyps.[298, 308]

Columnar Cell Carcinoma

This particular thyroid tumor was initially described by Evans, who described two cases of a clinically aggressive thyroid tumor occurring in men that had unique histologic features of papillary growth pattern and nuclear stratification.[310] LiVolsi described an additional feature in these tumors of prominent subnuclear vacuolation resembling early secretory endometrium.[23]

Based on the described clinical features, these tumors behave in a aggressive manner, show extrathyroidal extension, regional and distant metastasis, and a fatal outcome.[2, 23, 29, 311, 312]

Evans[313] described four cases of an encapsulated variant of columnar cell neoplasm; three of these tumors occurred in women. A thick capsule, ranging in size from 1.2 to 8.0 cm, surrounded all tumors, and three cases showed capsular invasion only. Follow-up on all these patients failed to reveal any evidence of recurrence or metastasis. Similar observations were reported by Wenig et al.[314] In this study, columnar cell carcinomas, which were encapsulated or confined to the thyroid, followed a favorable clinical course as compared with cases that showed extensive extrathyroidal extension.

Papillary Microcarcinoma

The thyroid microcarcinoma is defined by the World Health Organization as carcinoma 1 cm or less in greatest dimension.[151] Most of these tumors are found incidentally in two situations: thyroid examined at autopsy or histologic examination of thyroid lobe(s) resected for clinically evident benign lesions.[315–318] It is generally agreed that thyroid microcarcinoma is of benign biologic behavior, which is proved by high prevalence (up to 35%) of these lesions in autopsy studies.[316–317] However, up to 11% of thyroid microcarcinomas can exhibit lymph node metastases and local recurrences, which is found more commonly in multifocal and bilateral tumors as compared with unifocal tumors.[319] Thus, some authors have advocated that the unifocal tumors can be adequately treated by loboisthmusectomy, whereas total thyroidectomy is recommended for patients with multifocal tumors.[320, 321]

Lupoli et al[204] reported seven cases of familial papillary thyroid microcarcinoma. Five patients showed multifocal tumors, and vascular invasion was present in three patients. Local recurrence occurred in three patients, and one died of pulmonary metastases.

Radiation-Induced Pediatric Thyroid Cancer

External radiation to the head and neck increases the risk of PTC.[322–328] The first account of this occurrence was reported by Duffy and Fitzgerald in 1950[322]; this was followed by numerous reports confirming radiation as being one of the inducers of thyroid cancer.[322–328]

Recently, the literature on thyroid tumors contains several references to radiation-induced thyroid cancer seen in children after the Chernobyl disaster.[329–331] Nikiforov and Gnepp[330] published a detailed account of various forms of pediatric thyroid cancer seen in this population. In this report of 84 cases, papillary carcinoma was present in 83 patients and medullary carcinoma in 1. Among the histologic variants of PTC, solid variant was the most common, followed by follicular, classic, mixed, and diffuse sclerosing variants. In a similar study of 577 patients (358 children and 219 adolescents) who developed thyroid tumors after Chernobyl, Tronk et al[331] found that the majority of tumors were papillary carcinomas that showed follicular and solid growth patterns. These tumors were associated with a high frequency of lymph node metastases, venous invasion, and extrathyroidal extension.

In a retrospective 30-year analysis of pediatric thyroid cancer in the United Kingdom, the Cambridge authors noted a distinct histologic pattern they described as solid-follicular variant. Seen especially in very young children, this subtype has also been noted in the affected patients in the post-Chernobyl epidemic; it was referred to as solid if the majority of the tumors showed that morphologic feature.[329]

The solid variant of PTC is still an incompletely defined entity of undetermined biologic behavior among thyroid cancers.[2, 23, 29] It usually presents solid growth with infiltration into the surrounding thyroid parenchyma.[29] The tumor shows solid nests of tumor cells with nuclear features of PTC, separated by delicate-to-broad collagenous bands. Some tumors may show focal areas of follicular and papillary growth patterns. About 40% of these tumors show vascular invasion and extrathyroidal extension.[29, 332, 333]

The "solid" pattern described in children is most likely because of a "tight" microfollicle pattern. Solid PTC may be associated with FVPTC and usual PTC in primary tumors and metastases.[331, 333]

Some authors believe that presence of solid growth pattern suggests or represents areas of poorly differentiated carcinoma.[332, 334, 335] However, in the adult population, the meaning of solid growth pattern as related to prognosis is unknown. The solid growth/insular pattern can be seen in both papillary and nonpapillary cancers of the thyroid.[29, 333–335] We believe that these two are distinct patterns and deserve to be separated from each other; the areas of insular carcinoma usually show small round cells with scant cytoplasm arranged in well-defined nests that are separated from each other by loose connective tissue stroma containing a prominent vascular pattern.[23, 29, 335, 336] Foci of tumor necrosis are often noted. The solid pattern in PTC shows papillary cancer nuclei, whereas the insular carcinoma lacks the diagnostic nuclear features.[2, 23, 29, 331]

Diffuse Sclerosing Variant

This distinct variant of PTC is commonly found in children and adolescents.[337–341] Histologically, it is a papillary cancer that shows diffuse involvement of thyroid; additional diagnostic features include dense sclerosis, extensive squamous metaplasia, patchy to dense lymphocytic infiltrate, abundant psammoma bodies, and marked lymphatic permeation.[23, 29, 337, 338] This extensive lymphatic involvement is responsible for lymph node metastases present in almost all patients at the time of diagnosis.[337–341] Up to 25% of cases may show lung metastasis.[338–340] Some authors believe it is a clinically aggressive PTC.[338, 340] However, despite high incidence of lymph node and lung metastases, some reports indicate that these tumors demonstrate a clinical behavior similar to usual variants of PTC.[339, 341, 342] Fujimoto et al[343] studied 14 patients with diffuse sclerosing variant and found that all patients were alive and well (mean follow-up of 16 years). These authors suggested that this favorable outcome may be caused by the young age at the time of diagnosis.

Immunohistochemically, this variant shows dense accumulations of S-100 protein-positive dendritic/Langerhans' cells; it has been suggested that the presence of Langerhans' cells in usual PTC and the diffuse sclerosing variant may be responsible for a favorable prognosis.[342, 343]

Cytology of PTC

In our opinion, PTC is the only thyroid malignancy that can be diagnosed with confidence in cytology. However, some variants of PTC may pose some diagnostic difficulties.

The FNA specimen of PTC usually shows a cellular specimen consisting of tumor cells arranged in papillary groups, three-dimensional clusters or as single cells; the majority of the specimens show a combination of all patterns.[62, 344, 345] The background may show colloid, nuclear, or calcific debris; macrophages, and stromal fragments.[62, 344–347] The colloid in PTC is usually thick and is found as round-to-oval deposits; some authors have termed this "bubble gum colloid."[62, 344] The macrophages may be present in variable numbers; they are mainly seen in tumors, which are associated with a cystic component.[62, 348] Stromal fragments appear as strings of eosinophilic material either surrounded by or totally devoid of cells.[62, 344, 345] These are more common in cases that show extensive intra- and peritumoral sclerosis.[62, 346] Such cases usually give rise to less cellular aspirates.[346]

The diagnosis of PTC depends on the demonstration of nuclear features.[23, 29, 207, 208, 344–346, 349] The individual tumor cells are oval in shape, and the nuclei show elongation, membrane thickening, chromatin clearing, grooves, and inclusions[344–347] (see Fig. 4–5F). The nucleoli are small and eccentric.[62, 344]

Nuclear grooves and inclusions can be seen in other benign and malignant conditions of thyroid. These include Hashimoto's thyroiditis, nodular goiter, hyalinizing trabecular adenoma, Hürthle's cell tumors, and medullary carcinoma.[62, 175, 176, 349–352]

In our opinion, the diagnosis of PTC requires a constellation of these features.

The cytologic features of FVPTC have been reported by several authors.[276, 353–358] FNA specimens from this tumor may pose diagnostic difficulties because of its features that overlap with those of hyperplastic nodules or follicular neoplasm.[276, 356–358] This is usually because some FVPTC may resemble hyperplastic nodules, even in histologic features because of a mixture of small and large follicles and the paucity of nuclear features of papillary carcinoma.[276] The smears from FVPTC usually show tumor cells arranged in monolayer sheets, cellular groups, and microfollicles in a background of abundant watery colloid.[276, 355] Thick colloid can be seen in some cases; however, it is less frequently seen than in cases of the usual variant of PTC.[276] The individual tumor cells show nuclear elongation, chromatin clearing, and thick nuclear membranes; however, nuclear grooves and inclusions are not easily identifiable.[276, 356–358] We have noticed that chromatin clearing and nuclear membrane thickening are universal cytologic features of this tumor.[276] Thus, if one is faced with a lesion that shows both of these features and lacks others, then at least this suspicion should be mentioned in the cytology report.[276] At our institution, we usually diagnose such cases as "follicular derived neoplasm with features suspicious for PTC" and ask for an intraoperative consult (frozen section and touch preparation) for further characterization and definite surgical management. Up to 70% of our cases suspicious for PTC category turned out to be FVPTC.

Aspirates from the tall cell PTC variant usually show columnar or elongated cells with sharp borders, granular eosinophilic cytoplasm, and variably sized nuclei with nuclear features of PTC.[62, 359–361] Abelatif et al[359] reported an additional feature: presence of intraepithelial neutrophils in aspirates from cases of tall cell variant. This tumor can be confused with Hürthle's cell tumors on cytology due to eosinophilic cytoplasm; however, the nuclear features should help in differentiating between these two tumors.[62, 360, 361]

There are few reports on the cytologic features of Warthin's-like PTC. These tumors can show papillary fronds stuffed with lymphocytic infiltrates lined by cells with oncocytic cytoplasm and papillary cancer nuclei.[293, 294, 362]

Primary Epithelial Tumors: Follicular-Derived Nonpapillary Follicular Carcinoma

This well-differentiated, follicular-derived malignant tumor of the thyroid is characterized by follicle formation but without the nuclear changes of PTC.[2, 23, 29, 363–368] Follicular carcinoma accounts for 5% to 15% of all thyroid cancer; however, the high prevalence rates may be because of inclusion of some cases of follicular variant of papillary carcinoma.[367, 369, 370] This tumor is more common in iodine-deficient areas with prevalence rates up to 45% as compared with papillary cancer, which is more common in areas where iodine is used as a dietary supplement.[371–376]

Follicular carcinoma is more common in women and usually presents in an older age group.[23, 29, 363-368] The typical presentation is that of a solitary "cold" thyroid nodule.[366] This tumor grows slowly and metastasizes via the bloodstream; thus, bone and lung metastases are more common than papillary cancer.[2, 23, 29, 363-368, 377-381]

In some cases, the distant metastasis may be the first sign of the disease.[29, 366] Follicular carcinomas lack multifocality, do not invade lymphatics, and nodal metastases are very rare.[23, 363-368] Because of this, many surgeons and endocrinologists recommend removal of the affected lobe only.[382-384]

Two types of follicular carcinoma have been described in the literature: the encapsulated type, which grossly resembles an adenoma and is labeled as carcinoma on histologic demonstration of capsular and/or vascular invasion,[383-387] and the widely invasive type that diffusely infiltrates the affected lobe or the entire gland.[2, 23, 29, 388] These latter tumors can be either nonencapsulated or encapsulated with extensive capsular and vascular invasion.[388] The subtypes differ in their biologic behavior; the 10-year survival rates for the encapsulated type are 70% to 100% and for the widely invasive type 25% to 45%.[2, 23, 29, 366, 383-388]

On light microscopy, widely invasive follicular carcinoma can be easily identified on the basis of infiltrative margins and extensive vascular invasion.[388] The tumor usually grows as a combination of solid, trabecular, and follicular patterns.[366]

Diagnosing encapsulated follicular carcinoma is a difficult task for the surgical pathologist.[363, 364, 386, 389-391] This is because of the lack of consensus among experts in defining the diagnostic criteria. Various criteria that have been cited in the literature for the diagnosis of follicular carcinoma include invasion into the tumor capsule, through the tumor capsule, and into the capsular vessels.[23, 29, 364, 370, 386, 389-391] From this list, diagnosis solely based on capsular invasion is still debated among pathologists[364, 385, 386, 389] (some authors prefer the term "follicular neoplasm of undetermined malignant potential" for these tumors). Thus, the diagnosis of follicular carcinoma should be made only on the basis of vascular invasion.[363, 390-391] Khan and Perzin,[364] in their study of follicular tumors, found that capsular invasion without vascular invasion was associated with metastatic disease. Similarly, Evans[389] showed an association of metastasis with capsular invasion only. Yamashina[368] studied invasive characteristics of fourteen encapsulated follicular tumors by evaluating the entire circumference of the tumor capsule. He found that the tumors with capsular invasion or attenuation of the capsule also demonstrated foci of vascular invasion near or away from foci of capsular invasion.

In our practice, we designate encapsulated follicular tumors that show only capsular invasion as minimally invasive carcinoma (Fig. 4–6) and those with vascular invasion as angioinvasive grossly encapsulated follicular carcinomas. The angioinvasive tumors have the capacity to metastasize hematogenously to bone and lungs; about 50% of the patients die of tumor at 10 years' follow-up. Those lesions with only capsular invasion probably have a very slight (if any) chance of metastasizing.[2, 23, 29]

At present, no ancillary studies have helped in differentiating follicular adenomas from follicular carcinoma. Several studies have reported use of flow cytometric analysis in follicular neoplasms of thyroid, but such examinations are of limited value in the diagnosis of follicular carcinomas.[2, 29, 392] About 60% of the follicular carcinomas may show aneuploid populations; however, 27% of the follicular adenomas can exhibit DNA aneuploidy.[392] However, it has been shown that those histologically confirmed follicular carcinomas with diploid DNA content tend to have a better prognosis than the ones with aneuploid population.[392]

Advances in molecular biology techniques have provided much insight into the initiation and progression of thyroid carcinoma.[393, 394] Follicular thyroid carcinoma shows frequent loss of heterozygosity (LOH) on chromosome 10q and 3p as compared with follicular adenoma and papillary carcinoma, suggesting involvement of tumor suppressor genes.[395-397] Grebe et al[395] found additional LOH at 17p and suggested that this change might represent a late event in follicular thyroid carcinoma. The increase in frequency of LOH in follicular carcinomas as compared with papillary cancer suggests a fundamental difference in mechanisms controlling chromosomal stability and may be a cause of different biologic behaviors.[395-397] Follicular carcinomas have been shown to exhibit more frequently activated *ras* oncogene than other follicular-derived tumors.[261, 398] Karga et al[261] showed that the *ras* mutations in cases of follicular carcinoma were associated with bone metastases, suggesting a possible association with aggressive behavior.

Cytology of Follicular Neoplasm

The diagnostic term "follicular neoplasm" reflects the limitations of thyroid cytology.[62, 399-403] In our

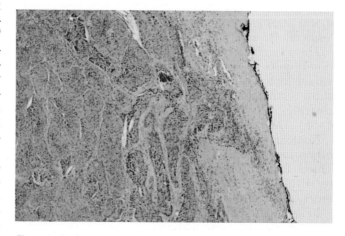

Figure 4–6. Follicular carcinoma with capsular invasion (minimally invasive follicular carcinoma).

view, this term should be considered as an indeterminate diagnosis in thyroid cytology because the diagnosis of follicular carcinoma is based only on the demonstration of capsular and/or vascular invasion at the tumor's periphery (not sampled by FNA).[364, 386] It has been shown that only up to 15% of cases diagnosed as "follicular neoplasm" are follicular carcinoma on histologic examination.[399, 403]

The FNA of a follicular neoplasm usually shows a cellular specimen consisting of a monotonous cell population with scant background colloid. The cells are usually arranged in three-dimensional groups and microfollicles with prominent nuclear overlapping. Some cases may show nuclear atypia; however, this is not a diagnostic criterion because benign adenomatous or hyperplastic nodules can show similar nuclear change.[399-402]

Hürthle's Cell Tumors

The oncocytic/oxyphilic cells of the thyroid are known as "Hürthle's cells."[2, 23, 29] It is now believed that thyroid oncocytes were first described by Askanazy in 1898[404] and that the cells described by Hürthle in the thyroid gland of dogs represent parafollicular or C cells.[405] Hürthle's cells are follicular in origin and express thyroglobulin and not calcitonin; ultrastructurally, they are similar to oncocytes in other organs.[23, 29] Earlier studies suggested that oncocytic change in thyroid follicular cells represented an end-point in the functional capacity of the thyroid follicular epithelium.[406] However, it has been shown by histochemical and immunohistochemical studies that Hürthle's cells show increased levels of oxidative enzymes and produce thyroglobulin.[407, 408]

Hürthle's cells exist in the thyroid as isolated cells lining follicles, as cellular aggregates, or as well-demarcated unencapsulated or partially encapsulated nodules.[2, 23, 29] These nodules are often multiple and, in some conditions such as Hashimoto's thyroiditis, the entire thyroid epithelium is replaced by such nodules.[23] Isolated random nuclear atypia and, occasionally, multinucleation are not rare in benign oncocytic lesions of the thyroid. Long-standing thyroiditis or Graves' disease as well as benign oncocytic nodules can show this change.[23, 29]

Hürthle's cell tumors of the thyroid are rare; however, they are interesting because of their histologic features, clinical behavior, and response to treatment.[409-421] Grossly, Hürthle's cell neoplasms are usually solitary lesions and can be distinguished from the surrounding thyroid parenchyma because of their mahogany-brown color. Some lesions may show partial or total infarction of the tumor because of previous FNA.[23, 29, 422-425] Post-FNA infarction is more commonly observed in Hürthle's cell tumors as compared with other follicular-derived neoplasms.[422-425] It has been postulated that post-FNA infarction in Hürthle's cell is due to their microvasculature (which is different from other non-neoplastic and neoplastic thyroid lesions)[422-425] and high

metabolic rate.[407-408] A high percentage of Hürthle's cell lesions are malignant (35%) as compared with non- Hürthle's follicular lesions. The other risk factors for malignancy in Hürthle's cell lesions include male sex and large size (lesions larger than 4 to 5 cm).[2, 23, 29, 418]

On light microscopy, Hürthle's cell tumors can show solid, trabecular, microfollicular, macrofollicular, and pseudopapillary growth patterns. Random nuclear atypia, multinucleation, and mitoses are common.[23, 29, 418]

Benign and malignant Hürthle's cell tumors are diagnosed according to the same criteria used for follicular adenomas and carcinomas.[23, 29, 363, 364, 382, 383, 388] Several authors have suggested that cellular atypia and mitotic activity in Hürthle's cell lesions can indicate malignancy[411, 415, 418]; however, follow-up data has failed to support this. Bronner and LiVolsi[171] defined a group of Hürthle's cell tumors as "atypical adenomas" on the basis of marked nuclear atypia, mitoses, spontaneous infarction, and necrosis without definite capsular or vascular invasion. Long-term (up to 13 years) follow-up of these lesions showed that these tumors behaved in a biologically benign fashion. Carcangui et al[409] classified some Hürthle's cell tumors as tumors of indeterminate malignant potential; all but one of their cases behaved as adenomas. Thus, the distinction between Hürthle's cell adenoma and carcinoma should solely depend on application of strict diagnostic criteria for invasive growth used for non-oncocytic follicular tumors.[23, 29, 364, 386, 389, 409, 426]

Hürthle's cell adenomas are encapsulated and lack invasion into the surrounding thyroid parenchyma or into the capsular vessels.[23, 29, 408, 417-421] The Hürthle cell carcinomas show capsular and/or vascular invasion.[23, 29, 407, 414, 418] Both benign and malignant Hürthle's cell neoplasms show thyroglobulin positivity; however, it is less intense than in usual follicular cells.[23, 29] They also stain positive for carcinoembryonic antigen (polyclonal CEA) and S-100 protein. Hürthle's cell neoplasms usually stain negative for keratins 5/6, 10, 16, 17 and 19.[23, 29, 161, 162, 427] Miettinen et al[161] found scattered cell reactivity for cytokeratin 19 in their cases of Hürthle's cell neoplasms; however, in our own experience, both benign and malignant Hürthle's cell tumors uniformly stain negative with cytokeratin 19.[155]

FNA has been an effective diagnostic tool in the management of thyroid nodules.[23, 29, 62-64] However, in cases of Hürthle's and non-Hürthle's follicular lesions, one can only render the cytologic diagnosis of follicular or Hürthle's cell neoplasm because the diagnosis of malignancy depends on demonstration of capsular and/or vascular invasion.[62-64, 428] FNA specimens of Hürthle's cell lesions (benign and malignant) usually show a cellular aspirate consisting of one cell population of Hürthle's cells in the background of scant colloid.[62] The cells can be arranged in cellular groups or as scattered single cells.[62-64, 428] Nuclear enlargement and pleomorphism are commonly observed.[23, 29, 418] Some authors have shown this to be more common in cases of Hürthle's cell carcinoma[429]; however, we believe that this is not a reproducible cytologic criterion because we have found it in benign Hürthle's cell lesions.

Flow cytometric analysis can be a useful prognostic indicator of malignant behavior in cases of Hürthle's cell carcinoma.[430] Aneuploidy in histologically proven Hürthle's cell carcinomas predicts metastasis and death. However, it is of no value in cases of benign Hürthle's cell lesions. Some (10% to 25%) oncocytic adenomas show aneuploid populations; thus, flow cytometry is of no value in differentiating benign from malignant Hürthle's cell tumors.[430, 431]

Hürthle's cell neoplasms exhibit a different set of genetic alterations than non-Hürthle's cell neoplasms, suggesting that these two tumor types represent separate entities.[432–435] Bouras et al[435] found a higher percentage of *ras* mutations for *Ha-ras* codon in Hürthle's cell carcinoma than in follicular carcinoma. Studies in chromosomal allelotyping of both follicular and Hürthle's cell tumors have also demonstrated an increase in allelic alterations in Hürthle's cell neoplasms when compared with follicular neoplasms (7.5% versus 23.3%).[432, 433] Hürthle's cell carcinomas also show significant differences in expression of TGF-α, TGF-β, IGF-1, and *N-myc* from follicular carcinoma.[434]

The biologic behavior of Hürthle's cell neoplasms is different from that of non-Hürthle's follicular neoplasms. Malignancy is more common in Hürthle's cell neoplasms (approximately 35%) as compared with that of follicular neoplasm (approximately 5%).[23, 29, 419–421] Lymph node and distant metastasis is more frequent in Hürthle's cell carcinomas than in follicular cancer (although much less common than in PTC).[23, 419–421] Rarely will these tumors show radioiodine uptake or only minimally so. This often leads to difficulties in treatment.[29, 415–417, 420]

Poorly Differentiated Thyroid Carcinoma

This entity remains controversial.[2, 23, 29, 332, 333] It has been suggested that clinical behavior of thyroid tumors diagnosed as poorly differentiated carcinoma falls between that of papillary carcinoma and of undifferentiated or anaplastic carcinoma.[2, 23, 194] In the literature, various authors have included morphologically diverse lesions into this category, giving rise to a heterogeneous group of tumors.[194, 332, 333, 436] The list of tumors cited under the heading of poorly differentiated carcinoma includes tall cell papillary carcinoma, columnar cell carcinoma, Hürthle's cell carcinoma, and insular carcinoma.[194, 332–334, 336, 414, 436–438] We believe that, because each of these tumors has been characterized pathologically and prognostically, these entities should be separated out in any diagnostic scheme.[2, 23, 29] Both papillary and follicular cancers can show areas of solid and trabecular growth—such areas can be associated with mitotic figures, abnormal

mitoses, and/or areas of spontaneous tumor necrosis (not in areas of FNA tracks); this should alert the pathologist to a tumor that may be dedifferentiating.[29, 194, 333, 334] However, the exact prognostic significance of such findings remains to be described. Nishida et al,[439] in their study of poorly differentiated thyroid cancers, noted that tumors with greater than 10% "poorly differentiated" areas had a significantly worse prognosis than those lesions with small foci of poorly differentiated growth. However, the authors included examples of insular and tall cell carcinomas as poorly differentiated, thus perpetuating the gathering of data from heterogeneous groups of tumors.[439]

Insular Carcinoma of Thyroid

Carcangui et al[336] described the features of this follicular-derived tumor in 1984 and named it as insular carcinoma because of its distinct histologic features of tumor cells arranged in well-formed nests or islands (insulae). They suggested that this thyroid tumor is similar to what had been described by Langhans in 1907 as "wuchernde struma."[440] Sakamoto et al[194] in 1983 designated a similar histologic picture as poorly differentiated carcinoma. However, as noted above, this term still needs to be defined. There are no exact figures available for the prevalence of this thyroid tumor; the reported prevalence rates vary among different geographic regions. The highest prevalence (5%) has been reported from Italy, whereas in United States it is much lower.[2, 23, 29, 335, 336, 438]

Insular carcinoma usually presents in an older age group but on the whole at slightly younger age than that of anaplastic carcinoma. The female-to-male ratio is about 2:1.

Grossly, these tumors are large, solid, and gray-white and may exhibit areas of necrosis. On light microscopy, the tumor cells are small, round, and monotonous and are arranged in well-defined clusters and nests (Fig. 4–7). The other features of this

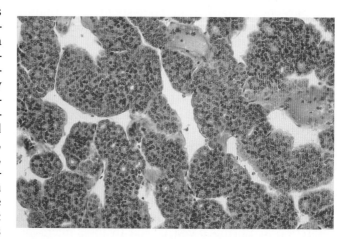

Figure 4–7. Insular carcinoma showing tumor nests (insulae) separated by prominent dilated vessels.

tumor are prominent vascularization, mitoses, and focal to large areas of coagulation necrosis. Vascular invasion is common. The tumors are diffusely positive for thyroglobulin, which helps to distinguish them from medullary carcinoma. Insular carcinoma behaves in an aggressive fashion: metastases are present in a majority of cases at the time of diagnosis; up to half of patients die of their tumors 1 to 8 years after therapy.[336, 438]

CALCITONIN CELL LESIONS OF THYROID

The calcitonin cells (C cells) are of neural crest origin, which has been proved by structural and embryologic studies.[441, 442] It has been proposed that they probably first migrate to the ultimobranchial body remnants before being incorporated into thyroid parenchyma.[441–445] In the normal gland, they are usually concentrated at the junction of the upper third and lower two-thirds of the lateral lobes.[445–448] They are usually unrecognizable on routine hematoxylin and eosin preparations; however, they can be identified by means of Grimelius' stain and immunohistochemical stains such as chromogranin A, synaptophysin, and neuron-specific enolase.[448–451] Immunostain for calcitonin, the hormone product of C cells, has become the immunostain of choice.[446–453] Calcitonin gene-related peptide (CGRP), somatostatin, gastrin-releasing peptide, and serotonin are other immunochemical markers that can localize the C cells.[454, 455]

Medullary Thyroid Carcinoma

Tumors of C cell origin are designated as medullary carcinomas; they comprise about 10% of all malignant thyroid tumors.[456–467] They are challenging as well as interesting because of their clinical presentation, familial origin, and association with other neuroendocrine lesions and morphologic spectrum.[456–488] To date, medullary cancer is the only thyroid tumor in which a possible precursor lesion—C cell hyperplasia—can be implicated.[2, 23, 29, 489, 490]

Historically, medullary carcinoma was considered as a variant of anaplastic carcinoma of thyroid.[491] Horn[492] in 1951 reported seven cases of this tumor as a distinctive morphologic variant of thyroid carcinoma; however, he did not use the term medullary carcinoma. Hazard and associates[493] were first to name this tumor and describe in detail its morphologic features, presence of amyloid, frequency of lymph node metastases, and its prognosis. Later, Williams[456] identified the cell of origin, which has led to a body of insight into the origin and pathogenesis of this lesion.

Most medullary carcinomas are sporadic[456–467, 494]; however, up to 20% are familial, inherited in an autosomal-dominant fashion with high penetrance.[468–488] These familial tumors can present either as a part of multiple endocrine neoplasia (MEN) syndrome type 2A (MEN IIA or Sipple's syndrome), type 2B (MEN IIb), MEN III (mucosal neuroma syndrome), or familial non-MEN medullary thyroid carcinoma.[468–488, 495–503]

Genetic abnormalities in familial medullary cancer syndromes have been mapped to the pericentromeric region of chromosome 10 by linkage analysis.[482, 504, 505] Following this discovery, mutations in *RET* proto-oncogene have been identified in more than 90% of the families with MEN-2, which can be used as a screening tool to diagnose and identify asymptomatic family members with this syndrome.[257, 258, 506] Analysis of *RET* in families with MEN-2A and familial medullary thyroid cancer have shown mutations in one of five cysteine codons in exon 10 and exon 11. These mutations are present in 95% of families with MEN-2A and in 85% of families with familial medullary thyroid carcinoma.[504–506] A point mutation at codon 918 (exon 16) has been identified in 95% of cases with MEN-2B.[257, 258, 506–508] Two additional novel mutations involving codon 768 (exon 13) and codon 804 (exon 14) have been discovered in cases of familial medullary thyroid cancer.[506, 509–511] It is recommended that first-degree relatives of a family member affected by one of the mentioned syndromes should have genetic testing; a positive result should be followed by prophylactic total thyroidectomy because no positives have been reported. This radical prophylaxis is usually performed at around 5 years of age because of early onset of disease; metastases can be found as early as 6 years of age.[506, 512, 513]

Sporadic medullary cancers can also exhibit *RET* mutations in the tumors. It has been shown that these mutations may affect the prognosis.[257, 506] The most common mutations in sporadic cases are seen in codon 918; the less common mutations involve cysteine codons and codons 768 and 883.[514–517] A small number (less than 5%) of sporadic cases of medullary cancer may turn out to be hereditary upon testing for *RET* mutations in the absence of family history, C cell hyperplasia, and multifocal tumors.[506]

The typical clinical presentation of medullary cancer is that of a firm, painless thyroid nodule; up to 50% of cases show nodal and 15% may present with distant metastases.[2, 23, 29, 457–460] Female predominance is seen in sporadic cases. The sporadic tumor is commonly seen at an older age (average age 45 years) than the familial forms (MEN 2a—27 years; MEN 2b—16 years).[2, 23, 29, 468–488, 494] As well as calcitonin, medullary carcinoma cells can also express other hormones, which include derivatives of pro-opiomelanocortin molecule (adrenocorticotropin hormone, melatonin-stimulating hormone, β-endorphin, and enkephalin), serotonin, glucagon, gastrin, and bombesin, among others.[453, 454, 518–521] This multiple hormone production may lead to a complicated clinical picture and difficulty in diagnosing the tumor accurately.

As previously mentioned, the familial forms of medullary cancer can present in different clinical settings. MEN type 2 or 2a or Sipple's syndrome consists of medullary thyroid cancer, C cell hyperplasia, adrenal pheochromocytoma, adrenal medullary hyperplasia, and parathyroid hyperplasia.[470–475] Almost all patients will have these lesions except parathyroid hyperplasia, which is seen in only one-thirdofcases.[502] Medullary thyroid carcinoma and C cell hyperplasia, pheochromocytoma, and adrenal medullary hyperplasia, mucosal neuromas, gastrointestinal ganglioneuromas, and musculoskeletal abnormalities characterize MEN type 2B.[485–487, 496–499] Medullary carcinoma in these cases is usually aggressive and leads to fatal outcome at an early age because of distant metastases; however, not all studies support this view of the aggressive behavior of medullary cancer in this setting.[494, 503, 512, 513, 522]

Grossly, the sporadic tumors are usually solitary lesions, whereas the familial are multiple and involve both lobes.[2, 23, 29, 494] They are usually located at the site of highest C cell concentration, i.e., the lateral upper two-thirds of the gland.[2, 23, 29, 446, 447, 457–460] The tumor size may range from very small to tumors that replace the entire thyroid.[457–460]

On light microscopy, medullary carcinoma can exhibit various growth patterns and mimic other thyroid tumors.[2, 23, 29, 523–530] Consequently, it is prudent to perform immunostains for calcitonin and/or CGRP to confirm the histologic impression.[531–534] The typical histologic picture of medullary carcinoma shows tumor cells arranged in trabecular, insular, or sheet-like growth patterns; however, in many cases there is a combination of all three patterns.[2, 23, 29, 457–460, 490] A dense collagenous or hyalinized material containing amyloid deposits usually separates the tumor cell nests; up to 80% of tumors will show presence of amyloid.[29, 490] The tumor cell can be oval, round, or spindle-shaped, with small round nuclei. The nuclear chromatin is finely granular as seen in neuroendocrine tumors with inconspicuous nucleoli[29, 458, 459, 531, 532] (Fig. 4–8A). In some cases, the tumor cells may resemble cells from a small cell carcinoma of the lung, whereas others may be composed entirely of spindle cells and can be confused with a thyroid tumor of mesenchymal or thymic origin.[23, 29, 525, 526, 530] A few cases of medullary carcinoma are composed of oncocytic cells and resemble Hürthle's cell carcinoma; such cases are classified as oncocytic variants.[29, 530] Mucin can also be noted in some tumors (about 10%).[527, 528]

Tumor necrosis and mitoses are rare in medullary cancer; however, large tumors may show areas of necrosis.[29, 471, 487]

Lymphatic invasion is common in medullary carcinoma; up to 50% of patients may show involvement of mediastinal and upper cervical nodes. The tumors may also show involvement of the extrathyroidal tissues by direct extension and involvement of the contralateral lobe by intraglandular metastases. The common sites for distant metastases include lung, bone, liver, and adrenals.[2, 23, 29, 457–460, 522, 532]

The diagnosis of medullary carcinoma must be established by performing immunostains. Calcitonin and CGRP represent the most sensitive markers for

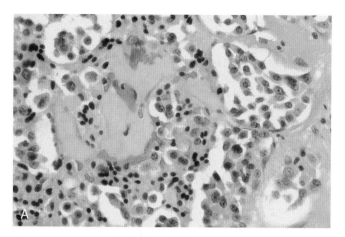

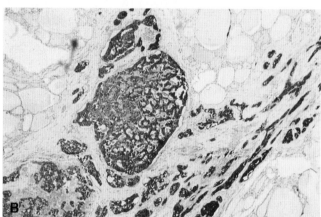

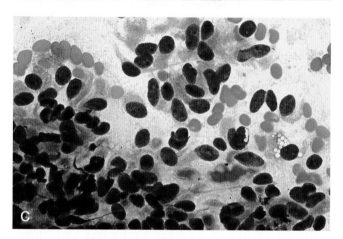

Figure 4–8. Medullary carcinoma showing tumor nests embedded in glassy eosinophilic stroma *(A);* the tumor cells staining positive for calcitonin immunostain *(B);* Diff-Quick stained thyroid FNA showing oval- to spindle-shaped tumor cells with scant cytoplasm from a case of medullary carcinoma *(C).*

these tumors, although they are not entirely specific because they can be found in endocrine tumors of nonthyroid origin (e.g., islet cell tumors)[455, 533–536] (see Fig. 4–8B). The number of calcitonin-positive tumor cells is variable among cases. The amyloid in medullary carcinoma also stains positive for calcitonin, which is related to the deposition of precursors of calcitonin molecule.[23, 29, 455, 533–535] Calcitonin-negative medullary cancer has been described (about 1.5% of cases), but these lesions are considered medullary thyroid cancer if they arise in a familial setting or are associated with C cell hyperplasia.[532, 534] All medullary carcinomas stain for CGRP.[455, 532, 534, 535] Medullary carcinomas also stain for cytokeratin, chromogranin A, neuron-specific enolase, and CEA.[533–535] It has been shown that immunoreactivity for calcitonin in 25% or fewer tumor cells and marked and positivity for CEA is associated with worse prognosis.[532]

Cytology of Medullary Carcinoma

FNA specimens from medullary carcinoma commonly show a cellular aspirate consisting of oval to spindle-shaped cells arranged mainly as single cells or loosely cohesive groups[62, 536–542] (see Fig. 4–8C). The individual tumor cells show ample granular cytoplasm, and up to 20% of cells demonstrate eosinophilic granules in Romanowsky-stained preparations.[62, 538, 541] The nuclei are usually placed eccentrically, giving a plasmacytoid appearance to tumor cells. The nuclear chromatin is similar to that seen in neuroendocrine tumors: coarse, clumped chromatin and inconspicuous nuclei. Some cases may show intranuclear inclusions and multinucleated cells.[537, 539] Amyloid may be observed in some cases as acellular material in the form of strings or as round-to-oval fragments.[540] Amyloid can be distinguished from colloid with a Congo red stain.[540] Positive stain for calcitonin confirms the diagnosis.[541, 542]

The differential diagnosis of medullary carcinoma in FNA specimens includes Hürthle's cell neoplasm, papillary carcinoma, metastatic neuroendocrine tumors, and plasmacytoma. Hürthle's cells usually show prominent nuclei and lack neuroendocrine chromatin pattern and cytoplasmic granules. Papillary carcinoma cells exhibit powdery chromatin, nuclear membrane thickening, grooves, and inclusions.[62, 538]

C Cell Hyperplasia

The familial forms of medullary cancer are characterized by multifocal and/or bilateral tumors and C cell hyperplasia.[2, 23, 29, 468–490] Currently, there is no uniform definition of C cell hyperplasia.[23, 29] Wolfe et al[446, 447] studied normal thyroids and found 4–10 C cells per low-power field in the central regions of upper and middle thirds of the lateral lobes. According to these authors, the normal C cells are arranged singly, whereas, multiple large clusters of C cells characterize the hyperplasia. Other studies have suggested the presence of more than 20 cells to indicate hyperplasia and fewer than 5 cells to suggest absence of hyperplasia.[543, 544] LiVolsi et al[544] suggested that 2 to 5 C cells with more than 50 cells per low-power field indicate hyperplasia.

It is generally accepted that there is a lack of definite criteria; that if C cell hyperplasia is suspected, sections should be submitted from the upper two-thirds of each lateral lobe; and that the presence of C cells in several clusters of more than six cells indicates hyperplasia.[2, 23, 448, 451, 544] C cell hyperplasia is not exclusively associated with familial medullary cancer because it has been described in autoimmune thyroiditis, hyperparathyroidism, and hypercalcemia because of other causes.[544, 545] It can also be seen in some cases of sporadic medullary carcinoma and follicular-derived tumors.[2, 23, 29, 546, 547] Some authors have shown that immunostains for polysialic acid component of neural adhesion molecule can distinguish primary from secondary C cell hyperplasia.[548] However, at present, genetic testing has proved an accurate method for identifying familial C cell lesions, lessening the burden to define familial cases based on histology.[512, 513]

MIXED MEDULLARY, FOLLICULAR, AND COMPOSITE TUMORS

These tumors show both parafollicular and follicular differentiation in the same tumor. Two tumors have been described under the heading of mixed carcinoma and composite carcinoma of thyroid.[549–556]

Mixed or intermediate tumors exhibit both medullary and follicular growth patterns or, rarely, admixed tumor cells with nuclear features of papillary carcinoma. The tumor cells show dual expression of calcitonin and thyroglobulin. The morphologic pattern and immunoprofile are retained in nodal metastases from these tumors.[549–555]

Apel et al[556] described composite tumor of thyroid: two distinct cell populations, thyroglobulin-positive papillary carcinoma, and calcitonin-positive medullary carcinoma characterize it. It is separated from mixed tumor on the basis that the follicular and parafollicular lineage can be demonstrated in two separate cell populations rather than in the same tumor cells, as in mixed tumors.

THYROID PARAGANGLIOMA

Paragangliomas of the thyroid are very rare. Only a limited number of cases have been reported in the pathology literature.[557–564] In the reported cases, most of the tumors ranged 1.5 to 10 cm, presented as a solitary mass, and occurred in women.[557–564] They present as circumscribed masses limited to the thyroid or can show extrathyroidal extension into the neighboring structures.[557–560, 564] Morphologically, they exhibit the typical nesting (Zellballen's) pattern seen in sites other than thyroid. The differential diagnosis of paraganglioma of thyroid includes medullary carcinoma, metastatic neuroendocrine neoplasms, hyalinizing trabecular adenoma, Hürthle's cell carcinoma, and insular carcinoma.[561, 564] Thyroid paragangliomas stain positive for neuron-specific enolase, chromogranin, synaptophysin, and S-100–positive sustentacular cells; the tumors are negative for thyroglobulin, EMA, keratins, calcitonin, and CEA. This immunoprofile is helpful in differentiating paragangliomas of the thyroid from the above-mentioned tumors.[561, 564] Distinguishing thyroid paraganglioma from metastasis of neuroendocrine tumors to thyroid may be difficult.[564] However, metastases to thyroid from neuroendocrine tumors are rarely solitary and circumscribed; they usually show lymphovascular invasion and areas of tumor necrosis.[23, 29, 564]

ANAPLASTIC CARCINOMA

Anaplastic carcinoma of the thyroid, although rare, is one of the most aggressive human tumors.[193, 565–573] It is usually seen in older patients and constitutes about 5% to 10% of all malignant tumors of thyroid.[193, 565–566, 570] It is more common in regions of endemic goiter.[193, 570] Clinically, it presents as a rapidly enlarging neck mass with compression symptoms and rapidly fatal outcome usually within months because of local progression and distant metastases. On light microscopy, it shows a cellular tumor with epithelial (squamoid), spindle, or giant cells or a combination of any component.[193, 567, 569, 571] The tumor cells display marked anaplasia, bizarre forms, and numerous mitoses; foci of tumor necrosis are common and may be extensive.[23, 29, 193, 567] Immunohistochemistry confirms the epithelial nature of the lesion; the tumor cells are keratin-positive and are usually negative for thyroglobulin and calcitonin. Some authors have shown that these tumors can exhibit thyroglobulin positivity and secrete thyroglobulin in tissue culture.[23, 29, 568, 569]

Usually, the diagnosis of anaplastic carcinoma of thyroid is not a problem, given its clinical presentation, microscopic picture, and immunohistochemical profile.[569] LiVolsi[23, 566] and, later, Wan et al[573] described a variant of anaplastic carcinoma that, on light microscopy, resembles Reidel's disease. The clinical presentation in the two patients reported by Wan et al was typical of an anaplastic carcinoma. On light microscopy, the tumors were paucicellular and showed large areas of sclerotic and infarcted tissue and spindle cells arranged in fascicular or storiform patterns. Bland cytologic features and rare mitotic figures characterized the individual spindle cells. The hypocellular areas were joined at their periphery by areas of higher cellularity that showed mild to moderate nuclear pleomorphism and increased mitoses. Vascular invasion was present in both cases, and one case showed lymph node metastases. Metastatic node was completely obliterated by hyalinized and infarcted tissue. Both cases stained positive for EMA and muscle-specific actin, and one case was positive for keratin.[573]

Paucicellular variant of anaplastic carcinoma can mimic Reidel's thyroiditis clinically and morphologically: presentation of a neck mass with compressive symptoms, sclerosis, spindle cell proliferation and lack of obvious anaplasia. These two entities can be differentiated from each other on the basis of tumor necrosis, presence of more cellular areas of tumor with diagnostic features of anaplastic carcinoma, vascular invasion, and metastasis.[123, 147, 574]

Cytology of Anaplastic Carcinoma

The aspirates from anaplastic carcinoma usually show epithelioid and spindle-shaped tumor cells, osteoclast-type giant cells with marked cellular pleomorphism, and anaplasia in a background of inflammation and necrosis.[575–578] Neutrophilic infiltration of the tumor cells is common.[62, 577] The nondiagnostic cases on FNA are common in these tumors because of extensive necrosis or sclerosis.[23, 62] However, when a thyroid aspirate in an older patient shows a necrotic and inflammatory background with rare pleomorphic cells, anaplastic carcinoma must be included in the differential diagnosis.[23, 62, 577]

SPINDLE CELL SQUAMOUS CARCINOMA OF THYROID

Primary squamous cell carcinomas of the thyroid are rare[579–586]; however, other thyroid neoplasms can exhibit focal or extensive squamous differentiation.[23, 29, 587, 588] Squamous metaplasia is most commonly seen in papillary carcinoma. Other thyroid tumors that can show squamous change include mucoepidermoid carcinoma, sclerosing mucoepidermoid carcinoma with eosinophilia, medullary carcinoma, carcinoma with thymus-like differentiation, anaplastic carcinoma, and, rarely, follicular adenoma and follicular carcinoma.[23, 29, 587, 589]

Bronner and LiVolsi[589] reported five cases of spindle cell squamous anaplastic carcinoma, which arose in association with tall cell variant of papillary carcinoma. The spindle cell component was similar to that seen in sarcomatoid squamous cell carcinomas of the oropharynx. All these tumors occurred in older patients (74 to 82 years), were large, and showed solid, cystic, and papillary areas on gross examination. On light microscopy, two distinct components comprising a tall cell variant of papillary carcinoma and spindle squamous cell anaplastic carcinoma were identified. The latter component consisted of islands of moderately to poorly differentiated squamous cell carcinoma admixed with anaplastic spindle cell areas. The anaplastic areas showed bizarre hyperchromatic nuclei with foci of necrosis and hemorrhage. Four cases in this series showed angioinvasion, and all showed extrathyroidal extension. Lymph node metastases were seen in two and were made up of the papillary component only. The squamous and the spindle cell components were negative for thyroglobulin and positive for high-molecular-weight cytokeratins.[589]

Anaplastic thyroid carcinoma is usually seen in combination with other well-differentiated thyroid carcinomas.[2, 23, 29, 565] This dedifferentiation may be focal or extensive to the levels where the entire tumor is composed of anaplastic component; however, extensive sampling of the tumor may still reveal foci of well-differentiated cancer at the periphery.[23, 29, 565]

Tumors with Thymic or Related Branchial Pouch Differentiation

Tumors placed in this group show histologic, immunohistochemical, and ultrastructural features that are consistent with thymic or related branchial pouch differentiation.

Intrathyroidal Thymoma

The incomplete descent or persistence of the cervical thymus may lead to thymic remnants in the neck tissues. This phenomenon can be observed in up to 21% of fetuses and newborns. Thymic tissue can be seen in 1.8% of thyroid glands. Usually, the thymic rests are seen closely abutting the thyroid capsule. Rarely, tumors may grow in these rests and can be mistaken for a thyroid primary tumor.[23, 590–593]

SETTLE

The term SETTLE (spindle epithelial tumor with thymus-like differentiation) was first introduced by Chan and Rosai in 1991.[594] Before this term, such tumors were designated as malignant teratoma of the thyroid and spindle cell tumor with mucous cysts.[595–597]

These tumors are common in children and young adults and usually present as a solitary circumscribed thyroid mass.[594, 598–600] Slow growth, late local recurrences, and distant metastasis (lung and kidney) characterize these tumors.[594]

FNA specimens from these tumors show spindle cells with scant cytoplasm, fine chromatin, and indistinct nucleoli arranged in tissue fragments or as scattered cells.[600] On light microscopy, the tumor is divided into incomplete lobules by thick sclerotic bands. The tumor cells show a mixture of spindle cells and epithelioid cells; however, the spindle cells usually predominate. The spindle cells exhibit bland nuclear cytologic features and are often arranged in a storiform configuration, whereas the epithelial cells show papillary, trabecular, or sheet arrangement. Occasionally, squamous differentiation reminiscent of Hassall's corpuscles can be seen. Cystic change can be noted on both gross and microscopic examination in some tumors; the cysts are usually small and are lined by squamous or columnar cells.[594, 596, 597] Interstitial mucin can be demonstrated in the majority of cases.[594, 596, 597, 600] Rarely, angiolymphatic invasion or invasion into the surrounding parenchyma can be identified.[594]

The spindle cells stain positive with cytokeratins, smooth muscle actin, and muscle-specific actin and stain negative with thyroglobulin and calcitonin.[594, 598]

Ultrastructurally, the tumor cells are encased by well-defined basal lamina and show tonofilaments and few desmosomes.[594, 600]

The differential diagnosis of SETTLE includes intrathyroidal thymoma; mesenchymal tumors of thyroid, especially synovial sarcoma; teratomas of thyroid gland, and anaplastic carcinoma.[594] Intrathyroidal thymomas usually occur in an older age group and are characterized by epithelial cells intermixed with lymphocytes.[590–593] Mesenchymal tumors are cytokeratin-negative. Anaplastic carcinoma occurs in older age and is characterized by rapid growth and fatal outcome.[23, 193, 570] SETTLE can arise in extrathyroidal soft tissue; therefore, it should be distinguished from synovial sarcoma. Cytokeratin immunoreactivity can be seen in synovial sarcoma; however, it would not contain mucous cysts, and mitotic figures would easily be found.[598, 600]

CASTLE

Miyachi et al[601] first described this entity as intrathyroidal thymoma because of its resemblance to thymoma. Chan and Rosai proposed the term CASTLE for carcinoma showing thymus-like differentiation.[594] The other terms used for this tumor include lymphoepithelioma-like carcinoma of the thyroid and intrathyroidal epithelial thymoma.[594, 601, 602]

CASTLE usually arises in the middle to lower third of the thyroid in adults 40 to 50 years of age and often extends into the extrathyroidal soft tissues. The tumors are circumscribed; well demarcated from the surrounding thyroid; and show a lobulated, firm, and gray cut surface. These tumors closely resemble thymic carcinoma by their histologic features and immunoprofile. The tumor cells show large nuclei with open chromatin pattern, prominent nucleoli, and abundant cytoplasm. Some tumors may show focal squamous change and perivascular lymphocytic infiltrates resembling lymphoepithelioma-like carcinoma of thymus[594, 603–607] (Fig. 4–9). Lymphoepithelioma-like carcinomas occurring in other sites

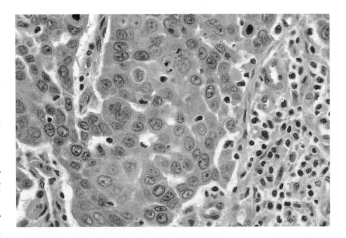

Figure 4–9. CASTLE showing groups of tumor cells in background of lymphocytic infiltrate.

such as the nasopharynx show a strong association with Epstein-Barr virus. Shek et al[608] found that CASTLE is negative for Epstein-Barr virus by in situ hybridization techniques (we have confirmed this finding in two cases). The tumor cells are positive for cytokeratin and negative for thyroglobulin and calcitonin.[594, 604] CASTLE has also shown to react with CD5 antibody similarly to thymic tumors[604, 609]; these results have confirmed the hypothesis of thymic differentiation of this tumor.[609] Similarly, bcl-2 and mcl-1 positivity has been demonstrated in both thymic carcinoma and CASTLE, which may represent an immunoprofile of malignant neoplasms with thymic differentiation.[610]

CASTLE usually progresses in a slow-growing fashion; late local recurrences are common and can be controlled by local excision and radiotherapy.[594]

Mucoepidermoid Carcinoma of the Thyroid Gland

Mucoepidermoid carcinoma of the thyroid gland is a rare tumor characterized by distinct morphologic features and indolent biologic behavior. It has generated much interest among pathologists because of its questionable cell of origin.[611]

Two types of thyroid tumors have been described under this heading: mucoepidermoid carcinoma and sclerosing mucoepidermoid carcinoma with eosinophilia.[612-622]

Mucoepidermoid Carcinoma

Mucoepidermoid carcinoma (MEC) is more common in woman and presents as painless solitary nodules.[611-617] Grossly, the tumors are predominantly solid but can display areas of cyst formation. Microscopically, the tumors are circumscribed and unencapsulated, with focal areas of infiltration at the edge, and show squamous differentiation and mucin production.[29, 611-617] The squamous cell component is arranged in solid sheets with horny, pearl formation, and the mucous cells line the duct- or gland-shaped component.[611-615] Occasionally, glandular spaces are filled with mucin and form mucous cysts.[29, 612-613] The tumor stroma is usually fibrotic and can exhibit foci of psammomatous calcification. Initially, MEC was reported as being negative for thyroglobulin; however, other authors (including ourselves) indicate these tumors are positive for thyroglobulin and cytokeratin and negative for calcitonin.[29, 611, 617]

Sclerosing Mucoepidermoid Carcinoma with Eosinophilia

Chan et al[618] reported eight cases of this low-grade tumor arising in association with Hashimoto's thyroiditis. Sclerosing mucoepidermoid carcinoma with eosinophilia (SMECE) is very similar in its clinical presentation and biologic behavior to MEC of the thyroid. However, SMECE can be separated from MEC on the basis of both morphologic and immunohistochemical features.

On light microscopy, there is squamous and glandular differentiation, and the tumor cells are arranged in narrow strands, anastomosing cords, and irregular groups. Occasionally, there is prominent mucin production and mucous cyst formation. The background of this tumor is as important diagnostically as the carcinomatous element: it is characterized by a prominent hyaline stroma and a mixed inflammatory infiltrate with prominent eosinophilia (Fig. 4–10). The surrounding thyroid shows chronic lymphocytic thyroiditis. The tumor cells are usually negative for thyroglobulin and calcitonin and positive for cytokeratins.[618-622]

Almost all MEC and SMECE cases reported in the literature and in our experience have pursued an indolent clinical course.[612-622] Lymph node metastases can occur, and some cases can show extrathyroidal extension and, rarely, distant metastases.[612-622]

FNA specimens of mucoepidermoid carcinoma of thyroid can show both squamous and glandular components with stromal fragments and a concomitant inflammatory infiltrate.[619, 621, 622] The prominence of squamous epithelium in FNA specimens can be mistaken for a primary or metastatic squamous carcinoma; on the other hand, the presence of lymphocytic infiltrate and stromal fragments can be mistaken for an inflammatory process such as Hashimoto's thyroiditis.[622, 623]

The origin of these tumors still needs to be determined. Initially, some authors suggested a possible origin from the ectopic salivary gland[612]; however, this hypothesis has never been proved. It has been reported that mucoepidermoid carcinoma usually shows neither C cell (calcitonin-negative) nor follicular (thyroglobulin-negative) differentiation by immunohistochemistry.[618, 620, 622] Wenig et al[611] reported thyroglobulin positivity in five of six cases, suggesting a follicular derivation.

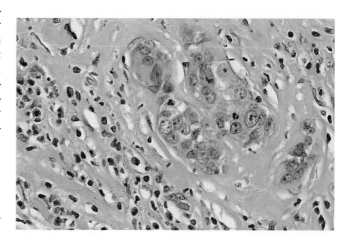

Figure 4-10. SMECE; tumor cells arranged in cords and nests in background of hyalinized stroma and eosinophilic infiltrate.

However, they did not separate cases of MEC and SMEC. We believe, despite the similar clinical features, that there are some distinct differences between these tumors. A majority of reported cases of SMECE fail to stain for thyroglobulin and calcitonin, arise in the background of Hashimoto's thyroiditis, and show a rich intratumoral eosinophilic infiltrate[618-622]; whereas MEC can express thyroglobulin and lack intratumoral eosinophils and a background of Hashimoto's thyroiditis.[612-617] Some authors have suggested that these tumors arise from ultimobranchial rests/solid cell nests seen mainly in lymphocytic thyroiditis.[613, 615, 618, 623] This hypothesis is based on the observation that ultimobranchial rests/solid cell nests show both squamous and glandular differentiation and that their immunoprofile is similar to that of SMECE. However, as mentioned above, some authors have shown thyroglobulin positivity in their cases of SMECE, whereas ultimobranchial rests/solid cell nests do not show any thyroglobulin positivity.[611] We have not been able to demonstrate thyroglobulin positivity in cases of SMECE.[622]

Other authors have suggested a possible relation to papillary carcinoma, thyroglossal duct, or C cells.[611, 616, 617]

We believe, until this debate comes to a conclusion, MEC and SMEC represent two distinct tumors that can be separated by histologic features and immunohistochemical profile. However, this distinction may be just academic because both these tumors behave in a similar fashion and, by this token, they may represent a spectrum of different morphologies.[611, 614, 618, 621]

The differential diagnosis of MEC and SMEC include fibrosing Hashimoto's thyroiditis, primary or metastatic squamous cell carcinoma, papillary carcinoma with squamous metaplasia, and Hodgkin's disease. Papillary carcinoma can show areas of squamous metaplasia and sclerosis[587, 588]; however, a diagnostic papillary component is always readily identifiable. Hyaline sclerosis and eosinophilic infiltrate seen in mucoepidermoid carcinoma can be mistaken for involvement of the thyroid by Hodgkin's disease.[622] The morphologic features, especially in a metastasis to neck lymph nodes, can be mistaken for a nodular sclerosis Hodgkin's disease. Immunostains for cytokeratins, CD30, and CD15 help differentiate these two entities.[622]

Primary Nonepithelial Tumors

Mesenchymal Tumors of the Thyroid Gland

Primary mesenchymal tumors of the thyroid are extremely rare.[2, 23, 29, 151] The diagnosis of a primary mesenchymal tumor in the thyroid should be made only after excluding metastases from another primary source because those are more common than a primary thyroid origin.[23, 29, 624]

Smooth Muscle Tumors of Thyroid

To date, less than 20 cases of benign and malignant primary smooth muscle tumors of the thyroid have been documented in the literature.[624-631]

Leiomyomas occur exclusively in women, present as a solitary encapsulated mass confined to the thyroid, and show histologic, immunohistochemical, and ultrastructural features consistent with smooth muscle origin. They are usually cured by lobectomy or partial thyroidectomy.[624-627]

Leiomyosarcomas are more common in older patients and do not show any specific gender predilection. Their presentation is usually that of a large mass with pleomorphism, mitoses, coagulative necrosis, and hemorrhage with infiltrative growth pattern on light microscopy.[624, 628-631] As mentioned, the diagnosis of primary malignant smooth muscle tumor of thyroid should be entertained only after primary tumor has been carefully excluded elsewhere.[624]

Tulbah et al[630] reported a case of leiomyosarcoma of thyroid in a child with congenital immunodeficiency disease. This tumor was found to express large amounts of Epstein-Barr virus messenger RNA similar to that seen in pediatric smooth muscle tumors associated with AIDS and/or after organ transplantation.

The differential diagnosis of primary leiomyosarcoma of thyroid includes anaplastic carcinoma and SETTLE. Anaplastic carcinoma can stain for both keratins and vimentin; however, the tumor cells are negative for smooth muscle actin, muscle-specific actin, and desmin.[631] SETTLE is usually a tumor of younger age group, shows bland cytologic features, and stains for cytokeratin.[594]

Solitary Fibrous Tumor

Solitary fibrous tumor is a mesenchymal tumor characterized by fibroblastic differentiation, and some cases may reveal focal or predominant myofibroblastic component. It stains positive with CD34. A majority of these tumors behave in benign fashion except for the pleural solitary fibrous tumor; 13% to 23% of tumors in that location are malignant.[632-634]

Fewer than 10 cases of solitary fibrous tumor of thyroid have been reported.[635-640] All have behaved in a benign fashion, with no local recurrences or distant metastasis.[635-640] On light microscopy, these tumors consist of spindle-shaped tumor cells and collagenous stroma without any pleomorphism or mitoses. In some instances, these tumors may be difficult to distinguish from hemangiopericytoma.[635, 639, 640] The tumor cells stain positive for CD34 and vimentin and are negative for cytokeratin, thyroglobulin, calcitonin, and S-100 protein. Ultrastructurally, these tumors show fibroblastic differentiation.[636, 637]

The differential diagnosis of solitary fibrous tumor of thyroid includes the same lesions mentioned previously for other spindle cell lesions.

Vascular Tumors

Vascular tumors of the thyroid are rare; some authors still debate their existence as true tumors rather than as a prominent vascular pattern in an otherwise benign or malignant thyroid tumor.[641] Nevertheless, recent reports have documented that these tumors do exist in their pure forms.[642-646]

The list of reported vascular tumors in thyroid includes hemangioma, epithelioid hemangioendothelioma, and angiosarcoma.[642-646]

Angiosarcoma of the thyroid is extremely rare and is almost unheard of in many parts of the world. The majority of cases have been reported from European Alpine regions, where it makes up approximately 4% of all thyroid malignancies. In these cases, it is usually seen in a gland affected by nodular goiter.[643]

Anaplastic carcinoma and poorly differentiated carcinoma of the thyroid can exhibit a prominent vascular pattern and should be included in the differential diagnosis for angiosarcoma of thyroid.[23, 29, 641] Angiosarcomas of the thyroid and other vascular tumors stain positive for factor VIII–related antigen and CD31 and are usually negative for keratin. On electron microscopy, Weibel-Palade bodies can be demonstrated only in well-differentiated lesions conforming to an endothelial origin. The angiosarcoma behaves in a manner similar to that of anaplastic carcinoma: persistent local disease, distant metastasis, and rapidly fatal outcome. Therefore, the differentiation between anaplastic carcinoma and angiosarcoma of the thyroid is only morphologic and probably of only academic interest.[641, 644-646]

Mucosa-Associated Lymphoid Tissue of the Thyroid

Primary thyroid lymphomas can present as small or large cell tumors and are usually of B cell phenotype.[647] Initially, it was suggested that they are of follicular center cell origin; however, it has been shown that primary lymphomas of the thyroid are variants of mucosa-associated lymphoid tissue (MALT).[648, 649] This is based on the facts that most thyroid lymphomas are immunophenotypically similar to maltomas in other sites; they lack the t(14;18) translocation seen in follicular cell lymphomas; when they propagate they often involve other extranodal sites, such as the gastrointestinal tract (also a MALT site); and they share the morphologic hallmark of MALT—the lymphoepithelial lesion.[649]

Recognition of MALT by immunophenotyping or molecular or cytogenetic analyses is important because other B cell lymphomas in the thyroid most likely represent secondary neoplasms and have a different clinical behavior. The 5-year survival in primary thyroid lymphomas of small cell type is very good (75%), and those showing plasmacytic differentiation (common in MALT) have an excellent prognosis (100%).[648-650]

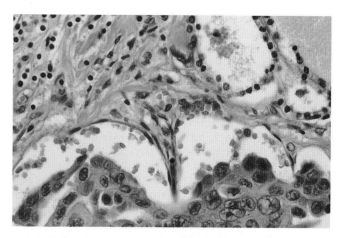

Figure 4–11. A case of metastatic non-small cell carcinoma of lung (lower half of photo) to thyroid.

SECONDARY (METASTATIC) TUMORS OF THE THYROID

Metastases to the thyroid are infrequent despite the gland's rich vascular supply.[651-656] The reported prevalence of secondary tumors of thyroid ranges 1.25% to 25%.[651, 656, 657] The most common tumors that metastasize to the thyroid gland include breast, lung, and renal cell carcinoma[651-656] (Fig. 4–11). In some cases, metastases to the thyroid can become manifest long after the detection of primary cancer; this scenario is most commonly encountered in renal cell carcinoma.[651, 654-656] However, a majority of these lesions are discovered within a short interval after detection of primary tumors.[651-660]

Metastases to the thyroid gland may pose diagnostic problems because (1) a majority of cases are asymptomatic and clinically undetectable[651-652, 656]; (2) the poorly differentiated cancers may be difficult to differentiate from poorly differentiated or anaplastic carcinomas of the thyroid, especially in FNA specimens[659-660]; (3) the metastatic tumor may be mistaken for a thyroid primary tumor if it presents as a solitary nodule and is detected long after the primary tumor[654, 656, 657]; and (4) rarely, the metastatic deposits may occur within a preexisting thyroid neoplasm, which can complicate the morphologic interpretation.[29, 661] In such cases immunohistochemical studies, including review of the primary tumor, is always helpful.[661]

Metastases to the thyroid gland usually indicate poor prognosis; however, in some cases, surgical excision of solitary metastases, such as from renal cell carcinoma, have proved to be curative.[654, 656]

References

1. Medvei VC: A history of endocrinology. In Kovacs K & Asa S, ed.: Functional Endocrinology. Blackwell Science, England, 1998, p. 1.
2. Murray D: The thyroid gland. In Kovacs K & Asa S, ed.: Functional Endocrinology. Blackwell Science, England, 1998, pp. 295–369.

3. Parry CH: Collections of the unpublished medical writings of the late Caled Hillier Parry. In Middlesworth LV, ed.: The Thyroid Gland: A Practical Clinical Treatise. Year Book Medical Publishers, Chicago, 1986, p. 1.
4. Von Basedow CA: Exopthalmos durch Hypertrophie des Zellgewebes in der Augenhoehle. In LiVolsi VA: Surgical Pathology of the Thyroid. WB Saunders, Philadelphia, 1990, p. xvi.
5. Hoyes AD, Kershaw DR: Anatomy and development of the thyroid gland. Ear Nose Throat J 1985; 64:318.
6. Kingsbury BF: Ultimobranchial body and thyroid gland in fetal calf. Am J Anat 1935; 56:44.
7. Janzer RC, Weber E, Hedinger C: The relation between solid cell nests and C-cells of the thyroid gland. Cell Tissue Res 1979; 197:295.
8. Yamaoka Y: Solid cell nests (SCN) in the human thyroid gland. Acta Pathol Jpn 1973; 23:493.
9. Williams ED, Toyn CE, Harach HR: The ultimobranchial gland and congenital thyroid abnormalities in man. J Pathol 1989; 159:135.
10. Thorpe-Beeston JG, Nicolaides KH, Felton CV, et al.: Maturation of the secretion of thyroid hormone and thyroid-stimulating hormone in the fetus. N Engl J Med 1991; 324:702.
11. Fisher DA, Klein AH: Thyroid development and disorders of thyroid function in newborn. N Engl J Med 1981; 304:702.
12. Baughman RA: Lingual thyroid and lingual thyroglossal tract remnants. Oral Surg Oral Med Oral Pathol 1972; 34:781.
13. Sauk JJ: Ectopic lingual thyroid. J Pathol 1970; 102:239.
14. Neinas FW, Gorman CA, Devine KD, et al.: Lingual thyroid clinical characteristics of 15 cases. Ann Intern Med 1973; 79:205.
15. Strickland AL, Macfie JA, Vanwyk JJ, et al.: Ectopic thyroid glands stimulating thyroglossal duct cysts. JAMA 1969; 208:307.
16. Kaplan M, Kauli R, Lubin E, et al. Ectopic thyroid gland. J Pediatr 1978; 92:205.
17. Walling AD: Ectopic thyroid tissue. Am Fam Phys 1987; 36:147.
18. Pollice L, Caruso G: Struma cordis: Ectopic thyroid goiter in the right ventricle. Arch Pathol 1986; 110:452.
19. Chanin LR, Greenberg LM: Pediatric upper airway obstruction due to ectopic thyroid: Classification and case reports. Laryngoscope 1988; 98:422.
20. Carpenter GR, Emery JL: Inclusions in the human thyroid. J Anat 1976; 122:77.
21. Weller GL: Development of the thyroid, parathyroid, and thymus gland in man. Contrib Embryol Carnegie Inst 1933; 141:93.
22. Gardner WR: Unusual relationship between thyroid gland and skeletal muscle in infants. Cancer 1956; 6:681.
23. LiVolsi VA: Surgical Pathology of the Thyroid. WB Saunders, Philadelphia, 1990.
24. Butler JJ, Tulinius H, Ibanez ML, et al.: Significance of thyroid tissue in lymph nodes associated with carcinoma of the head, neck or lung. Cancer 1967; 77:637.
25. Gerard-Marchant R: Thyroid follicle inclusions in cervical lymph nodes. Arch Pathol Lab Med 1964; 77:637.
26. Roth LM: Inclusions of non-neoplastic thyroid tissue within cervical lymph nodes. Cancer 1965; 18:105.
27. Klinck GH: Structure of the thyroid. In Hazard JB, Smith DE, eds.: The Thyroid. International Academy of Pathology Monograph. Williams & Wilkins, Baltimore, 1964, p. 1.
28. Meyer JS, Steinberg LS: Microscopically benign thyroid follicles in cervical lymph nodes. Cancer 1969; 24:301.
29. Rosai J, Carcangui ML, DeLellis RA: Atlas of Tumor Pathology: Tumors of the Thyroid Gland. Armed Forces Institute of Pathology, Washington, D.C., 1992.
30. MacMahon HE, Lee HY, Rivelis CF: Birefringent crystals in human thyroid gland. Acta Endocrinol 1968; 58:172.
31. Reid JD, Choi CH, Oldroyd NO: Calcium oxalate crystals in the thyroid: Their identification, prevalence, origin, and possible significance. Am J Clin Pathol 1987; 87:443.
32. Gibson W, Croker B, Cox C: C cell populations in normal children and young adults. Lab Invest 1989; 42:119.
33. Gibson WGH, Peng TC, Croker BP: Age-associated C cell hyperplasia in human thyroid. Am J Pathol 1982; 106:388.
34. Wolfe HJ, DeLellis RA, Voelkel EF, et al.: Distribution of calcitonin-containing cells in neonatal human thyroid gland: A correlation of morphology with peptide content. J Clin Endocrinol Metab 1975; 41:1076.
35. Heimann P: Ultrastructure of human thyroid: A study of normal thyroid, untreated and treated diffuse toxic goiter. Acta Endocrinol 1966; 53: 1.
36. Klinck GH, Oertel JE, Winship T: Ultrastructure of normal human thyroid. Lab Invest 1970; 22:2.
37. Vander JB, Gaston EA, Dawber TR: The significance of nontoxic thyroid nodules. Ann Intern Med 1968; 69:540.
38. Beckers C: Thyroid nodules. Clin Endocrinol Metab 1979; 8:181.
39. DeHaven JW, Sherwin RS: The thyroid nodule: Approach to diagnosis and therapy. Conn Med 1979; 43:761.
40. Hetzel BS: Iodine deficiency disorders (IDD) and their eradication. Lancet 1983; 2:1126.
41. Haneman G: Non-toxic goiter. Clin Endocrinol Metab 1979; 8:167.
42. Struder H, Peter HJ, Gerber H: Morphologic and functional changes in developing goiters. In Hall R, Kobberling J, eds.: Thyroid Disorders Associated with Iodine Deficiency and Excess. Raven Press, New York, 1987 p. 229.
43. Peter HJ, Studer H, Groscurth P: Autonomous growth, but not autonomous function in embryonic human thyroids: A clue to understanding autonomous goiter growth? J Clin Endocrinol Metab 1988; 66:968.
44. Ramelli F, Studer H, Bruggisser D: Pathogenesis of thyroid nodules in multinodular goiter. Am J Pathol 1982; 109:215.
45. Kraiem Z, Glaser B, Yigla M, et al.: Toxic multinodular goiter: A variant of autoimmune hyperthyroidism. J Clin Endocrinol Metab 1987; 65:659.
46. Brown RS, Jackson IMD, Pohl SL, et al.: Do thyroid-stimulating immunoglobulins cause nontoxic and toxic multinodular goiter? Lancet 1978; 1:904.
47. Peter HJ, Studer H, Smeds S: Pathogenesis of heterogeneity in human multinodular goiter. J Clin Invest 1985; 76:1992.
48. Peter HJ, Studer H, Forster R, et al.: The pathogenesis of "hot" and "cold" follicles in multinodular goiters. J Clin Endocrinol Metab 1982; 55:941.
49. Bigos ST, Ridgway EC, Kourides IA, et al.: Spectrum of pituitary alterations with mild and severe thyroid impairment. J Clin Endorcrinol Metab 1978; 46:317.
50. Carlson HE, Linfoot JA, Braunstein GD, et al.: Hyperthyroidism and acromegaly due to a thyrotropin- and growth hormone–secreting pituitary tumor. Am J Med 1983; 74:915.
51. Horn K, Erhardt F, Fahlbusch R, et al.: Recurrent goiter, hyperthyroidism, galactorrhea and amenorrhea due to a thyrotropin- and prolactin-producing pituitary tumor. J Clin Endocrinol Metab 1976; 43:137.
52. Tonacherra M, Sande JV, Parma J, et al.: TSH receptor and disease. Clin Endocrinology (Oxf) 1996; 44:621.
53. Struder H, Ramelli F: Simple goiter and its variants: Euthyroid and hyperthyroid. Endocr Rev 1982; 3:40.
54. Al-Moussa M, Berk JS: Histometry of thyroids containing few and multiple nodules. J Clin Pathol 1986; 39:483.
55. Namba H, Matsuo K, Fagin JA: Clonal composition of benign and malignant human thyroid tumors. J Clin Invest 1990; 86:120.
56. Hicks DG, LiVolsi VA, Neidlich JA, et al.: Clonal analysis of solitary follicular nodules in the thyroid. Am J Pathol 1990; 137:553.
57. Apel RL, Ezzat S, Bapat BV, et al.: Clonality of thyroid nodules in sporadic goiter. Diagn Mol Pathol 1995; 4:113.
58. Kopp P, Kimura ET, Aeschimann S, et al.: Polyclonal and monoclonal thyroid nodules coexist within human multinodular goiters. J Clin Endocrinol Metab 1994; 79:134.
59. Ashcraft MW, Van Herle AJ: Management of the thyroid nodule: Scanning techniques, thyroid suppressive therapy and fine-needle aspiration. Head Neck Surg 1981; 3:297.
60. Silverman JF, West RL, Larkin EW, et al.: The role of fine-needle aspiration biopsy in the rapid diagnosis and management of thyroid neoplasm. Cancer 1986; 57:1164.
61. Nunez C, Mendelsohn G: Fine-needle aspiration and needle biopsy of the thyroid gland. Pathol Annu 1989; 24:16.

62. Kini SR: Guides to Clinical Aspiration Biopsy Thyroid, 2nd ed. Igaku-Shoin, New York, 1996.

63. Klemi JP, Joensuu H, Nylamo E: Fine-needle aspiration biopsy in the diagnosis of thyroid nodules. Acta Cytol 1991; 35:434.

64. Baloch Z, Sack MJ, Yu GH, et al.: Fine-needle aspiration thyroid: An institutional experience. Thyroid 1998; 8:565.

65. Erdogan MF, Kamel N, Aras D, et al.: Value of re-aspirations in benign nodular thyroid disease. Thyroid 1998; 8:1087.

66. Thomas JO, Adeyi OA, Nwachokor FN, et al.: Fine needle aspiration cytology in mangement of thyroid enlargement: Ibadan experience. East Afr Med J 1998; 75:657.

67. Hamburger JI: Fine needle biopsy diagnosis of thyroid nodules: Perspective. Thyroidology 1988; 1:21.

68. Goellner JR, Gharib H, Grant CS, et al.: Fine needle aspiration cytology of the thyroid, 1980–1986. Acta Cytol 1987; 31:587.

69. Marketos SG, Eftychiadis A, Koutras DA: The first recognition of the association between goiter and exophthalmos. J Endocrinol Invest 1983; 6:401.

70. Hennemann G: Historical aspects about the development of our knowledge of Morbus Basedow. J Endocrinol Invest 1991; 14:617.

71. Burman KD, Baker JR: Immune mechanisms in Graves' disease. Endocr Rev 1985; 6:183.

72. Farid NR: Immunogenetics of autoimmune thyroid disorders. Endocrinol Metab Clin North Am 1987; 16:229.

73. Schicha H, Emrich D, Schreivogel I: Hyperthyroidism due to Graves' disease and due to autonomous goiter. J Endocrinol Invest 1985; 8:399.

74. Spjut HJ, Warren WD, Ackerman LV: Clinical-pathologic study of 76 cases of recurrent Graves' disease, toxic (nonexophthalmic) goiter, and nontoxic goiter. Am J Clin Pathol 1957; 27:367.

75. Johnson JR: Adenomatous goiters with and without hyperthyroidism. Arch Surg 1949; 59:1088.

76. Smith BR, Hall R: Thyroid stimulating immunoglobulins in Graves' disease and due to autonomous goiter. J Endocrinol Invest 1985; 8:399.

77. Bech K: Immunological aspects of Graves' disease: Importance of thyroid-stimulating immunoglobulins. Acta Endocrinol (Copenh) 1983; 254:1.

78. Solomon DH, Kleeman KE: Concepts of pathogenesis of Graves' disease. Adv Intern Med 1976; 22:273.

79. Furmaniak J, Nakajima Y, Hashim FA, et al.: The TSH receptor: Structure and interaction with autoantibodies in thyroid disease. Acta Endocrinol (Copenh) 1987; 281:157.

80. Skillern PG: Genetics of Graves' disease. Mayo Clin Proc 1972; 47:848.

81. Sawin CT: Theories of causation of Graves' disease: A historical perspective. Endocrinol Metab Clin North Am 1998; 27:63.

82. Stenszky V, Kozma L, Balazs C, et al.: The genetics of Graves' disease: HLA and disease susceptibility. J Clin Endocrinol Metab 1985; 61:735.

83. Brix TH, Kyvik KO, Hegedus L: What is the evidence of genetic factors in the etiology of Graves' disease? A brief review. Thyroid 1998; 8:627.

84. Watson PF, Pickerill AP, Davies R, et al.: Analysis of cytokine gene expression in Graves' disease and multinodular goiter. J Clin Endocrinol Metab 1994; 79:355.

85. Chang DCS, Wheeler MH, Woodcock JP, et al.: The effect of preoperative Lugol's iodine on thyroid blood flow in patients with Graves' hyperthyroidism. Surgery 1987; 8:439.

86. Carnell NE, Valente WA: Thyroid nodules in Grave's disease: Classification, characterization, and response to treatment. Thyroid 1998; 8:647.

87. Jayaram G, Singh B, Marwaha RK: Graves' disease: Appearance in cytologic smears from fine needle aspirates of the thyroid gland. Acta Cytol 1989; 33:36.

88. Myren J, Sivertssen E: Thin needle biopsy of the thyroid gland in the diagnosis of thyrotoxicosis. Acta Endocrinol 1962; 39:431.

89. Nilsson G: Marginal vacuoles in fine needle aspiration biopsy smears of toxic goiters. Acta Pathol Microbiol Scand [A] 1972; 80:289.

90. Smith JF: The pathology of the thyroid in the syndrome of sporadic goiter and congenital deafness. Q J Med 1960; 29:297.

91. Moore GH: The thyroid in sporadic goitrous cretinism. Arch Pathol Lab Med 1962; 74:35.

92. Bataskis JG, Nishiyama RH, Schmidt RW: "Sporadic goiter sydrome": A clinicopathologic analysis. Am J Clin Pathol 1963; 30:241.

93. Kennedy JS: The pathology of dyshormonogenetic goiter. J Pathol 1969; 99:251.

94. Barsano CP, DeGroot LG: Dyshormonogenetic goiter. Baillieres Clin Endocrinol Metab 1979; 8:145.

95. Lever EG, Medeiros-Neto GA, DeGroot LJ: Inherited disorders of thyroid metabolism. Endocr Rev 1983; 4:213.

96. Fisher DA, Klein AH: Thyroid development and disorders of thyroid function in the newborn. N Engl J Med 1981; 304:702.

97. Cooper DS, Axelrod L, DeGroot LJ, et al.: Congenital goiter and the development of metastatic follicular carcinoma with evidence for a leak of nonhormonal iodide: Clinical, pathological, kinetic and biochemical studies and a review of the literature. J Clin Endodrinol Metab 1981; 52:294.

98. Vickery AL: The diagnosis of malignancy in dyshormonogenetic goiter. J Clin Endocrinol Metab 1981; 10:317.

99. Fadda G, Baloch Z, LiVolsi VA: Dyshormonogenetic goiter. Intl J Surg Pathol 1999; 7:125.

100. Volpe R: Acute and subacute thyroiditis. Pharmacal Ther 1976; 1:171.

101. Volpe R: Acute suppurative thyroiditis. In Werner SC, Ingbar SH, eds.: The Thyroid. Harper & Row, New York, 1971, p. 849.

102. Burhans EC: Acute thyroiditis. Surg Gynecol Obstet 1928; 47:478.

103. Kakuda K, Kanokogi M, Mitsunobu M, et al.: Acute mycotic thyroiditis. Acta Pathol Jpn 1983; 33:147.

104. Hajjar ET, Salti IS: Tuberculosis of the thyroid. Lebanese Med J 1973; 26:273.

105. Leers WD, Dussault J, Mullens JE, et al.: Suppurative thyroiditis: An unusual case caused by Actinomyces naeslundi. Can Med Assoc 1969; 101:714.

106. Dan M, Garcia A, von Westrap C: Primary actinomycosis of the thyroid, mimicking carcinoma. J Otolaryngol 1984; 12:109.

107. Gallant JE, Enriquez RE, Cohen KL, et al.: Pneumocystis carinii thyroiditis. Am J Med 1988; 84:303.

108. Frank TS, LiVolsi VA, Connor AM: Cytomegalovirus infection of the thyroid in immunocompromised adults. Yale J Biol Med 1987; 60:1.

109. Bauchet LJ: De la thyroidite (goitre aigu) et du goitre enflamme (goitre chronique enflamme). Gaz Hebd Med Chir 1857; 4:19.

110. Hazard JB: Thyroiditis: A review. Am J Clin Pathol 1955; 25:289.

111. Bastenie PA, Bonnyns M, Neve P: Subacute and chronic granulomatous thyroiditis. In Bastenie PA, Erman AM, eds.: Thyroiditis and Thyroid Function: Clinical, Morphological, and Physiological Studies. Pergamon Press, Oxford, UK, 1972, p. 69.

112. Greene JN: Subacute thyroiditis. Am J Med 1971; 51:97.

113. DeQuervain F: Die akute nicht eiterige thyroiditis und die Beteiligung der Schilddruse an akuten intoxikationen und infektionen überhaupt. Mitt Grenzgeb Med Chir 1904; 6:1.

114. DeQuervain F, Giordanengo G: Die akute und subakute nicht eiterige thyreoditis. Mitt Grenzgeb Med Chir 1936; 44:538.

115. Eylan E, Zmucky R, Sheba C: Mumps virus and subacute thyroiditis: Evidence of a casual association. Lancet 1957; 1:1062.

116. Vople R, Row VV, Ezrin C: Circulating viral and thyroid antibodies in subacute thyroiditis. J Clin Endocrinol Metab 1967; 27:1275.

117. Goldman J, Bochna AJ, Becker FO: St. Louis encephalitis and subacute thyroiditis. Ann Intern Med 1977; 87:250.

118. Dorfman SG, Cooperman MT, Nelson RI, et al.: Painless thyroiditis and transient hyperthyroidism without goiter. Ann Int Med 1977; 86:24.

119. Steinberg FU: Subacute granulomatous thyroiditis: A review. Ann Intern med 1960; 52:1104.

120. Volpe R: The pathology of thyroiditis. Hum Pathol 1978; 9:429.

121. Lindsay S, Dailey ME: Granulomatous or giant cell thyroiditis. Surg Gynecol Obstet 1954; 98:197.

122. Carney JA, Moore SB, Northcutt RC, et al.: Palpation thyroiditis (multifocal granulomatous thyroiditis) Am J Clin Pathol 1975; 64:639.
123. Rose E, Royster HP: Invasive fibrous thyroiditis (Reidel's struma). JAMA 1961; 176:224.
124. Best TB, Burwell MS, Volpe R: Reidel's thyroiditis associated with Hashimoto's thyroiditis, hypoparathyroidism and retroperitoneal fibrosis. J Endocrinol Invest 1991; 13:13.
125. Taubenberger JK, Merino MJ, Medeiros J: A thyroid biopsy with histologic features of both Reidel's thyroiditis and the fibrosing variant of Hashimoto's thyroiditis. Hum Pathol 1992; 23:1072.
126. Julie C, Vieillefond A, Desligneres S, et al.: Hashimoto's thyroiditis associated with Reidel's thyroiditis and retroperitoneal fibrosis. Pathol Res Pract 1997; 193:573.
127. Baloch ZW, Saberi M, LiVolsi VA: Simultaneous involvement of thyroid by Reidel's disease and fibrosing Hashimoto's thyroiditis: A case report. Thyroid 1998; 4:337.
128. Hashimoto H: Zur Kenntnis der lymphomatosen Veränderungen der Schilddruse (struma lymphomatosa). Arch Klin Chir 1912; 97:219.
129. Fisher DA, Beall GN: Hashimoto's thyroiditis. Pharmacol Ther 1976; 1:445.
130. Woolner LB, McConahey WM, Beahrs OH: Struma lymphomatosa (Hashimoto's disease) and related thyroidal disorders. J Clin Endocrinol Metab 1959; 19:53.
131. Bastenie PA, Erman AM, eds.: Thyroiditis and Thyroid Function: Clinical, Morphological, and Physiological Studies. Pergamon Press, Oxford, UK, 1972.
132. Marshall SF, Meissner WA, Smith DC: Chronic thyroiditis. N Engl J Med 1948; 238:758.
133. Vickery AL, Hamlin E: Struma lymphomatosa (Hashimoto's thyroiditis). N Engl J Med 1961; 264:226.
134. Weetman AP: Autoimmune thyroiditis: Predisposition and pathogenesis. Clin Endocrinol (Oxf) 1992; 36:307.
135. Iwatani Y, Amino N, Mori H, et al.: T lymphocyte subsets in autoimmune thyroid diseases and subacute thyroiditis detected with monoclonal antibodies. J Clin Endocrinol Metab 1982; 56:251.
136. Londei M, Bottazo GF, Feldman M: Human T cell clones from autoimmune thyroid glands: Specific recognition of autologous thyroid cells. Science 1984; 228:85.
137. Yagi Y, Sato E, Yagi S: Population of T-lymphocytes in various kinds of thyroid disease. Endocrinol Jpn 1983; 30:113.
138. Berho M, Suster S: Clear nuclear changes in Hashimoto's thyroiditis: A clinicopathologic study of 12 cases. Ann Clin Lab Sci 1995; 25:513.
139. Williams ED: Malignant lymphoma of the thyroid. Clin Endocrinol Metab 1981; 10:83.
140. Kato I, Tajima K, Suchi T, et al.: Chronic lymphocytic thyroiditis as a risk factor of B-cell lymphoma in the thyroid gland. Jpn J Cancer Res 1984; 53:2515.
141. Jayram G, Marwaha RK, Gupta RK, et al.: Cytomorphologic aspects of thyroiditis: A study of 51 cases with functional, immunological and ultrasonographic data. Acta Cytol 1986; 31:687.
142. Kumarasinghe MP, De Silva S: Pitfalls in cytological diagnosis of autoimmune thyroiditis. Pathology 1999; 31:1.
143. Ravinsky E, Safneck JR: Differentiation of Hashimoto's thyroiditis from thyroid neoplasms in fine needle aspirates. Acta Cytol 1988; 32:854.
144. Katz SM, Vickery AL: The fibrous variant of Hashimoto's thyroditis. Hum Pathol 1974; 5:161.
145. Harach HR, Willimas ED: Fibrous thyroiditis: An immunopathological study. Histopathology 1983; 7:739.
146. Reidel BMKL: Die chronische, zur Bildung eisenharter Tumoren führende Entzündung der Schilddruse. Verh Dtsch Ges Chir 1896; 25:101.
147. Beierwalters WH: Thyroiditis. Ann N Y Acad Sci 1965; 124:586.
148. Schwaegerle SM, Bauer TW, Esseltyn CB: Reidel's thyroiditis. Am J Clin Pathol 1988; 90:715.
149. Thomson JA, Jackson IMD, Duguid WP: The effect of steroid therapy on Reidel's thyroiditis. Scott Med J 1968; 13:13.
150. Mitchinson MJ: Retroperitoneal fibrosis revisited. Arch Pathol Lab Med 1986; 110:784.
151. Hedinger C, Williams ED, Sobin LH: Histological Typing of Thyroid Tumours: WHO International Histological Classification of Tumours, 4th ed. Springer-Verlag, Berlin, 1988.
152. Chu KC, Kramer BS: Cancer patterns in the United States. In Greenwald P, Kramer BS, Weed DL, eds.: Cancer prevention and control. Marcel Dekker, New York, 1995, p. 37.
153. Ron E, Modan B: Thyroid. In Schottenfield D, Fraumeni JF, eds.: Cancer Epidemiology and Prevention. WB Saunders, Philadelphia, 1982, p. 837.
154. Taylor S: Clinical features of thyroid tumors. Clin Endocrinol Metab 1979; 8:209.
155. Baloch ZW, Abraham S, Roberts S, et al.: Expression of differential cytokeratins in follicular variant of papillary carcinoma: An immunohistochemical study and its diagnostic utility. Hum Pathol 1999; 10:1166.
156. Permanetter W, Nathrath WBL, Löhrs U: Immunohistochemical analysis of thyroglobulin- and keratin-benign and malignant thyroid tumors. Virchows Arch 1982; 398:221.
157. Buley ID, Gatter KC, Heryet A, et al.: Expression of intermediate filament proteins in normal and diseased thyroid glands. J Clin Pathol 1987; 40:136.
158. Schelfhout LJDM, Van Muijen GNP, Fleuren GJ: Expression of keratin 19 distinguishes papillary thyroid carcinoma from follicular carcinoma and follicular thyroid adenoma. Am J Clin Pathol 1989; 92:654.
159. Rapheal SJ, McKeown-Eyssen G, Asa SL: High-molecular-weight cytokeratin and cytokeratin-19 in the diagnosis of thyroid tumors. Mod Pathol 1994; 47:295.
160. Miettinen M, Lehto V-P, Franssila K, et al: Expression of intermediate filaments in thyroid and thyroid tumors. Lab Invest 1984; 50:262.
161. Miettinen M, Kovatich AJ, Kärkkäinen P: Keratin subsets in papillary and follicular thyroid lesions: A paraffin section analysis with diagnostic implications. Virchows Arch 1997; 431:407.
162. Fonseca E, Nesland JM, Höie J, et al.: Patterns of expression of intermediate cytokeratin filaments in the thyroid gland: An immunohistochemical study of simple and stratified epithelial-type cytokeratins. Virchows Arch 1997; 430:239.
163. Pollina L, Pacini F, Fonatanini G, et al.: bcl-2, p53 and proliferating cell nuclear antigen expression is related to the degree of differentiation in thyroid carcinomas. Br J Cancer 1996; 73:139.
164. Basolo F, Pollina L, Fonatanini G, et al.: Apoptosis and proliferation in thyroid carcinoma: Correlation with bcl-2 and p53 protein expression. Br J Cancer 1997; 75:537.
165. Ho Y, Tseng SC, Chin TY, et al.: P53 gene mutation in thyroid carcinoma. Cancer Lett 1996; 103:57.
166. Branet F, Caron P, Camallieres M, et al.: bcl-2 proto-oncogene expression in neoplastic and non-neoplastic thyroid tissue. Bull du cancer 1996; 83:213.
167. Van Hoeven KH, Kovatich AJ, Miettinen M: Immunocytochemical evaluation of HBME-1, CA 19-9, and CD-15 (Leu-M1) in fine-needle aspirates of thyroid nodules. Diag Cytopathol 1998; 18:93.
168. Sack MJ, Astengo-Osuna C, Lin BT, et al.: HBME-1 immunostaining in thyroid fine-needle aspirations: A useful marker in the diagnosis of carcinoma. Mod Pathol 1997; 10:668.
169. Bounacer A, Wicker R, Caillou B, et al.: High prevalence of activating ret proto-oncogene rearrangements in thyroid tumors from patients who had received external radiation. Oncogene 1997; 15:1263.
170. Hazard JB, Kenyon R: Atypical adenoma of the thyroid. Arch Pathol Lab Med 1954; 58:554.
171. Bronner MP, LiVolsi VA: Oxyphilic (Askanazy/Hürthle cell) tumors of the thyroid: Microscopic features predict biologic behavior. Surg Pathol 1988; 2:137.
172. Carney J, Ryan J, Goellner J: Hyalinizing trabecular adenoma of the thyroid gland. Am J Surg Pathol 1987; 11:583.
173. McCluggage W, Sloan J: Hyalinizing trabecular carcinoma of the thyroid gland. Histopathology 1996; 28:357.
174. Molberg K, Albores-Saavedra J: Hyalinizing trabecular carcinoma of the thyroid gland. Hum Pathol 1994; 25:192.
175. LiVolsi VA, Gupta PK: Thyroid fine-needle aspiration: Intranuclear inclusions, nuclear grooves and psammoma bodies–paraganglioma-like adenoma of the thyroid. Diagn Cytopathol 1991; 8:82.

176. Akin MR, Nguyen GK: Fine-needle aspiration biopsy cytology of hyalinizing trabecular adenomas of the thyroid. Diagn Cytopathol 1999; 20:90.

177. Rothenberg HJ, Goellner JR, Carney JA: Hyalinizing trabecular adenoma of the thyroid gland: Recognition and characterization of its cytoplasmic yellow body. Am J Surg Pathol 1999; 23:118.

178. Bronner M, LiVolsi V, Jennings T: PLAT: Paraganglioma-like adenomas of the thyroid. Surg Pathol 1988; 1:383.

179. Chetty R, Beydoun R, LiVolsi V: Paraganglioma-like (hyalinizing trabecular) adenoma of the thyroid revisited. Pathology 1994; 26:429.

180. Li M, Rosai J, Carcangui M: Hyalinizing trabecular adenoma of the thyroid: A distinct tumor type or a pattern of growth? Evaluation of 28 cases. Mod Pathol 1995; 8;54.

181. Sambade C, Franssila K, Cameselle-Teijeiro J, et al.: Hyalinizing trabecular adenoma: A misnomer for a pecular tumor of the thyroid gland. Endocr Pathol 1991; 2:83.

182. Fonseca E, Nesland JM, Sobrinho-SimoÂes M: Expression of stratified epithelial-type cytokeratins in hyalinizing trabecular adenomas support their relationship with papillary carcinomas of the thyroid. Histopathology 1997; 31:330.

183. Rigaud C, Peltier F, Bogomoletz WV: Mucin-producing microfollicular adenoma of the thyroid. J Clin Pathol 1985; 38:277.

184. Carcangui ML, Sibley RK, Rosai J: Clear cell change in primary thyroid tumors: A study of 38 cases. Am J Surg Pathol 1985; 9:705.

185. Alsop JE, Yerbury PJ, O'Donnell PJ, et al.: Signet-ring cell microfollicular adenoma arising in a nodular ectopic thyroid: A case report. J Oral Pathol 1986; 15:518.

186. Harach HR, Virgilli E, Soler G, et al.: Cytopathology of follicular tumours of the thyroid with clear cell change. Cytopathology 1991; 2:125.

187. Vigliani R, Galliano D, Iandolo M: Signet-ring-cell adenoma of the thyroid: Description of a case and review of the literature. Pathologica 1994; 86:206.

188. Brisigotti M, Lorenzini P, Alessi A, et al.: Mucin-producing adenoma of thyroid gland. Tumori 1986; 72:211.

189. Gherardi G: Signet ring cell "mucinous" thyroid adenoma: A follicle cell tumour with abnormal accumulation of thyroglobulin and peculiar histochemical profile. Histopathology 1987; 11:317.

190. Schroder S, Bocker W: Signet-ring-cell thyroid tumors: Follicle cell tumors with arrest of folliculogenesis. Am J Surg Pathol 1985; 9:619.

191. Livolsi VA: Well differentiated thyroid carcinoma. Clin Oncol 1996; 8:281.

192. Tubiana M, Schlumberger M, Rougier P, et al.: Long-term results and prognostic factors in patients with differentiated thyroid carcinoma. Cancer 1985; 55:794.

193. Carcangui ML, Steeper T, Zampi G, et al.: Anaplastic thyroid carcinoma: A study of 70 cases. Am J Clin Pathol 1985; 83:135.

194. Sakamoto A, Kasai N, Sugano H: Poorly differentiated carcinoma of the thyroid: A clinicopathologic entity for a high risk group of papillary and follicular carcinoma. Cancer 1983; 52:1849.

195. Meissner WA, Adler A: Papillary carcinoma of the thyroid: A study of the pathology of two hundred twenty-six cases. Arch Pathol Lab Med 1958; 66:518.

196. Vickery AL: Thyroid papillary carcinoma: Pathological and philosophical controversies. Am J Surg Pathol 1983; 7:797.

197. Vickery AL, Carcangui ML, Johannssen JV, et al.: Papillary carcinoma. Semin Diagn Pathol 1985; 2:90.

198. Rosai J, Zampi G, Carcangui ML: Papillary carcinoma of the thyroid. Am J Surg Pathol 1983; 7:809.

199. Carcangui ML, Zampi G, Pupi A, et al.: Papillary carcinoma of the thyroid: A clinicopathologic study of 244 cases treated at the University of Florence, Italy. Cancer 1985; 55:805.

200. Carcangui ML, Zampi G, Rosai J: Papillary thyroid carcinoma: A study of its many morphologic expressions and clinical correlates. Pathol Annu 1985; 20:1.

201. Stigt JA, Vasen HF, van der Linde K, et al.: Thyroid carcinoma as first manifestation of familial adenomatous polyposis. Netherlands J Med 1996; 49:116.

202. Bell B, Mazzaferri EL: Familial adenomatous polyposis (Gardner's syndrome) and thyroid carcinoma: A case report and review of the literature. Dig Dis Sci 1993; 38:185.

203. Harach HR, Williams GT, Williams ED: Familial adenomatous polyposis–associated thyroid carcinoma: A distinct type of follicular cell neoplasm. Histopathology 1994; 25:549.

204. Lupoli G, Vitale G, Caraglia M, et al.: Familial papillary thyroid microcarcinoma: A new clinical entity. Lancet 1999; 353:637.

205. Mazzaferri EL, Young RL, Oertel JE: Papillary thyroid carcinoma: The impact of therapy in 576 patients. Medicine 1977; 137:553.

206. Chan JK: Papillary carcinoma of the thyroid: Classical and variants. Histol Histopathol 1990; 5:241.

207. Hapke MR, Dehner LP: The optically clear nucleus: A reliable sign of papillary carcinoma of the thyroid? Am J Surg Pathol 1979; 3:31.

208. Johannessen JV, Gould VE, Jao W: The fine structure of human thyroid cancer. Hum Pathol 1978; 9:385.

209. Echeverria OM, Hernandez-Pando R, Vazquez-Nin GH: Ultrastructural, cytochemical, and immunocytochemical study of nuclei and cytoskeleton of thyroid papillary carcinoma. Ultrastruc Pathol 1998; 22:185.

210. Chan JK, Saw D: The grooved nucleus: A useful diagnostic criterion of papillary carcinoma of the thyroid. Am J Surg Pathol 1986; 10:672.

211. Deligeorgi-Piloti H: Nuclear crease as a cytodiagnostic feature of papillary thyroid carcinoma in fine needle aspiration biopsies. Diagn Cytopathol 1987; 3:307.

212. Scopa CD, Melachrinou M, Saradopoulou C: The significance of grooved nucleus in thyroid lesions. Mod Pathol 1993; 3:307.

213. Kaneko C, Shamoto M, Niimi H, et al.: Studies on intranuclear inclusions and nuclear grooves in papillary thyroid cancer by light, scanning electron and transmission electron microscopy. Acta Cytol 1996; 40:417.

214. Tunio GM, Hirota S, Nomura S, et al.: Possible relation of osteopontin to the development of psammoma bodies in human papillary thyroid cancer. Arch Pathol Lab Med 1998; 122:1087.

215. LiVolsi VA: Papillary neoplasms of the thyroid: Pathologic and prognostic features. Am J Clin Pathol 1992; 97:426.

216. Lida F, Yonekura M, Miyakawa M: Study of intraglandular dissemination of thyroid cancer. Cancer 1969; 24:764.

217. Russell WO, Ibanez M, Clark R, et al.: Thyroid carcinoma: Classification, intraglandular dissemination and clinicopathologic study based upon whole organ sections of 80 thyroid glands. Cancer 1963; 16:1425.

218. Fialkow PJ: The origin and development of human tumor studies with cell markers. New Engl J Med 1974; 291:26.

219. Sugg SL, Ezzat S, Rosen IB, et al.: Distinct multiple RET/PTC gene rearrangements in multifocal papillary thyroid neoplasia. J Clin Endocrinol Metab 1998; 83:4116.

220. Demeure MJ, Clark OH: Surgery in the treatment of thyroid cancer. Endocrinol Metab Clin North Am 1990; 19:663.

221. DeGroot LJ, Kaplan EL, McCormick M, et al.: Natural history treatment and course of papillary thyroid carcinoma. J Clin Endocrinol Metab 1990; 71:414.

222. Hay ID, Grant CS, Taylor WF, et al.: Ipsilateral lobectomy versus bilateral lobar resection in papillary thyroid carcinoma: A retrospective analysis of surgical outcome using a novel prognostic scoring system. Surgery 1987; 102:1088.

223. Hay ID: Nodal metastases from papillary thyroid carcinoma. Lancet 1986; 2:1283.

224. Noguchi S, Noguchi A, Murakami N: Papillary carcinoma of the thyroid II: Value of prophylactic lymph node dissection. Cancer 1970; 26:1061.

225. Hoie J, Stenwig AE, Kullman G, et al: Distant metastases in papillary thyroid cancer: A review of 91 patients. Cancer 1988; 61:1.

226. Ruegemer JJ, Hay ID, Bergstralh EJ, et al.: Distant metastases in differentiated thyroid carcinoma: A multivariate analysis of prognostic variables. J Clin Endocrinol Metab 1988; 67:501.

227. Dockhorn-Dvornickzak B, Frank WW, Schröder S, et al.: Patterns of cytoskeletal proteins in human thyroid gland and thyroid carcinoma. Differentiation 1987; 35:53.

228. Nishimura R, Yokose T, Mukai K: S-100 protein is a differentiation marker in thyroid carcinoma of follicular cell origin: An immunohistochemical study. Pathol Int 1997; 47:673.

229. Diaz NM, Mazoujian G, Wick MR: Estrogen-receptor protein in thyroid neoplasms: An immunohistochemical analysis of papillary carcinoma, follicular carcinoma, and follicular adenoma. Arch Pathol Lab Med 1991; 115:1203.

230. Lewy-Trenda I: Estrogen receptors in the malignant and benign neoplasms of the thyroid. Polski Merkuriusz Lekarski 1998; 5:80.

231. Khan A, Baker SP, Patwardhan NA, et al.: CD57 (Leu-7) expression is helpful in diagnosis of the follicular variant of papillary thyroid carcinoma. Virchows Arch 1998; 432:427.

232. Lai ML, Rizzo N, Liguori C, et al.: Alpha-1-antichymotrypsin immunoreactivity in papillary carcinoma of the thyroid gland. Histopathology 1998; 33:332.

233. Gu J, Daa T, Kashima K, et al.: Expression of splice variants of CD44 in thyroid neoplasms derived from follicular cells. Pathol Int 1998; 48:184.

234. Ensinger C, Obrist P, Bacher-Stier C, et al.: Beta 1-integrin expression in papillary thyroid carcinoma. Anticancer Res 1998; 18:33.

235. Arps H, Sablotny B, Dietal M, et al.: DNA cytophotometry in malignant thyroid tumors. Virchows Arch 1988; 413:319.

236. Cusick EL, Macintosh CA, Krukowski ZH, et al.: Comparison of flow cytometry with static densitometry in papillary thyroid carcinoma. Br J Surg 1990; 77:913.

237. Metaye T, Kraimps JL, Goujon JM, et al.: Expression, localization, and thyrotropin regulation of cathepsin D in human thyroid tissue. J Clin Endocrinol Metab 1997; 82:3383.

238. Basolo F, Pollina L, Pacini F, et al.: Expression of the Mr 67,000 laminin receptor is an adverse prognostic indicator in human thyroid cancer: An immunohistochemical study. Clin Cancer Res 1996; 1:1777.

239. Kameyama K: Expression of MMP-1 in the capsule of thyroid cancer: Relationship with invasiveness. Path Res Pract 1996; 192:20.

240. Nakamura H, Ueno H, Yamashita K, et al.: Enhanced production and activation of progelatinase A mediated by membrane-type 1 matrix metalloproteinase in human papillary thyroid carcinoma. Cancer Res 1999; 59:467.

241. Fusco A, Grieco N, Santoro M, et al.: A new oncogene in human thyroid papillary carcinomas and their lymph-nodal metastases. Nature 1987; 328:170.

242. Jhiang SM, Sagartz JE, Tong Q, et al.: Targeted expression of the ret/PTC1 oncogene induces papillary thyroid carcinomas. Endocrinology 1996; 137:375.

243. Santoro M, Chiappetta G, Cerrato A, et al.: Development of thyroid papillary carcinomas secondary to tissue-specific expression of the RET/PTC1 oncogene in transgenic mice. Oncogene 1996; 12:1821.

244. Jhiang SM, Cho Y, Furminger TL: Thyroid carcinoma in RET/PTC transgenic mice: Recent results. Can Res 1998; 154:265.

245. Fisher AH, Bond JA, Taysavang P, et al.: Papillary thyroid carcinoma oncogene (RET/PTC) alters the nuclear envelope and chromatin structure. Am J Pathol 1998; 153:1443.

246. Takahashi M: The role of the ret proto-oncogene in human disease. Nagoya J Med Sci 1997; 60:23.

247. Lam AK, Montone KT, Nolan KA, et al.: Ret oncogene activation in papillary thyroid carcinoma: Prevalence and implication on the histological parameters. Hum Pathol 1998; 29:565.

248. Soares P, Fonseca E, Wynford-Thomas D, et al.: Sporadic ret-rearranged papillary carcinoma of the thyroid: A subset of slow growing, less aggressive thyroid neoplasms. J Pathol 1998; 185:71.

249. Williams GH, Rooney S, Thomas GA, et al.: RET activation in adult and childhood papillary thyroid carcinoma using a reverse transcriptase-n-polymerase chain reaction approach on archival-nested material. Br J Cancer 1996; 74:585.

250. Sugg SL, Ezzat S, Zheng L, et al.: Oncogene profile of papillary carcinoma. Surgery 1999; 125:46.

251. Wirrtschafter A, Schmidt R, Rosen D, et al.: Expression of RET/PTC fusion gene as a marker for papillary carcinoma in Hashimoto's thyroiditis. Laryngoscope 1997; 107:95.

252. Kusafukha T, Puri P: The ret proto-oncogene: A challenge to our understanding of disease pathogenesis. Ped Surg Int 1997; 12:11.

253. Pisarchik AV, Ermak G, Fomicheva V, et al.: The ret/PTC1 rearrangement is a common feature of Chernobyl-associated papillary thyroid carcinoma from Belarus. Thyroid 1998; 8:133.

254. Jossart GH, Greulich KM, Siperstein AE: Molecular and cytogenetic characterization of a t(1;10;21) translocation in human papillary thyroid cancer cell line TPC-1 expresssing the ret/H4 chimeric transcript. Surgery 1995; 118:1018.

255. Fugazzola L, Pierotti MA, Vigano E: Molecular and biochemical analysis of RET/PTC4, a novel oncogenic rearrangement between RET and ELE1 genes, in a post-Chernobyl papillary thyroid cancer. Oncogene 1996; 13:1093.

256. Klugbauer S, Deidchik EP, Lengfelder E, et al.: Detection of a novel type of RET rearrangement (PTC5) in thyroid carcinomas after Chernobyl and analysis of the involved RET-fused gene RFG5. Cancer Res 1998; 58:198.

257. Quadro L: Frequent RET protooncogene mutations in multiple endocrine neoplasia type 2a. J Clin Endocrinol Metab 1994; 79:590.

258. Hofstra RMW: A mutation of RET protooncogene associated with MEN2b and sporadic medullary carcinoma. Nature 1994; 367:375.

259. Tallini G, Santoro M, Helie M, et al.: Ret/PTC oncogene activation defines a subset of papillary carcinomas lacking evidence of progression to poorly differentiated or undifferentiated tumor phenotypes. Clin Cancer Res 1998; 4:287.

260. Challeton C, Bounacer A, Du Villard JA, et al.: Pattern of ras and gsp oncogene mutations in radiation-associated human thyroid tumors. Oncogene 1995; 11:601.

261. Karga H, Lee JK, Vickery Al Jr, et al.: Ras oncogene mutations in benign and malignant thyroid neoplasms. J Clin Endocrinol Metabol 1991; 73:832.

262. Ezzat S, Zheng L, Kolenda J, et al.: Prevalance of activating ras mutations in morphologically characterized thyroid nodules. Thyroid 1996; 6:409.

263. Russo D, Arturi F, Schlumberger M, et al.: Activating mutations of the TSH receptor in differentiated thyroid carcinomas. Oncogene 1995; 11:1907.

264. Soars P, Sambade C, Sobrinho-Simões M: Expression of C-erb B2 in tumours and tumour-like lesions of the thyroid. Inter J Cancer 1994; 56: 459.

265. Akslen LA, Varhaug JE: Oncoproteins and tumor progression in papillary thyroid carcinoma. Cancer 1995; 76:1543.

266. Haugen DR, Akslen LA, Varhaug JE, et al.: Expression of c-erbB-3 and c-erbB-4 proteins in papillary thyroid carcinomas. Cancer Res 1996; 56:1184.

267. Sugg SL, Ezzat S, Zheng L, et al.: Cytoplasmic staining of erbB-2 but not mRNA levels correlates with differentiation in human thyroid neoplasia. Clin Endocrinol 1998; 49:629.

268. Samman NA, Schultz PN, Hickey RC, et al.: The results of various modalities of treatment of well differentiated thyroid carcinoma: A retrospective review of 1599 patients. J Clin Endocrinol Metab 1992; 75:714.

269. Samel S, Kaufer C: Need for thyroidectomy in differentiated thyroid cancers. Langenbecks Arch Surg 1995; 380:260.

270. Schlumberger MJ: Papillary and follicular thyroid carcinoma. New Engl J Med 1998; 338:297.

271. Fujimoto Y, Sugitani I: Postoperative prognosis of intrathyroidal papillary thyroid carcinoma: Long term (35–45) follow-up study. Endocrin J 1998; 45:475.

272. Henry JF, Gramatica L, Denizot A, et al.: Morbidity of prophylactic lymph node dissection in the central neck area in patients with papillary thyroid carcinoma. Langenbecks Arch Surg 1998; 383:167.

273. LiVolsi VA: Unusual variants of papillary thyroid carcinoma. Adv Endocrinol Metab 1995; 6:39.

274. Lindsay S: Carcinoma of the thyroid gland: A clinical and pathological study of 293 patients at the University of California Hospital. Charles C Thomas, Springfield, IL, 1960.

275. Chen TKK, Rosai J: Follicular variant of thyroid papillary carcinoma: A clinicopathologic study of six cases. Am J Surg Pathol 1997; 1:123.

276. Baloch ZW, Gupta PK, Yu GH, et al.: Follicular variant of papillary carcinoma: Cytologic and histologic correlation. Am J Clin Pathol 1999; 111:216.

277. Albores-Saavedra J, Gould E, Vardaman C, et al.: The macrofollicular variant of papillary thyroid carcinoma: A study of 17 cases. Hum Pathol 1991; 22:1195.

278. Albores-Saavedra J, Housini I, Vuitch F, et al.: Macrofollicular variant of papillary thyroid carcinoma with minor insular component. Cancer 1997; 80:1110.

279. Hawk WA, Hazard JB: The many appearances of papillary carcinoma of the thyroid. Cleve Clin Q 1976; 43:207.

280. Flint A, Davenport RD, Llyod RV: The tall cell variant of papillary carcinoma of the thyroid gland. Arch Pathol Lab Med 1991; 115:196.

281. Ostrowski ML, Merino MJ: Tall cell variant of papillary thyroid carcinoma: A reassessment and immunohistochemical study with comparison to the usual type of papillary carcinoma of the thyroid. Am J Surg Pathol 1996; 20:964.

282. Ruter A, Nishiyama R, Lennquist S: Tall-cell variant of papillary thyroid cancer: Disregarded entity? World J Surg 1997; 21:15.

283. Ruter A, Dreifus J, Jones M, et al.: Overexpression of p53 in tall cell variants of papillary thyroid carcinoma. Surgery 1996; 120:1046.

284. Roque L, Clode AL, Gomes P, et al.: Cytogenetic findings in 31 papillary thyroid carcinomas. Genes Chromosomes Cancer 1995; 13:157.

285. Beckner M, Heffess CS, Oertel JE: Oxyphil papillary thyroid carcinomas. Am J Clin Pathol 1995; 103:280.

286. Sobrinho-SimoÃes MA, Nesland JM, Holm R: Hürthle cell and mitochondrion-rich papillary carcinoma of the thyroid gland. Ultrastruc Pathol 1985; 8:131.

287. Wu PS-C, Hay ID, Hermann MA, et al.: Papillary thyroid carcinoma (PTC), oxyphil cell type: A tumor misclassified by the world health organization (WHO). Clin Res 1991; 39:279.

288. Berho M, Suster S: The oncocytic variant of papillary carcinoma of the thyroid: A clinicopathologic study of 15 cases. Hum Pathol 1997; 28:47.

289. Berger N, Borda A, Bizollon MH: Thyroid papillary carcinoma and its variants. Arch Anat Cytol Pathol 1998; 46:45.

290. Hager J, Hofstader F: Familial occurrence of oncocytic carcinoma of the thyroid gland during pregnancy. Zentrum allgemein Pathol Pathol Anat 1979; 123:56.

291. Barbutto D, Carcangui ML, Rosai J: Papillary Hürthle cell neoplasms of the thyroid gland: A study of 20 cases. Lab Invest 1987; 56:5.

292. Apel RL, Asa SL, LiVolsi VA: Papillary Hürthle cell carcinoma with lymphocytic stroma: "Warthin-like tumor" of the thyroid. Am J Surg Pathol 1995; 19:810.

293. Fadda G, Mule A, Zannoni GF, et al.: Fine needle aspiration of a Warthin-like thyroid tumor: Report of a case with differential diagnostic criteria vs. other lymphocytic-rich thyroid lesions. Acta Cytol 1998; 42:998.

294. Vera-Sempere FJ, Prieto M, Camanas A: Warthin-like tumor of the thyroid: A papillary carcinoma with mitochondrion-rich cells and abundant lymphoid stroma: A case report. Pathol Res Pract 1998; 194:341.

295. Chan JK, Carcangui ML, Rosai J: Papillary carcinoma of thyroid with exuberant nodular fasciitis-like stroma: Report of three cases. Am J Clin Pathol 1991; 95:309.

296. Michael M, Chlumska A, Fakan F: Papillary carcinoma of thyroid with exuberant nodular fasciitis-like stroma. Histopathology 1992; 21:577.

297. Terayama K, Toda S, Yonemitsu N, et al.: Papillary carcinoma of the thyroid with exuberant nodular fasciitis-like stroma. Virchows Arch 1997; 431:291.

298. Hizawa K, Iida M, Yao T, et al.: Association between thyroid cancer of cribriform variant and familial adenomatous polyposis. J Clin Path 1996; 49:611.

299. Civitelli S, Tanzini G, Cetta F, et al.: Papillary thyroid carcinoma in three siblings with familial adenomatous polyposis. Int J Colorectal Dis 1996; 11:34.

300. Colletta G, Sciacchitano S, Palmirotta R, et al.: Analysis of adenomatous polyposis coli gene in thyroid tumours. Br J Cancer 1994; 70:1085.

301. Zeki K, Spambalg D, Sharifi N, et al.: Mutations of the adenomatous polyposis coli gene in sporadic thyroid neoplasms. J Clin Endocrinol Metab 1994; 79:1317.

302. Ono C, Iwama T, Mishima Y: A case of familial adenomatous polyposis complicated by thyroid carcinoma, carcinoma of the ampulla of vater and adrenocortical adenoma. Jpn J Surg 1991; 21:234.

303. Perrier ND, van Heerden JA, Goellner JR, et al.: Thyroid cancer in patients with familial adenomatous polyposis. World J Surg 1998; 22:738.

304. Bulow C, Bulow S: Is screening for thyroid carcinoma indicated in familial adenomatous polyposis? The Leeds Castle Polyposis Group. Int J Colorectal Dis 1997; 12:240.

305. Burgess JR, Duffield A, Wilkinson SJ, et al.: Two families with an autosomal dominant inheritance pattern for papillary carcinoma of the thyroid. J Clin Endocrinol Metab 1997; 82:345.

306. Cetta F, Toti P, Petracci M: Thyroid carcinoma associated with familial adenomatous polyposis. Histopathology 1997; 31:231.

307. van der Linde K, Vasen HF, van Vliet AC: Occurrence of thyroid carcinoma in Dutch patients with familial adenomatous polyposis: An epidemiological study and report of new cases. Eur J Gastroenterol Hepatol 1998; 10:777.

308. Soravia C, Sugg SL, Berk T, et al.: Familial adenomatous polyposis-associated thyroid cancer: A clinical, pathological, and molecular genetics study. Am J Clin Pathol 1999; 154:127.

309. Cetta F, Chiapetta G, Melillo RM, et al.: The ret/ptc1 oncogene is activated in familial adenomatous polyposis-associated thyroid papillary carcinomas. J Clin Endocrinol Metab 1998; 83:1003.

310. Evans HL: Columnar-cell carcinoma of the thyroid: A report of two cases of an aggressive variant of thyroid carcinoma. Am J Clin Pathol 1986; 85:77.

311. Sobrinho-Simões M, Nesland J, Johannessen J: Columnar-cell carcinoma: Another variant of poorly differentiated carcinoma of the thyroid. Am J Clin Pathol 1988; 89:264.

312. Ferreiro JA, Hay ID, Lloyd RV: Columnar-cell carcinoma of the thyroid: Report of three additional cases. Hum Pathol 1996; 27:1156.

313. Evans HL: Encapsulated columnar-cell neoplasm of the thyroid: A report of four cases suggesting a favorable prognosis. Am J Surg Pathol 1996; 20:1205.

314. Wenig BM, Thompson LDR, Adair CF, et al.: Thyroid papillary carcinoma of columnar cell type. Cancer 1998; 82:740.

315. Harach HR, Fransilla KO, Wasenius VM: Occult papillary carcinoma of the thyroid a "normal" finding in Finland: A systematic autopsy study. Cancer 1985; 56:531.

316. Lang W, Borrusch H, Bauer L: Occult carcinoma of the thyroid: Evaluation of 1,020 sequential autopsies. Am J Clin Pathol 1988; 90:72.

317. Hubert JP, Kiernan PD, Beahrs OH, et al.: Occult papillary carcinoma of the thyroid. Arch Surg 1980; 115:394.

318. Baudin E, Travagli JP, Ropers J, et al.: Microcarcinoma of the thyroid gland: The Gustave-Roussy Institute experience. Cancer 1998; 83:553.

319. Strate SM, Lee EL, Childers JH: Occult papillary carcinoma of the thyroid with distant metastases. Cancer 1984; 54:1093.

320. Rossi RL, Cady B, Silverman ML, et al.: Current results of conservative surgery for differentiated thyroid carcinoma. World J Surg 1986; 10:612.

321. Vickery AL, Wang CA, Walker AM: Treatment of intrathyroidal papillary carcinoma of the thyroid. Cancer 1987; 60:587.

322. Duffy BJ, Fitzgerald PJ: Cancer of the thyroid in children: A report of 28 cases. J Clin Endocrinol Metab 1950; 10:1296.

323. Clark DE: Association of irradiation with cancer of the thyroid in children and adolescents. JAMA 1955; 159:1007.

324. Hayles AB, Johnson LM, Beahrs OH, et al.: Carcinoma of the thyroid in children. Am J Surg 1963; 106:735.

325. Welch JW: Malignant disease of the thyroid in children. Int Surg 1966; 45:176.

326. Winship T, Rosvoll RV: Thyroid carcinoma in childhood: Final report on a 20 year study. Clin Proc Children's Hosp Washington DC. 1970; 26:327.

327. Kaplan MM, Garnick MB, Gelber R, et al.: Risk factors for thyroid abonormalities after neck irradiation for childhood cancer. Am J Med 1983; 74:272.

328. Harach HR, Willimas ED: Chidhood thyroid cancer in England and Wales. Br J Cancer 1995; 72:777.

329. Furmanchuk AW, Averkin JI, Egloff B, et al.: Pathomorphological findings in thyroid cancer of children from the Republic of Belarus: A study of 86 cases occurring between 1986 ("post-Chernobyl") and 1991. Histopathology 1992; 21:401.

330. Nikiforov Y, Gnepp DR: Pediatric thyroid cancer after the Chernobyl disaster: Pathomorphologic study of 84 cases (1991–1992) from the Republic of Belarus. Cancer 1994; 74:748.

331. Tronk MD, Bogdanova TI, Komissarenko IV, et al.: Thyroid carcinoma in children and adolescents in Ukraine after the Chernobyl nuclear accident: Statistical data and clinicomorphologic characteristics. Cancer 1999; 86:149.

332. Papotti M, Micca B, Favero A, et al.: Poorly differentiated thyroid carcinomas with primordial cell component: A group of aggressive lesions sharing insular, trabecular, and solid patterns. Am J Surg Pathol 1993; 17:291.

333. Pilloti S, Collini P, Manzari A, et al.: Poorly differentiated forms of papillary thyroid carcinoma: Distinctive entities or morphologic patterns? Semin Diagn Pathol 1995; 12:249.

334. Ashfaq R, Vuitch F, Delgado R, et al.: Papillary and follicular carcinomas with an insular component. Cancer 1994; 73:416.

335. Flynn SD, Forman BH, Stewart AF, et al.: Poorly differentiated (insular) thyroid carcinoma of the thyroid gland: An aggressive subset of differentiated thyroid neoplasms. Surgery 1988; 104:963.

336. Carcangui ML, Zampi G, Rosai J: Poorly differentiated (insular) thyroid carcinoma: A reinterpretation of Langhan's wuchernde struma. Am J Surg Pathol 1984; 8:655.

337. Chan JKC, Tsui MS, Tse CH: Diffuse sclerosing variant of papillary carcinoma of the thyroid: A histological and immunohistochemical study of three cases. Histopathology 1987; 11:191.

338. Carcangui ML, Bianchi S: Diffuse sclerosing variant of papillary thyroid carcinoma: Clinicopathologic study of 15 cases. Am J Surg Pathol 1989; 13:1041.

339. Macak J, Michal M: Diffuse sclerosing variant of papillary thyroid carcinoma. Ceskoslovenska Patologie 1993; 29:6.

340. Hayashi Y, Sasao T, Takeichi N, et al.: Diffuse sclerosing variant of papillary carcinoma of the thyroid: A histopathological study of four cases. Acta Pathol Jpn 1990; 40:193.

341. Gomez-Morales M, Alvaro T, Munoz M, et al.: Diffuse sclerosing papillary carcinoma of the thyroid: Immunohistochemical analysis of the local host response. Histopathology 1991; 18:427.

342. Schroder S, Bay V, Dumke K: Diffuse sclerosing variant of papillary thyroid carcinoma: S-100 protein immunohistochemistry and prognosis. Virchows Arch 1990; 416:447.

343. Fujimoto Y, Obara T, Ito Y, et al.: Diffuse sclerosing variant of papillary carcinoma of the thyroid: Clinical importance, surgical treatment, and follow-up study. Cancer 1990; 66:2306.

344. Kini SR, Miller JM, Hamburger JI, et al.: Cytopathology of the papillary carcinoma of the thyroid by fine needle aspiration. Acta Cytol 1980; 24:511.

345. Miller TR, Bottles K, Holly EA, et al.: A step-wise logistic regression analysis of papillary carcinoma of the thyroid. Acta Cytol 1986; 30: 285.

346. Leung C-S, Hartwick RWJ, Bedard YC: Correlation of cytologic and histologic features in variants of papillary carcinoma of the thyroid. Acta Cytol 1993; 37:645.

347. Tabbara SO, Acoury N, Sidaway MK: Multinucleate giant cells in thyroid neoplasms: A cytologic, histologic and immunohistochemical study. Acta Cytol 1996; 40:1184.

348. Goellner JR, Johnson DA: Cytology of cystic papillary carcinoma of the thyroid. Acta Cytol 1982; 26:797.

349. Francis IM, Das DK, Shiekh ZA, et al.: Role of intranuclear grooves in the diagnosis of papillary thyroid carcinoma: A quantitative assessment on fine needle aspiration smears. Acta Cytol 1995; 30:409.

350. Caraway NP, Sneige N, Samaan NA: Diagnostic pitfalls in thyroid fine-needle aspiration: A review of 394 cases. Diagn Cytopathol 1993; 9:345.

351. Fiorella RM, Isley W, Miller LK, et al.: Multinodular goiter of the thyroid mimicking malignancy: Diagnostic pitfalls in fine-needle aspiration biopsy. Diagn Cytopathol 1993; 9:351.

352. Hall TL, Layfield LJ, Philippe A, et al.: Sources of diagnostic error in fine needle aspiration of the thyroid. Cancer 1989; 63:718.

353. Hugh JC, Duggan MA, Chang-Poon V: The fine-needle aspiration appearance of the follicular variant of thyroid papillary carcinoma: A report of three cases. Diagn Cytopathol 1988; 4:196.

354. Harach HR, Zusman SB: Cytologic findings in the follicular variant of papillary carcinoma of the thyroid. Acta Cytol 1992; 36:142.

355. Gallagher J, Oertel YC, Oertel JE: Follicular variant of papillary carcinoma of the thyroid: Fine-needle aspirates with histologic correlation. Diagn Cytopathol 1997; 16:207.

356. Sidaway KS, Del Vecchio DM, Knoll SM: Fine-needle aspiration of thyroid nodules: Correlation between cytology and histology and evaluation of discrepant cases. Cancer 1997; 81:253.

357. Zacks JF, de Las MA, Beazley RM: Fine-needle aspiration cytology diagnosis of colloid nodule versus follicular variant of papillary carcinoma of the thyroid. Diagn Cytopathol 1998; 18:87.

358. Hirokawa M, Shimizu M, Terayama K, et al.: Macrofollicular variant of papillary thyroid carcinoma: Report of a case with fine needle aspiration biopsy findings. Acta Cytol 1998; 42:1441.

359. Abelatif OS, Peters SB, LiVolsi VA: Intraepithelial neutrophils: A portent of aggressive behavior in FNAs of papillary thyroid carcinoma. Endocr Pathol 1996; 6:123.

360. Armando GD, Fernando CG, Norma O, et al.: Tall cell variant of papillary thyroid carcinoma: A cytohistologic correlation. Acta Cytol 1997; 41:672.

361. Therese B, DiTomasso JP, Ramzy I, et al.: Tall cell variant of papillary thyroid carcinoma: Cytologic features and differential diagnostic considerations. Diagn Cytopathol 1997; 17:25.

362. Baloch Z, LiVolsi VA: Fine-needle aspiration cytology of papillary Hürthle carcinoma with lymphocytic stroma "Warthin-like tumor" of the thyroid. Endocr Pathol 1998; 9:287.

363. Fransilla KO, Ackerman LV, Brown CL, et al.: Follicular carcinoma. Semin Diagn Pathol 1985; 2:101.

364. Khan N, Perzin KH: Follicular carcinoma of the thyroid: An evaluation of the histologic criteria used in diagnosis. Pathol Anuu 1983; 18:221.

365. Williams ED: Pathology and natural history. In Duncan W, ed.: Thyroid Cancer. Springer-Verlag, Berlin, 1980, p. 47.

366. Brennan MD, Bergstrahl EJ, van Heerden JA, et al.: Follicular thyroid cancer treated at the Mayo Clinic, 1946 through 1970: Initial manifestations, pathologic findings, therapy and outcome. Mayo Clin Proc 1991; 66:11.

367. Johannessen JV, Sobrinho-Simões M: Well-differentiated thyroid tumors: Problems in diagnosis and understanding. Pathol Annu 1983; 18:255.

368. Yamashina M: Follicular neoplasms of the thyroid: Total circumferential evaluation of the fibrous capsule. Am J Surg Pathol 1992; 16:392.

369. Cady B, Sedgwick CE, Meissner WA, et al.: Changing clinical pathologic, therapeutic and survival patterns in differentiated thyroid carcinoma. Ann Surg 1976; 184:541.

370. LiVolsi VA, Asa SL: The demise of follicular carcinoma of the thyroid gland. Thyroid 1994; 4:233.

371. Cuello C, Correa P, Eisenberg H: Geographic pathology of thyroid carcinoma. Cancer 1969; 23:230.

372. Harach HR, Escalante DA, Onativia A, et al.: Thyroid carcinoma and thyroiditis in an endemic goiter before and after iodine prophylaxis. Acta Endocrinol (Copenh) 1985; 108:55.

373. Hofstadter F: Frequency and morphology of malignant tumours of the thyroid before and after the introduction of iodine prophylaxis. Virchows Arch 1980; 385:263.

374. Wahner HW, Cuello C, Correa P, et al.: Incidence of thyroid carcinoma in an endemic goiter area. Am J Med 1966; 40:58.

375. Fukunaga FH, Yatani R: Geographic pathology of occult thyroid carcinomas. Cancer 1975; 36: 1095.

376. Williams ED, Doniach I, Bjarnson O, et al.: Thyroid cancer in an iodine rich area. Cancer 1977; 39:215.

377. Lang W, Choritz H, Hundeshagen H: Risk factors in follicular thyroid carcinomas: A retrospective follow-up study covering a 14 year period with emphasis on morphological findings. Am J Surg Pathol 1986; 10:246.

378. Cady B, Rossi R, Silverman M, et al.: Further evidence of the validity of risk group definition in differentiated thyroid carcinoma. Surgery 1985; 98:1171.

379. Cady B, Sedgwick CE, Meissner WA, et al.: Risk factor analysis in differentiated thyroid cancer. Cancer 1979; 43:810.

380. Crile G, Pontius KI, Hawk WA: Factors influencing the survival of patients with follicular carcinoma of the thyroid gland. Surg Gynecol Obstet 1985; 160:409.

381. Shaha AR, Loree TR, Shah JP: Prognostic factors and risk group analysis in follicular carcinoma of the thyroid. Surgery 1995; 18:1131.

382. Buckwalter JA, Thomas CG: Selection of surgical treatment for well dedifferentiated thyroid carcinomas. Ann Surg 1972; 176:565.

383. Schmidt RJ, Wang CA: Encapsulated follicular carcinoma of the thyroid: Diagnosis, treatment and results. Surgery 1986; 100;1068.

384. Lida F: The fate and surgical significance of adenoma of the thyroid gland. Surg Gynecol Obstet 1974; 136:536.

385. Lang W, Georgii G: Minimal invasive cancer in the thyroid. Clin Oncol 1982; 1:527.

386. Lang W, Georgii G, Stauch G, et al.: The differentiation of atypical adenomas and encapsulated follicular carcinomas in the thyroid gland. Virchows Arch 1980; 385:25.

387. Hazard JB, Kenyon R: Encapsulated angioinvasive carcinoma (angioinvasive adenoma) of the thyroid gland. Am J Clin Pathol 1954; 24:755.

388. Silverberg SG, Hutter RVP, Foote FW: Fatal carcinoma of the thyroid: Histology, metastases and causes of death. Cancer 1970; 25:792.

389. Evans HL: Follicular neoplasms of the thyroid. Cancer 1984; 54:535.

390. Meissner WA: Follicular carcinoma of the thyroid: Frozen section diagnosis. Am J Surg Pathol 1977; 1:171.

391. Harach HR, Jasani B, Williams ED: Factor VIII as a maker of endothelial cells in follicular carcinoma of the thyroid. J Clin Pathol 1977; 36:1051.

392. Hruban RH, Huvos AG, Traganos F, et al.: Follicular neoplasms of the thyroid in men older than 50 years of age: A DNA flow cytometric study. Am J Clin Pathol 1990; 94:527.

393. Baxter ID: Advaces in molecular biology: Potential impact on diagnosis and treatment of disorders of the thyroid. Med Clin North Am 1991; 75:41.

394. Gagel RF: An overview of molecular abnormalities leading to thyroid carcinogenesis: A 1993 perspective. Stem Cells 1997; 15:7.

395. Grebe SK, McIver B, Hay ID, et al.: Frequent loss of heterozygosity on chromosomes 3p and 17p without VHL and p53 mutations suggests involvement of unidentified tumor suppressor genes in follicular thyroid carcinoma. J Clin Endocrinol Metab 1997; 82:3684.

396. Ward LS, Brenta G, Medvedovic M, et al.: Studies of allelic loss in thyroid tumors reveal major differences in chromosomal instability between papillary and follicular carcinomas. J Clin Endocrinol Metab 1998; 83:525.

397. Segev DL, Saji M, Phillips GS: Polymerase chain reaction–based microsatellite polymorphism analysis of follicular and Hürthle cell neoplasms of the thyroid. J Clin Endocrinol Metab 1998; 83:2036.

398. Lemoine NR, Mayall ES, Wyllie FS, et al.: Activated ras oncogenes in human thyroid cancers. Cancer Res 1988; 48:4459.

399. Gharib H, Goellner JR, Zinsmeister AR, et al.: Fine-needle aspiration biopsy of the thyroid: The problem of suspicious cytologic findings. Ann Intern Med 1984; 101:25.

400. Kini SR, Miller JM, Hambuerger JI, et al.: Cytopathology of follicular lesions of the thyroid gland. Diagn Cytopathol 1985; 1:123.

401. Ravinsky E, Safneck JR: Fine needle aspirates of follicular lesions of the thyroid gland: The intermediate-type smear. Acta Cytol 1990; 34:813.

402. Linzie BM, Lenel JC, Thomas PA, et al.: Fine needle aspiration (FNA) of follicular thyroid lesions: Logistic regression analysis to separate adenoma, carcinoma, and goiter. Modern Pathol 1995; 8:42.

403. Schlinkert RT, van Heerden JA, Goellner JR, et al.: Factors that predict malignant thyroid lesions when fine-needle aspiration is "suspicious for follicular neoplasm." Mayo Clin Proc 1997; 72:913.

404. Askanazy M: Pathologisch-anatomische beiträge zur kenntnis des morbus basedowii, insbesondere über die dabeiaufretende muskelekrankung. Dtsch Arch Klin Med 1898; 61:118.

405. Hürthle K: Beitrage zur kenntnis des sekretionsvorgänges in der Schilddruse. Arch Physiol 1894; 56:1.

406. Heimann P, Ljunggren JG, Lowhagen T, et al.: Oxyphilic adenoma of the human thyroid: A morphological and biochemical study. Cancer 1973; 31:246.

407. Tremblay G: Histochemical study of cytochrome oxidase and adenosine triphosphatase in Askanazy cell (Hürthle cells) of the human thyroid. Lab Invest 1962; 11;514.

408. Tremblay G, Pearse AGE: Histochemistry of oxidative enzyme systems in the human thyroid with special reference to Askanazy cells. J Pathol Bacteriol 1960; 80:353.

409. Carcangui ML, Bianchi S, Savino D, et al.: Follicular Hürthle cell tumors of the thyroid gland. Cancer 1991; 68:1944.

410. Grant CS, Barr D, Goellner JR, et al.: Benign Hürthle cell tumors of the thyroid: A diagnosis to be trusted? World J Surg 1988; 12:488.

411. González-Cámporá R, Herrero-Zapatero A, et al.: Hürthle cell and mitochondrion-rich cell tumors. Cancer 1986; 57:1154.

412. Har-El G, Hadar T, Segal K, et al.: Hürthle cell carcinoma of the thyroid gland: A tumor of moderate malignancy. Cancer 1986; 57:1613.

413. Heppe H, Armin A, Calandra DB, et al.: Hürthle cell tumors of the thyroid gland. Surgery 1985; 98:1162.

414. Papotti M, Torchio B, Grassi L, et al.: Poorly differentiated oxyphilic (Hürthle cell) carcinoma of the thyroid. Am J Surg Pathol 1996; 20:686.

415. Rosen IB, Luk S, Katz I.: Hürthle cell tumor behavior: Dilemma and resolution. Surgery 1985; 98:777.

416. Thompson NW, Dunn EL, Batsakis JG, et al.: Hürthle cell lesions of the thyroid gland. Surg Gynecol Obstet 1974; 139:555.

417. Tollefsen HR, Shah JP, Huvos AG: Hürthle cell carcinoma of the thyroid. Am J Surg 1975; 130:390.

418. Bronner MP: Hürthle cell lesions of the thyroid. Path Case Rev 1997; 2:200.

419. Caplan RH, Abellera RM, Kisken WA: Hürthle cell tumors of the thyroid gland. JAMA 1985; 251:3114.

420. Gosain AK, Clark OH: Hürthle cell neoplasms. Arch Surg 1984; 119:151.

421. Gundry SR, Burney RE, Thompson NW, et al.: Total thyroidectomy for Hürthle cell neoplasm of the thyroid. Arch Surg 1983; 118:529.

422. LiVolsi VA, Merino MJ: Worrisome histologic alterations following fine-needle aspiration of the thyroid (WHAFFT). Pathol Annu 1994; 29:99.

423. Layfield LJ, Lones MA: Necrosis in thyroid nodules after fine-needle aspiration biopsy. Acta Cytol 1991; 35:427.

424. Jayram G, Aggarwal S: Infarction of thyroid nodule: A rare complication following fine needle aspiration. Acta Cytol 1989; 33:940.

425. Baloch ZW, LiVolsi VA: Post-FNA histologic alteration of thyroid: Revisited. Am J Clin Pathol 1999; 112:311.

426. Tallini G, Carcangui ML, Rosai J: Oncocytic neoplasms of the thyroid gland. Acta Pathol Jpn 1992; 42:305.

427. Johnson TL, Llyod RV, Burney RE, et al.: Hürthle cell thyroid tumors: An immunohistochemical study. Cancer 1987; 59:107.

428. McIvor NP, Freeman JL, Rosen I, et al.: Value of fine-needle aspiration in the diagnosis of Hürthle cell neoplasms. Head Neck 1993; 15:335.

429. Pambuccian SE, Becker RL Jr, Ali SZ, et al.: Differential diagnosis of Hürthle cell neoplasms on fine-needle aspirates: Can we do better with morphometry? Acta Cytol 1997; 41:197.

430. Grant CS, Hay ID, Ryan JJ, et al.: Diagnostic and prognostic utility of flow cytometric DNA measurements in follicular thyroid tumors. World J Surg 1990; 14:283.

431. Bronner MP, Clevenger CV, Edmonds PR, et al.: Flow cytometric analysis of DNA content in Hürthle cell adenomas and carcinomas of the thyroid. Am J Clin Pathol 1988; 89:764.

432. Zedenius J, Wallin G, Svensson A, et al.: Allelotyping of follicular thyroid tumors. Hum Genet 1995; 96:27.
433. Segev DL, Saji M, Phillips GS, et al.: Polymerase chain reaction–based microsatellite polymorphism analysis of follicular and Hürthle cell neoplasms of the thyroid. J Clin Endocrinol Metab 1998; 83:2036.
434. Masood S, Auguste LJ, Westerband A, et al.: Differential oncogenic expression in thyroid follicular and Hürthle cell carcinomas. Am J Surg 1993; 166:366.
435. Bouras M, Bertholon J, Dutrieux-Berger N, et al.: Variability of Ha-ras (codon 12) proto-oncogene mutations in diverse thyroid cancers. Eur J Endocrinol 1998; 139:209.
436. Sakamoto A: Poorly differentiated carcinoma of the thyroid: An aggressive type of tumor arising from thyroid follicular epithelium. Curr Topics Pathol 1997; 91:49.
437. Ohori NP, Schoedel KE: Cytopathology of high-grade papillary thyroid carcinomas: Tall-cell variant, diffuse sclerosing variant and poorly differentiated papillary carcinoma. Diagn Cytopathol 1999; 20:19.
438. Rodriguez JM, Parilla P, Moreno A, et al.: Insular carcinoma: An infrequent subtype of thyroid cancer. J Am Coll Surg 1998; 187:503.
439. Nishida T, Katayama S, Tsujimoto M, et al.: Clinicopathological significance of poorly differentiated thyroid carcinoma. Am J Surg Pathol 1999; 23:205.
440. Langhans T: Über die epithelialen formen der malignen struma. Virchows Arch Pathol Anat 1907; 189:69.
441. Pearse AGE, Polak JM: Cytochemical evidence for the neural crest origin of mammalian ultimobranchial C-cells. Histochemie 1976; 27:96.
442. Weston JA: The regulation of normal and abnormal neural crest cell development. Adv Neurol 1981; 29:77.
443. Godwin MC: Complex IV in the dog with special emphasis on the relation of the ultimobranchial body to the interfollicular cells in the postnatal glands. Am J Anat 1937; 60:299.
444. Ito M, Kameda Y, Tagawa T: An ultrastructural study of the cysts in chicken ultimobranchial glands, with special reference to C-cells. Cell Tissue Res 1986; 246:39.
445. Roediger WEW: The oxyphil and C-cells of the human thyroid gland. Cancer 1975; 36:688.
446. Wolfe HJ, DeLellis RA, Voelkel EF, et al.: Distribution of calcitonin-containing cells in the normal neonatal human thyroid gland: A correlation of morphology with peptide content. J Clin Endocrinol Metab 1975; 41:1076.
447. Wolfe HJ, Voelkel EF, Tashjian AH: Distribution of calcitonin-containing cells in the normal adult human thyroid gland: A correlation of morphology and peptide content. J Clin Endocrinol Metab 1974; 38:688.
448. McMillian PJ, Hooker WM, Deftos LJ: Distribution of calcitonin-containing cells in the human thyroid. Am J Anat 1974; 140:73.
449. Pearse AGE: Common cytochemical and ultrastructural characteristics of cells producing polypeptide hormones (the APUD series) and their relevance to thyroid and ultimobranchial C-cells and calcitonin. Proc R Soc Lond [Biol] 1968; 170:71.
450. Gibson WCH, Peng TC, Croker BP: C-cell nodules in adult human thyroid: A common autopsy finding. Am J Clin Pathol 1980; 73:347.
451. DeLellis RA, Wolfe HJ: Pathobiology of the human calcitonin (C) cell: A review. Pathol Annu 1981; 16:25.
452. Nunez EA, Gershon MD: Thyrotropin-induced thyroidal release of 5-hydroxytryptamine and accompanying ultrastructural changes in parafollicular cells. Mol Endocrinol 1989; 3:2101.
453. O'Toole K, Fenoglio-Preiser C, Pushparaj N: Endocrine changes associated with the human aging process III: Effect of age on the number of calcitonin immunoreactive cells in the thyroid gland. Hum Pathol 1985; 16:991.
454. Sunday ME, Wolfe HJ, Ross BA, et al.: Gastrin-releasing peptide gene expression in developing hyperplastic and neoplastic thyroid C-cells. Endocrinology 1988; 122:51.
455. Zajac JD, Penshchow J, Mason T, et al.: Identification of calcitonin and calcitonin gene–related peptide messenger ribonucleic acid in medullary thyroid carcinomas by hybridization histochemistry. J Clin Endocrinol Metab 1986; 62:1037.
456. Williams ED: Histogenesis of medullary carcinoma of the thyroid. J Clin Pathol 1966; 19:114.
457. Fletcher JR: Medullary (solid) carcinoma of the thyroid gland. Arch Surg 1970; 100:257.
458. Dunn EL, Nishiyama RH, Thompson NW: Medullary carcinoma of the thyroid gland. Surgery 1973; 73:848.
459. Corvin TR: Medullary carcinoma of the thyroid. Surg Gynecol Obstet 1974; 138:453.
460. Hill CS, Ibanez ML, Samaan NA, et al.: Medullary (solid) carcinoma of the thyroid gland: An analysis of the MD Anderson Hospital experience with patients with tumor, its special features and its histogenesis. Medicine (Baltimore) 1973; 52:141.
461. Freeman D: Medullary carcinoma of the thyroid gland: A clinicopathological study of 33 patients. Arch Pathol Lab Med 1965; 80:575.
462. Gonzalez-Licea A, Hartman WH, Yardley JH: Medullary carcinoma of the thyroid gland. Am J Clin Pathol 1968; 49:512.
463. Gordon PR, Huvos AG, Strong EW: Medullary carcinoma of the thyroid gland. Am J Clin Pathol 1968; 49:512.
464. Ibanez ML, Cole VW, Russell WO, et al.: Solid carcinoma of the thyroid gland: Analysis of 53 cases. Cancer 1967; 20:706.
465. Keynes WM, Till AS: Medullary carcinoma of the thyroid. Q J Med 1971; 159:443.
466. Sizemore GW: Medullary carcinoma of the thyroid gland. Semin Oncol 1987; 54:89.
467. Tashjian AH, Melvin KEW: Medullary carcinoma of the thyroid gland. N Engl J Med 1968; 279:279.
468. Hillyard CJ, Evans IMA, Hill PA, et al.: Familial medullary thyroid carcinoma. Lancet 1978; 1:915.
469. Williams ED: A review of 17 cases of carcinoma of the thyroid and pheochromocytoma. J Clin Pathol 1965; 18:288.
470. Sipple JH: The association of pheochromocytoma with carcinoma of the thyroid gland. Am J Med 1961; 31:163.
471. Bigner SH, Cox EB, Mendelsohn G, et al.: Medullary carcinoma of the thyroid in the multiple endocrine neoplasia IIA syndrome: Am J Surg Pathol 1981; 5:459.
472. Catalona WJ, Engelman K, Ketcham AS, et al.: Familial medullary thyroid carcinoma, pheochromocytoma and parathyroid adenoma (Sipple's syndrome). Cancer 1971; 28:1245.
473. Cushman P: Familial endocrine tumors. Am J Med 1962; 32:352.
474. Huang SN, McLeish WA: Pheochromocytoma and medullary carcinoma of the thyroid. Cancer 1968; 21:302.
475. Ljungberg O, Cederquist E, Von Studnitz E: Medullary thyroid carcinoma and pheochromocytomas: A familial chromaffinosis. Br Med J 1967; 1:279.
476. Manning PC, Molnar GD, Black BM, et al.: Pheochromocytoma, hyperparathyroidism and thyroid carcinoma occurring coincidentally. N Engl J Med 1963; 268:68.
477. Melvin KEW, Tashjian AH, Miller HH: Studies in familial medullary thyroid carcinoma. Recent Prog Horm Res 1972; 28:399.
478. Sarosi G, Doe RP: Familial occurrence of parathyroid adenomas, pheochromocytoma, and medullary carcinoma of the thyroid with amyloid stroma (Sipple's syndrome). Ann Intern Med 1968; 68:1305.
479. Schimke RN: Multiple endocrine adenomatosis syndromes. Adv Intern Med 1976; 21:249.
480. Schimke RN, Hartman WH: Familial amyloid producing medullary thyroid carcinoma and pheochromocytoma: A distinct genetic entity. Ann Intern Med 1965; 63:1027.
481. Schimke RN, Hartman WH, Prout TE, et al.: Syndrome of bilateral pheochromocytoma, medullary thyroid carcinoma and multiple neuromas. N Engl J Med 1979; 279:1.
482. Baylin SB, Hsu SH, Gann DS, et al: Inherited medullary thyroid carcinoma: A final monoclonal mutation in one of multiple clones of susceptible cells. Science 1978; 199:429.
483. Bartlett RD, Myall RWT, Bean LR, et al.: A neuroendocrine syndrome: Mucosal neuromas, pheochromocytoma and medullary thyroid carcinoma. Oral Surg Oral Med Oral Pathol 1971; 31:206.
484. Block MA, Horn RC, Miller JM, et al.: Familial medullary carcinoma of the thyroid. Ann Surg 1967; 166:403.
485. Brown RS, Colle E, Tashjian AH: The syndrome of multiple mucosal neuromas and medullary thyroid carcinoma in childhood. J Pediatr 1975; 86:77.

486. Cunliffe WJ, Judgson P, Fulthorpe JJ, et al.: A calcitonin-secreting medullary thyroid carcinoma associated with mucosal neuromas, marfanoid features, myopathy, and pigmentation. Am J Med 1970; 48:120.

487. Fassina AS, Scapinello A, Pelizzo MR, et al.: Medullary thyroid carcinoma in multiple endocrine neoplasia type II syndromes. Tumori 1985; 71:397.

488. Steiner AL, Goodman AD, Powers SR: Study of a kindred with pheochromocytoma, medullary thyroid carcinoma, hyperparathyroidism and Cushing's disease: Multiple endocrine neoplasia type 2. Medicine (Baltimore) 1968; 47:371.

489. Jansson S, Hansson G, Salander H, et al.: Prevalence of C-cell hyperplasia and medullary thyroid carcinoma in a consecutive series of pheochromocytoma patients. World J Surg 1984; 8:493.

490. Ram MD, Rao, KN, Brown L: Hypercalcitoninemia, pheochromocytoma and C-cell hyperplasia: A new variant of Sipple's syndrome. JAMA 1978; 239:2155.

491. Laskowski J: Carcinoma hyalinicum thyroideae. Nowotory 1957; 7:23.

492. Horn RC: Carcinoma of the thyroid: Description of a distinctive morphological variant and report of seven cases. Cancer 1951; 4:697.

493. Hazard JB, Hawk WA, Crile G: Medullary (solid) carcinoma of the thyroid: A clinicopathologic entity. J Clin Endocrinol Metab 1959; 19:152.

494. Block MA, Jackson CE, Greenawald KA, et al.: Clinical characteristic distinguishing hereditary from sporadic medullary thyroid carcinoma: Treatment implications. Arch Surg 1980; 115:142.

495. Khairi MRS, Dexter RN, Burzynski NJ, et al.: Mucosal neuroma, pheochromocytoma and medullary thyroid carcinoma: Multiple endocrine neoplasia type 3. Medicine (Baltimore) 1975; 54:89.

496. Carney JA, Hales AB: Alimentary tract manifestations of multiple endocrine neoplasia, type 2b. Mayo Clin Proc 1977; 52:543.

497. Deschryver-Keckemeti K, Clouse RE, Goldstein MN, et al.: Intestinal ganglioneuromatosis: A manifestation of overproduction of nerve growth factor? N Engl J Med 1983; 308:635.

498. Carney JA, Hales AB, Pearse AGE, et al.: Abnormal cutaneous innervation in multiple endocrine neoplasia, type 2b. Ann Intern Med 1981; 94:262.

499. Carney JA, Sizemore GW, Hales AB: Multiple endocrine neoplasia, type 2b. Pathobiol Annu 1978; 8:105.

500. Carney JA, Sizemore GW, Sheps SG: Adrenal medullary disease in multiple endocrine neoplasia, type 2. Am J Clin Pathol 1976; 66:279.

501. Carney JA, Sizemore GW, Tyce GM: Bilateral adrenal medullary hyperplasia in multiple endocrine neoplasia, type 2: The precursor of bilateral pheochromocytoma. Mayo Clin Proc 1975; 50:3.

502. Carney JA, Roth SI, Heath H, et al.: The parathyroid glands in multiple endocrine neoplasia, type 2b. Am J Pathol 1980; 99:387.

503. Norton JA, Froome BA, Farrell RE, et al.: Multiple endocrine neoplasia tye IIb: The most aggressive form of medullary thyroid carcinoma. Surg Clin North Am 1979; 59:109.

504. Mathew CGP, Chin KS, Easton DF, et al.: A linked genetic marker for multiple endocrine neoplasia type 2A on chromosome 10. Nature 1987; 328:527.

505. Simpson NE, Kidd KK, Goodfellow PJ, et al.: Assignment of multiple endocrine neoplasia type 2A to chromosome 10 by linkage. Nature 1987; 328:528.

506. Eng C: The Ret proto-oncogene in multiple endocrine neoplasia type 2 and Hirschsprung's disease. New Engl J Med 1996; 335:943.

507. Eng C, Smith DP, Mulligan LM, et al.: Point mutation within the tyrosine kinase domain of the RET proto-oncogene in multiple endocrine neoplasia type 2B and related sporadic tumors. Hum Mol Genet 1994; 3:237.

508. Carlson KM, Dou S, Chi D, et al.: A single missense mutation in the tyrosine kinase catalytic domain of the RET protooncogene is associated with multiple endocrine neoplasia type 2B. Proc Natl Acad Sci U S A 1994; 91:1579.

509. Eng C, Smith DP, Mulligan LM, et al.: A novel point mutation in the thyrosine kinase domain of the RET proto-oncogene in sporadic medullary thyroid carcinoma and in the family with FMTC. Oncogene 1995; 10:509.

510. Bolino A, Schuffenecker I, Luo Y, et al.: RET mutaions in exons 13 and 14 of FMTC patients. Oncogene 1995; 10:2415.

511. Chiefari E, Russo D, Giuffrida D, et al.: Analysis of RET proto-oncogene abnormalities in patients with MEN-2A, MEN 2B, familial or sporadic medullary thyroid carcinoma. J Endocrinol Invest 1998; 21:358.

512. Lips CJM, Lansvater RM, Hoppener JWM, et al.: Clinical screening as compared with DNA analysis in families with multiple endocrine neoplasia type 2A. N Engl J Med 1994; 331:828.

513. Wells SA Jr, Chi DD, Toshima K, et al.: Predictive DNA testing and prophylactic thyroidectomy in patients at risk for multiple endocrine neoplasia type 2A. Ann Surg 1994; 220:237.

514. Zedenius J, Larsson C, Bergholm U, et al.: Mutations of codon 918 in the RET proto-oncogene correlate to the poor prognosis in sporadic medullary thyroid carcinomas. J Clin Endocrinol Metab 1995; 80:3088.

515. Eng C, Mulligan LM, Healy CS, et al.: Heterogenous mutation of the RET proto-oncogene in subpopulations of medullary thyroid carcinoma. Cancer Res 1996; 56:2167.

516. Huang CN, Wu SL, Chang TC, et al.: RET protooncogene mutations in patients with apparently sporadic medullary thyroid carcinoma. J Formosan Med Assoc 1998; 97:541.

517. Shan L, Nakamura M, Nakamura Y, et al.: Somatic mutations in the RET protooncogene in Japanese and Chinese sporadic medullary thyroid carcinomas. Jpn J Cancer Res 1998; 89:883.

518. Kakudo K, Miyauchi A, Ogihara T, et al.: Medullary carcinoma of the thyroid with ectopic ACTH syndrome. Acta Pathol Jpn 1982; 32:793.

519. Szijj I, Csapo Z, Laslo FA, et al.: Medullary cancer of the thyroid gland associated with hypercorticism. Cancer 1969; 4:167.

520. Williams ED, Karim SMM, Sandler M: Prostaglandin secretion by medullary carcinoma of the thyroid: A possible cause of the associated diarrhea. Lancet 1968; 1:22.

521. Williams ED, Morales AM, Horn RC: Thyroid carcinoma and Cushing's syndrome. J Clin Pathol 1968; 21:129.

522. Saad MF, Ordonez NG, Rashid RK, et al.: Medullary carcinoma of the thyroid: A study of the clinical features and prognostic factors in 161 patients. Medicine (Baltimore) 1984; 63:319.

523. Sambade C, Baldaque-Faria A, Cardoso-Oliveira M, et al.: Follicular and papillary variants of medullary carcinoma of the thyroid. Pathol Res Pract 1984; 98:184.

524. Kakudo K, Miyauchi A, Ogihara T, et al.: Medullary carcinoma of the thyroid: Giant cell type. Arch Pathol Lab Med 1978; 102:445.

525. Mendelsohn G, Baylin SB, Bigner SH, et al.: Anaplastic variants of medullary thyroid carcinoma: A light microscopic and immunohistochemical study. Am J Surg Pathol 1980; 4:333.

526. Martinelli G, Bazzocchi F, Govoni E, et al.: Anaplastic type of medullary thyroid carcinoma: An ultrastructural and immunohistochemical study. Virchows Arch 1983; 400:61.

527. Landon G, Ordonez NG: Clear cell variant of medullary carcinoma of the thyroid. Hum Pathol 1985; 16:844.

528. Zaatari GS, Saigo PE, Huvos AG: Mucin production in medullary carcinoma of the thyroid. Arch Pathol Lab Med 1983; 107:70.

529. Marcus JN, Dise CA, LiVolsi VA: Melanin production in a medullary thyroid carcinoma. Cancer 1982; 49:2518.

530. Dominguez-Malagon H, Delgado-Chavez R, Torres-Najera M, et al.: Oxyphil and squamous variants of medullary thyroid carcinoma. Cancer 1989; 63:1183.

531. Bergholm V, Adami H-O, Auer G, et al.: Histopathologic characterists and nuclear DNA content as prognostic factors in medullary thyroid carcinoma. Cancer 1989; 64:135.

532. Schroder S, Bocker W, Baisch H, et al.: Prognostic factors in medullary thyroid carcinoma: Survival in relation to age, sex, stage, histology, immunocytochemistry, and DNA content. Cancer 1988; 61:806.

533. DeLellis RA, Rule AH, Spiler F, et al.: Calcitonin and carcinoembryonic antigen as tumor markers in medullary thyroid carcinoma. Am J Clin Pathol 1978; 70:587.

534. Holm R, Sobrinho-SimoÃes M, Nesland JM, et al.: Medullary carcinoma of the thyroid gland: An immunocytochemical study. Ultrastruct Pathol 1985; 8:25.

535. Sikri KL, Varndell IM, Hamid QA, et al.: Medullary carcinoma of the thyroid: An immunocytochemical and histochemical study of 25 cases using eight separate markers. Cancer 1985; 56:2481.

536. Geddie BT, Bedard YC, Strawbridge HT: Medullary carcinoma of the thyroid in fine-needle aspiration biopsies. Am J Clin Pathol 1984; 82:552.

537. Kini SR, Miller JM, Hambuerger JI, et al.: Cytopathologic features of medullary carcinoma of the thyroid. Arch Pathol Lab Med 1984; 108:156.

538. Forrest CH, Frost FA, de Boer WB, et al.: Medullary carcinoma of the thyroid: Accuracy of diagnosis of fine-needle aspiration cytology. Cancer 1998; 84:295.

539. Henry JF, Denizot A, Puccini M, et al.: Latent subclinical medullary thyroid carcinoma: Diagnosis and treatment. World J Surg 1998; 22:752.

540. Halliday BE, Silverman JF, Finley JL: Fine-needle aspiration cytology of amyloid associated with nonneoplastic and malignant lesions. Diagn Cytopathol 1998; 18:270.

541. Collins BT, Cramer HM, Tabatowski K, et al.: Fine needle aspiration of medullary carcinoma of the thyroid: Cytomorphology, immunocytochemistry and electron microscopy. Acta Cytol 1995; 39:920.

542. Bose S, Kapila K, Verma K: Medullary carcinoma of the thyroid: A cytological, immunocytochemical, and ultrastructural study. Diagn Cytopathol 1992; 8:28.

543. Perry A, Molberg K, Albores-Saavedra J: Physiologic versus neoplastic C-cell hyperplasia of the thyroid: Separation of distinct histologic and biologic entities. Cancer 1996; 77:750.

544. LiVolsi VA, Feind CR, LoGerfo P, et al.: Demonstration by immunoperoxidase staining of hyperplasia of parafollicular cells in the thyroid gland in hyperparathyroidism. J Clin Endocrinol Metab 1973; 37:550.

545. Guyetant S, Wion-Barbot N, Rousselet MC, et al.: C-cell hyperplasia associated with chronic lymphocytic thyroiditis: A retrospective quantitiative study of 112 cases. Hum Pathol 1994; 25:514.

546. Albores-Saavedra J, Monforte H, Nadji M, et al.: C-cell hyperplasia in thyroid tissue adjacent to follicular cell tumors. Hum Pathol 1988; 19:795.

547. Chan JKC, Tse CH: Solid cell nest–associated C-cells: Another possibile explanation for C-cell hyperplasia adjacent to follicular cell tumors. Hum Pathol 1989; 20:498.

548. Komminoth P, Roth J, Saremasiani P, et al.: Polysialic acid of the neural cell adhesion molecule in the human thyroid: A marker for medullary carcinoma and primary C-cell hyperplasia: An immunohistochemical study on 79 thyroid lesions. Am J Surg Pathol 1994; 18:399.

549. Pfaltz M, Hedinger CE, Muhlethaler JP: Mixed medullary and follicular carcinoma of the thyroid. Virchows Arch 1983; 400:53.

550. Hales M, Rosenau W, Okerlund MD, et al.: Carcinoma of the thyroid with a mixed medullary and follicular pattern: Morphological, immunohistochemical, and clinical laboratory studies. Cancer 1982; 50:1352.

551. Holm R, Sobrinho-SimoÃes M, Nesland JM, et al.: Concurrent production of calcitonin and thyroglobulin by the same neoplastic cells. Ultrastruct Pathol 1986; 10:241.

552. Albores-Saavedra J, de la Mora TG, de la Torre-Rendon F, et al.: Mixed medullary papillary carcinoma of the thyroid: A previously unrecognized variant of thyroid carcinoma. Hum Pathol 1990; 21:1151.

553. Sobrinho-SimoÃes M: Mixed medullary and follicular carcinoma of the thyroid. Histopathology 1993; 23:287.

554. Ogawa H, Kino I, Arai T: Mixed medullary-follicular carcinoma of the thyroid: Immunohistochemical and electron microscopic studies. Acta Pathol Jpn 1989; 39:67.

555. LiVolsi VA: Mixed carcinoma: A real entity? Lab Invest 1987; 57:237.

556. Apel RL, Alpert LC, Rizzo A, et al.: A metastasizing composite carcinoma of the thyroid with distinct medullary and papillary components. Arch Pathol Lab Med 1994; 118:1143.

557. Ermulovich I: Chemodectoma of the thyroid gland simulating nodular goiter. Probl Endokrinol (Mosk) 1968; 14:53.

558. Haegert DG, Wang MS, Farrer PA, et al.: Non-chromaffin paraganliomatosis manifesting as a cold thyroid nodule. Am J Clin Pathol 1974; 6:561.

559. Isaicev BA, Chraibman MM: Chemodectoma simulating a tumor of the thyroid gland. Klin Khir 1970; 5:45.

560. Mitsudo SM, Grajower MM, Balbi H, et al.: Malignant paraganglioma of the thyroid gland. Arch Pathol Lab Med 1987; 1111:378.

561. Brownlee RE, Shockley WW: Thyroid paraganglioma. Ann Otol Rhinol Laryngol 1992; 101:293.

562. de Vries E, Watson CG: Paraganglioma of the thyroid. Head Neck 1989; 11:462.

563. Lack EE, Cubilla AL, Woodruff JM: Paraganglioma of the head and neck region: A pathologic study of tumors from 71 patients. Cancer 1979; 10:191.

564. LaGuette J, Matias-Guiu X, Rosai J: Thyroid paraganglioma: A clinicopathologic and immunohistochemical study of three cases. Am J Surg Pathol 1997; 21:748.

565. Wychulis AR, Beahrs OH, Woolner LB: Papillary carcinoma with associated anaplastic carcinoma in the thyroid gland. Surg Gynecol Obstet 1965; 120:28.

566. Kapps DS, LiVolsi VA, Sanders MM: Anaplastic carcinoma following well-differentiated thyroid cancer: Etiologic considerations. Yale J Biol Med 1982; 55:521.

567. Aldinger KA, Samaan NA, Ibanez M, et al.: Anaplastic carcinoma of the thyroid: A review of 84 cases of spindle cell and giant cell carcinoma of the thyroid. Cancer 1978; 41:2267.

568. Nel CJC, van Heerden JA, Goellner JR: Anaplastic carcinoma of the thyroid: A clinicopathologic study of 82 cases. Mayo Clin Proc 1985; 60:51.

569. LiVolsi VA, Brooks JJ, Arendash-Durand B: Anaplastic thyroid tumors: Immunohistochemistry. Am J Clin Pathol 1987; 87:434.

570. Venkatesh YS, Ordonez NG, Schultz PN, et al: Anaplastic carcinoma of the thyroid: A clinicopathologic study of 121 cases. Cancer 1990; 66:321.

571. Rosai J, Saxen EA, Woolner L: Undifferentiated and poorly differentiated carcinoma. Semin Diagn Pathol 1985; 2:123.

572. Spires JR, Schwartz MR, Miller RH: Anaplastic thyroid carcinoma: Association with differentiated thyroid cancer. Arch Otolaryngol Head Neck Surg 1988; 114:40.

573. Wan S-K, Chan JKC, Tang S-K: Paucicellular variant of anaplastic thyroid carcinoma: A mimic of Reidel's thyroiditis. Am J Clin Pathol 1996; 105:388.

574. Chan JKC, Tsang WYW: Endocrine malignancies that may mimic benign lesions. Semin Diagn Pathol 1995; 12:45.

575. Schneider V, Frable WJ: Spindle and giant cell carcinoma of the thyroid: Cytologic diagnosis by fine needle aspiration. Acta Cytol 1980; 24:184.

576. Lee JS, Lee MC, Park CS, et al: Fine needle aspiration cytology of anaplastic carcinoma with osteoclast-like giant cells of the thyroid: A case report. Acta Cytol 1996; 40:1309.

577. Us-Krasovec M, Golouh R, Auersperg M, et al.: Anaplastic thyroid carcinoma in fine needle aspirates. Acta Cytol 1996; 40:953.

578. Burt AD, Kerr DJ, Brown IL, et al.: Lymphoid and epithelial markers in small cell anaplastic thyroid tumors. J Clin Pathol 1985; 38:893.

579. Hang TY, Assor D: Primary squamous cell carcinoma of the thyroid gland: A report of four cases. Am J Clin Pathol 1971; 55:93.

580. Kampsen EB, Jager N, Max MH: Squamous cell carcinoma of the thyroid: A report of two cases. J Surg Oncol 1977; 9:567.

581. Saito K, Tomotsune Y, Yamamoto K, et al.: A case of primary squamous cell carcinoma of the thyroid associated with marked neutrophilia and hypercalcemia. J Jpn Soc Int Med 1979; 68:1466.

582. Harada T, Shimaoka K, Yakumaru K, et al.: Squamous cell carcinoma of the thyroid gland: Transition from adenocarcinoma. J Surg Oncol 1982; 19:36.

583. Segal K, Sidi J, Abraham A, et al.: Pure squamous cell carcinoma and mixed adenosquamous cell carcinoma of the thyroid gland. Head Neck Surg 1984; 6:1035.

584. Riddle PE, Dincsoy HP: Primary squamous cell carcinoma of the thyroid associated with leucocytosis and hypercalcemia. Arch Pathol Lab Med 1987; 111:373.

585. Simpson WJ, Carruthers J: Squamous cell carcinoma of the thyroid gland. Am J Surg 1988; 156:44.

586. Chaudhary RK, Barnes EL, Myers EN: Squamous cell carcinoma arising in Hashimoto's thyroiditis. Head Neck 1994; 16:582.

587. Matsuura M, Kawashima M, Tateno K, et al.: Three cases of thyroid cancer, including a component of squamous cell carcinoma. Jpn J Cancer Clin 1989; 35:1043.

588. Katoh R, Sakamoto A, Kasai N, et al.: Squamous differentiation in thyroid carcinoma: With special reference to histogenesis of squamous cell carcinoma of the thyroid. Acta Pathologica Japonica 1989; 39:306.

589. Bronner MP, LiVolsi VA: Spindle cell squamous carcinoma of the thyroid: An unusual anaplastic tumor associated with tall cell papillary cancer. Mod Pathol 1991; 4:637.

590. Martin JME, Randhawa G, Temple WJ: Cervical thymoma. Arch Pathol Lab Med 1986; 110:354.

591. Harach HR, Day ES, Fransilla KO: Thyroid spindle cell tumor with mucous cysts: An intrathyroidal thymoma? Am J Surg Pathol 1985; 9:525.

592. Takahashi H, Ono H, Nagai I: A case of intrathyroidal thymoma presenting as a thyroid mass. J Jpn Assoc Thoracic Surg 1991; 39:351.

593. Oh YL, Ko YH, Ree HJ: Aspiration cytology of ectopic cervical thymoma mimicking a thyroid mass: A case report. Acta Cytol 1998; 42:1167.

594. Chan JKC, Rosai J: Tumors of the neck showing thymic or related branchial pouch differentiation: A unifying concept. Hum Pathol 1991; 22:349.

595. Kingsley DPE, Elton A, Bennett MH: Malignant teratoma of the thyroid: Case report and a review of the literature. Br J Cancer 1968; 22:7.

596. Yamashita H, Murakami N: Cervical thymoma and incidence of cervical thymus. Acta Pathologica Japonica 1983; 33:189.

597. Harach HR, Day ES, Franssila KO: Thyroid spindle cell tumor with mucous cysts: An intrathyroid thymoma? Am J Surg Pathol 1985; 9:525.

598. Hofman P, Mainguene C, Michiels JF, et al.: Thyroid spindle epithelial tumor with thymus-like differentiation (the "SETTLE" tumor): An immunohistochemical and electron microscopic study. Eur Arch Otorhinolaryngol 1995; 252:316.

599. Chetty R, Goetsch S, Nayler S, et al.: Spindle epithelial tumour with thymus-like element (SETTLE): The predominantly monophasic variant. Histopathology 1998; 33:71.

600. Su L, Beals T, Bernacki EG, et al.: Spindle epithelial tumor with thymus-like differentiation: A case report with cytologic, histologic, immunohistologic, and ultrastructural findings. Mod Pathol 1997; 10:510.

601. Miyauchi A, Kuma K, Matsuzuka F, et al.: Intrathyroidal epithelial thymoma: An entity distinct from squamous cell carcinoma of the thyroid. World J Surg 1985; 9:128.

602. Miyachi A, Ishikawa H, Maeda M, et al.: Intrathyroidal epithelial thymoma: A report of six cases with immunohistochemical and ultrastructural studies. Endocr Surg 1989; 6:289.

603. Kakudo K, Mori I, Tamaoki N, et al.: Carcinoma of possible thymic origin presenting as a thyroid mass: A new subgroup of squamous cell carcinoma of the thyroid. J Surg Oncol 1988; 138:187.

604. Dorfmann DM, Shahsafaei A, Miyauchi A: Intrathyroidal epithelial thymoma (ITET)/carcinoma showing thymus-like differentiation (CASTLE) exhibits CD5 immunoreactivity: New evidence for thymic differentiation. Histopathology 1998; 32:104.

605. Ahuja AT, Chan ES, Allen PW, et al.: Carcinoma showing thymic-like differentiation (CASTLE tumor). Am J Neuroradiol 1998; 19:1225.

606. Damiani S, Filotico M, Eusebi V: Carcinoma of the thyroid showing thymus-like features. Virchows Arch 1991; 418:463.

607. Jochum W, Padberg BC, Schroder S: Lymphoepithelial carcinoma of the thyroid gland: A thyroid gland carcinoma with thymus-like differentiation. Pathologie 1994; 15:361.

608. Shek TW, Luk IS, Ng IO, et al.: Lymphoepithelioma-like carcinoma of the thyroid gland: Lack of evidence of association with Epstein-Barr virus. Hum Pathol 1996; 27:851.

609. Berezowski K, Grimes MM, Gal A, et al.: CD5 immunoreactivity of epithelial cells in thymic carcinoma and CASTLE using paraffin-embedded tissue. Am J Clin Pathol 1996; 106:483.

610. Dorfmann DM, Shahsafaei A, Miyauchi A: Immunohistochemical staining for bcl-2 and mc1-1 in intrathyroidal epithelial thymoma (ITET)/carcinoma showing thymus-like differentiation (CASTLE) and cervical thymic carcinoma. Mod Pathol 1998; 11:989.

611. Wenig BM, Adair CF, Heffess CS: Primary mucoepidermoid carcinoma of the thyroid gland: A report of six cases and a review of the literature of a follicular epithelial-derived tumor. Hum Pathol 1995; 26:1099.

612. Rhatigan RM, Roque JL, Bucher RL: Mucoepidermoid carcinoma of the thyroid gland. Cancer 1977; 39:210.

613. Franssila KO, Harach HR, Wasenius VM: Mucoepidermoid carcinoma of the thyroid. Histopathology 1984; 8:847.

614. Mizukami Y, Matsubara F, Hashimoto T, et al.: Primary mucoepidermoid carcinoma in the thyroid gland: A case report including ultrastructural and biochemical study. Cancer 1984; 53:1741.

615. Sambade C, Franssila K: Mucoepidermoid carcinoma of the thyroid revisited. Surg Pathol 1990; 3:271.

616. Arezzo A, Patetta R, Ceppa R, et al.: Mucoepidermoid carcinoma of the thyroid gland arising from a papillary epithelial neoplasm. Am Surg 1998; 64:307.

617. Cameselle-Teijeiro J, Febles-Perez C, Sobrinho-Simões M: Papillary and mucoepidermoid carcinoma of the thyroid with anaplastic transformation: A case report with histologic and immunohistochemical findings that support a provocative histogenetic hypothesis. Path Res Pract 1995; 191:1214.

618. Chan JKC, Albores-Saavedra J, Battofora H, et al.: Sclerosing mucoepidermoid thyroid carcinoma with eosinophilia. Am J Surg Pathol 1991; 15:438.

619. Bondenson L, Bondenson AG: Cytologic features in fine-needle aspirates from a sclerosing mucoepidermoid thyroid carcinoma with eosinophilia. Diagn Cytopathol 1996; 15:301.

620. Sim SJ, Ro JY, Ordonez NG, et al.: Sclerosing mucoepidermoid carcinoma with eosinophilia of the thyroid: Report of two patients, one with distant metastasis, and review of the literature. Hum Pathol 1997; 28:1091.

621. Geisinger KR, Steffee CH, McGee RS, et al.: The cytomorphologic features of sclerosing mucoepidermoid carcinoma of the thyroid gland with eosinophilia. Am J Clin Path 1998; 109:294.

622. Solomon AC, Baloch ZW, Salhany KE, et al.: Sclerosing mucoepidermoid carcinoma with eosinophilia of the thyroid gland: Presentation mimicking Hodgkins disease. Arch Pathol Lab Med 2000; 124:446.

623. Dube VE, Joyce GT: Extreme squamous metaplasia in Hashimoto's thyroiditis. Cancer 1971; 27:434.

624. Thompson L, Wenig B, Adair C, et al.: Primary smooth muscle tumors of the thyroid gland. Cancer 1997; 79:579.

625. Hendrick J, Tuscaloosa A: Leiomyoma of the thyroid gland: Report of case. Surgery 1957; 42:597.

626. Andrion A, Bellis D, Delsedine L, et al.: Leiomyoma and neurilemoma: Report of two unusual non-epithelial tumors of the thyroid gland. Virchows Arch 1988; 413:367.

627. Biankin SA, Cachia AR: Leiomyoma of the thyroid gland. Pathology 1999; 31:64.

628. Lida Y, Katoh R, Yoshioka M, et al.: Primary leiomyosarcoma of the thyroid gland. Acta Pathologica Japonica 1993; 43:71.

629. Chetty R, Clark SP, Dowling JP: Case report: Leiomysarcoma of the thyroid: Immunohistochemical and ultrastructural study. Pathology 1993; 25:203.

630. Tulbah A, Dayel F, Fawaz I, et al.: Epstein-Barr virus–associated leiomyosarcoma of the thyroid in a child with congenital immunodeficiency: A case report. Am J Surg Pathol 1999; 23:473.

631. Kawahara E, Nakanishi I, Terahata S, et al.: Leiomyosarcoma of the thyroid gland: A case report with a comparative study of five cases of anaplastic carcinoma. Cancer 1988; 62:2558.

632. Chan JKC: Solitary fibrous tumor: Everywhere, and a diagnosis in vogue. Histopathology 1997; 31:568.

633. Hanau CA, Miettinen M: Solitary fibrous tumor: Histological and immunohistochemical spectrum of benign and malignant variants presenting at different sites. Hum Pathol 1995; 26:440.

634. Goodland JR, Fletcher CDM: Solitary fibrous tumor arising at unusual sites: Analysis of a series. Histopathology 1991; 19:515.

635. Camselle-Teijeiro J, Varela-Duran J, Fonseca E, et al.: Solitary fibrous tumor of the thyroid. Am J Clin Pathol 1994; 101:537.

636. Cameselle-Teijeiro J, Varela-Duran J: CD34 and thyroid fibrous tumor. Am J Surg Pathol 1995; 19:1096.

637. Taccagni G, Sambade C, Nesland J, et al.: Solitary fibrous tumor of the thyroid: Clinicopathological, immunohistochemical and ultrastructural study of three cases. Virchows Arch 1993; 422:491.

638. Kie JH, Kim JY, Park YN, et al.: Solitary fibrous tumor of the thyroid. Histopathology 1997; 30:365.

639. Brunnemann R, Ro J, Ordonez N, et al.: Extrathoracic localized fibrous tumor: A clinicopathologic review of 20 cases. Mod Pathol 1997; 10:8.

640. Villaschi S, Macciomei MC: Solitary fibrous tumor of the perithyroid soft tissue: Report of a case simulating a thyroid nodule. Ann Ital Chir 1996; 67:89.

641. Mills SE, Gaffey MJ, Watts JC, et al.: Angiomatoid carcinoma and "angiosarcoma" of the thyroid gland: A spectrum of endothelial differentiation. Am J Clin Pathol 1994; 102:322.

642. Egloff B: The hemangioendothelioma of thyroid. Virchows Arch 1983; 400:119.

643. Hedinger C: Geographic pathology of thyroid diseases. Pathol Res Pract 1981; 171:285.

644. Tanda F, Massarelli G, Bosincu L, et al.: Angiosarcoma of the thyroid: A light, electron microscopic and histoimmunologic study. Hum Pathol 1988; 19:742.

645. Eusebi V, Carcangui ML, Dina R, et al.: Keratin-positive epithelioid angiosarcoma of thyroid: A report of four cases. Am J Surg Pathol 1990; 14:737.

646. Klinck GH: Hemangioendothelioma and sarcoma of the thyroid. In Hedinger CE, ed.: Thyroid Cancer. Springer-Verlag, Berlin, 1969, p. 60.

647. Campagno J, Oertel JE: Malignant lymphoma and other lymphoproliferative disorders of the thyroid gland. Am J Clin Pathol 1980; 74:1.

648. Harris NJ: Extranodal lymphoid infiltrates and mucosa-associated lymphoid tissue (MALT). Am J Surg Pathol 1991; 15:879.

649. Salhany KE, Pietra GG: Extranodal lymphoid disorders. Am J Clin Pathol 1993; 99:472.

650. van de Rijn M, Salhany KE: Lymphoid neoplasms of the thyroid. Pathol Case Rev 1997; 2:218.

651. Willis RA: Metastatic tumors in the thyroid gland. Am J Pathol 1931; 7:187.

652. Rice CO: Microscopic metastases in the thyroid gland. Am J Pathol 1934; 10:407.

653. Czech JM, Lichtor TR, Carney JA, et al.: Neoplasms metastatic to the thyroid gland. Surg Gynecol Obstet 1982; 155:503.

654. Madore P, Lan S: Solitary metastasis from clear-cell renal cell carcinoma. Can Med Assoc J 1975; 112:719.

655. Nakhjavani MK, Gharib H, Goellner JR: Metastasis to the thyroid gland: A report of 43 cases. Cancer 1997; 79:574.

656. Lam KY, Lo CY: Metastatic tumors of the thyroid gland: A study of 79 cases in Chinese patients. Arch Pathol Lab Med 1998; 122:37.

657. Ivy HK: Cancer metastatic to the thyroid: A diagnostic problem. Mayo Clin Proc 1984; 59:856.

658. McCabe DP, Farrar WB, Petkov TM: Clinical and pathologic correlations in disease metastatic to the thyroid gland. Am J Surg 1985; 150:519.

659. Chaco MS, Greenbaum E, Moussouris HF: Value of aspiration cytology of the thyroid in metastatic disease. Acta Cytol 1987; 31:705.

660. Smith SA, Gharib H, Goellner JR: Fine-needle aspiration: Usefulness for diagnosis and management of metastatic carcinoma to the thyroid. Arch Intern Med. 1987; 147:311.

661. Baloch ZW, LiVolsi VA: Tumor to tumor metastases to follicular variant of papillary carcinoma of thyroid. Arch Pathol Lab Med 1999; 123:703.

5

The Parathyroid Glands

Robyn L. Apel and Sylvia L. Asa

THE NORMAL PARATHYROID GLAND

Embryology

The embryologies of the parathyroid glands, the thymus, and the thyroid gland are intimately associated[1] as they all develop from the branchial pouches of the pharynx.[1] The inferior glands and thymus arise from the third branchial pouch, and the superior parathyroid glands and the ultimobranchial body, which gives rise to the parafollicular C cells of the thyroid, are derived from the fourth pouch. The parathyroid glands are first recognized as thickenings in the ventrolateral wall of their respective pouches in the 7.1-mm fetus.[1] The superior parathyroid glands are usually located near the midportion of the posterior surface of the thyroid lobes, close to the point where the inferior thyroid artery crosses the recurrent laryngeal nerve. The inferior parathyroid glands descend through the neck with the thymus, most often to the lower pole of the thyroid; however, they may be found anywhere along their course of descent, from high in the neck down into the thorax.

Anatomy, Histology, and Ultrastructure

Gross Anatomy

In adults, the parathyroid glands are soft, flat, ovoid, or reniform-shaped organs, although occasionally they may be bi- or multilobed glands. The color of the glands reflects largely the extent of stromal fat and ranges from red-brown to yellow-tan as the fat content increases.[2] The sizes and weights of parathyroid glands vary both within and between individuals.[3] Normal glands measure 4 to 9 mm in length, 2 to 4 mm in width, and 0.5 to 2 mm in thickness.[4-6] The weight of a normal gland is usually less than 40 mg,[3, 5, 6] but higher values have been reported,[7-9] and up to 103 mg has been considered

normal,[2, 3, 5, 8-10] so that 70 mg is a more realistic value against which to assess the presence of glandular enlargement of individual parathyroid glands.[7] Gland weights are influenced by gender, race, health status, age, and stromal fat content. Healthy black patients are said to have heavier parathyroid glands compared with white patients.[5, 8] Fat content varies with age and amount of body fat. Other aspects of health status and gender have inconsistent impact on parathyroid gland weight.[5, 8, 11] Because of the influence of fat content, some investigators have suggested that parenchymal weight should be used to assess parathyroid gland sizes,[10, 12] but this is not practical for surgical pathologists.

The majority of people have four parathyroid glands[13-15]; supernumerary glands have been found in 5% of subjects.[16, 17] Additional glands may be found along the normal parathyroid migratory pathways or in abnormal positions, most commonly within the thymic tongue and mediastinum. True supernumerary parathyroid glands must be distinguished from split, bi- or multilobed glands, or small rudimentary cell clusters associated with otherwise normal glands; these occurred in 8% of cases in one large autopsy series.[2, 16] It is rare to have fewer than four parathyroid glands[13, 18]; reports of this in up to 7% of the population[14, 15, 18] may represent difficulty in locating these small organs.

Complete agenesis of the parathyroid glands is rare. Partial or complete failure of parathyroid development is usually associated with abnormal development of the thymus and thyroid C cells, a complex known as DiGeorge's syndrome.[19]

The embryologic migration of the parathyroid glands results in a wide range of normal locations of these structures. This variability is important during attempted removal of diseased glands but also during any surgery on the neck, when they can be inadvertently damaged or removed. The longer migratory pathway of the inferior glands results in greater variability in their localization. Sixty-one percent of inferior glands are found inferior, posterior,

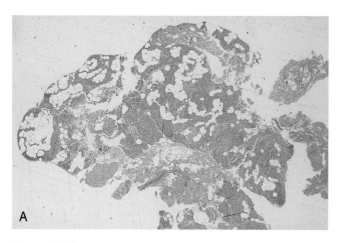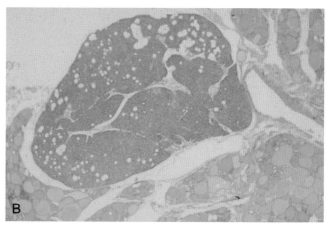

Figure 5–1. The range of normal cellularity is wide in patients with no evidence of parathyroid dysfunction. *A,* The usual ratio of fat to parenchymal cells in an adult is 1:1. *B,* This parathyroid gland has abundant cellularity and scant stromal fat; this appearance is typical for younger patients but may also be found in adults.

or lateral to the lower pole of the thyroid.[16] They may also be located behind any portion of the thyroid; within the thyroid parenchyma or thymus; at the bifurcation of the common carotid arteries even above the "superior" parathyroid glands; in a paratracheal location; or in the anterior, superior, or posterior mediastinum.[16, 17, 20, 21] The superior glands are generally found within 1 cm of their "classic" site, which is within the fibrous tissue adjoining the posterior edge of the thyroid to the pharynx, where the inferior thyroid artery crosses the recurrent laryngeal nerve.[13] Occasionally, the superior glands may be located within the thyroid capsule, or rarely they may be embedded within the thyroid parenchyma or in the retropharyngeal or retroesophageal space.[21] Unusual migratory patterns tend to be bilateral, with 70% to 80% of cases showing symmetry.[2] Parathyroid tissue has also been identified in "ectopic" sites, including the vaginal wall, submucosa of the eosophagus, hypopharynx, and within the vagus nerve or paraganglion.[12, 22–26]

The parathyroid glands are usually supplied by the inferior thyroid arteries, although their blood supply may be via the superior thyroid arteries or the anastomosing plexus between these vessels.[20, 27, 28] The venous drainage parallels that of the thyroid gland, with veins draining into the thyroid venous plexus on the anterior surface of the thyroid gland.[20] Lymph collects in a subcapsular plexus and then drains, with the thyroid lymphatic vessels, into the inferior deep cervical and paratracheal lymph nodes and ultimately into the thoracic and right lymphatic ducts.[20]

The nerve supply of the parathyroid glands is derived from the sympathetic trunk, either directly from the superior or middle cervical sympathetic ganglia, or from the plexus surrounding the superior and inferior thyroid arteries.[20]

Microscopic Anatomy

The parathyroid glands are delineated by thin layers of fibrous connective tissue[28] that extend into the glands, dividing them into ill-defined lobules of parenchymal cells. The lobularity is more evident in adults[9] and may not be apparent in children.[6] The fibrous trabecula are usually not dense, but occasionally the perivascular connective tissue is dense and hyaline.[28] The fibrous tissue does not form a well-defined capsule, and small irregular nests of parathyroid cells are occasionally seen outside the gland in the surrounding soft tissues.[9]

Parenchymal cells and fat cells constitute the main components of the parathyroid glands (Fig. 5–1). The parenchymal-to-fat ratio varies throughout life; children have less fat, and the fat component increases up to ages 25 to 30 years when fat constitutes 10% to 25% of gland volume.[3] Some authors have shown no correlation between age and the amount of stromal fat.[9] Traditionally, a 50:50 parenchymal cell–to–fat cell ratio has been said to be normal for adults; however, this is probably an overestimation of the amount of fat in adult glands.[9] A more realistic estimation of the amount of fat is 10% to 17%.[9, 11, 29] Although the parenchymal cell–to–fat cell ratio is used to determine the functional status of parathyroids, the ratio is inaccurate because of the variability between individuals[9] and because of the variable fat distribution within single glands; the polar regions contain more stromal fat, whereas the central areas are usually more cellular.[16, 28] There is also often variability in the amount of fat present in the glands of any one individual; this can vary as much as from less than 10% of the stroma in one gland to 50% in another.[9] Small biopsy samples of normal parathyroid glands can therefore vary from predominantly parenchymal cells to predominantly fat cells or varying proportions of the two cell types; multiple sections are required to accurately estimate the correct ratio in any given gland.[30] This raises serious concerns about the validity of histopathologic examination of one or a few sections of parathyroid glands to evaluate parenchymal cell–to–fat cell ratios.[3, 30]

Like other endocrine organs, the parathyroid glands are supplied by a rich capillary network.

Within the gland or lobules, the parenchymal cells are arranged in sheets, cords, and nests around the capillary framework. Occasional nodules may be present and tend to be less than 1 mm in diameter, although they may measure up to 4 mm.[9] Parenchymal cells may form acinar or follicular structures that contain eosinophilic material that resembles colloid and stains with the periodic acid–Schiff (PAS) technique.[28] This material can also demonstrate the staining characteristics of amyloid and is immunoreactive for parathyroid hormone (PTH), suggesting that this material may be hormone-derived amyloid, as in other endocrine tumors.[31, 32] Various cystic structures have been described on the surface and deep within the parathyroid glands (Fig. 5–2A); many are irregular in shape have a variable lining of parenchymal cells, flattened cells, or fibrous tissue, and contain faintly-staining material[28] The histogenesis of these structures is not known, although some may represent vestigial remnants of embryologic structures. They may be related to clinically significant cysts that rarely occur within the parathyroid glands.[1, 28]

Parenchymal cells can exhibit three distinct morphologic variations: chief cells, oxyphil cells, and clear cells. They are admixed singly, in groups, or as nodules. Chief cells, averaging 8 μm in diameter, are generally polygonal with amphophilic-to-slightly-eosinophilic cytoplasm and small, round-to-oval central nuclei with dense coarse chromatin (see Fig. 2B).[28] In formalin-fixed tissues, the cytoplasm of chief cells often appears vacuolated.[6] Eighty percent of chief cells in resting adult glands contains intracytoplasmic neutral lipids, compared with 30% to 40% of these cells in glands in children.[33] Chief cells are typically well glycogenated, and when the cytoplasmic glycogen is abundant, the cytoplasm is clear in routine histologic sections; hence the term "clear cells." Although clear cells are the principal cell type in embryos and fetuses, their predominance declines after birth.[28] These cells tend to be slightly larger than chief cells, with an average cell diameter of 10

μm.[28] These cells differ from the water-clear Wasserhelle cells described in the disorder water-clear cell hyperplasia, where the clear cytoplasm is due not to glycogen but to numerous membrane-bound vacuoles.[34] Water-clear cells have not been described in the ultrastructure of normal human parathyroid glands.[34] Oxyphil cells appear generally in adolescence, although they are occasionally present in children. They are believed to increase in number with increasing age,[28] although some investigators have shown no correlation between the percentage of oxyphil cells and age.[9] These cells may form nodules that, when large, can be impossible to distinguish from oxyphil adenomas.[6] Oxyphil cells are generally larger than chief cells (7 to 18 μm in diameter, average 11 μm) and have well-defined cell borders with abundant granular eosinophilic cytoplasm. Their nuclei have been variably described as both larger and smaller than those of chief cells,[6, 28] but they typically appear pyknotic. Some oxyphil cells have less eosinophilic cytoplasm and represent transitional oxyphil cells. Nuclear atypia and mitotic figures are not usually seen in normal parathyroid glands.[9]

Histochemistry and Immunohistochemistry

Glycogen and neutral lipids are common cytoplasmic constituents of parathyroid chief cells. Quantitation of these products roughly reflects a cell's secretory activity because both substances are more plentiful in resting cells than in hyperfunctioning cells.[29, 35] Routine histochemical stains, such as PAS with and without diastase predigestion (PAS-D), oil-red O, or Sudan IV, or ultrastructural examination may be used to determine the abundance of these substances.

Oxyphil cells are oncocytes that contain numerous, often abnormal, mitochondria that are rich in oxidative enzymes.[36] It has been suggested that oncocytes reflect a mitochondrial cytopathy related to

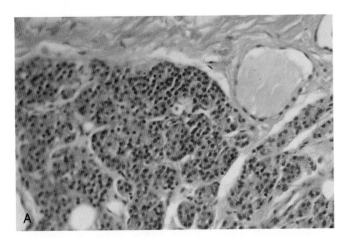
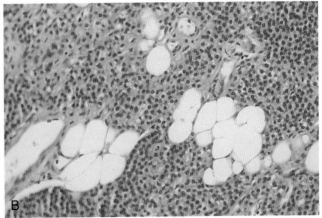

Figure 5-2. A, The normal adult parathyroid is composed of chief cells with scattered oxyphils and may contain follicle-like cysts with colloid-like material in the lumen. *B,* The gland is composed of a mixture of chief cells and oxyphils, with adipocytes scattered throughout the parenchyma.

aging.[37] Histochemical techniques that detect respiratory enzymes have identified defects in staining for cytochrome-c-oxidase in parathyroid oncocytic cells and, to a greater degree, in parathyroid hyperplasia as opposed to adenomas.[37] This defect is not apparent in all oxyphilic cell clusters, suggesting that there may be different mechanisms of oncocytic transformation.[37]

Keratins 8, 18, and 19 (molecular weight [MW] 52K, 45K, and 40k, respectively) have been identified in all types of parathyroid parenchymal cells by immunohistochemistry.[38] Oxyphil cells exhibit less intense, more delicate, fibrillary staining of the cytoplasm compared with chief cells.[38] The high MW keratins typical of stratified epithelia are not present in parathyroid tissues.[38] Vimentin has been detected only in the stromal components of the parathyroid glands.[38] The presence of various neuroendocrine markers has been assessed in parathyroid glands. Neurofilaments are not detected in normal parathyroid tissue; neuron-specific enolase is to a variable degree.[38, 39] Chromogranin A (also known as secretory protein-1) is costored with PTH in the secretory granules of the parathyroid glands (Fig. 5–3), and both peptides are cosecreted under conditions of decreased extracellular calcium.[40–44] Immunohistochemical staining is positive in most parathyroid cells but cannot distinguish normal from abnormal parathyroid tissue[45] nor can relative levels of chromogranin A messenger RNA (mRNA) transcripts.[46] Although S-100 protein is strongly positive in these glands of rats and rabbits, only focal positivity has been identified in normal and adenomatous human parathyroid glands.[39]

Potential immunohistochemical markers useful in identifying tissues as parathyroid in nature are antibodies against PTH and a calcium-sensing receptor.[47] Various antibodies, differing in their specificities for the intact, amino, or mid or carboxy terminals, are available for the detection of PTH and yield cytoplasmic positivity that is usually less intense in oxyphils.[48, 49] Difficulties may arise when parenchymal cells store relatively small amounts of PTH.[6] Ultrastructural staining localizes PTH largely to secretory granules and less in aggregated sacs of rER; the Golgi complex is negative.[49] Monoclonal antibodies against a calcium-sensing receptor are also available and may prove valuable in confirming parathyroid differentiation.[7, 50, 51] These receptors are also expressed in renal proximal tubular cells and placental cells. Immunohistochemical studies have identified positivity in normal, suppressed, adenomatous, and hyperplastic parathyroid tissue as well as in metastatic deposits of parathyroid carcinoma.[7, 50]

Ultrastructural Anatomy

The parathyroid glands, like other endocrine organs, contain a rich network of fenestrated capillaries. The parenchymal cells are surrounded by well-formed basal laminae and are connected by small desmosomes and terminal bars.[52] The ultrastructural form of parathyroid cells varies with their level of hormone production and secretion.[34, 52] Only 20% of chief cells is in the hormone-producing phase at any given time in normal adults.[4] Functional activity is associated with smaller cells that exhibit greater tortuosity of plasma membranes, electron-dense cytoplasm due to the proximity of organelles, and decreased amounts of glycogen and lipid.[34, 52] Forming secretory granules concentrate in the vicinity on the Golgi apparatus. They measure 50 to 150 nm in diameter and are generally round with a central electron-dense core and lucent halo surrounded by a limiting membrane.[6, 34] Mature secretory granules measure 100 to 500 nm in diameter and vary in size and shape. They are extremely electron-dense and are surrounded by a closely applied limiting membrane without a lucent halo.[34] In contrast to functionally active cells, resting cells are larger with relatively straight cell membranes and abundant lipid and glycogen.[34, 49, 52] The rER and free ribosomes are dispersed throughout the cytoplasm, and secretory and prosecretory granules are scarce.

Oxyphil cells are larger than chief cells, and their cytoplasm is filled with numerous mitochondria that may be enlarged and dilated.[34, 52] Glycogen granules and free ribosomes are interspersed between the mitochondria, and rER, Golgi's complexes, secretory granules, and lipid inclusions are poorly developed. Transitional oxyphil cells demonstrate morphologic characteristics intermediate between chief cells and oxyphil cells.[34, 52]

Molecular Anatomy

Molecular techniques, such as PTH mRNA in situ hybridization (ISH), have been used to evaluate parathyroid function at a cellular level.[53–56] In normal parathyroid glands, PTH mRNA expression is

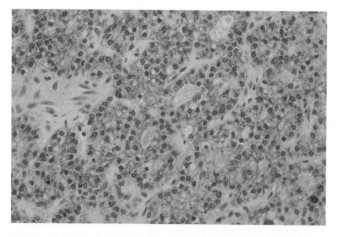

Figure 5–3. Immunohistochemical staining documents the presence of chromogranin A in a paraffin section of formalin-fixed tissue of normal parathyroid (avidin-biotin peroxidase technique).

confined to a small proportion of cells, commonly aggregated into small groups.[53] In hyperplastic and adenomatous glands the proportion of cells exhibiting PTH mRNA production is greatly increased, whereas the level of expression of any individual cell is unchanged.[53] Stronger expression is seen in cells with large vesicular nuclei than in those with small dark nuclei,[53] and oxyphil cells have markedly reduced PTH mRNA. Chromogranin mRNA is also expressed in human parathyroid cells.[46]

Physiology

Biosynthesis of Parathyroid Hormone

The PTH polypeptide is encoded by a gene on the short arm of chromosome 11 (11p15).[57, 58] Within the parathyroid cells, a large 115–amino acid precursor molecule, preproparathyroid hormone (preproPTH), is synthesized and processed via a 90–amino acid intermediate precursor, proparathyroid hormone (proPTH), to form the native secretory 1-84 PTH. The biologic actions of PTH are classically attributed to amino acids 1-34 region; the N-terminal region is often referred to as the "active" fragment and the C-terminal region is described as the "inactive" fragment. However, different regions, such as 1–27, 1–34, 30–34, and 53–84, are each responsible for different biologic activities of PTH on target organs due to interactions with distinct receptors.[59] N-terminal and C-terminal fragments of PTH are formed in the peripheral circulation, liver, and kidneys; C-terminal fragments may also be secreted directly from the parathyroid glands.[6] This immunoheterogeneity of intact and fragmented PTH molecules circulating in the peripheral blood has been largely responsible for the difficulties in developing specific immunoassays to measure PTH.[60, 61] Renal failure accentuates differences between techniques measuring intact PTH and midregion and C-terminal PTH fragments, as the kidneys are believed to play a role in the metabolism of carboxy and possibly midregion fragments.[60]

Actions of Parathyroid Hormone

Calcium homeostasis is the primary function of PTH. Along with calcitonin and calcitriol (1,25 [OH]$_2$D$_3$), PTH maintains serum calcium levels through direct and indirect actions on the bones, kidneys, and intestinal tract.

The skeletal effects of PTH are due to bone resorption and inhibition of bone formation.[62] Although the multinucleated osteoclast appears to be the major effector of PTH-mediated localized bone resorption, osteoclasts do not express PTH receptors, and their actions are mediated through osteoblasts.[63–67] How osteoblasts stimulate osteoclastic bone resorption is not completely understood, but bone-resorbing factors, such as prostaglandin E$_2$, lymphokines, and growth factors, may be released from osteoblasts in a paracrine fashion.[68, 69] PTH also causes osteoblasts to contract, exposing underlying mineral to osteoclasts,[70] and osteoblasts secrete collagenases and neutral proteases that facilitate degradation of osteoid matrix.

In the kidneys, PTH acts on proximal tubular cells to inhibit reabsorption of phosphate and on the distal convoluted tubule to enhance tubular reabsorption of calcium.[71] PTH also regulates conversion of 25-hydroxycholecalciferol to 1,25-dihydroxycholecalciferol and other metabolites of vitamin D by stimulating 1α-hydroxylase enzymatic activity.[69] 1,25-dihydroxycholecalciferol promotes absorption of calcium from the gastrointestinal tract.[72] This active vitamin D metabolite also exerts negative feedback on parathyroid cells through the vitamin D nuclear receptor, decreasing transcription rates of preproPTH and inhibiting secretion of PTH.[73]

Regulation of Parathyroid Hormone

Parathyroid cells store relatively small amounts of preformed hormone but are capable of responding to minor fluctuations in calcium concentrations by rapidly altering the rate of hormone secretion and by altering more slowly the rate of hormone synthesis.[73] Calcium is the most important physiologic regulator of PTH biosynthesis and secretion. Decreasing extracellular concentrations of calcium stimulates secretion of PTH that acts on target organs to restore the serum calcium concentration to within a narrow range. In the presence of a low-serum calcium concentration, newly formed PTH may bypass storage in secretory granules and be released directly into the circulation.[73] When circulating calcium levels are elevated, amino acid uptake by the parathyroid cells, synthesis of preproPTH, conversion to PTH, and secretion of stored hormone are inhibited.[6, 73] Although PTH is responsible for extracellular calcium homeostasis, it seems that the intracellular concentration of calcium is ultimately the regulator of PTH.[74] At least two mechanisms allow the parathyroid cell to sense extracellular calcium levels: calcium-selective channels and secondary messengers that release intracellular stores of calcium when stimulated by extracellular calcium[75] and a selective calcium-sensing receptor.[47]

In addition to calcium, various other agents, such as dopamine, epinephrine, isoproterenol, prolactin, divalent cations, potassium, lithium, fluoride, adenosine triphosphate, vitamin D, PG F$_{2a}$, glucocorticoids, estrogen, and osmolarity can modulate PTH secretion.[74–77] A number of potential mechanisms have been explained. Some of these agents influence PTH secretion through changing intracellular calcium concentrations, whereas others do not.[75] Secondary messengers also implicated include adenyl cyclase–activated cyclic adenosine 3′,5′-monophosphate (cAMP) and inositol phosphates as part of signal transduction pathways generating inositol triphosphate, diacylglycerol, and protein kinase C.[74, 75, 77] The regulation of PTH secretion is obviously complex and potentially involves many pathways, in addition to the well-established calcium/adenyl cyclase/cAMP mechanism. Although the parathyroid glands are innervated, the role of neural control of physiologic function of the glands is unknown.

Parathyroid Hormone-Related Peptide

PTH-related peptide (PTHrP) is a hormone produced by many normal tissues and some malignant neoplasms. As its name suggests, this peptide is closely related to PTH, both structurally and in evolution.[78, 79] The gene that encodes PTHrP is on the short arm of chromosome 12 and is thought to have evolved from the PTH gene on chromosome 11.[80] The two hormones share some structural homology and, at least in some organs, they appear to interact with the same receptors.[81-84] In bone and kidney, PTHrP and PTH result in identical biologic effects, stimulating bone resorption and promoting calcium reabsorption and phosphorus excretion in the kidneys.[81, 85, 86]

PTHrP is produced by such diverse tissues as skin keratinocytes, lactating mammary tissue, uteroplacental tissues, adrenal cortex and medulla, pancreatic islet cells, thyroid follicular epithelium, adenohypophysis, testicular Leydig's cells, ovarian granulosa and theca cells, bone marrow, stomach mucosa, heart, kidney, lung, smooth and skeletal muscle, fetal liver, brain, lymphocytes, and parathyroid glands.[87-92]

Adult parathyroid glands express PTHrP mRNA, but secretion by these glands has not been identified.[93] PTHrP mRNA and protein are identified in parathyroid adenomas and carcinomas and in hyperplastic glands of patients with chronic renal failure.[87, 93-95] The amount of PTHrP mRNA detected in adenomas is variable, but even in cases where a high level of PTHrP mRNA has been expressed, only small amounts of PTHrP protein were immunoreactive; this may reflect poor translational efficiency of the PTHrP mRNA or rapid processing or degradation of the PTHrP to a form not detectable by the immunoassays used.[95]

The function of PTHrP in most normal tissues is currently unknown. Its wide distribution in normal tissues suggests that it may fulfill diverse physiologic roles in many biologic processes, such as cell growth and differentiation, reproduction, lactation, vasoregulation, smooth-muscle relaxation, and calcium metabolism,[73, 96] its diversity may result from its action as a polyhormone, or it may represent a precursor for different peptides.[59, 78] It has been suggested that PTHrP plays a crucial endocrine role in fetal mineral metabolism, functioning as the fetal PTH.[72] It may be responsible for maintaining a fetal-to-maternal calcium gradient by stimulating placental calcium transport.[90, 97, 98] PTHrP is also a potent relaxant of smooth muscle, and in blood vessels it acts to regulate vascular tone.[99] PTHrP possesses β-transforming growth factor activity, which is not the case for PTH.[100] Lactation, however, appears to be the only physiologically normal situation in which plasma levels of PTHrP are elevated.[101]

When PTHrP is present in the circulation in greater quantities than the usual low levels, such as when secreted by malignant tumors, hypercalcemia may result. In these circumstances, the term humoral hypercalcemia of malignancy (HHM) is used.[102-104] Only a minority of cancers that express PTHrP, as detected by immunohistochemistry and ISH, are associated with hypercalcemia.[83, 87, 105] Tumor-specific post-translational modification of PTHrP may be important in producing specific molecular forms of PTHrP with hypercalcemic activity, or other modifying factors may be required.[83, 87, 106] Further work is required to explain the mechanisms involved in the development of PTHrP-induced HHM.

ADDITIONAL PATHOLOGIC EXAMINATION TECHNIQUES

Fine-Needle Aspiration Biopsy

Fine-needle aspiration (FNA) biopsies may be used in combination with noninvasive radiologic techniques to assess parathyroid lesions preoperatively. Image guided FNA biopsy is particularly valuable in patients undergoing reoperations for persistent hypercalcemia where the anatomy is distorted.[107, 108] The parathyroid origin of aspirated material can be established by cytologic examination combined with immunocytochemistry and/or by radioimmunoassays for PTH.[109, 110]

The morphologic distinction of parathyroid from thyroid follicular epithelial cells or lymphocytes can be difficult.[108, 111-125] The cellularity of parathyroid aspirates may be scant to moderately cellular.[123] Architectural features aid in distinguishing parathyroid from thyroid cells: epithelial cells arranged in a perivascular pattern around capillary cores, an overall organoid or trabecular architecture with frequent microacini,[123] or thick cohesive cell groups with frayed edges[116] are typical of parathyroid, whereas thyroid nodules tend to produce evenly spaced "honeycomb" sheets.[117] However, both can form follicles with colloid-like material.[108, 116, 119] In general, benign parathyroid cells tend to be slightly smaller and have less cytoplasm than thyroid follicular epithelium.[123] Parathyroid cells tend to have uniform, round-to-oval nuclei with granular, evenly distributed, chromatin and small single nucleoli,[123] however, they can be variable with hyperchromatic, coarsely granular chromatin, and multiple large nucleoli.[116] The cytoplasm may have a pink hue with fine blue granularity on Diff-Quik[123] or may be pale and vacuolated, amphophilic, or abundant and granular consistent with oxyphil cells that are easily misinterpreted as thyroid Hürthle's cells.[6]

Paravacuolar cytoplasmic granules and hemosiderin-laden macrophages are not common in parathyroid lesions but are seen frequently in thyroid.[123] Occasionally, a parathyroid gland is embedded within or is in close association with the thyroid, and the aspiration tract may penetrate both tissues.[126]

Special stains, such as the Sevier-Munger silver stain, can detect argyrophilic granules in the parathyroid cell cytoplasm.[112] Immunoperoxidase stains for PTH,[127] thyroglobulin, and chromogranin A[128] may be useful. Positive staining for chromogranin A, in conjunction with negative staining for thyroglobulin, strongly supports parathyroid origin. Although chromogranin A is not as specific as PTH, it is often technically easier to use.[123] Parathyroid cells, thyroid parafollicular C cells, and medullary carcinomas are all chromogranin A–positive; however, distinction is usually not difficult, because parafollicular C cells constitute a very small component of the thyroid gland and therefore do not pose a diagnostic problem. Medullary carcinomas exhibit characteristic FNA features, including a predominantly dispersed cell population, eccentric nuclei, and tails of cytoplasm.[123]

Lesions composed of parathyroid cells on cytology cannot be further classified as hyperplasia, adenoma, or carcinoma,[116, 119, 123] despite claims to the contrary.[115, 129] However, FNA cytology may be of value to confirm metastases in patients with persistent hyperparathyroidism following "curative" surgery for parathyroid carcinoma. CT-guided FNA has been used to distinguish occult bone metastasis from a localized lytic brown tumor of hyperparathyroidism.[130]

FNA cytology can be used to diagnose a parathyroid cyst.[131] The aspirate from a cyst is characterized by a few macrophages and groups of small cells consistent with parathyroid cells. Markedly elevated PTH levels are measured in aspirated fluid,[123] whereas aspirates from nonparathyroid lesions contain PTH levels below normal serum levels.[109]

FNA can cause fragments of parathyroid tissue to be disseminated throughout the neck,[107, 132] this has raised concern about this procedure, but it remains a theoretical risk.

Clonality studies of hyperplastic parathyroid glands have revealed monoclonality in glands from patients with secondary hyperparathyroidism and sporadic primary hyperparathyroidism.[133] Because of potential significance in the management of patients, it has been suggested that in the future clonality may be determined on ultrasound-guided FNA biopsy specimens,[134] as has been described for parathyroid adenomas.[135]

Intraoperative Frozen Sections and Fat Stains

Because of the lack of well defined histologic criteria for the major pathologic entities affecting the parathyroid glands, the role of intraoperative histopathologic examination of these glands is often limited to identification of the tissue.[136–140] However, using careful gross inspection with gland weights, hematoxylin and eosin–stained frozen and permanent sections, and possibly stains for the assessment of cytoplasmic fat content, the pathologist can make a significant contribution to the management of patients with parathyroid disease.[3, 7, 141, 142]

An important caveat is the need for a thorough appreciation of the wide variability among normal parathyroid glands, in relation to size, weights, and histologic characteristics. Interpretation of parathyroid pathology requires knowledge of the patient's personal or family history of other endocrine disorders as well as the number of enlarged glands; their size, consistency, and color; and the anatomic site from which tissue has been obtained.

The initial assessment entails gross inspection. Surrounding fat should be removed from the submitted glands prior to weighing and measuring. Characteristics such as the external appearance, color, and consistency should be noted. Abnormal parathyroid glands are generally larger (5 mm to 8 cm, weighing 0.4 to 120 mg), reddish-brown, of slightly firmer consistency, and noncompressible with rounded edges; normal glands are smaller (generally less than 40 mg but may weigh up to 70 mg); oval or bean-shaped; yellow-tan; and soft, flat, and compressible.[138] If an adenoma is suspected clinically, the gland should be inspected thoroughly for any attached pale tan tissue, which may represent a rim of compressed tissue outside the adenoma capsule. As this is most often found at the vascular pole of the gland, it is helpful if the surgeon marks this area with a suture so that it can be included in sections for microscopy. Some authors promote touch preparations to examine parathyroids at intraoperative consultation.[143] Sections submitted for histologic examination should include any normal tissue and the capsule of abnormal nodules. If fat stains are to be utilized, they must be obtained from frozen tissue or imprints[129] at the time of intraoperative consultation, when samples may also be fixed for electron microscopy or frozen for molecular studies.

The identification of tissue as parathyroid is usually not difficult, although in small biopsy samples the distinction between thyroid, lymphoid tissue, thymic epithelial cells, and parathyroid can be a challenge. Follicle formation can lead to erroneous identification of parathyroid as thyroid tissue; clear and oncocytic cell lesions can also occur in the thyroid gland. Lymphoid cells have less cytoplasm and more clumped chromatin than do parathyroid cells. Hassall's corpuscles establish the presence of thymic tissue. Lipoadenomas are frequently composed of abundant adipose tissue, rendering assessment by standard frozen sections difficult.[144]

The diagnosis of parathyroid pathology can be difficult or impossible at the time of surgery. The variation in size and parenchymal cell–to–fat cell ratios can lead to erroneous interpretation.[3, 30] The helpful diagnostic features and the pitfalls in the recognition of parathyroid hyperplasia, carcinoma, and adenoma are addressed later. The distinction of adenoma from hyperplasia can rarely be made by examining only one parathyroid gland; in such circumstances, the pathologist may be able to state only that the tissue is hypercellular.[141, 145, 146] Examination of a second gland frequently allows accurate distinction.[146] Fat stains may give supportive evidence.

The rationale for assessing cytoplasmic lipid content with fat stains is that in normal or suppressed parathyroid parenchyma, the parathyroid chief cells demonstrate abundant intracytoplasmic neutral lipid droplets, whereas in hyperfunctioning tissue, including adenoma, hyperplasia, or carcinoma, the cytoplasm of chief cells is essentially devoid of droplets of intracytoplasmic neutral lipid (Fig. 5–4).[147] In the majority (more than 80%) of cases, these observations are true.[35, 148, 149]

The value of fat stains in distinguishing between adenoma and hyperplasia is controversial. Both lesions are hyperfunctioning and therefore are expected to have reduced intracellular fat. Fat stains, however, may highlight a rim of normal tissue, the cells of which would typically contain greater amounts of fat compared with the adjacent adenoma cells. Alternatively, a diagnosis of adenoma is also supported if a second gland has abundant intracellular fat, suggesting that it is not hyperplastic. However, some investigators have identified inconsistencies in the amount of cytoplasmic fat.[147, 148, 150, 151] Just as determining the amount of stromal fat is difficult because of an irregular distribution within single glands, the interpretation of fat stains is sometimes difficult because of variability in the amount of cytoplasmic fat throughout an individual gland.[150, 152] Interestingly, in nodular hyperplasia the compact nodules of chief cells are often devoid of fat, whereas the compressed parenchyma contains fat droplets of varying size and number, sometimes to the same extent as uninvolved parathyroid tissue from patients with adenomas.[148] This can be misleading, misinterpreting such tissue as a rim around

an adenoma. It does, however, suggest that the nodules represent autonomously hyperfunctioning foci within intervening stroma that remain responsive to elevated serum calcium.[148]

Two stains for fat, Sudan IV and oil-red O, have been used with varying results.[140] Some investigators report similar results with these two stains: Sudan IV is said to yield more intense staining that is easier to interpret[35, 150]; others prefer oil-red O as the fat dye[148] because it produces less loss of small fat droplets, deeper staining, and greater distinction between hyperfunctioning and uninvolved parathyroid tissue.[148] Others prefer aqueous osmium carmine.[140]

Opinions about the value and role of fat stains in the assessment of parathyroid pathology vary from strong advocates or cautious supporters to those who feel that these histochemical stains are not justified in the routine assessment of parathyroid pathology.[147] Clearly, fat stains, like other investigative techniques available, must not be interpreted in isolation.

Density Gradients

Density gradient techniques measure the densities of whole parathyroid glands, and as the density is related linearly to the parenchymal cell content, this can be used as an indicator of relative parenchymal cell mass, enabling the distinction between normal and abnormal glands.[12] The underlying principle is that parenchymal cells and fat cells have different densities, that normal glands contain appreciable quantities of extra- and intracellular fat, and that adenomatous or hyperplastic glands contain less fat. The approach is objective, rapid, and reproducible. If the total gland weight is also known, the approximate parenchymal weight can be calculated.

Density gradients have been applied intraoperatively to assess biopsy samples of enlarged glands and of apparently normal glands.[153, 154] The tissue sam-

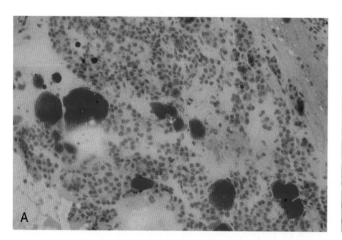
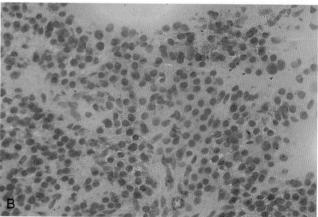

Figure 5–4. The oil-red O fat stain is useful for distinguishing suppressed normal parathyroid parenchyma from hyperactive parathyroid adenoma or hyperplasia. *A,* There is abundant fat, both in adipocytes and in the cytoplasm of parathyroid cells within the compressed normal tissue adjacent to an adenoma. *B,* In contrast, in the adenoma, the cells are almost devoid of fat, with only scattered small droplets of intracytoplasmic neutral lipid.

ples are floated in test tubes of high-density 20% or 25% mannitol or Percoll equilibrated with sodium chloride to isoosmotic conditions; the densities are determined when each sample sinks. In single-gland disease, the denser abnormal specimen sinks while the normal tissue continues to float. In multiglandular disease, the two specimens sink at the same or similar densities. The density differences of various glands of an individual patient are easier to examine[153] than are defined ranges of normal.[154] However, the reported studies have short postoperative follow-up periods and/or poor documentation of the gross and histologic appearances of the parathyroid glands.[155]

DNA Cytometry

A number of studies have reported the use of static and flow cytometry in the analysis of parathyroid disease. In this area, however, even the definition of "normal" is controversial. Some investigators have reported that normal glands are diploid,[156] whereas others have found some normal glands to have small tetraploid populations.[157–159] Among morphologically classified adenomas, there is a high incidence of polyploidy or aneuploidy. Some investigators have found that as many as 80% of adenomas and some hyperplasias have tetraploid peaks,[157, 158] but this may reflect technical artefact due to failure to disperse cell aggregates.[156] In various series, 8% to 21% of adenomas exhibit tetraploidy, and 3% to 25% display aneuploidy. Aneuploidy and tetraploidy may be more frequent in carcinomas than in adenomas; however, because of significant overlap, these characteristics are not useful for accurately distinguishing two entities.[156, 159–162] It has been speculated that the subpopulation of hyperplasias and adenomas with aneuploid or tetraploid profiles may represent a subset of parathyroid tumors that could evolve into carcinomas if allowed to progress.[159]

The use of Feulgen-stained sections for tissue cytometry is reported to be more reliable; aneuploidy is detected in a subpopulation of carcinomas but not in adenomas, and carcinomas have a higher mean nuclear DNA content than do adenomas or normal glands. This form of DNA cytometry has the advantage that it can be performed on 4-μm paraffin sections or on FNA specimens[163]; however, the purported accuracy remains to be proved. Using this method, a finding of more than 2% tetraploid cells is said to strongly favor the diagnosis of adenoma over hyperplasia.[164]

In one study, the mean S-phase fraction of normal glands was 1.2% compared with 0.8% in hyperplasia, 1.5% in adenomas, and 6% in carcinomas; these data led the authors to suggest that an S-phase fraction greater than 4% supported a diagnosis of carcinoma regardless of ploidy.[156]

Although these techniques may not yield accurate diagnostic information, it appears that once a diagnosis of malignancy is established, ploidy may have prognostic significance. Aneuploid carcinomas appear to follow a more aggressive course than do diploid carcinomas.[165]

HYPERPARATHYROIDISM: CLINICAL FEATURES

Primary Hyperparathyroidism

Etiology and Pathogenesis

Primary hyperparathyroidism (PHP) is a common disease characterized by inappropriately elevated PTH secretion relative to the serum calcium level, in the absence of a known stimulus for PTH hypersecretion.[166] Approximately 80% to 90% (range 6% to 95%) of PHP is attributed to parathyroid adenoma, 10% to 15% (1.0% to 84%) to parathyroid hyperplasia, and a small minority (1% to 5%) to parathyroid carcinomas.[110, 138, 145, 146, 149, 167–178] Very rarely, PHP is associated with a parathyroid cyst.[179–182]

The cause of PHP is unknown. The cell membranes of normal parathyroid cells detect alterations in ambient extracellular calcium levels, which are reflected by changes in intracellular calcium concentrations; ultimately, it is the cytoplasmic calcium concentration that regulates PTH secretion.[75] Abnormal parathyroid cells from patients with PHP are relatively insensitive to ambient extracellular calcium levels. In vitro calcium-mediated suppressibility of PTH secretion from adenomas and hyperplastic (primary and secondary) glands exhibits a wide continuum among the three tissue types, indicating that altered set point is an underlying pathogenetic factor[183] due to altered expression of the calcium-sensing receptor.[50, 184] The rate of PTH secretion by cells of parathyroid adenomas in vitro is substantially lower than from cells obtained from hyperplastic glands, implying that in adenomas an increase in absolute cell numbers, as well as alterations in the degree of calcium responsiveness, may prove to be important.[183]

Radiation to the head and neck has been implicated as an etiologic factor in the development of parathyroid hyperplasia and neoplasia.[185–197] The delay between radiation exposure and the development of clinical PHP is often great; in one large series the shortest lag period was 20 years after radiation exposure, and in this series approximately 5% of exposed patients subsequently developed PHP.[189, 190] Studies of atomic bomb survivors have also shown greater than expected rates of hyperparathyroidism,[198, 199] with some suggestion of decreasing risk with increasing age at exposure.[198] Hyperparathyroidism has also been reported following radioactive iodine therapy for Graves' disease.[200]

Coexistence of PHP and thyroid tumors and of Hashimoto's thyroiditis and hypothyroidism have been reported in humans and in experimental models.[201–203] In a rat model of propylthiouracil-induced hypothyroidism, 95% of the animals developed parathyroid hyperplasia with a 30% mean increase in circulating PTH levels.[204] Adenoma formation did not result, but this may reflect the short time course of the study.

To help unravel the pathogenesis and cause of parathyroid lesions, investigators have assessed the clonality of enlarged parathyroid glands. Although early studies using glucose-6-phosphate dehydrogenase (G6PD) isoenzyme inactivation profiles did not prove clonality,[205, 206] subsequent studies using more sophisticated molecular approaches have reported that most, if not all, adenomas are monoclonal and that multiglandular hyperplastic glands in secondary hyperplasia are polyclonal.[207–209]

Genetic mutations have been detected in both sporadic and familial cases of PHP. One of the familial syndromes in which PHP is a major component is multiple endocrine neoplasia type I (MEN-I, or Wermer's syndrome). This disorder exhibits autosomal-dominant transmission with variable penetrance. Members of affected kindreds develop synchronous or metachronous proliferative endocrine lesions, involving most commonly the parathyroid glands, pancreatic islets, and anterior pituitary.[210] Occasional associated lesions include bronchial and gastrointestinal neuroendocrine tumors, adrenal cortical neoplasms, thyroid follicular neoplasms, and lipomas. The parathyroid glands typically demonstrate chief cell hyperplasia of both the nodular and diffuse types, although adenomas and carcinomas have been reported in individuals with MEN-I.[31, 211–213] Unequal involvement of the four parathyroid glands by nodular hyperplasia may be responsible for some of the diagnoses of solitary or multiple adenomas. Inheritance of a single locus on chromosome 11q13 is responsible for the development of the MEN-I syndrome.[214, 215] Pancreatic endocrine tumors and hyperplastic and adenomatous parathyroid tissues from these patients have exhibited loss of heterozygosity (LOH) of part of chromosome 11, resulting in inactivation of both copies of the MEN-I gene; these findings are consistent with a tumor suppressor function for the menin protein expressed by this gene.[214, 216–218] Although the histology of the parathyroid glands in MEN-I–associated hyperparathyroidism is classically described as parathyroid hyperplasia, the molecular studies are consistent with multiple monoclonal proliferations.[216] The gene responsible for MEN-I was mapped to the long arm of chromosome 11 (11q13) based on LOH at the locus in tumors associated with this syndrome,[214, 215] and the gene was cloned in 1997.[219] In keeping with Knudson's two-hit hypothesis for tumorigenesis in hereditary cancers,[220] the product of the MEN-I gene, *menin,* is a tumor suppressor gene (TSG).[221] More than 250 inherited inactivating germline mutations have been reported in kindreds with this syndrome, with LOH indicating loss of the normal allele in the pancreatic endocrine tumors, pituitary adenomas, and enlarged parathyroid glands of affected patients.[222, 223] This TSG was an obvious candidate gene implicated in the more common sporadic parathyroid adenomas, and indeed 5% of

sporadic parathyroid adenomas exhibit allelic loss of this region of chromosome 11, with mutation of the remaining allele.[224, 225]

Other genes at 11q13 have been implicated in parathyroid tumorigenesis, including *cyclin D1, SEA, Bcl-1, FAU, hst, INT2,* and *FOLR.*[226, 227] The PRAD1 pericentromeric inversion of chromosome 11 involving the PTH gene regulatory region and the cyclin D1 coding region results in upregulated expression of the cell cycle regulator, implicating this molecular mechanism as a cause of cell proliferation in a subpopulation of parathyroid adenomas.[228, 229] Another 11q13 rearrangement involving the *PTH* gene and the *INT2* gene that encodes a member of the fibroblast growth factor family has also been reported in isolated nonfamilial parathyroid adenomas.[207, 208] A parathyroid mitogenic factor with similarities to basic fibroblast growth factor (bFGF) has been identified in the plasma of patients with MEN-I.[230] Immunohistochemistry has also identified bFGF more frequently in hyperplastic glands from patients with MEN-I than non-MEN-associated hyperplastic glands[231]; however whether bFGF plays a significant role in the development of parathyroid hyperplasia, especially in MEN-I, has yet to be determined.

Other familial syndromes with hyperparathyroidism may shed light on the pathogenesis of this disorder. Parathyroid disease occurs in more than half of patients with MEN-IIA,[6] suggesting that mutations of the *ret* proto-oncogene may be important. MEN-II is characterized by the development of medullary carcinoma of the thyroid and pheochromocytoma. The syndrome is subtyped by the associated features. In MEN-IIA, the affected individuals have a normal appearance. In contrast, patients with MEN-IIB have a characteristic appearance with thickened lips, mucosal ganglioneuromatosis, and a marfanoid habitus. Clinically apparent parathyroid disease is more rare in patients with MEN-IIB than in those with MEN-IIA. MEN-IIA and -IIB are both dominantly inherited familial syndromes due to inheritance of an activated oncogene; different mutations in the same gene are responsible for the two variants of the syndrome. The gene responsible, the *RET* proto-oncogene, located at 10q11.2,[232–235] encodes a transmembrane tyrosine kinase receptor that has a large extracellular ligand-binding domain that includes a cysteine-rich segment, a transmembrane domain, and an intracytoplasmic tyrosine kinase domain.[236, 237] The receptor is the signaling partner of several related ligands in the glial-derived nerve growth factor (GDNF) family that form trimeric complexes with GDNF receptors, which do not signal, and *RET.*[238–240] More than 95% of patients with MEN-IIA have mutations affecting five codons in the extracellular cysteine-rich ligand-binding domain (codons 609, 611, 618, and 620; especially 634); each case involves a base pair substitution that replaces a cysteine with another amino acid.[232, 241–245] There are some genotypic-phenotypic correlations; for example, patients with Cys634Arg or Cys634Y mutations are those who develop parathyroid disease. In contrast to the genetic abnormalities found in MEN-IIA, more than 90% of patients with MEN-IIB have a base pair substitution within the intracellular tyrosine kinase domain (codon 918).[243, 246–248] Patients with familial medullary thyroid carcinoma, unassociated with other endocrine neoplasia, have mutations similar to those with MEN-IIA without parathyroid disease.[242–244] It is striking that sporadic medullary thyroid carcinomas and pheochromocytomas exhibit *RET* mutations similar to those of familial disease, and usually codon 918 mutations[246, 248]; however, *RET* mutations rarely play a part in the pathogenesis of sporadic parathyroid tumors.[249, 250]

The hyperparathyroidism-jaw tumor syndrome is a familial disorder in which parathyroid tumors are associated with renal polycystic disease, hamartomas, Wilm's tumor, or papillary renal cell carcinomas as well as ossifying fibromas[251, 252]; the latter may be misdiagnosed as "brown tumors" because of hyperparathyroidism. Almost one-third of patients with this rare form of parathyroid disease have parathyroid carcinomas, suggesting that the gene implicated is important for malignant transformation in this gland. This autosomal-dominant disease has been mapped to a putative TSG at 1q21-32 that exhibits LOH in the tumors of these patients.[253, 254] A subpopulation of affected patients has no parathyroid disease, and a variant of isolated parathyroid disease maps to the same genetic locus.

Other isolated familial hyperparathyroidism (FH) has been linked to the MEN-I locus as a putative variant of that disorder.[255–259] Nonendocrine disorders may be associated with FH; for example, two siblings have been reported with colonic carcinoma and primary parathyroid hyperplasia.[260] Pathologically parathyroid glands from patients with isolated FH may exhibit chief cell hyperplasia or adenomas.[211, 261]

Two classical TSGs have been implicated in malignant transformation of sporadic parathyroid neoplasms. The retinoblastoma gene *(Rb)* is a cell-cycle inhibitor that has been reported to be reduced or absent in parathyroid carcinomas.[262] Loss of one *Rb* allele at 11q13 is common in parathyroid carcinomas and is associated with loss of expression of the Rb protein detected by immunohistochemistry,[262] presumably by mutation of the remaining allele. This event appears to be responsible for metastatic potential, because the same Rb allelic deletion is present in primary tumor and in each metastasis.[262] Although allelic loss of the *Rb* gene was identified in one of 19 adenomas, there was positive immunohistochemical staining of the Rb protein, indicating there was not functional inactivation of the gene in any adenomas.[262]

Although *p53* mutations are the most common genetic alterations in human cancer, they do not appear to be a primary event in neoplastic transformation of the parathyroid glands.[263] Like Rb loss, *p53* loss appears to be responsible for malignant transformation in a subset of parathyroid carcinomas.[264] A missense mutation in the *p53* gene has been reported in one parathyroid adenoma.[265] The majority of *p53* gene mutations in human tumors occur in evolutionary conserved regions, primarily exons 5–8[266–268]; however, in parathyroid carcinomas the mutations appear to occur outside these regions.[264]

The most frequent genomic alterations in parathyroid adenomas are deletions on chromosomes 11, 17, and 22. Deletions of 1p and 17 were thought to be restricted to carcinomas[225]; however, extensive losses of chromosome 1 have been reported in up to 40% of adenomas.

p27[kip1] is another cell-cycle regulator; it is a cyclin-dependent kinase inhibitor that regulates transition from the G1 to the S1 phase of the cell cycle. Loss or downregulation of p27 has been implicated in the pathogenesis of endocrine tumors, including parathyroid neoplasms.[269] Parathyroid hyperplasias have three times more p27-positive cells than do parathyroid adenomas, suggesting that p27 immunostaining may be useful in distinguishing between these two conditions.[269] Moreover, there is progressive lowering of p27 labeling indices in the progression from normal (89.6 +/− 1.4) to hyperplasia (69.6 +/− 7.5), adenoma (56.8 +/− 3.4), and carcinoma (13.9 +/− 2.6).[270]

The pathogenetic relationship between parathyroid hyperplasia and adenoma is unresolved. Are they discrete entities or do they represent different stages of the same process? The difficulties in distinguishing the features of each disorder histologically, their occasional coexistence,[271, 272] lower serum calcium levels associated with hyperplasia compared with adenomas,[273] younger ages for patients with hyperplasia,[273] results of clonality studies,[133] and similar genetic abnormalities identified in both lesions suggest that the two diseases may be different phenotypic expressions of the same disorder, which are related temporally.

Epidemiology

PHP is a common disease,[274] although its incidence is difficult to determine. In one health survey, 1% of the adult population had hypercalcemia attributed to PHP; the prevalence approximated 3% in women older than 60 years and was markedly higher in women than in men.[275] Others quote incidence figures such as 1 in every 1000 individuals and up to 1 in every 500 women older than 45 years.[171] In one city, the average annual incidence has been determined to be 51.1 +/− 9.6 cases per 100,000 population.[276] Although PHP is primarily a disease of middle-aged and elderly women, it may afflict people of a wide age range, for example 13–88 years (mean, 58 years).[171, 273] The age and sex incidence of parathyroid adenomas reflects that of PHP generally. Parathyroid carcinoma occurs with approximately equal frequency in females and males.[175, 177, 213, 277–279] The age range of occurrence is broad; for example, 23 to 83 years in one series with a median age of 52 years for women and 45 years for men.[279] Therefore, although it is said to occur about one decade earlier than benign hyperparathyroidism,[4, 280] this is an unreliable variable for suspecting malignancy.

Clinical Manifestations

Since the advent of biochemical screening, hyperparathyroidism is typically not heralded by the classic complications of hypercalcemia (Table 5–1). The majority of patients with PHP are now detected on routine biochemistry testing. However, on detailed retrospective questioning, very few patients are truly asymptomatic; most experience vague complaints, especially of a psychiatric or neuromuscular nature, such as personality changes, backache, lassitude, anemia, and impaired concentration.[169, 171, 274, 281] Even patients with only mild, vague symptoms can have significant morbidity from osteoporosis and premature mortality from cardiovascular disease. The clinical manifestations experienced by patients with PHP generally do not differ in relation to the underlying disorder.

Biochemical studies cannot distinguish between the associated pathologic entities. Unexplained sustained elevation of the serum calcium level remains the mainstay in the diagnosis[169]; however, the calcium level may not be greatly elevated, and it may fall within the upper limit of the normal range.[274] Measurement of immunoreactive PTH levels demonstrates an absolute or relative elevation of PTH.[274] When PHP is mild, provocative tests may be useful. In some patients, radiologic analysis of the terminal phalanges of the hands may reveal subperiosteal bone resorption.

Radiologic Investigations

The success of surgical treatment of hyperparathyroidism depends to a great degree on locating the hyperfunctioning parathyroid tissue. Because of the importance of localization, various preoperative imaging methods have been used, including noninvasive techniques of ultrasonography, computed tomographic scanning, magnetic resonance imaging, positron emission tomography, radionucleotide scintigraphy (Fig. 5–5) and thermography, and invasive procedures such as arteriography, venography with selective sampling for PTH, imaging-guided biopsy/aspiration, and intraoperative ultrasonography. Intraoperative localization of radionucleotides has proved valuable. The myriad of techniques reflects the lack of consensus about the value of preoperative localization and the lack of a clearly superior technique. No single method seems capable of detecting all glands under all circumstances of varying size and location. Some investigators believe that for patients who have not had previous thyroid or parathyroid surgery, none of the

Table 5–1. Manifestations of Hyperparathyroidism

Bone	Diffuse osteopenia, subperiosteal bone resorption, dissecting osteitis, osteitis fibrosa cystica (brown tumors), pain, pathologic fractures, "salt and pepper" skull, absence of lamina dura.
Renal	Calculi (recurrent), nephrocalcinosis, renal insufficiency, polyuria, polydipsia.
Gastrointestinal	Peptic ulcers, pancreatitis, anorexia, vomiting, nausea, weight loss, constipation, abdominal pain.
Cardiovascular	Hypertension, bradycardia, tachycardia, arrhythmias, cardiac arrest, digitalis sensitivity.
Neuromuscular	Fatigue, lethargy, muscle weakness with fiber atrophy, myopathy, hyporeflexia.
Ocular	Conjunctivitis, corneal calcification (band keratopathy).
Neuropsychiatric	Headache, apathy, delirium, stupor, coma, depression, neurotic behavior, hallucinations, paranoia, psychosis, personality changes, anxiety, failing memory, impaired concentration.
Dermatologic	Soft-tissue calcification, cutaneous vascular calcification, ulceration (most common on the buttocks and extremities).
Hypercalcemic crisis	Mental depression ranging from mild lassitude to stupor, and coma precipitated by further elevation in serum calcium levels due to enforced bed rest, associated with acute renal failure; rapidly fatal course.

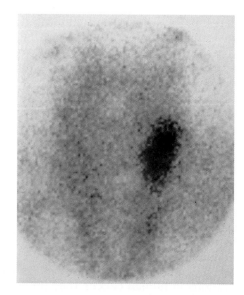

Figure 5–5. ^{99m}Tc-sestamibi scanning is helpful for localizing parathyroid lesions. Imaging of the neck 2 hours after injection identified a large abnormal parathyroid gland on the left.

radiologic approaches are as sensitive or specific for the localization of abnormal parathyroid glands as an experienced surgeon, who can achieve cure rates of 92% to 98% at the initial operation without localization techniques.[113, 142, 171, 282–284] There appears to be virtually universal agreement that both invasive and noninvasive localization procedures are warranted in the setting of repeat parathyroid surgery, which is associated with lower success rates, longer procedures, and greater complication rates.[21, 24, 107, 110, 113, 285–291] In this setting, noninvasive imaging studies are generally less sensitive due to scarring, obscuration of normal tissue planes, and greater likelihood of residual abnormal parathyroid tissue being located in ectopic or aberrant sites.[21, 113, 288, 292]

Treatment

Surgical parathyroidectomy is the only definitive cure for PHP and is recommended both for all symptomatic patients who are operative candidates and for many asymptomatic patients; the procedure carries low morbidity and mortality rates.[110, 293, 294] It has even been recommended as the best management strategy for patients older than 75 years who have hyperparathyroidism.[178]

Classically, parathyroid adenomas are treated by removal of the single enlarged gland; parathyroid hyperplasia by subtotal parathyroidectomy removing three and one-half glands. Traditionally, parathyroid surgery entails bilateral neck exploration, with visualization of all glands with/without biopsy sampling of some or all of the glands.[139, 145, 171, 288, 295] Numerous controversies exist, however. For the surgical treatment of hyperplasia, some surgeons purport conservative surgery, removing only the largest gland(s) over the more radical subtotal parathyroidectomy.[138, 139, 142, 288, 296–298] Supporters of the lesser operation advocate that the recurrence rate of hypercalcemia is not increased and that there is a lower rate of iatrogenic hypoparathyroidism. This approach has received support from those who apply intraoperative imaging to lateralize and localize the culprit gland.[299, 300] In this era of "minimally invasive surgery," the parathyroid glands have not been spared from attempted removal by endoscopic surgery.[301] Removal of a single gland without biopsy of at least one other gland can compromise definitive diagnosis[138, 142, 282, 296]; however, some investigators believe that microscopic hyperplasia is of no clinical consequence.[138, 171, 174, 282, 296]

Some studies have concluded that rapid intraoperative measurement of intact (1–84) PTH may be of value in guiding the extent of surgical exploration needed[302]; however, others have found the technique lacking.[303]

Parathyroid autotransplantation is most often used in the management of patients undergoing repeat parathyroid surgery, patients with secondary hyperparathyroidism or FH, and patients during radical thyroid operations.[21, 171, 304, 305] The role of autotransplantation during uncomplicated primary exploration for PHP is controversial.[171, 305, 306] Following total parathyroidectomy, fresh or cryopreserved fragments of parathyroid tissue are implanted into the muscles or subcutaneous tissues of the forearm or the sternocleidomastoid muscle.[305, 307, 308] The advantages include a lower incidence of persistent hypercalcemia in cases with multiglandular disease and the relative ease of managing graft-dependent hypercalcemia should it occur.

Although surgery results in at least a 90% cure rate in nonfamilial cases of PHP, treatment is less successful in patients with MEN-associated hyperparathyroidism. Even with subtotal parathyroidectomy, patients with familial disease have recurrence rates of approximately 50% within 10 years of surgery.[309] Rates of postoperative hypocalcemia are also greater in patients with MEN-I compared with nonfamilial PHP.[309] Consequently, if the diagnosis of MEN-I has been made, total parathyroidectomy and autotransplantation are advocated by some surgeons at the initial operation. Such an aggressive surgical approach is advocated in this subgroup of patients, regardless of the gross and histologic appearances of the parathyroid glands, which must all be identified for a successful outcome.

Even in the hands of experienced parathyroid surgeons, persistent (recurrent hypercalcemia within 6 to 12 months) or recurrent hyperparathyroidism (after 6 to 12 months) may occasionally occur in patients with sporadic PHP.[310–313] Surgical failure most commonly stems from an incorrect diagnosis; most commonly, failure to distinguish multiglandular disease from solitary abnormal glands, resulting in inadequate surgery.[21, 288] Other reasons for failed surgical treatment include an inability to localize the abnormal tissue due to technical inexperience or the presence of a microadenoma, supernumerary glands, or glands in ectopic locations.[17] Recurrent disease may be caused by regrowth of partially removed abnormal glands in situ or after transplantation into the neck or forearm. Recurrent or metastatic parathyroid carcinoma may also be responsible for the reappearance of hypercalcemia. Parathyromatosis is a term applied to multiple rests of hyperfunctioning parathyroid tissue scattered throughout the fibrofatty tissues of the neck and mediastinum.[110, 312, 313] It is stated to be a rare cause of failed surgical treatment of hyperparathyroidism. The origin of these disseminated rests of benign parathyroid tissue has been attributed to rupture of gland capsules with seeding of the operative field during previous surgeries, or overgrowth of parathyroid rests remaining after ontogenesis.[312, 313] This condition is likely to be most significant in patients with renal failure who have an increased risk of developing physiologically significant hypertrophy of residual parathyroid tissue.[312] In addition, as many as 0.5% to 11% of patients with failed prior operations will be found to have familial benign (hypocalciuric) hypercalcemia rather than hyperparathyroidism.[132, 171, 314]

In addition to failed treatment, other surgical complications include recurrent laryngeal nerve damage, wound infections, and hematoma formation.

Parathyroid carcinoma is managed optimally by surgery. The best initial surgical approach, however, is controversial. Wide en bloc resection incorporating any involved structures is generally advocated[175, 177, 213, 301]; however, some surgeons include an ipsilateral hemithyroidectomy and ipsilateral radical neck dissection. The value of a radical neck dissection is questionable in view of the low frequency of regional lymph node metastases.[175] The most frequent causes of death in patients with parathyroid carcinoma are complications of hypercalcemia. As serum calcium levels are directly related to tumor bulk, it is important to reduce this surgically if possible, even when cure is unlikely.[4] Medical management techniques for hypercalcemia include mithramycin, calcitonin, estrogens, saline, and furosemide or phosphates; however, these methods are often only transiently beneficial. Although less effective than surgery, some parathyroid lesions may be ablated by injection of contrast material through an angiographic catheter into the artery supplying the gland or by percutaneous injection of alcohol into the gland itself.[21, 113]

Treatment with radiotherapy has been largely unsuccessful.[4, 176] All chemotherapeutic regimens have failed to show significant benefit in lowering serum calcium or prolonging life.[176, 213]

Secondary Hyperparathyroidism

Etiology and Pathogenesis

The term secondary hyperparathyroidism (SHP) refers to parathyroid hyperplasia in response to a chronic low serum calcium level. The most common setting is chronic renal failure. The mechanisms responsible for stimulating PTH synthesis and secretion and parathyroid cell hyperplasia in chronic renal failure patients involve a relative or absolute decrease in plasma calcitriol, a decrease in plasma-ionized calcium, and an increase in plasma phosphorus.[134] SHP may also be attributed to lack of vitamin D due to dietary deficiency or abnormal metabolism, malabsorption syndromes, tissue resistance to vitamin D, severe hypomagnesemia, and pseudohypoparathyroidism.[6]

The parathyroid glands most commonly show multiglandular hyperplasia of mixed cell types; they cannot reliably be distinguished, microscopically or macroscopically, from parathyroid glands removed from patients with primary parathyroid hyperplasia or tertiary hyperparathyroidism (THP).[3, 133, 315] Upregulated expression of transforming growth factor-alpha mRNA and protein has been identified in parathyroid tissue from patients with severe SHP.[316] Parathyroid tissue also expresses epidermal growth factor receptor, indicating a possible autocrine growth-promoting mechanism in the development of SHP. The proliferative process has been considered to be polyclonal; however, it has been shown that patients with refractory uremic hyperparathyroidism may develop at least one monoclonal parathyroid tumor that usually cannot be identified morphologically.[133] These findings may have implications for management because parathyroid autografts are often performed as part of subtotal parathyroidectomy.

It is expected that in SHP, if the stimulus for PTH secretion is removed, parathyroid gland function would revert to normal.[317] However, it appears that the expected suppression of parathyroid gland function to increasing calcium levels is only relative.[4] In both PHP and SHP, the inhibitory effect of calcium on PTH release is blunted; it is thought that this is due to increases in parathyroid gland mass[318] and that a calcium-sensing defect is a late rather than early consequence of renal SHP.[250] The increased parathyroid cell mass in SHP regresses very slowly after successful renal transplantation,[319] predominantly by apoptosis.[320] Variability in the reversibility of the hyperparathyroidism may reflect polyclonality as compared with the emergence of monoclonal disease.[134]

Clinical Manifestations

Clinically, SHP is characterized by elevated serum PTH, alkaline phosphatase, and calcium levels; enlarged parathyroid glands; bone disease; and metastatic calcification.[321] The renal osteodystrophy that is typical of this disorder is due to the combined effects of excessive PTH and deficiency of vitamin D metabolites, resulting in features of both osteitis fibrosa cystica and osteomalacia, respectively.[322] Patients suffer from bone pain, pathologic fractures, and deformities. Metastatic calcification with extensive deposits of calcium in viscera, blood vessels, and soft tissues around joints is also typical of SHP. These deposits respond poorly to treatment. Calciphylaxis, which is characterized by ischemic necrosis of skin, muscles, and subcutaneous fat, may rarely develop in patients with chronic renal failure and SHP.[323]

Treatment

SHP may be treated medically; for example, with dietary restriction of phosphorus, administration of phosphate binders, calcium supplementation, and intermittent vitamin D therapy.[324]

Early administration of 1α-hydroxycholecalciferol (alfacalcidol) to patients with mild-to-moderate renal failure has been reported to suppress PTH secretion and to favorably alter the natural course of renal bone disease.[325] With disease progression, medical therapy of SHP may no longer be effective. Intraglandular injections of ethanol into the largest gland(s) under ultrasound guidance has been used to restore the responsiveness to calcitriol therapy by reducing the functioning parathyroid cell mass.[326] Surgery is the optimal long-term treatment.[327] Generally, a subtotal parathyroidectomy or a total parathyroidectomy, with autotransplantation of a portion of the parathyroid gland into neck or arm muscles or abdominal subcutaneous fat, is performed.[304] Complications of parathyroid grafts include failure of the graft to remain viable, resulting in hypoparathyroidism. Alternatively, because of the persistent stimulus, the transplanted tissue can undergo marked hyperplasia, causing recurrent hyperparathyroidism.

Tertiary Hyperparathyroidism

Most patients with SHP due to renal failure have calcium levels depressed below the normal range. If the calcium level is normal or slightly elevated, THP may be suspected. THP is a condition that occurs in the setting of SHP when parathyroid function becomes autonomous; that is, the parathyroid gland or glands continue to hyperfunction despite the stimulus being removed. Three criteria are generally required to establish the diagnosis: (1) documented renal disease with hypocalcemia followed (2) by hypercalcemia in spite of renal dialysis or transplantation and (3) subsequent return to normocalcemia with parathyroidectomy.[328] The mechanisms leading to the development of THP are unknown. It has been suggested that the error is in the calcium set point.[329] The underlying disorder is controversial. It is variously stated that there is parathyroid hyperplasia, an adenoma, or one or more adenomas on a background of hyperplasia.[315, 330, 331] This controversy is not surprising, given the difficulty in distinguishing hyperplasia from adenoma that would be complicated by a mixed process. Molecular studies have suggested that progression to THP is associated with allelic loss on chromosome 11,[332] consistent with a monoclonal tumor arising in the setting of parathyroid hyperplasia. The increased proliferative activity in SHP may heighten the cumulative risk for DNA mutations and the emergence of monoclonal neoplasms[333]; uremic patients have impaired capacity for DNA repair.[334] However, the genetic abnormalities contributing to parathyroid tumorigenesis in SHP have not been confirmed.[133, 134] Heterogeneous and multiple processes may be involved, including amplification of cyclin D1 and phosphorylation of the retinoblastoma gene product.[254] Rarely, parathyroid carcinoma may develop in the setting of SHP.[335, 336] The potential oncogenes and tumor suppressor genes that play a role in this process are discussed in the development of PHP.

Familial Benign Hypercalcemia (Familial Hypocalciuric Hypercalcemia) and Neonatal Hyperparathyroidism

Familial benign (hypocalciuric) hypercalcemia (FBH) is an autosomal-dominant condition that is fairly common but infrequently diagnosed.[337–339] It must be considered in the differential diagnosis of PHP; biochemically, it can be difficult to distinguish the two conditions.[340] FBH is a fairly common cause of persistent hypercalcemia following subtotal parathyroidectomy for presumed PHP. FBH is characterized by lifelong hypercalcemia of a degree comparable to that of typical PHP[341]; the hypercalcemia often starts in childhood. In contrast to PHP, in FBH symptoms and signs of hypercalcemia are rare.[260] More than one-third of patients are asymptomatic, and the remainder develop vague mild symptoms such as fatigue, weakness, mental symptoms, arthralgias, polyuria, polydipsia, and headaches; these symptoms are usually so mild that medical attention is not sought.[338] Biochemically, patients have a low urinary excretion of calcium relative to serum calcium levels; half have elevated serum magnesium concentrations, and renal function is well maintained.[338] The PTH levels are generally lower than in typical PHP,[342, 343] although they may be greater than normal[343, 344] or normal.[342]

One form of autosomal-dominant FBH has been found to result from a heterozygous state of inactivating mutations in the gene encoding the calcium-sensing receptor.[345, 346] Neonatal hyperparathyroidism (NH) is the consequence of homozygosity for inactivating mutations of these receptors. The kidneys are more sensitive to exogenous and endogenous PTH[347, 348] but, in addition, parathyroid gland dysfunction is an integral feature of the disorder.[337]

Unlike sporadic PHP, the raised calcium levels are very difficult to correct in FBH, and subtotal and total parathyroidectomies often give unsatisfactory results.[338, 349]

Pathologically, mild parathyroid hyperplasia has been described in the glands of these patients, whereas other researchers have reported that the majority of the glands are indistinguishable from normal parathyroid glands.[350–352]

Various other conditions have been associated with FBH in different kindreds; for example, chondrocalcinosis, pancreatitis, severe NH, and less often adult onset diabetes mellitus, cardiovascular disease, and lymphocytic thyroiditis.[338, 344, 353] The association with NH is interesting; in some infants with NH, one or both parents have FBH, suggesting that NH is the most severe phenotype of FBH and may be related to the homozygous state.[337] Not all cases of NH occur in kindreds with FBH. The diagnosis of FBH is particularly difficult to make in small families. Marx and associates listed the following features most helpful in the diagnosis: "hypercalcemia in many relatives without other features of MEN-I; recognition of hypercalcemia before the age of ten years in some members; hypercalcemia without hypercalciuria; and abnormal serum calcium levels after parathyroidectomy."[337]

NH may occur as a very rare primary disorder or secondary to maternal hypoparathyroidism.[354] Neonates with severe PHP have a life-threatening disorder characterized by hypercalcemia, muscular hypotonia, skeletal abnormalities, and failure to thrive.[337, 353, 355, 356] Typically, the symptoms of severe hypercalcemia develop during the 1st week of life. Radiologic assessment may show severe demineralization, subperiosteal resorption, pathologic fractures, and renal calcinosis.[6, 354] If this condition is not recognized, it is usually fatal within 7 months of birth.[354] The treatment of choice is total parathyroidectomy, although this may be unsuccessful in lowering the calcium level. The excised glands are of normal size or are enlarged.[357] Histologically, the glands demonstrate diffuse chief cell hyperplasia.[355, 356] One neonate with this disorder was found to have an abnormality of PTH secretory control with a high set point for secretory suppression by calcium.[358]

PATHOLOGY OF HYPERPARATHYROIDISM

Parathyroid Adenoma

Definition

Definitive criteria for the diagnosis of parathyroid adenoma are lacking. Histopathology frequently provides definitive diagnoses; however, proliferative lesions of the parathyroid glands are one realm of anatomic pathology lacking precise diagnostic criteria. By definition, an adenoma is a benign neoplastic proliferation, involving only one, or rarely two, parathyroid glands. However, in practice, it is difficult to distinguish adenoma, localized or asymmetrical hyperplasia, and carcinoma. All studies reporting epidemiologic statistics, evaluating imaging techniques, and unraveling genetic mechanisms are flawed by the lack of a gold standard against which to define these entities.

The most universal criterion used to diagnose parathyroid adenoma is involvement of a single gland. However, it is impossible to be certain of the number of diseased glands present, usually determined by the surgeon. Moreover, parathyroid glands can also be enlarged falsely on gross examination; for example, if normal parathyroid tissue is intermingled with thymic tissue.[172] Some studies have concluded that solitary parathyroid gland enlargement does not exclude hyperplasia, as up to 30% to 75% of patients with hyperplasia exhibit only one enlarged gland on gross, radiologic, and/or functional examination by selective venous sampling.[172, 359] Pathologists traditionally have not, therefore, distinguished parathyroid adenoma from hyperplasia if only one gland is submitted for pathologic examination.[146, 168, 360–363] In contrast, studies that have examined the significance of microscopic or occult hyperplasia diagnosed on biopsy alone have indicated that this feature is unimportant,[137, 364] indicating that resection of the single dominant gland in these patients is curative. Therefore, the identification of solitary gland enlargement alone cannot consistently distinguish adenoma from hyperplasia.

Another important criterion for the diagnosis of adenoma is the presence of a rim of compressed normal or atrophic parathyroid tissue around a discrete nodular lesion. This feature is identifiable only in approximately 50% to 60% of adenomas; even when identified, this feature is not entirely reliable.[6] Any enlarging mass in a parathyroid gland, whether neoplastic or hyperplastic, will cause compression of the surrounding tissues, and even a condensed fibrous capsule may be formed.[261, 360, 362, 365] Fat stains—to demonstrate more intracytoplasmic lipid in cells in the surrounding rim as opposed to within the nodular lesion—are useful to highlight true capsules and compressed rims around adenomas. Another controversy surrounding parathyroid adenomas is the existence of double or multiple adenomas, concurrently or sequentially. The reported prevalence is approximately 1% to 4% of cases of PHP.[138, 139, 174, 288] Many researchers, however, are skeptical about the possible occurrence of double adenomas.[6, 363] The alternative explanation is that the multiglandular involvement is due to asymmetric pseudoadenomatous or nodular hyperplasia. Many of the reported cases give inadequate pathologic data, family histories, and/or follow-up to exclude PHP. Harness and associates[174] have defined criteria that they believe identify the rare patient with non familial PHP caused by double adenomas:

1. More than one enlarged gland that is histologically hypercellular.
2. Operative confirmation that the remaining glands are normal in size.
3. No clinical evidence or family history of MEN syndromes or familial parathyroid disease.
4. Permanent cure of hypercalcemia by excision of the enlarged glands.

The application of these criteria requires clinicopathologic correlation but, unfortunately, what constitutes "hypercellularity" and "normal size" are not uniformly agreed upon, and hence the diagnosis of double adenomas is still questionable.

Gross Anatomy

Parathyroid adenomas may develop in any site where normal parathyroid tissue has been described. Ninety percent of adenomas arises in the superior and inferior glands in the neck, and 10% occurs within ectopic or supernumerary glands.[6]

Adenomas range in size. They may measure from less than 6 mm to approximately 10 cm. Weights may vary from less than 100 mg to several grams.[295, 366–368] They are typically round or oval nodules that are sharply demarcated from the surrounding tissues with rounded-off smooth edges due to the increased parenchymal mass (Fig. 5–6).[32] Occasionally, they are lobated.[6] Because of reduced stromal fat, adenomas are red-brown. Close gross inspection of the parathyroid gland may reveal a yellow-tan or light brown remnant of normal

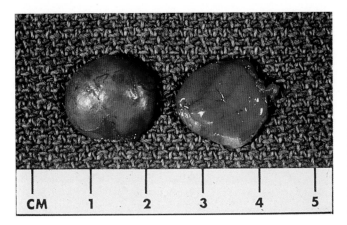

Figure 5-6. The gross appearance of a parathyroid adenoma is characteristic; these tumors are usually smooth and well encapsulated (left). Due to the reduction in stromal fat, they have a red-brown cut surface (right).

parathyroid tissue, most often at the vascular pole, beside the adenoma.[152] However, this normal rim is identified only in 50% to 60% of adenomas.[6] Larger adenomas tend to replace entire glands.[4] The cut surface of an adenoma may reveal a circumscribed nodule surrounded by a thin capsule, or the enlarged gland may have a homogeneous surface. Larger lesions may exhibit degenerative features such as hemorrhage, cystic change, fibrosis, and calcification. Occasionally, severe degeneration can result in complete cystification, and the walls may be thickened and adhere to the surrounding soft tissues.[6] A parathyroid adenoma has been described in association with a branchial cleft cyst, highlighting their common embryologic origins.[369]

Microscopic Anatomy

Parathyroid adenomas are typically encapsulated lesions, with complete, thick, lamellated, fibrous capsules.[172] Intrathyroidal hyperplastic parathyroid nodules, however, can develop thick capsules. If a rim of normal tissue is present outside an adenoma, the intervening capsule is sometimes indistinct or even absent (Fig. 5–7).[6]

Within adenomas, the cells are variably arranged into solid sheets, cords, acinar structures, and nodules (Fig. 5–8A). These architectural patterns are often intermixed (see Fig. 5–8B). Some adenomas are dominated by a follicular or acinar pattern, producing an appearance resembling thyroid parenchyma (see Fig. 5–8C). Some follicles even contain PAS-positive homogeneous eosinophilic colloid-like material; however, immunohistochemical stains for thyroglobulin are negative.[6] Sometimes the eosinophilic material is laminated and focally calcified, resembling psammoma bodies. Parathyroid adenomas frequently possess a florid yet delicate capillary network. The parenchymal cells may aggregate around the capillaries to form pseudorosettes. One author

has noted that most adenomas possess a plexiform branching vascular pattern, with vessels with thick hyaline walls or of a sinusoidal type.[172] True papillae with fibrovascular cores rarely occur in parathyroid lesions,[222, 370] but can lead to a misdiagnosis of papillary carcinoma of thyroid on FNA biopsy.[122] The cells in papillary parathyroid adenomas lack the classic cytologic features of papillary carcinoma, are immunoreactive for parathyroid hormone, are immunonegative for thyroglobulin, and lack psammoma bodies.[222, 370]

Parathyroid adenomas are composed predominantly of tightly packed chief cells, often intermingled with oxyphil and clear cells. The chief cells are often enlarged, and their nuclei show greater variability in size than chief cells in normal parathyroid glands (see Fig. 5–8A). Their cell margins are often indistinct, and the cells have pale eosinophilic cytoplasm. Oxyphil cells and transitional oxyphil cells may predominate in some tumors (see Fig. 5–8D); however, they are usually scattered diffusely or arranged in poorly demarcated nodules best seen on low power examination. Clear cells with sharp cell membranes and abundant glycogen may be similarly distributed (Fig. 5–8E). There does not appear to be any significance to the predominance of one cell type or the admixture with nodular clustering of cell types within adenomas.

Most chief cells have central, relatively small dark nuclei. Sometimes there is marked nuclear pleomorphism focally or throughout the adenoma (Fig. 5–9). These bizarre enlarged hyperchromatic single or multinucleated cells are not evidence of malignancy but are thought to be a degenerative feature. Some authors have stated that mitoses never occur in parathyroid adenomas[4] and, if present, one should suspect malignancy. However, several studies have identified mitotic figures in parathyroid adenomas and hyperplasia,[371, 372] most cases have had less

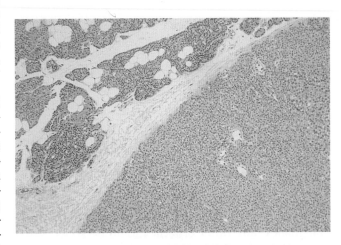

Figure 5-7. A parathyroid adenoma is uniform, devoid of stromal fat, and readily distinguished from the rim of compressed normal gland that contains abundant stromal fat. The adenoma cells are larger and more homogeneous than the cells of the normal gland.

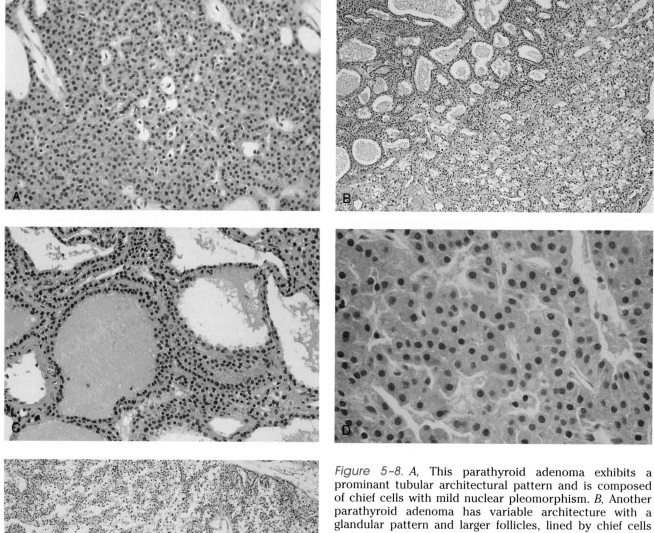

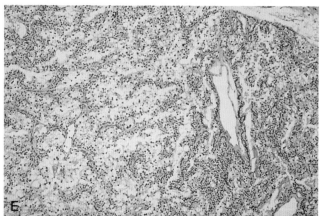

Figure 5–8. A, This parathyroid adenoma exhibits a prominant tubular architectural pattern and is composed of chief cells with mild nuclear pleomorphism. *B,* Another parathyroid adenoma has variable architecture with a glandular pattern and larger follicles, lined by chief cells and clear cells. *C,* This parathyroid adenoma forms follicles that resemble thyroid and store colloid-like material. The tumor cells are relatively monomorphic chief cells with centrally placed, hyperchromatic nuclei, pale eosinophilic cytoplasm, and indistinct cell borders. *D,* An oxyphilic adenoma is characterized by large polygonal cells with abundant granular eosinophilic cytoplasm and hyperchromatic nuclei that can show mild-to-moderate amounts of pleomorphism. *E,* This parathyroid adenoma is composed mainly of large clear cells with sharp cell membranes; glycogen is abundant in such tumors.

than 1 mitotic figure per 10 high power fields (HPF); some have more than this number. The most mitotically active adenoma in a series had 4 mitoses per 10 HPFs.[372] Mitotic figures alone, therefore, cannot be regarded as evidence of malignancy. Their presence should heighten awareness of the possibility of malignancy, and other criteria should be sought.

Parathyroid adenomas generally contain sparse stroma. Stromal fat tends to be absent or minimal within adenomas. If a rim of compressed parathyroid tissue is present outside an adenoma, it is typically composed of smaller, more uniform parathyroid cells

intermingled with abundant stromal fat (see Fig. 5–7). If fat is present within a parathyroid nodule, it does not exclude the diagnosis of an adenoma; if present, the fat cells may be dispersed or in small clusters.[32] Stroma within adenomas may also, rarely, contain focal aggregates of amyloid.

The chief cells of most adenomas contain no or only small amounts of cytoplasmic lipid.[35, 140, 148] Exceptions do occur. Some adenomas are composed of clear cells containing significant intracellular lipid. Sometimes, these lipid-bearing cells are only focally present; occasionally, they are abundant and

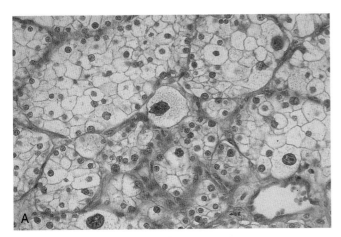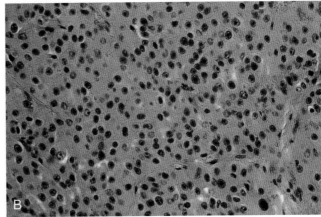

Figure 5–9. A, A large clear-cell adenoma is characterized by polyhedral cells with marked vacuolation of the cytoplasm and a honeycomb appearance. There is marked nuclear pleomorphism that does not predict malignancy. *B,* Nuclear pleomorphism is seen in many oncocytic adenomas.

throughout the adenoma.[152] Fat stains can also highlight differences between cells within adenomas and outside them. Classically, they reveal more abundant and coarser cytoplasmic fat vacuoles in the cells of the rim than in the adenoma cells.[6]

Larger parathyroid adenomas may exhibit degenerative features, such as cystic change, fibrosis, hemosiderin deposition, necrosis, foreign body reactions, and cholesterol deposits. Fibrous bands resembling those described as a diagnostic feature of parathyroid carcinoma occasionally occur in adenomas; such extensive fibrosis is usually a degenerative feature and is associated with the other degenerative features listed previously. Calcification and ossification may, rarely, be present in the capsules of large adenomas.

Precise histologic criteria are not applied universally to the diagnosis of adenoma. One set of criteria suggested by Ghandur-Mnaymneh and Kimura[172] follows. They diagnose a mass lesion as an adenoma if all of the following features are present:

1. A benign neoplasm that grows by pushing the surrounding stromal and parenchymal cells in a broad front; i.e., no stromal fat cells within the mass.
2. Expansile growth, producing a circumscribed lesion that is distinctly demarcated from the surrounding tissues at all points.
3. Lack of a lobular pattern, which is present in normal or hyperplastic glands.

These criteria tend to be stricter than those applied by most authors who would accept some fat. In one autopsy study of unselected patients dying over the age of 50 years with no abnormal calcium or phosphorus levels or metabolic or renal diseases, 16 of 20 patients had hypercellular parathyroid glands, and 7 of these were said to fulfill classic criteria of adenomas.[373] This variability in a presumably normal population confirms the non-

specificity of single morphologic features in the evaluation and classification of proliferative lesions of the parathyroid glands.

Parathyroid Glands Associated with an Adenoma

The nonadenomatous parathyroid glands accompanying an adenoma are generally indistinguishable from glands of normocalcemic individuals in terms of their size, weights, and color.[168] Occasionally, they may be smaller with lower average glandular and parenchymal weights.[374] The chief cells may be indistinguishable from those in glands from normocalcemic patients, or they may be smaller with more uniform nuclei, and often there is abundant intracellular fat reflecting suppressed endocrine secretory activity. More abundant stromal fat may also be present. In contrast to the expected findings, some authors have noted microscopic evidence of hyperplasia in normal-sized glands accompanying adenomas[137]; however, the criteria on which this diagnosis has been made are not detailed. Different series report favorable surgical outcomes whether these patients are treated by single gland removal or subtotal parathyroidectomy.[137, 364] Perhaps this represents the involuting hyperplasia that preceded development of an adenoma.

Using flow cytometry, 71% of the parathyroid glands accompanying adenomas have been found to have a diploid profile, and 29% have had tetraploid peaks reflecting cells in G2 and M phases of cell cycle, as is seen in hyperplastic and adenomatous parathyroid tissue.[157] Ultrastructurally, different patterns have also been described. Some studies report that chief cells in glands accompanying adenomas exhibit features of reduced secretory activity,[375] and others have noted features of hormonal hyperactivity despite a "normal" intracytoplasmic lipid profile with fat stains and a "normal" histologic appearance.[376] This evidence supports the opinion that many adenomas in fact represent asymmetrical hyperplasia.[157]

Special Investigations

Immunohistochemical analysis may be useful in distinguishing a parathyroid adenoma from a thyroid nodule, particularly when the architecture of the adenoma is predominantly follicular. Chromogranin A (parathyroid secretory protein 1) is identified in most normal and neoplastic chief cells, and PTH has been demonstrated in adenomas by this technique.[49, 377] Alternatively, in situ hybridization may be used to give more consistent evidence of PTH production by identifying PTH mRNA.[53] Monoclonal antibodies directed against a calcium receptor have been shown to uniformly and intensely stain normal human parathyroid tissues.[50] Adenomas, however, produced a clearly reduced intensity of staining[378]; oxyphil adenomas, in particular, gave a very weak staining pattern.

Low-molecular-weight cytokeratins (MW 52, 45, 40 kD) have been identified immunohistochemically in parathyroid adenomas; chief cells stain more strongly than oxyphils.[38] Some adenomas coexpress neurofilaments and cytokeratins, with positive staining for neurofilaments occurring in some cells in one-third of adenomas.[38] Vasoactive intestinal polypeptide, neurotensin, substance-P, gastrin-releasing peptide, calcitonin, and calcitonin gene-related peptide have all been detected in extracts of sporadic human parathyroid adenomas.[379] Potential roles in regulating PTH synthesis and release and parathyroid replication have been postulated for some of these peptides; however, it is uncertain whether the neuropeptides are synthesized by associated nerves or adenoma cells.[379] The biologic significance of these results is not known.

Immunohistochemical staining for the retinoblastoma (Rb) protein may be useful in the distinction between parathyroid carcinomas, which may be Rb protein–negative, and parathyroid adenomas, which are Rb protein–positive.[262] A positive result is regarded as a heterogeneous pattern of nuclear staining throughout representative sections of the tumor. The intensity of a positive staining reaction can vary as the levels of Rb protein are cell-cycle-dependent[380]; some adenomas exhibit weak nuclear staining, probably reflecting different mitotic rates.[262] Positive immunohistochemical staining for the p53 protein also favors a diagnosis of carcinoma rather than adenoma, although molecular studies of p53 mutations are more reliable in this differential diagnosis.[381] One study correlated high p53 immunohistochemical detection with high preoperative calcium levels of more than 1.5 mmol/L; the suggestion that this reflects a relationship between altered serum calcium regulation in hyperparathyroidism and the p53 tumor suppressor gene requires further investigation.[252]

Immunostaining for MIB-1, an antibody that labels the cell cycle–associated antigen Ki-67 in paraffin sections, has also shown differential staining patterns for benign and malignant parathyroid glands; lesions with a proliferative fraction of greater than 5% behave aggressively.[382, 383]

Parathyroid adenomas have been shown to have a varied chromosome content by static and flow cytometry; they are most commonly diploid, but varying frequencies of tetraploidy and aneuploidy have been reported.[156–158, 162] Some of the variability may be due to different histologic criteria used to classify the lesions analyzed. These studies are not able to distinguish reliably among normal, adenomatous, or carcinomatous parathyroid tissue. It is not known whether the subpopulation of adenomas with tetraploid or near-tetraploid profiles may represent a subset of parathyroid tumors that could evolve into carcinomas if allowed to progress.[159]

Due to the association between parathyroid adenomas and functional hyperactivity, one would expect electron microscopic assessment of adenomas to reveal increased synthetic and secretory activity. It is often not possible to determine whether individual cells are in a resting or synthetic state.[363] Most cells in adenomas appear by ultrastructural analysis to have lost integration of their synthetic and secretory functions.[384] Specific ultrastructural features reported to occur more frequently in adenomas include complex indigitations of plasma membranes, pleomorphic mitochondria, extensive rER and large Golgi's complexes with more vesicles.[6] The number of prosecretory and mature secretory granules, however, are said not to be increased.[263, 384] Microvillous formation has been detected on the surface of adenoma cells when there is severe hypercalcemia but not with lower serum calcium levels; it was suggested that this feature correlates with the degree of synthetic activity.[385] Molecular studies support the ultrastructural suggestion that the endocrine function of individual cells is variable; occasional cells demonstrate very strong PTH mRNA signals,[53] and many cells contain less PTH mRNA than nonadenomatous cells in the rim surrounding adenomas.

Certain ultrastructural features have been reported to suggest the diagnosis of adenoma; for example, ribosomal-lamellar complexes, which are cylindrical structures composed of spiral or concentric lamellae studded with ribosomes, and groups of centrioles.[363] The value of these features needs clarification. Annulate lamellae and intracytoplasmic microlumina have also been interpreted by some as ultrastructural markers of adenomas[34, 386, 387]; however, they have also been seen in hyperplastic glands.[363]

Electron microscopy has also been used to depict the endocrine activity of chief cells in apparently normal glands associated with enlarged glands in an attempt to aid the adenoma-hyperplasia diagnostic dilemma. It was found that even when light microscopy suggests endocrine suppression, ultrastructural examination may reveal chief cell activity, rendering a diagnosis of hyperplasia rather than adenoma.[363] It has been suggested that "microscopic hyperplasia" present in normal-sized glands is not of clinical significance; consequently, the value of determining isolated "ultrastructural hyperplasia" is not known.

Variants of Adenoma

Oncocytic Adenomas

Oncocytic adenoma is a rare subtype of adenoma (4.4% to 8.4% of adenomas) that is composed predominantly (more than 80% to 90%) or exclusively of oxyphil cells.[173, 388] Initially, oxyphil cells were considered to be incapable of secreting PTH, and hence it was thought that oxyphil adenomas were clinically nonfunctional.[389] There have been a number of reports of oxyphil adenomas associated with hyperparathyroidism.[173, 360, 388, 390, 391] This association has been explained by oxyphil adenomas containing a mixed population of cell types and that the hyperactivity is due to these other cell types.[392] Various other studies have shown that classic oxyphil cells are capable of PTH synthesis and secretion.[173, 377, 390] These tumors constitute approximately 3% to 8% of lesions associated with PHP.[173, 388] Like typical adenomas, they occur more frequently in women and are found most often in the 6th or 7th decade (range 28 to 82 years).[173, 360, 388] Most patients are asymptomatic, even if the tumor is functioning, or they experience symptoms associated with mild to moderate hypercalcemia, such as depression, nervous disorders, renal lithiasis, and hypertension.[360, 388] They have been detected almost exclusively in the neck.[173, 360, 377, 388] Grossly, the tumors tend to be large and have been reported to range in size from 0.2 to 61 g (average 1.1 to 2.8 g); they are soft, spherical, ellipsoid, lobulated, or nodular, and range in color from light tan to dark orange-brown or mahogany.[173, 360, 377, 388] The color is generally not pronounced enough to allow distinction from typical chief cell adenomas.[388] Microscopically, the adenomas are composed predominantly of polygonal cells with abundant brightly eosinophilic granular cytoplasm and small, round, central hyperchromatic nuclei (see Fig. 5–8D and 5–9B). The cells are arranged in solid sheets, anastomosing cords, and acini. Moderate nuclear pleomorphism is present in some lesions. Mitotic figures are very rare. Transitional oxyphil cells with less deeply eosinophilic cytoplasm are present in variable numbers. Fat stains show reduced cytoplasmic fat as per typical adenomas.[360, 388] Immunohistochemical staining for the mitochondrial respiratory enzyme, cytochrome c oxidase, is intense,[388] and a positive reaction for PTH has been reported.[48, 49] Numerous mitochondria are densely packed throughout the cytoplasm on ultrastructural examination (Fig. 5–10); these are round to elongated and sometimes tortuous and have numerous cristae and a variably electron-dense matrix. The nuclei are round with mild peripheral chromatin condensation and occasional nucleoli. Similar amounts of rER, Golgi's apparatus,

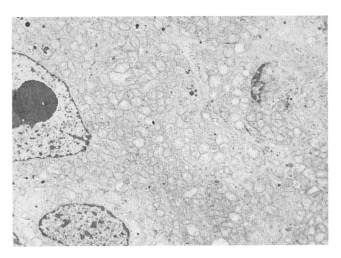

Figure 5–10. On electron microscopy, oxyphilic tumors are composed of oncocytes, cells with numerous densely packed, round-to-elongated mitochondria that have prominant cristae. Scattered subcellular organelles are recognized, including secretory granules, lysosomes, short profiles of rough endoplasmic reticulum, and glycogen particles.

and secretory granules have been identified in cells of oxyphil cell adenomas as in cells of chief cell adenomas; the amount of glycogen, however, is inversely correlated with the number of mitochondria.[393] The transitional oxyphil cells contain fewer mitochondria, more frequent rER, and more numerous prosecretory and secretory granules compared with oxyphil cells.

Lipoadenomas

Lipoadenoma is another rare subtype of adenoma that was first described in 1958 as a parathyroid hamartoma.[394] The initial description was of a nonfunctioning mass; subsequent reports documented that these lesions can be responsible for PHP.[395–400] Although they are usually located in the neck, lipoadenomas have been found in the superior[395] and posterior mediastinum.[396] The lesion comprises a lobulated yellow-tan mass composed of nests, acini, and cords of chief cells and occasional oxyphil and clear cells, intimately associated with large areas of adipose tissue and/or myxoid stroma. They are typically surrounded by a thin fibrous capsule and can vary in weight from 0.5 to 420 g.[32] Sometimes, a rim of normal parathyroid tissue is present at the periphery. The term "parathyroid adenomas with stromal components" has been proposed for these neoplasms to encompass those that contain myxomatous stroma, metaplastic bone, or other mesenchymal elements.[401]

The term "lipothymoadenoma of the parathyroid" has been coined for a variant of this entity, which is a rare cause of PHP.[402] The lesion was identified in the superior mediastinum; it consisted of a 7-cm partially cystic mass that was incompletely encapsulated and composed of mature adipose tissue, scattered nests of thymic tissue including well-developed Hassall's corpuscles, scattered inflammatory cells, and strands and nests of parathyroid clear cells. Despite the close embryologic association of the inferior parathyroid glands and the thymus, it was believed that the lesion was best classified as a neoplasm rather than as a hamartoma or malformation, given the encapsulation, autonomous function, and coexistent normal parathyroid glands.[402]

Large Clear-Cell (Light Chief-Cell) Adenoma

Histologic examination of adenomas associated with PHP occasionally reveals an adenoma composed almost entirely of polyhedral cells with marked vacuolation of the cytoplasm (see Figs. 5–8E and 5–9A).[403] PAS staining with and without diastase predigestion and/or electron microscopy demonstrates that the honeycomb appearance of the cytoplasm seen by light microscopy is due to abundant glycogen accumulation. Electron microscopic examination of this type of adenoma from a patient with MEN-I syndrome exhibited unusual forms of ER, annulate lamellae, and rail-like configurations, in continuity with conventional rER; neither feature correlated with endocrine activity or growth rates.[404] This subtype of adenoma is not of any clinical significance.

Water-Clear Cell Adenomas

Water-clear cell adenomas have been described.[405] Their existence was initially doubted, and many authors believed that they likely represented large clear-cell adenomas with glycogen accumulation rather than tumors composed of true water-clear cells whose glycogen-free cytoplasm was filled with membrane-bound vesicles. However, a report has brought this rare entity to attention,[110] and the entity is now accepted.

Atypical Adenoma

Atypical adenoma is the term used to describe parathyroid adenomas that exhibit atypical cytologic features without definite evidence of malignancy; that is, vascular and/or soft-tissue invasion or metastases.[406] The malignant potential of atypical adenomas in terms of recurrent or metastatic behavior is uncertain. These lesions may exhibit conspicuous mitoses, adherence to surrounding tissues, trabecular cellular arrangements, capsular invasion, or broad fibrous bands.[6] One such lesion consisted of a multifocal spindle-cell proliferation that was mitotically active, averaging 8 mitoses per 10 HPFs within an otherwise typical parathyroid adenoma.[407] Areas of transition between the spindled cells and more typical rounded parathyroid cells were present. DNA cytometry has shown that atypical adenomas may be diploid, diploid with evidence of proliferation, or tetraploid.[163]

Differential Diagnosis

Parathyroid adenomas need to be distinguished from parathyroid hyperplasia and parathyroid carcinoma; the difficulty of these differential diagnoses and helpful features have been discussed.

Parathyroid lesions associated with hypercalcemia and elevated PTH levels are relatively easily determined to be parathyroid in differentiation; however, nonfunctional parathyroid tumors need to be distinguished from thyroid nodules, particularly as parathyroid tissue can occur within the thyroid capsule and even within the thyroid parenchyma. Thyroid lipoadenomas with a microfollicular pattern and abundant adipose tissue can also bear a striking resemblance to parathyroid lesions. As mentioned in the light microscopic appearance of parathyroid adenomas, occasionally a follicular pattern may predominate, and colloid-like material and psammoma body-like structures may be present.[126] Deeper sectioning usually reveals areas more typical of parathyroid tissue; that is, small cells with central, round nuclei and dense chromatin with eosinophilic, oxyphilic, or clear cytoplasm arranged in cords, nests, or solid sheets. Crystals of calcium oxalate monohydrate within the lumina of follicles favor a thyroid origin as opposed to a parathyroid lesion.[408] PAS-D staining for glycogen and immunohistochemical stains for PTH, calcium receptor, chromogranin A, and thyroglobulin are all useful in distinguishing follicular thyroid tissue from parathyroid tissue. Molecular studies can reveal PTH synthesis by identifying PTH mRNA. These investigations can also be used to distinguish oxyphilic parathyroid adenomas from Hürthle's cell thyroid nodules.

On FNA biopsy, one case of parathyroid adenoma was misdiagnosed as a papillary thyroid carcinoma because of the presence of papillary structures.[118] True papillae rarely occur in parathyroid adenomas,[222, 370] and nuclear grooves, intranuclear cytoplasmic pseudoinclusions, and thyroglobulin immunoreactivity should readily distinguish papillary thyroid carcinomas.

Thyroid C-cell lesions also need to be considered in the differential diagnosis of parathyroid adenomas. Medullary carcinoma cells generally have finely granular eosinophilic cytoplasm, larger and more vesicular nuclei, and immunohistochemical positivity for calcitonin, calcitonin gene-related peptide, and carcinoembryonic antigen, in addition to chromogranin-A positivity.

Parathyroid Carcinoma

Definition

Parathyroid carcinoma is a rare malignant neoplasm derived from the parenchymal cells of the parathyroid glands. It has been reported to be responsible for 0.1% to 5.0% of cases of PHP.[4, 6, 175–177, 213, 301, 409]

It remains uncertain whether parathyroid carcinomas arise in preexisting benign parathyroid lesions.[272, 409] There are occasional reports of carcinomas arising in the setting of primary parathyroid hyperplasia[410]; some of these have occurred in the setting of FH.[212, 411] Patients with SHP have also developed carcinomas.[335, 336] The rarity of these cases questions the significance of a hyperplasia-neoplasia progression. Reports claiming carcinomas arising in preexisting adenomas are complicated by the diagnostic difficulties involved in distinguishing hyperplasia, adenomas, and carcinomas and recurrent hyperparathyroidism after inadequate treatment of patients with hyperplasia and adenomas. Familial parathyroid carcinoma has been reported in the absence of preceding hyperplasia.[412] The constitutional karyotypes from this kindred were normal. Three clones of tumor cells, each with different chromosomal abnormalities [a reciprocal translocation between chromosomes 3 and 4 46,XY,t(3;4); trisomy 7 47,XY +7; a pericentric inversion in chromosome 9 46,XY,inv(9) (p24q12)] were identified from tissue removed from one patient at different operations for local recurrences. Tumor tissue from two other patients lacked chromosomal abnormalities. The significance of these mutations is not yet known, but such rare familial tumor syndromes may lead to the identification of new growth-regulating genes. Patients with hyperparathyroid–jaw tumor syndrome also develop parathyroid carcinoma.[251–254]

Only rare patients with parathyroid carcinoma have a history of prior neck irradiation.[177, 409, 413] One carcinoma developed 53 years after neck irradiation for exophthalmic goiter,[409] and another developed in a parathyroid gland already chronically stimulated because of chronic renal failure, approximately 3 years after neck irradiation for laryngeal carcinoma.[413] The etiologic significance of prior irradiation, however, is not known.

Morphologic features diagnostic of malignancy in parathyroid lesions are difficult to define, identify, and apply. In one series of 40 patients with metastatic parathyroid cancer, as many as 50% were thought to have benign disease by the surgeon and by the pathologist at the initial operation.[279] Metastases are the only certain sign of malignancy; however, metastatic behavior is rare at presentation.[175] Many other purported features of parathyroid carcinoma, such as adherence to surrounding tissues, local invasion, vascular invasion, fibrous bands dividing the lesion, trabecular cellular arrangement, and mitoses, may be present to some extent in benign tumors or are easily misinterpreted. As discussed later, each of these features is of value in the morphologic assessment of malignancy in parathyroid lesions, but no single feature is pathognomonic of malignancy, other than a metastasis.

Gross Anatomy

Parathyroid carcinomas are characteristically large tumors, with as many as 32% to 50% being palpable

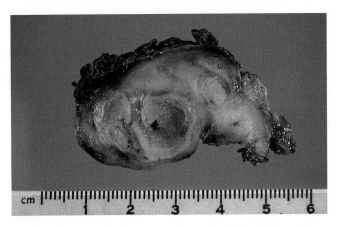

Figure 5–11. Parathyroid carcinoma tends to exhibit fibrosis, necrosis, and invasion with adherence to surrounding structures.

on presentation.[175, 176] The tumors may measure 1.5 to 6 cm in diameter, with a mean of 3 cm.[175] Although the average weights of carcinomas are reported to be greater than those of adenomas, there appears to be great overlap; carcinomas range from 0.6 to 110 g, with the majority weighing between 2 and 10 g; adenomas range from 0.05 to 120 g.[295, 366–368, 409] Carcinomas usually arise in the upper or lower parathyroid glands,[175] although they can occur in ectopic supernumerary glands; for example, in the mediastinum.[414] The majority of parathyroid carcinomas are firm or hard in consistency and gray-white, as opposed to adenomas, which tend to be soft and tan.[175, 213, 409] Adherence of the lesion to surrounding tissues (Fig. 5–11) is common,[213, 409] and this may be noted by the surgeon attempting to excise the gland.[176] However, surgeons' opinions regarding the presence of macroscopic infiltration by the tumor has been shown not to correlate with histologic evidence of microscopic infiltration.[415] Previous surgery renders this feature unreliable, because postoperative fibrosis can cause benign glands to be adherent. Similarly, previous hemorrhage into an adenoma may be associated with fibrosis and adherence to adjacent structures.[4, 409] In the absence of hemorrhage or previous surgery, long-term follow-up of cases exhibiting adherence is recommended as many of these tumors behave as carcinomas.[4] Some carcinomas, however, are encapsulated, are easily removed surgically, and are grossly indistinguishable from an adenoma.[6, 175]

Metastases at the time of presentation are unusual, but they rarely may be found in regional lymph nodes.[175, 279] Parathyroid carcinoma is more often associated with widespread local infiltration, with invasion into contiguous structures such as thyroid, strap muscles, and the recurrent laryngeal nerve. When advanced, however, metastases may be found in the lungs, bone, cervical and mediastinal lymph nodes, liver, and occasionally in kidney, adrenal glands, and pancreas.[32, 175, 176, 279, 280] Pulmonary metastases are by far the most common distant metastases.[279]

Microscopic Anatomy

The amount of cellular differentiation can vary both within and between parathyroid carcinomas, ranging from adenoma-like tumors to anaplastic lesions.[6, 32] Parathyroid carcinomas are usually composed mainly of chief cells; however, oxyphil and transitional oxyphil cells may be found and may even predominate.[279, 416] In general, tumor cells in parathyroid carcinomas tend to be larger than those in adenomas and have greater mean diameters (carcinomas: 8.1 +/− 1.4 μm; adenomas: 5.8 +/− 0.8 μm), but there is substantial overlap in the range of nuclear diameters.[213, 417] The nuclear-to-cytoplasmic ratio is generally increased; nucleoli may be inconspicuous to prominent (Fig. 5–12A), and the cytoplasm may be clear, amphophilic, or eosinophilic, even within different regions of the same malignant neoplasm. Cellular atypia is often minimal in parathyroid carcinomas, with the cells having a uniform cytologically bland appearance, although there is usually some amount of hyperchromasia and variability in nuclear size.[176, 213] Nuclear pleomorphism is more typical of parathyroid adenomas, although some carcinomas exhibit marked pleomorphism and anaplasia (see Fig. 5–12B).[6, 7] In one series of 40 metastatic parathyroid cancers, 65% of tumors was described as exhibiting "severe nuclear atypia."[279]

Although the presence of mitoses has been purported to be the single most important criterion for the diagnosis of parathyroid carcinoma,[280] the value of this feature is debated. In addition, mitotic counting has many difficulties. Eighty to one hundred percent of parathyroid carcinomas demonstrate mitoses,[6, 176, 213, 279, 409] although they may not be numerous. In fact, lesions with no mitoses have been associated with recurrent or metastatic disease or have resulted in the patient's demise.[280] Carcinoma should be considered if abnormal mitotic figures in particular are identified.[409] Mitotic figures may also be found in hyperplastic and adenomatous parathyroid tissues with more than 1 per 10 HPFs being reported in up to 20% of benign proliferative parathyroid lesions.[371, 372] Mitoses have been noted in 71% of parathyroid adenomas in a series.[372] Although mitotic counts may be of limited value in distinguishing benign and malignant lesions, they may provide important prognostic information by identifying a clinically more aggressive subgroup of parathyroid carcinomas. Among metastatic carcinomas, frequent mitoses (>5 per HPF) have been described as occurring "often," although exact quantitative details were not included.[279] Among carcinomas selected on the basis of invasive growth, local recurrence, and/or distant metastases, mitotic rates in excess of 5 per 50 HPFs, macronucleoli, and necrosis (see Fig. 5–12C) were associated with tumors that were more aggressive in terms of recurrent or metastatic disease.[161] Another study compared carcinomas diagnosed on histologic grounds only, without clinical evidence of malignant behavior, and carcinomas with histologic and clinical features of malignancy (distant metastases and/or recurrences); mitotic counts were signifi-

cantly greater in the clinically aggressive group (3.75 mitoses per 10 HPFs versus 0.5 mitoses per 10 HPFs in the "morphology only" carcinomas; $p < .01$).[382] There was no significant difference between the "morphology only" carcinomas and parathyroid adenomas or hyperplasias. Interestingly, other than the constant presence of extensive vascular invasion in the aggressive carcinomas, no other morphologic feature distinguished these two groups of tumors.[382] When counting mitotic figures in individual cases, the limitations of this technique must be considered. Inaccuracies in mitotic counts arise if tissues are poorly fixed, fixation is delayed, or sections are cut thickly or overstained.[418] True parenchymal cell mitoses must be distinguished from pyknotic nuclei and mitoses in the stromal components of the neoplasm.[280]

The architectural arrangement of tumor cells in parathyroid carcinomas is variable even within single lesions. The tumors may form large sheets or be arranged in trabecular or pseudorosette patterns, with cells oriented in a regular fashion around thin-walled blood vessels (see Fig. 5–12D) or central noncellular areas.[409] These two patterns have been described as suggestive of malignancy[409]; however, nuclear palisading may also be present in hyperplasia and adenomas.[6] A predominantly solid growth pattern has been noted to be more typical within metastatic parathyroid cancers than a trabecular growth pattern, which occurred only in 20% of such cases.[279]

Thick fibrous bands, mitotic activity, capsular and vascular invasion, and trabecular cellular architecture have been described as principle features distinguishing carcinomas from adenomas.[280, 409] Suspicion of carcinoma should be aroused if the fibrous trabeculae that irregularly subdivide the tumor are composed of dense, hyaline collagenous tissue rather than loose connective tissue.[409] Dense fibrous bands were described in up to 90% of cases of carcinoma in one series.[280] These bands may extend from the surrounding capsule and penetrate the tumor; capsules of parathyroid carcinomas tend to be thicker than those of adenomas of a similar size.[280] Loose, fibrous trabecula and dense fibrosis associated with hemosiderin and chronic inflammation reflecting degenerative changes may be present in adenomas.[280, 409]

Invasive behavior is a feature of malignacy. Parathyroid carcinomas tend to infiltrate in tongue-like protrusions into the encapsulating fibrous tissue and sometimes through the capsule into the surrounding soft tissues, thyroid parenchyma (see Fig. 5–12E), nerves, or esophagus. Local invasion is more common at presentation than lymph node metastases.[4] In the series reported by Wynne and associates, all cases had infiltration into the fibrous capsule, and most had involvement of surrounding tissues, but the frequency of these features depend on the criteria used for the classification of a lesion as a carcinoma.[213] Although tumors were occasionally adherent to the thyroid gland, invasion of the latter was not common.[213] True capsular invasion needs to be distinguished from pseudoinvasion, which may be seen in large adenomas of long standing where there may have been prior hemorrhage with consequent fibrosis and "trapping" of nests of tumor cells within the capsule.[4] Vascular invasion has been reported in approximately 10% to 15% of parathyroid carcinomas (see Fig. 5–12E and F).[280] Some regard this feature as "virtually diagnostic of malignancy,"[6] and others have identified it in large but otherwise typical adenomas and have not considered it diagnostic of malignancy.[409] To fulfill the criteria of vascular invasion, some authors require at least partial attachment to the wall of the vascular channel[6] or associated thrombosis, and others define it as positive only if present outside the

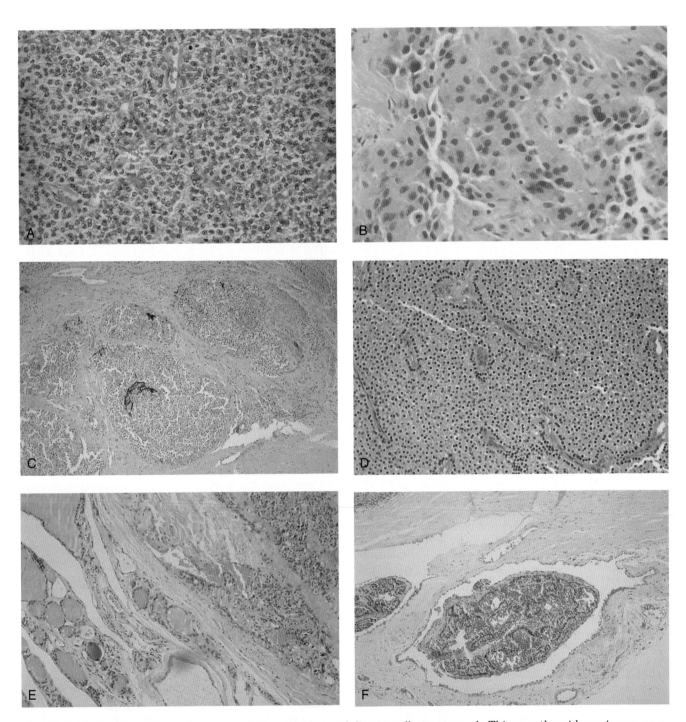

Figure 5-12. Parathyroid carcinomas exhibit marked variability in cell structure. *A,* This parathyroid carcinoma composed of chief cells shows nuclear crowding and enlargement with hyperchromasia and prominent nucleoli but minimal pleomorphism. *B,* This parathyroid carcinoma is composed of large, incohesive, and less well differentiated oxyphils with focal marked nuclear atypia. *C,* Parathyroid carcinomas are characterized by a solid architectural growth pattern with formation of thick, fibrous bands and focal tumor necrosis. *D,* This parathyroid carcinoma exhibits a solid architectural growth pattern with palisading around vascular channels. *E,* Parathyroid carcinomas invade into adjacent thyroid parenchyma, and vascular involvement is diagnostic of malignancy. *F,* Unequivocal vascular invasion with associated thrombus predicts malignant behavior with metastatic spread.

vicinity of the neoplasm.[4] Perineural invasion by parathyroid carcinoma is rarely identified but again suggestive of malignancy if present. Focal necrosis was recorded in nearly 50% of metastatic parathyroid cancers in one series,[279] and the presence of otherwise unexplained necrosis should alert one to search for other histologic features of malignancy.

Special Investigations

In addition to simple mitotic counts, a number of other measures of proliferative activity have been used to study parathyroid tumors, including flow cytometric DNA analysis and monoclonal antibodies to components of proliferating cells. Ploidy studies have identified parathyroid carcinomas that are diploid (5/15 cases), aneuploid (6/15 cases), and tetraploid (4/15 cases).[156] It has been suggested that carcinomas that are aneuploid behave more aggressively than those that are diploid.[165] Carcinomas have been reported to have a higher mean nuclear DNA content than adenomas or normal glands.[163] Because of the overlap of results, however, ploidy is generally not helpful in the differential diagnosis of parathyroid carcinoma and adenoma.[160] In contrast, S-phase fractions may be helpful. One group reported that the mean S-phase fractions in parathyroid carcinoma is 6% compared with 1.2% in normal glands, 1.5% in adenomas, and 0.8% in secondary hyperplasia; therefore, a diagnosis of carcinoma can be made if the mean S-phase fraction is greater than 4% and the DNA index is over 1.2, regardless of ploidy results.[156]

Another technique used to assess proliferative activity of tumors is immunohistochemical staining with the monoclonal MIB-1 antibody, which detects the cell cycle–associated marker, the Ki-67 antigen, in paraffin sections. A study has shown that the mean tumor proliferative fraction (TPF), expressed as the number of Ki-67–positive nuclei per 1000 cells, is significantly greater in parathyroid carcinomas in comparison to normal, hyperplastic, and adenomatous parathyroid glands (TPF 60.5 in carcinomas, 0.8 in normal glands, 26.0 in hyperplasias, 32.8 in adenomas).[382] In addition to being diagnostically useful for distinguishing carcinomas from adenomas, the results of this study suggest that MIB-1 staining may also yield prognostic information, as it was also found to discriminate between clinically aggressive carcinomas and histologically invasive but clinically indolent tumors.[382] The authors concluded that tumors with a TPF lower than 50 were always associated with benign behavior, and a TPF greater than 60/1000 cells was indicative of aggressive behavior; the intermediate scores between 50 to 60 were of indeterminate behavior, with both benign and aggressive lesions having such counts.[382] Another group found that Ki-67 is useful in distinguishing parathyroid adenoma from carcinoma, although the group found overlaps in the proliferative indices in these two diseases.[419] Additional studies are needed to determine the reliability of proliferation markers to distinguish carcinoma from adenoma.

Another special technique used in recent years to discriminate between benign and malignant tumors, including parathyroid lesions, is the enumeration of nucleolar organizer regions (NOR), highlighted by silver stains that produce nuclear black dots (AgNORs) due to the argyrophilia of the acidic nonhistone proteins associated with the loops of ribosomal RNA. The mean number of AgNORs in hyperplastic and adenomatous glands has been found not to differ significantly from counts in normal parathyroid glands. In comparison, a significantly greater number was found in carcinomatous parathyroid glands, and there was greater variability in the size and configuration of the dots.[221, 420] Although occasionally the aggregation of chromatin in the nuclei of parathyroid carcinoma cells may interfere with the interpretion of AgNOR stains, this approach may be another technique to help distinguish benign and malignant parathyroid lesions.[221, 420]

Immunohistochemical staining for the protein products of tumor suppressor genes may also be useful diagnostically; for example, parathyroid carcinomas are reported to lack staining for the Rb protein, and there is positive staining in adenomas.[262] Lack of Rb immunostaining reflects functional inactivation of both Rb alleles, which is said to be important in the pathogenesis of parathyroid carcinomas.[262] These data remain to be verified. In our experience, parathyroid carcinomas with proven metastases can be Rb protein–immunoreactive. Although p53 mutations occur much less frequently than loss of Rb gene function in parathyroid carcinomas, p53 mutation has not been identified in parathyroid adenomas; consequently, it may, along with Rb inactivation, be a potentially useful molecular marker for carcinoma of the parathyroids. Although immunohistochemical staining for p53 protein often implies the presence of a mutant p53 protein with a prolonged half-life,[421] this technique is less reliable than molecular studies, as nuclear staining may reflect accumulated wild-type p53 protein.[381, 422]

Ultrastructural examination of parathyroid carcinomas has been limited. No specific features at the electron microscopic level have been found to be diagnostic of parathyroid carcinoma. However, some suggest that an "angry nucleus" with electron-dense clumps of chromatin dispersed throughout the karyoplasm is suggestive of malignancy,[409] whereas others describe enlarged nuclei with prominent and frequently multiple nucleoli and focal loss of nucleolemma with intracytoplasmic spill of nuclear material occurring in carcinomas but not in adenomas.[423] These features, however, need to be confirmed as markers of malignancy. Long-spacing collagen has been identified in one case of parathyroid carcinoma as a nonspecific finding.[424] Others describe hypertrophic and homogeneously electron-dense nucleoli and "disorganization" of cytoplasmic organelles.[363]

As these special techniques generally fail to distinguish parathyroid adenomas from nonaggressive parathyroid carcinomas, they do not aid the resolution of this histopathologic diagnostic dilemma.

The solution will most likely require a multiparametric approach using such analyses as traditional morphology, proliferative markers, and DNA studies including genetic studies to detect mutations in oncogenes and tumor suppressor genes.[418]

Differential Diagnosis

The distinction between parathyroid carcinoma and parathyroid adenoma is very difficult; a definitive diagnosis of carcinoma can really only be made in the presence of metastases, vascular or capsular invasion, or infiltrative growth through the surrounding capsule into the adjacent tissues. Other features such as mitoses, acellular fibrous bands, a trabecular growth pattern, and gross adherence to surrounding tissues can suggest the diagnosis of carcinoma, but without the definitive criteria this diagnosis should not be made, as all of these features are occasionally seen in benign parathyroid lesions. Atypical mitoses and perineural invasion are uncommon but again highly suggestive of carcinoma. In the absence of definitive criteria of malignancy, the presence of the above features may warrant the diagnosis of atypical adenoma to indicate uncertain malignant potential.

Three clinical circumstances in which benign parathyroid tissue can have an infiltrative growth pattern and mimic carcinoma are (1) intraoperative spillage of benign parathyroid tissue, (2) hyperplasia of parathyroid rests remaining after ontogenesis, occurring particularly in the setting of chronic renal failure, and (3) parathyroid autografts being embedded in arm and neck muscles following total parathyroidectomy. When benign parathyroid tissue has been "spilled" in the operative field, multiple implants of parathyroid tissue may grow; histologically, these implants have lacked prominent mitotic activity and vascular invasion despite the infiltrative growth.[425] Parathyroid autotransplants, when removed because of graft-induced hyperparathyroidism, have exhibited nodular hyperplasia with focal nuclear pleomor-

phism, occasional mitotic figures, and a distinctly invasive growth pattern with small nests and islands of vascularized parathyroid tissue growing into the adjacent tissues.[426] In patients with true locally recurrent carcinomas, in addition to extensive soft-tissue infiltration, there is typically vascular invasion and prominent mitotic activity.[6]

Parathyroid carcinomas, particularly nonfunctioning tumors, need to be distinguished from thyroid carcinomas, of both follicular and C-cell origin, and other malignancies, such as renal cell carcinoma. Amyloid has even been reported in one case of an intrathyroidal nonfunctioning parathyroid carcinoma.[427] The correct diagnosis was reached using immunohistochemistry; the tumor cells were immunoreactive for PTH, and there was no staining with antibodies to thyroglobulin and calcitonin. These immunohistochemical stains can also be used to distinguish parathyroid carcinomas with a follicular architecture from follicular thyroid carcinomas and oxyphilic parathyroid carcinomas from Hürthle's cell thyroid tumors.

Prognosis

Parathyroid carcinoma usually pursues an indolent course, typified by prolonged survival with numerous local recurrences and metastatic behavior late in the disease.[213] Multiple recurrences many years after treatment are not uncommon, despite being normocalcemic after the initial resection.[213, 277] In one study, two groups of patients with recurrent disease were noted, those whose recurrence was an early manifestation and those whose recurrence was after a long disease-free interval (overall 228 months, median 33 months).[279] Early recurrences generally indicated a poor prognosis.[279, 428] Morbidity and mortality from parathyroid carcinoma are generally attributable to complications of severe hypercalcemia (Fig. 5–13).[278] Metastases have been reported in only 30% of patients with parathyroid carcinoma.[280] Nonfunctioning carcinoma may be a more

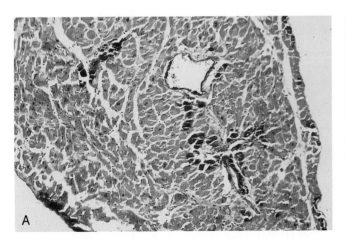
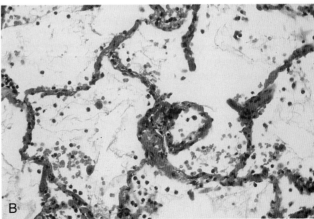

Figure 5–13. Patients with disseminated parathyroid carcinoma develop severe refractory hypercalcemia that can result in calcinosis of heart *(A)* and *(B)*. The cause of death is usually attributed to these complications.

aggressive disease with larger primary lesions, more invasive behavior, and more frequent metastases out of the neck; however, this apparent aggressive behavior may only reflect later detection of the neoplasm.[278] The 5-year survival rate in various series ranges from 30% to 69%.[175, 277, 279, 280]

Chief Cell Hyperplasia

Definition

Chief cell hyperplasia describes a proliferative condition of the parathyroid parenchymal cells that results in an absolute increase in parenchymal cell mass and weight. The proliferation typically involves all four parathyroid glands. The involvement is often not uniform, and it may manifest as gross enlargement of one, two, three, or four glands. Two patterns have been described, diffuse hyperplasia, which is rather uncommon and results in uniformly enlarged glands, and the far more frequent pattern, nodular hyperplasia, in which the increased parenchymal cells form nodular aggregates and asymmetrically enlarged glands. The disorder can occur in a variety of settings; PHP, SHP, THP, and FH, including in association with MEN syndromes. Classically, it has been said that 10% to 15% of cases of PHP are attributed to chief cell hyperplasia; however, based on a lack of consistent diagnostic criteria, a wide range of frequencies have been quoted, from 1.3% to 84%.[172] The prevalence appears to increase with age.[6] Approximately 20% to 30% of patients with chief cell hyperplasia have FH or one of the MEN syndromes.[46] The stimulus inducing parenchymal cell proliferation is unknown in PHP and FH; in SHP, hypocalcemia induces increased PTH secretion. The clinicopathologic features, including the etiology, epidemiology, and clinical manifestations in relation to each of the above settings were discussed in the section on Hyperparathyroidism: Clinical Features.

Gross Anatomy

As previously mentioned, chief cell hyperplasia is an abnormality of all parathyroid glands. The natural course of the hyperplasia may be a very slow progression, and one, two, three, or four glands may be enlarged at any one time.[172] The discrepancy in size between the glands may be great, sometimes resulting in very large glands in association with one or two normal-sized glands (Fig. 5–14). Consequently parathyroid hyperplasia is occasionally indistinguishable from an adenoma on gross inspection. The lower glands are reported to be more often enlarged than the upper glands; ectopic parathyroid tissue and intrathyroidal and mediastinal glands (Fig. 5–15) may also be hyperplastic.[137, 172, 429] In a series of 441 patients with PHP, only about 15% of patients with parathyroid hyperplasia had four symmetrically enlarged glands. The majority of these cases were wa-

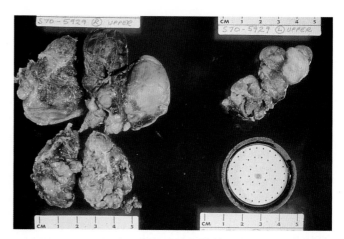

Figure 5–14. Parathyroid hyperplasia usually results in asymmetrical enlargement of all four glands, with striking variation in size. In this case, the left lower gland is normal; the others are markedly enlarged and infiltrative.

ter-clear cell hyperplasia (see Microscopic Anatomy) or were associated with MEN syndromes.[273]

Hyperplastic glands may be round to oval or be irregular in shape. Like adenomas, they are soft and red-brown. Generally, the cut surface is homogenous, although occasionally nodularity may be evident grossly.

Microscopic Anatomy

Parathyroid glands afflicted by chief cell hyperplasia contain an increased number of parenchymal cells; chief cells are the predominant cell type, hence the terminology. Oxyphil and transitional oxyphil cells, however, are commonly present and may be abundant. Clear cells may also be admixed among the other cell types.

Stromal fat cells, the other major component within parathyroid glands, are typically reduced in

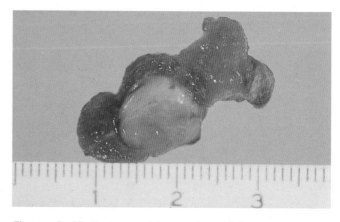

Figure 5–15. Patients with parathyroid hyperplasia may have ectopic or supernumerary glands that require resection to alleviate the clinical symptoms. In this patient, an intrathyroidal parathyroid gland is obviously enlarged with nodular hypercellularity.

hyperplastic glands. The irregular distribution of fat within single glands and the difficulty in defining the amount of fat consistent with a normal gland makes this diagnostic feature of questionable practical value unless markedly abnormal. A 50:50 parenchymal-cell-to-fat-cell ratio was once considered normal for parathyroid glands in adults; from autopsy studies without parathyroid disease, it appears that normal glands in adults can have as little as 10% to 17% stromal fat.[11, 29] Occasionally, hyperplastic glands can contain abundant stromal fat; the term lipohyperplasia was coined for these cases.[430] In the original description, most of these glands were massively enlarged, weighing 100 to 200 mg. Biopsy specimens from hyperplastic glands may be composed predominantly of adipose tissue or of parenchymal cells, depending on the site of the biopsy. This feature in glands with abundant fat complicates the diagnosis and emphasizes the importance of the gross appearance of all parathyroid glands.

Diffuse chief cell hyperplasia is characteristically composed of solid masses of cells with minimal-to-absent stromal fat. (Fig. 5–16A). In contrast, nodular chief cell hyperplasia, also termed adenomatous or pseudoadenomatous hyperplasia, is characterized by circumscribed nodules of cells (Fig. 5–16B), each nodule composed of a single cell type; less stromal fat is generally present within the nodules, compared with the internodular and perinodular zones. The parenchymal cells are arranged in solid sheets, cords, micronodules, acinar structures or, most commonly, a mixture of all patterns. Nodules may be solitary or multiple. The nodules may be surrounded by fibrous connective tissue, mimicking a capsule, or demarcated by predominance of different cell types or patterns. Large thick-walled blood vessels with fibromuscular walls, as described in normal glands, are also present in hyperplastic parathyroid glands.[172]

The chief cells within hyperplastic glands are often enlarged with large nuclei and mild nuclear variability. Marked nuclear pleomorphism is more characteristic of parathyroid adenomas; however, occasional enlarged hyperchromatic nuclei may be present in hyperplastic glands.[362] The cytoplasmic fat content within these hyperplastic cells is generally reduced; the degree of reduction is generally not uniform throughout the gland. Sometimes the cells within discrete nodules contain less fat than the cells in the intervening parenchyma. If stromal fat cells are also more frequent in the intervening zones, these areas can mimic a "normal compressed rim" around a parathyroid adenoma. Sometimes hyperplastic parathyroid cells can contain abundant cytoplasmic fat. Mitotic figures may be frequent in hyperplastic glands.[371, 372] One report noted mitoses in 80% of cases of PHP and SHP, with the majority (60%) having less than 1 mitotic figure per 10 HPFs.[372] However, up to 5 per 10 HPFs were seen in one case of chief cell hyperplasia in a patient with MEN-2.[372] When hyperplastic glands become markedly enlarged, cysts and other degenerative features, such as fibrosis and hemosiderin deposition, may be seen. These features make the distinction of infiltrative hyperplasia from carcinoma difficult.

Two histologic features helpful in distinguishing hyperplasia and adenoma are a clearly defined lobular arrangement and a lack of circumscription within hyperplastic glands.[172] In chief cell hyperplasia, the parenchymal tissue lacks sharp delineation, and it infiltrates surrounding tissues. When this irregularity at the periphery of glands is pronounced, the term parathyromatosis[431] has been applied; it refers to multifocal aggregates of hyperplastic parathyroid cells distributed within the soft tissues surrounding a hyperplastic parathyroid gland. It is thought that these clusters of cells may arise from stimulation of embryonic nests of parathyroid cells that are scattered throughout the neck and mediastinum

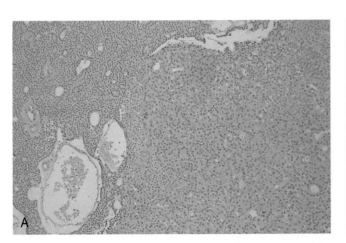 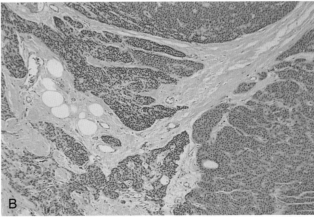

Figure 5–16. A, In diffuse chief cell hyperplasia, the gland is composed of solid masses of cells of a single cell type. B, Circumscribed nodules in this case of nodular hyperplasia resemble adenomatoid lesions. This patient had involvement of several glands. Hyperplastic parathyroid glands can exhibit marked fibrosis, which may make the distinction from infiltrating carcinoma difficult.

during development. They are thought to be inconspicuous normally, but they enlarge during diffuse hyperplasia of the parathyroid glands. The term parathyroma is also applied to scattered nests of benign parathyroid tissue around an operative field, where prior spillage of parathyroid tissue is the attributed cause.

Secondary parathyroid hyperplasia cannot be distinguished from primary hyperplasia, although at least early in the disorder there is a greater tendency for the glands to be more uniform in size.[32] As the disease progresses, asymmetry becomes more evident. The amount of glandular enlargement tends to reflect the severity of the underlying process.[6] The largest glands are seen in patients whose disease started in childhood.[432] There are also no unique pathologic features that are characteristic of THP. In fact, there is controversy over the most common-associated disorder; for example, hyperplasia of a diffuse or nodular type combined diffuse and nodular hyperplasia, adenomas, or multiple adenomas on a background of hyperplasia.[330, 331] In fact, the most striking feature observed in a study of 31 parathyroid glands from 11 patients with THP was the "extreme variability," both morphologically and functionally, as indicated by PTH immunoreactivity.[433] In this study, the authors noted that the spectrum of morphologic changes were very similar to those described in patients with primary chief cell hyperplasia with and without evidence of MEN syndromes; only more prominent degenerative changes and greater gland weights seemed peculiar to THP.[433] Ultrastructurally, the majority of cells show evidence of high secretory activity.[328, 393]

Special Investigations

Studies of proliferative activity have been performed on parathyroid glands from patients with renal hyperparathyroidism, including analysis of autotransplantation grafts that have been associated with recurrent graft-induced hyperparathyroidism. Using an antiproliferating cell nuclear antigen (PCNA) antibody, proliferative activity has been shown to be significantly greater in nodular hyperplastic glands than in diffusely hyperplastic glands.[434] In this study, all cases where there was graft-induced recurrent hyperparathyroidism, the graft had been taken from nodular tissue.[434] In another study, nodular foci in both adenomas and hyperplasias exhibited consistently higher PCNA or MIB-1 labeling than diffuse areas.[435] These results support the previously empirical surgical approach where the smallest diffusely hyperplastic parathyroid gland is used for graft autotransplantation.

Electron microscopic examination of most parathyroid glands with chief cell hyperplasia confirms the presence of an admixture of parenchymal cell types. The cells are in an active stage of endocrine secretion with hypertrophic Golgi's apparatus, abundant rER, scarce cytoplasmic lipid, and prominent interdigitations of plasma membranes.[363, 393]

It has been suggested that electron microscopy may aid in the adenoma-hyperplasia diagnostic dilemma, especially when only one enlarged gland and one normal-sized gland are available for assessment; ultrastructural examination may reveal chief cell secretory activity in the small gland, rendering a diagnosis of hyperplasia that may have been unexpected from the gross and light microscopic examinations.[363] Cinti and associates[363] believe that hyperplasia modifies parathyroid cells in a progressive fashion and that grossly enlarged glands show greater ultrastructural alterations than glands of normal size exhibiting mild or early hyperplasia; disappearance of intracytoplasmic lipid is not an early phenomenon. In view of the controversy concerning the significance of hyperplasia when identified only at the light microscopic level, it seems unlikely that hyperplasia only detectable at the ultrastructural level will aid in the practical management of patients.

Both diploidy and aneuploidy have been identified in parathyroid glands from patients with sporadic PHP and MEN-1–associated hyperparathyroidism; the incidence of aneuploidy was significantly greater in MEN-associated glands.[436, 437]

Differential Diagnosis

The distinction between chief cell hyperplasia and adenoma can be difficult. Some surgeons make the distinction purely on visualization of the glands; they equate solitary gland enlargement with an adenoma, and they interpret multigland enlargement as hyperplasia or, rarely, multiple adenomas. Histologically, the distinction cannot be made if only one gland is available for assessment, as both conditions can cause an identical microscopic picture. Biopsies of other glands to assess the parenchymal cellularity and the parenchymal cell-to-fat-cell ratio is not infallible, as stromal fat is often irregularly distributed throughout normal and hyperplastic glands. In isolation, the pathologist cannot often make the distinction unless the pathologic changes are marked. The most reliable diagnosis can be reached by using a team approach; the surgeon needs to visualize all glands and relay information about the size, color, and consistency of all glands to the pathologist, who, using this knowledge in combination with light microscopic features, possibly fat stains, and sometimes ultrastructural examination, will reach the correct diagnosis.

Parathyroid hyperplasia is particularly difficult to diagnose in children as their normal glands are cellular and contain very little stromal fat. The diagnosis requires total glandular weights.[6]

Another diagnostic dilemma is distinguishing mild hyperplastic parathyroid glands from normal glands, as there is wide variability in what constitutes a normal gland. Histologic features that appear to indicate abnormality are cytologic atypia, more generalized chief cell nodularity, and diminished intracytoplasmic lipid.[9]

Water-Clear (Wasserhelle) Cell Hyperplasia

Definition

Water-clear cell hyperplasia is a rare disorder of the parathyroid glands that was first described in 1934.[438] The frequency of this condition as a cause of PHP has declined in recent decades, although a constant annual incidence has been reported.[273, 439] It occurs as a sporadic nonfamilial disorder,[146, 440] and an association with blood group O has been noted.[441] In contrast with other forms of PHP, there is no predominance in women.[439, 441, 442] In one study, 81% had chief cell hyperplasia, and 19% had water-clear cell hyperplasia; patients with the clear-cell type tend to be older.[146, 439] Water-clear cell hyperplasia is generally associated with higher serum calcium levels, and patients often have pronounced symptoms.[146, 273, 439] Approximately 90% of patients with water-clear cell hyperplasia have renal stones, in comparison with 43% to 53% of patients with chief cell hyperplasia.[146, 442] Impaired renal function is particularly common.[439] Patients are also more likely to develop a hypercalcemic crisis.[439]

Gross Anatomy

Parathyroid glands exhibiting this type of hyperplasia are usually markedly enlarged. All glands are enlarged in most patients, although the size of each of the glands can vary. Grossly, they cannot be distinguished confidently from glands with chief cell hyperplasia, although suggestive features include considerably larger, heavier glands[146]; frequently, more than 5 to 10 g of tissue is resected at surgery.[146, 439] The upper glands are often larger than the lower glands,[439] and the parathyroid glands tend to be irregular in shape and form pseudopods.[146] They are soft, and their color has been vividly described as dark-brown, chocolate-brown, and mahogany.[4, 6, 32, 146] Cystic degeneration is common.

Microscopic Anatomy

Histologically, water-clear cell hyperplasia is characterized by diffuse sheets of water-clear cells with virtual absence of other cell types, including fat cells. The cells may be arranged in acini, follicles, papillae, and trabeculae; nodules are rarely seen. Degenerate cysts lined by clear cells and containing proteinaceous material and degenerate cells are common. The water-clear cells are large, measuring 10 to 40 μm in diameter.[145] They are polygonal cells with distinct cell membranes. Occasionally, they fuse into multinucleated forms. The nuclei are small and tend to be polar, oriented preferentially toward the adjacent stroma and blood vessels.[359] They contain dense chromatin and are typically uniform in appearance, although isolated enlarged hyperchromatic nuclei may be present. On high power examination, the cytoplasm may be seen to contain tiny vacuoles. Cytoplasmic lipid is not present; however, moderate amounts of glycogen may be identified. Water-clear cells need to be distinguished from chief cells containing abundant glycogen (clear cells); parathyroid hyperplasia has never been reported to consist exclusively of this type of clear cell. The histologic appearance of water-clear cell hyperplasia bears a resemblance to that of renal cell carcinoma.

Special Investigations

Electron microscopic examination reveals that the cytoplasm is filled with numerous membrane-bound vacuoles that measure up to 0.8 μm. It is thought that these vacuoles are probably derived from the vesicles of the Golgi complex.[443] Dense material in some vacuoles may represent PTH. It has been suggested that individual water-clear cells may have low endocrine activity and that the severe hypercalcemia is due to the large mass of cells.[439] In keeping with this suggestion, the concentration of PTH per mg of fresh tissue has been found to be 1000 times lower than in normal glands or in adenomas.[444] An alternate explanation is that this reflects low storage of PTH and a high rate of secretion.[4]

It has been suggested that chief cell hyperplasia may represent an early stage of water-clear cell hyperplasia[146]; because of the differences in frequency and the lack of an intermediate morphologic pattern, this seems unlikely.

HYPOPARATHYROIDISM: CLINICAL FEATURES

Hypoparathyroidism

Hypoparathyroidism is largely a functional clinical disorder characterized by hypocalcemia and hyperphosphatemia secondary to a deficiency of PTH. The clinical manifestations may be subtle and the diagnosis delayed. Subclinical disease may be revealed by eliciting facial and carpal muscular contractions by tapping the facial nerve (Chvostek's sign) or applying a blood pressure cuff around the arm (Trousseau's sign), respectively. When hypoparathyroidism is overt, patients experience paresthesia, tetanic muscular spasms of the hands and feet, laryngeal stridor, convulsions, mental changes ranging from irritability to depression and frank psychosis, basal ganglia calcification with extrapyramidal symptoms, raised intracranial pressure with papilloedema, electrocardiographic changes such as prolongation of the QT interval and T-wave changes, and cataract formation.[445]

Hypoparathyroidism may occur as a transient acute phenomenon or as a chronic disease. Transient impairment of parathyroid function occurs not uncommonly after parathyroid or thyroid surgery.[168]

The resultant hypocalcemia is usually mild and may not require treatment, although occasionally calcium supplements and/or vitamin D may be necessary for days to months for symptomatic relief. Mild hypoparathyroidism has been described following [131]Iodine therapy for hyperthyroidism.[446, 447]

Chronic hypoparathyroidism is a rare disorder and may occur as iatrogenic, developmental, idiopathic (autoimmune), or infiltrative disorders or in a group of disorders called pseudohypoparathyroidism.[4] Iatrogenic complications are the most common cause of chronic hypoparathyroidism; inadvertent removal or damage of the parathyroid glands may occur during neck surgery.[168, 445] It may occur as a complication of radical thyroid surgery, bilateral radical cervical lymph node dissections, or overzealous surgery for parathyroid hyperplasia or parathyroid adenoma. Excessive parathyroid tissue may be removed, or the blood supply may be interrupted, resulting in atrophy, scarring, or infarction.[448]

Agenesis of the parathyroid glands is rare. The glands may completely or partially fail to develop in isolation or, more often, in combination with other derivatives of the third and fourth branchial pouches, that is, the thymus and thyroid C cells. The classic symptom complex, termed DiGeorge's syndrome, manifests in neonatal life and consists of absence of cell-mediated immunity, hypoparathyroidism, and congenital defects of the heart and great vessels.[19, 449] Partial DiGeorge's syndrome is the term that describes the condition when some parathyroid tissue and C cells are present.[19]

Familial hypoparathyroidism is rarely the result of an inherited mutation of the calcium-sensing receptor, a gain-of-function mutation that renders the receptor more sensitive to activation by calcium.[450]

Hypoparathyroidism may also occur as an autoimmune disorder called idiopathic hypoparathyroidism. It most commonly affects children or young adults but may develop at any age.[445, 451] Pathologically, the parathyroid glands, if detectable, may be completely replaced by fat, or they may be atrophic and infiltrated by fat with focal aggregates of lymphocytes and plasma cells.[451–454] In some cases, the minute atrophic glands have not been identifiable at postmortem examination,[451] and in others the glands have been completely replaced by fat. Focal infiltration by lymphocytes and plasma cells (Fig. 5–17) with fibrosis, glandular atrophy, or fatty replacement have also been described.[452, 454] Normal or hypoplastic glands have been identified in some patients with this disorder.[455] Blizzard and coworkers[456] found antibodies in 38% of 74 patients with idiopathic hypoparathyroidism. Cytotoxic antibodies capable of causing lysis of bovine chief cells have been identified in patients with autoimmune hypoparathyroidism.[457] However, several other investigators have not been able to demonstrate parathyroid autoantibodies.[458] One possible explanation that has been given for these discrepant results is that mitochondrial reactive autoantibodies in certain sera may react with mitochondria-rich oxyphil cells in parathyroid tissues, giving a

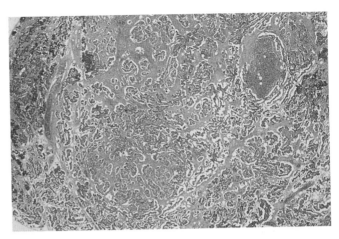

Figure 5–17. Chronic parathyroiditis is characterized by a chronic lymphoplasmacytic infiltrate that can be associated with extensive stromal fibrosis and that ultimately results in glandular atrophy.

false impression of the presence of specific antiparathyroid autoantibodies.[458]

Idiopathic hypoparathyroidism is a rare disease, but its association with other endocrine autoimmune diseases is well documented in human autoimmune polyendocrinopathy or polyendocrine autoimmune syndrome.[458] Patients with such disorders may also have antibodies directed against the ovaries, adrenal glands, thyroid gland, and other tissues, resulting in ovarian failure, Addison's disease, Hashimoto's thyroiditis, hypothyroidism, diabetes mellitus, pernicious anemia, and mucocutaneous candidiasis.[451, 456] If the disease manifests before 6 months of age, it is often an X-linked recessive disorder, whereas many other affected families exhibit an autosomal-recessive inheritance pattern.[445] Some cases have had their onset immediately following acute viral infections.[451] Families have also been described with idiopathic hypoparathyroidism and seizures developing in infancy, without the association of other autoimmune diseases or candidiasis.[459] Reports implicate activating mutations of the calcium-sensing receptors as the cause of autosomal-dominant hypocalcemia.[450]

The parathyroid glands may also be destroyed or replaced by infiltrates, such as metastatic malignancy, amyloid, and iron (hemochromatosis). However, it is very rare that sufficient parathyroid tissue is replaced to cause clinical hypoparathyroidism. In excess of 70% of the parathyroid tissue must be lost before parathyroid function is compromised.

Chronic hypoparathyroidism requires life-long treatment with supplemental calcium and vitamin D and necessitates frequent monitoring of urinary and serum calcium levels to prevent complications.[460] Successful transplantation of cultured allogeneic parathyroid cells would be an attractive alternative; however, at present grafts function for only up to 1 year.[460]

Pseudohypoparathyroidism and Pseudopseudohypoparathyroidism

Pseudohypoparathyroidism (pseudoHP) comprises a group of disorders characterized by renal and skeletal resistance to the physiologic effects of PTH. Two subtypes of pseudoHP have been described, each differing slightly in their pathophysiology. In 1942 Albright and associates[461] proposed that the hypocalcemia and hyperphosphatemia typical of the disease were due to target organ resistance to PTH rather than PTH deficiency. The actions of PTH are mediated by stimulating the synthesis of cAMP by adenylate cyclase. PseudoHP type 1 is characterized by failure to increase urinary excretion of cAMP and phosphate in response to PTH,[462] implicating a defect in the hormone receptor–adenylate cyclase signal pathway. Guanine nucleotide–binding proteins (G proteins) couple receptors to adenylate cyclase.[463] In one form of the disease (pseudoHP type 1a), there is reduced activity of the Gsγ protein.[464, 465] As the G protein is not tissue-specific, these patients are also resistant to the actions of other hormones that act by stimulating adenylate cyclase.[466] Many of these patients have the phenotype termed Albright's hereditary osteodystrophy.[461] Affected individuals are short and stocky in stature, with short necks, round facies, short metacarpals and metatarsals, abnormal dentition, mental retardation, cataracts, and soft-tissue calcification.[461] In pseudoHP type 1b, the patients have a normal appearance, normal G-protein activity, and in most instances are resistant to PTH only.[466] Mutations of the PTH receptor, adenylate cyclase, or proteins that would alter the response to PTH may be implicated and have occasionally been identified in pseudoHP type 1a.[467] PseudoHP type II is characterized by marked increases in urinary excretion of cAMP but not of phosphate in response to PTH.[468] In one patient with pseudoHP type II and Sjögren's syndrome, the block in PTH-induced phosphaturia appeared to be caused by an antirenal tubular plasma membrane autoantibody.[469] The parathyroid glands in patients with pseudoHP have been described as normal in appearance[470] or as showing diffuse hyperplasia.[432]

Pseudopseudohypoparathyroidism is an inherited disorder; a sex-linked dominant mode of transmission has been suggested.[445] Some members of affected kindreds exhibit the characteristic phenotypic appearance of pseudoHP but lack the PTH-unresponsiveness; that is, they are short with round facies, brachydactyly, and normal serum calcium and phosphate levels.[445, 471]

PATHOLOGY OF MISCELLANEOUS LESIONS OF THE PARATHYROID GLANDS

Chronic Parathyroiditis

Precise diagnostic criteria have not been defined for chronic parathyroiditis. Lymphocytic infiltration to varying degrees has been reported in up to 10% of parathyroid glands examined at postmortem in patients with normal parathyroid gland function.[472] These infiltrates are commonly sparse, focal, and well-circumscribed in a perivascular distribution and are not associated with parenchymal destruction. Clinically chronic parathyroiditis is more often associated with hypoparathyroidism as opposed to overactivity of the parathyroid glands. Some patients with this condition are afflicted with other autoimmune disease; in other patients chronic parathyroiditis-induced hypoparathyroidism occurs in isolation.[473]

Rare cases of chronic parathyroiditis have been described in association with parathyroid hyperplasia with and without hyperparathyroidism,[474–476] one patient had MEN-1.[476] The parathyroid glands in these cases were characterized by nodules and strands of parenchymal cells separated by hyaline and loose fibrous stroma diffusely infiltrated by numerous plasma cells and lymphocytes, including scattered lymphoid follicles with germinal centers. The lymphoid infiltrate was composed of a mixed population of T and B cells.[476] Areas of parenchymal cell destruction were evident, and it was suggested that these associations may represent an auto-immune phenomenon, similar to Hashimoto's thyroiditis.[476] In two of the four reported cases of parathyroid hyperplasia associated with chronic parathyroiditis in which antiparathyroid antibodies were sought, none were detected.[474, 476] In two patients, infiltrating lymphocytes were confined to adenomatous tissue.[477] In one tumor there was also considerable fibrosis and atrophy of the adenomatous tissue. It has been suggested that this may represent a tumor-specific autoimmune reaction.[477]

Another interesting constellation of pathologic features was reported in a man with PHP. He had two enlarged inferior parathyroid glands that histologically exhibited diffuse features of chronic parathyroiditis and widespread oxyphilic cell change, focal parenchymal cell atrophy, and small cysts lined by respiratory-type epithelium and focal squamous epithelium.[478] Lymphoid tissue was intimately associated with the epithelial linings, and the appearance was reminiscent of branchial cleft cysts. Similar branchial cleft-like cysts have been reported in the thyroid in association with autoimmune thyroiditis,[479, 480] and it is possible that this association in the parathyroid glands may prove to be an autoimmune phenomenon.

Parathyroid Cyst

Although microscopic cysts in the parathyroid glands are relatively common, cysts large enough to produce a significant mass are rare. Preoperatively, they are frequently mistaken for cystic thyroid nodules or branchial cleft or thyroglossal duct cysts.

The majority present as asymptomatic neck masses, although occasional patients complain of respiratory distress, dysphagia, or hoarseness.[481] PHP has rarely been reported[131, 179, 181]; two patients have even presented with a hyperparathyroid crisis.[181] These cysts have been described more commonly in women,[482, 483] and they occur in the neck and mediastinum.[179, 181, 484–486] They may arise in any of the parathyroid glands but are more common in the lower glands.[481] They may measure up to 10 cm in diameter[181] and may be loosely attached to the thyroid. Dissection from this organ poses little difficulty. They are unilocular with a smooth, gray-white, thin, translucent wall. Occasional foci of yellow-tan tissue, representing parathyroid parenchyma, may be recognized grossly in the cyst wall.[481] The contents of these cysts are often clear and serous,[487] although some are described to contain straw-colored, bloody, or opalescent fluid. It has been reported that the fluid is rich in PTH.[131, 181, 487]

Microscopically, the wall is composed of fibrous and adipose tissue lined by a single layer of compressed cuboidal or columnar epithelium, which may have clear glycogen-rich or amphophilic cytoplasm. The diagnosis depends on the presence of entrapped islands of typical parathyroid tissue within the wall. Smooth muscle fragments have also been described in the wall of some cysts.[488] Rarely, thymic tissue may be present, particularly in parathyroid cysts of the mediastinum; the term third pharyngeal pouch cysts has been applied to these cysts.[486]

The origin of parathyroid cysts is not known. They may arise from multiple sources. Postulated theories include developmental and degenerative origins. Developmentally, they may arise through cystic change in either remnants of the branchial pouches or the canals of Kursteiner, which are rudimentary gland-like structures found within fetal parathyroid glands and thought to arise from the parathyroid gland or thymic anlage.[1, 28] More common microcysts may coalesce to form clinical lesions or enlarge due to fluid accumulation.[488] Cystic degeneration within adenomas and hyperplastic glands has also been proposed as the source of some parathyroid cysts; this may explain the rare occurrence of hyperfunctioning parathyroid cysts.[4, 179, 181] Nonfunctioning parathyroid cysts may be successfully treated by FNA.[487]

Secondary Tumors

The parathyroid glands may be involved by secondary malignancies through direct extension or metastases. Such malignant destruction is rarely associated with hypoparathyroidism as this requires loss of more than 70% of parathyroid parenchyma.[489] Nineteen of 160 patients (11.9%) dying with cancer had metastatic disease in at least one parathyroid gland at postmortem examination.[489] Breast carcinoma was the most common of these malignancies;

in another series of patients with disseminated breast carcinoma, 6% had parathyroid involvement.[490] The other sites of origin in decreasing order of frequency were blood (leukemia), skin (melanoma), lung, and soft tissues.[489]

Other

Parathyroid Gland Morphology in Nonparathyroid Hormone-Mediated Hypercalcemia

Hypercalcemia may be caused by many conditions: hyperparathyroidism is the most common; the second is malignancy. Hypercalcemia is the most common paraneoplastic syndrome[7]; humoral hypercalcemia of malignancy occurs in patients with no skeletal involvement by tumor but rather arises from the humoral actions of tumor-derived factors, largely PTHrP, which produces a generalized increase in osteoclastic bone resorption. Other causes of hypercalcemia include sarcoidosis, vitamin D intoxication, hyperthyroidism, immoblization, thiazide diuretics, and vitamin A intoxication.[6] Occasionally, these patients are mistakenly thought to have PHP and undergo parathyroidectomy. Glands from these patients are similar to normal parathyroid glands in size and ratios of parenchymal cells to stromal fat cells, with neither atrophy nor hyperplasia.[491]

Patients with familial benign hypercalcemia are also sometimes mistakenly thought to have hyperparathyroidism. No consistent histologic findings have been identified in the parathyroid glands of these patients; some investigators have described enlarged or normal-weight glands with increased or reduced parenchymal cell area.[351, 352] The majority of glands in this clinical setting, however, appear to be indistinguishable from normal, despite the functional abnormality. Surgical pathologists, therefore, need to consider the possible absence of parathyroid disease when asked to examine parathyroid glands at frozen section in patients with hypercalcemia.

Incidental Parathyroid Enlargement in Patients with Normal Parathyroid Gland Function

Occasionally during neck surgery, enlarged parathyroid glands (110 to 1000 mg) are found incidentally in normocalcemic patients with normal PTH levels[166]; these glands may exhibit parenchymal hypercellularity, reduced cytoplasmic fat content, and scarce stromal fat cells. It has been postulated that in such cases there is a functional disturbance in parathyroid physiology characterized by abnormal calcium regulation of intracellular calcium concentrations; altered calcium receptors have been detected on the surface of parathyroid cells by immunohistochemical staining.[7, 50, 51] These cases may represent a biochemically subclinical stage of PHP.

Multisystem Diseases

Parathyroid glands may be affected secondarily in a number of disorders; however, the diagnosis does not generally depend on pathologic examination of the parathyroid glands. For example, in Pompe's disease,[492] deficiency of a lysosomal enzyme leads to intralysosomal glycogen storage in multiple organs including heart, liver, skeletal muscles, and endocrine organs, such as the parathyroid glands.

CONCLUSION

Despite the small anatomic size of the parathyroid glands, it is clearly apparent that there is a rapidly growing wealth of literature covering clinical and pathologic topics, reflecting the myriad of unexplained and poorly understood aspects surrounding this vital endocrine organ. In particular, the molecular basis of parathyroid hyperplasia and neoplasia is an area of exciting research, which may unravel some of the mystery regarding the pathogenesis of parathyroid disease. Consistent diagnostic criteria for parathyroid hyperplasia versus adenoma versus carcinoma need to be identified. Without a reproducible gold standard, further investigations are impeded.

References

1. Gilmour JR. The embryology of the parathyroid glands, the thymus and certain associated rudiments. J Path Bact 1937; 45:507.
2. Grimelius L, Åkerström G, Johansson H, et al.: Anatomy and histopathology of human parathyroid glands. Pathol Annu 1981; 16:1.
3. Grimelius L, Åkerström G, Bondeson L, et al.: The role of the pathologist in diagnosis and surgical decision making in hyperparathyroidism. World J Surg 1991; 15:698.
4. LiVolsi VA: Pathology of the parathyroid glands. In Barnes L, ed.: Surgical Pathology of the Head and Neck. New York, Marcel Dekker, Inc. 1985, p. 1487.
5. Ghandur-Mnaymneh L, Cassady J, Hajianpour MA, et al.: The parathyroid gland in health and disease. Am J Pathol 1986; 125:292.
6. DeLellis RA: Atlas of Tumor Pathology–Tumors of the Parathyroid Gland, 3 ed. Washington, D.C.: Armed Forces Institute of Pathology, 1993.
7. Shelling DH: The Parathyroids in Health and Disease. St. Louis: C.V. Mosby, 1935.
8. Dufour DR, Wilkerson SY: Factors related to parathyroid weight in normal persons. Arch Pathol Lab Med 1983; 107:167.
9. Saffos RO, Rhatigan RM, Urgulu S: The Normal parathyroid and the borderline with early hyperplasia: A light microscopic study. Histopathology 1984; 8:407.
10. Åkerström G, Grimelius L, Johansson H, et al.: The parenchymal cell mass in normal human parathyroid glands. Acta Path Microbiol Scand 1981; 89:367.
11. Dufour DR, Wilkerson SY: The normal parathyroid revisited: Percentage of stromal fat. Hum Pathol 1982; 13:717.
12. Åkerström G, Grimelius L, Johansson H, et al.: Estimation of the parathyroid parenchymal cell mass by density gradients. Am J Pathol 1980; 99:685.
13. Wang C: The anatomic basis of parathyroid surgery. Ann Surg 1976; 183:271.
14. Heinbach WF: Study of the number and location of the parathyroid glands in man. Anat Rec 1933; 57:251.
15. Gilmour JR: The gross anatomy of the parathyroid glands. J Path Bact 1938; 46:133.
16. Åkerström G, Malmaeus J, Bergström R: Surgical anatomy of human parathyroid glands. Surgery 1984; 95:14.
17. Hooghe L, Kinnaert P, Van Geertruyden J: Surgical anatomy of hyperparathyroidism. Acta Chir Belg 1992; 92:1.
18. Alveryd A: Parathyroid glands in thyroid surgery; anatomy of parathyroid glands; postoperative hypoparathyroidism–identification and autotransplantation of parathyroid glands. Acta Chir Scand 1968; 38:91.
19. Robinson HB: Di George's or the III-IV pharyngeal pouch syndromes: Pathology and a theory of pathogenesis. In Rosenberg HS, Bolande RP, eds.: Perspectives in Pediatric Pathology, vol 2. Chicago, Year Book Medical Publishers, 1975, p. 173.
20. Moore KL: Clinically Oriented anatomy. Baltimore/London, Williams & Wilkins, 1980.
21. Carty SE, Norton JA: Management of patients with persistent or recurrent primary hyperparathyroidism. World J Surg 1991; 15:716.
22. Lack EE, Delay S, Linnoila RI: Ectopic parathyroid tissue within the vagus nerve: Incidence and possible clinical significance. Arch Pathol Lab Med 1988; 112:304.
23. Doppman JL, Shawker TH, Fraker DL, et al.: Parathyroid adenoma within the vagus nerve. AJR Am J Roentgenol 1994; 163:943.
24. Billingsley KG, Fraker DL, Doppman JL, et al.: Localization and operative management of undescended parathyroid adenomas in patients with persistent primary hyperparathyroidism. Surgery 1994; 116:982.
25. Michal M: Ectopic parathyroid within a neck paraganglia. Histopathology 1993; 22:85.
26. Kurman RJ, Prabha AC: Thyroid and parathyroid glands in the vaginal wall: Report of a case. Am J Clin Pathol 1973; 59:503.
27. Jander HP, Diethelm AG, Russinovich NA: The parathyroid artery. AJR Am J Roentgenol 1980; 135:821.
28. Gilmour JR: The Normal histology of the parathyroid glands. J Path Bact 1939; 48:187.
29. Dekker A, Dunsford HA, Geyer SJ: The normal parathyroid gland at autopsy: The significance of stromal fat in adult patients. J Pathol 1979; 128:127.
30. Grimelius L, Åkerström G, Johansson H, et al.: Estimation of parenchymal cell content of human parathyroid glands using the image analyzing computer technique. Am J Pathol 1978; 93:793.
31. Harach HR, Jasani B: Parathyroid hyperplasia in multiple endocrine neoplasia type 1: A pathological and immunohistochemical reappraisal. Histopathology 1992; 20:305.
32. Grimelius L, Åkerström G, Johansson H, et al.: The parathyroid glands. In Kovacs K, Asa SL, eds.: Functional Endocrine Pathology. Boston, Blackwell Scientific Publications, 1991, p. 375.
33. Abu-Jawdeh GM, Roth SI: Parathyroid glands. In Sternberg SS, ed.: Histology for Pathologists. New York, Raven Press, 1992, p. 311.
34. Altenähr E: Ultrastructural pathology of parathyroid glands. Curr Top Pathol 1972; 56:1.
35. Roth SI, Gallagher MJ: The rapid identification of "normal" parathyroid glands by the presence of intracellular fat. Am J Pathol 1976; 84:521.
36. Bedetti CD: Immunocytochemical demonstration of cytochrome C oxidase with an immunoperoxidase method: A specific stain for mitochondria in formalin-fixed and paraffin-embedded human tissues. J Histochem Cytochem 1985; 33:446.
37. Müller-Höcker J: Random cytochrome-C-oxidase deficiency of oxyphil cell nodules in the parathyroid gland: A mitochondrial cytopathy related to cell aging? Path Res Pract 1992; 188:701.
38. Miettinen M, Clark R, Lehto V-P, et al.: Intermediate-filament proteins in parathyroid glands and parathyroid adenomas. Arch Pathol Lab Med 1985; 109:986.
39. Zabel M, Dietel M: S-100 protein and neuron-specific enolase in parathyroid glands and C-cells of the thyroid. Histochemistry 1987; 86:389.

40. Cohn DV, Morrissey JJ, Shofstall RE, et al.: Cosecretion of secretory protein-1 and parathormone by dispersed bovine parathyroid cells. Endocrinology 1982; 110:625.

41. Cohn DV, Zangerle R, Fischer-Colbrie R, et al.: Similarity of secretory protein I from parathyroid gland to chromogranin A from adrenal medulla. Proc Natl Acad Sci U S A. 1982; 79:6056.

42. Iacangelo A, Affolter HU, Eiden LE, et al.: Bovine chromogranin A sequence and distribution of its messenger RNA in endocrine tissues. Nature 1986; 32:382.

43. MacGregor RR, Hinton DA, Ridgeway RD: Effects of calcium on synthesis and secretion of parathyroid hormone and secretory protein I. Am J Physiol 1988; 255:E299.

44. Ikeda K, Arnold A, Mangin M, et al.: Expression of transcripts encoding a parathyroid hormone-related peptide in abnormal parathyroid tissues. J Clin Endocrinol Metab 1989; 69:1240.

45. Wilson BS, Lloyd RV: Detection of chromogranin in neuroendocrine cells with a monoclonal antibody. Am J Pathol 1984; 115:458.

46. Levine MA, Dempsey MA, Helman LJ, et al.: Expression of chromogranin-A messenger ribonucleic acid in parathyroid tissue from patients with primary hyperparathyroidism. J Clin Endocrinol Metab 1990; 70:1668.

47. Brown EM, Gamba G, Riccardi D, et al.: Cloning and characterization of an extracellular Ca(2+)-sensing receptor from bovine parathyroid. Nature 1993; 366:575.

48. Futrell JM, Roth SI, Su SP, et al.: Immunocytochemical localization of parathyroid hormone in bovine parathyroid glands and human parathyroid adenomas. Am J Pathol 1979; 94:615.

49. Pesce C, Tobia F, Carli F, et al.: The sites of hormone storage in normal and diseased parathyroid glands. Histopathology 1989; 15:157.

50. Juhlin C, Åkerström G, Klareskog L, et al.: Monoclonal antiparathyroid antibodies revealing defect expression of a calcium receptor mechanism in hyperparathyroidism. World J Surg 1988; 12:552.

51. Juhlin C, Holmdahl R, Johansson H, et al.: Monoclonal antibodies with exclusive reactivity against parathyroid cells and tubule cells of the kidney. Proc Natl Acad Sci U S A 1987; 84:2990.

52. Capen CC, Roth SI: Ultrastructural and functional relationships of normal and pathologic parathyroid cells. In Sommers SC, ed.: Endocrine Pathology Decennial 1966–75. New York, Appleton, Century, Crofts, 1975; p. 267.

53. Kendall CH, Roberts PA, Pringle JH, et al.: The expression of parathyroid hormone messenger RNA in normal and abnormal parathyroid tissue. J Pathol 1991; 165:111.

54. Baba H, Kishihara M, Tohman M, et al.: Identification of parathyroid hormone messenger ribonucleic acid in an apparently non-functioning parathyroid carcinoma transformed from a parathyroid carcinoma with hyperparathyroidism. J Clin Endocrinol Metab 1986; 62:247.

55. Yamamoto M, Igarashi T, Muramatsu M, et al.: Hypocalcemia increases and hypercalcemia decreases the steady-state level of parathyroid hormone messenger RNA in the rat. J Clin Invest 1989; 83:1053.

56. Naveh-Many T, Friedlaender MM, Mayer H, et al.: Calcium regulates parathyroid hormone messenger ribonucleic acid (mRNA), but not calcitonin mRNA in vivo in the rat: Dominant role of 1,25-dihydroxyvitamin D. Endocrinology 1989; 125:275.

57. Naylor SL, Sakaguchi AY, Szoka P, et al.: Human parathyroid hormone gene (PTH) is on short arm of chromosome 11. Somatic Cell Genet 1983; 9:609.

58. Zabel BU, Kronenberg HM, Bell GI, et al.: Chromosome mapping of genes on the short arm of human chromosome 11: parathyroid hormone gene is at 11p15 together with the genes for insulin, c-Harvey-ras 1, and beta-hemoglobin. Cytogenet Cell Genet 1985; 39:200.

59. Mallette LE: The Parathyroid polyhormones: New concepts in the spectrum of peptide hormone action. Endocr Rev 1991; 12:110.

60. Goltzman D, Gomolin H, DeLean A, et al.: Discordant disappearance of bioactive and immunoreactive parathyroid hormone after parathyroidectomy. J Clin Endocrinol Metab 1984; 58:70.

61. Goltzman D, Bennett HP, Koutsilieris M, et al.: Studies of the multiple molecular forms of bioactive parathyroid hormone

and parathyroid hormone-like substances. Recent Prog Horm Res 1986; 42:665.

62. Wong G: Skeletal actions of parathyroid hormone. Miner Electrol Metab 1982; 8:188.

63. Chambers TJ: The cellular basis of bone resorption. Clin Orthop 1980; 151:283.

64. Chambers TJ, Revell PA, Fuller K, et al.: Resorption of bone by isolated rabbit osteoclasts. J Cell Sci 1984; 66:383.

65. Pliam NB, Nyiredy KO, Arnaud CD: Parathyroid hormone receptors in avian bone cells. Proc Natl Acad Sci U S A 1982; 79:2061.

66. Silve CM, Hradek GT, Jones AL, et al.: Parathyroid hormone receptor in intact embryonic chicken bone: Characterization and cellular localization. J Cell Biol 1982; 94:379.

67. McSheehy PMJ, Chambers TJ: Osteoblastic cells mediate osteoclastic responsiveness to parathyroid hormone. Endocrinology 1986; 118:824.

68. Vaes G: Cellular biology and biochemical mechanism of bone resorption: A review of recent developments on the formation, activation, and mode of action of osteoclasts. Clin Orthop 1988; 231:239.

69. de Vernejoul MC, Horowitz M, Demignon J, et al.: Bone resorption by isolated chick osteoclasts in culture is stimulated by murine spleen cell supernatant fluids (osteoclast-activating factor) and inhibited by calcitonin and prostaglandin E2. J Bone Min Res 1988; 3:69.

70. Rodan GA, Martin TJ: Role of osteoblasts in hormonal control of bone resorption-A hypothesis. Cal Tiss Int 1981; 33:349.

71. Sutton RA, Dirks JH: Renal handling of calcium. Fed Proc 1978; 37:2112.

72. Mallette LE: Regulation of blood calcium in humans. Endocrinol Metab Clin North Am 1989; 18:601.

73. Capen CC, Rosol TJ: Pathobiology of parathyroid hormone and parathyroid hormone-related protein. In LiVolsi VA, DeLellis RA, eds.: Pathobiology of the Parathyroid and Thyroid Glands. Baltimore, Williams and Wilkins, 1993, p. 1.

74. Åkerström G, Rastad J, Ljunghall S, et al.: Cellular physiology and pathophysiology of the parathyroid glands. World J Surg 1991; 15:672.

75. Pocotte SL, Ehrenstein G, Fitzpatrick LA: Regulation of parathyroid hormone secretion. Endocr Rev 1991; 12:291.

76. Aurbach CD: Regulation of secretion of parathyroid hormone. Adv Nephrol 1982; 11:131.

77. Brown EM, LeBoff MS, Oetting M, et al.: Secretory control in normal and abnormal parathyroid tissue. Recent Prog Horm Res 1987; 43:337.

78. Ratcliffe WA: Editorial: parathyroid hormone-related protein and hypercalcaemia of malignancy. J Pathol 1994; 173:79.

79. Orloff JJ, Wu TL, Stewart AF: Parathyroid hormone-like proteins: Biochemical responses and receptor interactions. Endocr Rev 1989; 10:476.

80. Mangin M, Webb AC, Dreyer BE: Identification of a cDNA encoding a parathyroid hormone-like protein from a human tumor associated with humoral hypercalcemia of malignancy. Proc Natl Acad Sci U S A 1988; 85:597.

81. Martin TJ, Suva LJ: Parathyroid hormone-related protein in hypercalcaemia of malignancy. Clin Endocrinol 1989; 31:631.

82. Nissenson RA, Diep D, Strewler GJ: Synthetic peptides comprising the amino-terminal sequence of a parathyroid hormone-like protein from human malignancies: Binding to parathyroid hormone receptors and activation of adenylate cyclase in bone cells and kidney. J Biol Chem 1988; 263:12866.

83. Rabbani SA, Mitchell J, Roy DR, et al.: Influence of the amino terminus on in vitro and in vivo biological activity of synthetic parathyroid hormone-like peptides of malignancy. Endocrinology 1988; 123:2709.

84. Orloff JJ, Wu TL, Heath HW, et al.: Characterization of canine renal receptors for the parathyroid hormone-like protein associated with humoral hypercalcemia of malignancy. J Biol Chem 1989; 264:6097.

85. Ebeling PR, Adams WR, Moseley JM, et al.: Actions of synthetic parathyroid hormone-related protein (1–34) on the isolated rat kidney. J Endocrinol 1989; 120:45.

86. Rosol TJ, Capen CC, Horst RL: Effects of infusion of human parathyroid hormone-related protein (1–40) in nude mice: Histomorphometric and biochemical investigations. J Bone Min Res 1988; 3:699.

87. Asa SL, Henderson J, Goltzman D, et al.: Parathyroid hormone-like peptide in normal and neoplastic human endocrine tissues. J Clin Endocrinol Metab 1990; 71:1112.

88. Donahue HJ, Fryer MJ, Eriksen EF, et al.: Differential effects of parathyroid hormone and its analogues on cytosolic calcium ion and cAMP levels in cultured rat osteoblast-like cells. J Biol Chem 1988; 263:13522.

89. Kramer S, Reynolds FH Jr, Castillo M, et al.: Immunological identification and distribution of parathyroid hormone-like protein polypeptides in normal and malignant tissues. Endocrinology 1991; 128:1927.

90. Rodda CP, Kubota M, Heath JA: Evidence for a novel parathyroid hormone-related protein in fetal lamb parathyroid glands and sheep placenta: Comparisons with a similar protein implicated in humoral hypercalcaemia of malignancy. J Endocrinol 1988; 117:261.

91. Loveridge N, Caple IW, Rodda C, et al.: Evidence for a parathyroid hormone-related protein in fetal parathyroid glands of sheep. J Exp Physiol 1988; 73:781.

92. Thiede MA: The mRNA encoding a parathyroid hormone-like peptide is produced in mammary tissue in response to elevations in serum prolactin. Mol Endocrinol 1989; 3:1443.

93. Ikeda K, Weir EC, Mangin M: Expression of messenger ribonucleic acids encoding a parathyroid hormone-like peptide in normal human and animal tissues with abnormal expression in human parathyroid adenomas. Mol Endocrinol 1989; 2:1230.

94. Danks JA, Ebeling PR, Hayman JA, et al.: Immunohistochemical localization of parathyroid hormone-related protein in parathyroid adenoma and hyperplasia. J Pathol 1990; 161:27.

95. Docherty HM, Ratcliffe WA, Heath DA, et al.: Expression of parathyroid hormone-related protein in abnormal human parathyroids. J Endocrinol 1991; 129:431.

96. Burton PBJ, Moniz C, Quirke P, et al.: Parathyroid hormone-related peptide: Expression in fetal and neonatal development. J Pathol 1992; 167:291.

97. Pitkin RM: Calcium metabolism in pregnancy and the perinatal period: a review. Am J Obstet Gynecol 1985; 15:99.

98. Care AD, Abbas SK, Pickard DW, et al.: Stimulation of ovine placental transport of calcium and magnesium by mid-molecule fragments of human parathyroid hormone-related protein. Exp Physiol 1990; 75:605.

99. Roca-Cusachs A, Dipette DJ, Nickols GA: Regional and systemic hemodynamic effects of parathyroid hormone-related protein: Preservation of cardiac function and coronary and renal flow with reduced blood pressure. J Pharmacol Exp Ther 1991; 256:110.

100. Insogna KL, Stewart AF, Morris CA, et al.: Native and a synthetic analogue of the malignancy-associated parathyroid hormone-like protein have in vitro transforming growth factor–like properties. J Clin Invest 1989; 83:1057.

101. Grill V, Hillary J, Ho PMW, et al.: Parathyroid hormone-related protein: a possible endocrine function in lactation. Clin Endocrinol 1992; 37:405.

102. Moseley JM, Kubota M, Diefenbach-Jagger H, et al.: Parathyroid hormone-related protein purified from a human lung cancer cell line. Proc Natl Acad Sci U S A 1987; 84:5048.

103. Strewler GJ, Stern PH, Jacobs JW, et al.: Parathyroid hormone-like protein from human renal carcinoma cells: Structural and functional homology with parathyroid hormone. J Clin Invest 1987; 80:1803.

104. Weir EC, Burtis WJ, Morris CA, et al.: Isolation of 16,000-dalton parathyroid hormone-like proteins from two animal tumors causing humoral hypercalcemia of malignancy. Endocrinology 1988; 123:2744.

105. Henderson JE, Shustik C, Kremer R, et al.: Circulating concentrations of parathyroid hormone-like peptide in malignancy and hyperparathyroidism. J Bone Min Res 1990; 5:105.

106. Goltzman D, Bennett HP, Koutsilieris M, et al.: Studies of the multiple molecular forms of bioactive parathyroid hormone and parathyoid hormone-like substances. Recent Prog Horm Res 1986; 42:665.

107. Clark OH, Stark DD, Gooding GAW, et al.: Localization procedures in patients requiring reoperation for hyperparathyroidism. World J Surg 1984; 8:509.

108. Gooding GA, Clark OH, Stark DD, et al.: Parathyroid aspiration biopsy under ultrasound guidance in the postoperative hyperparathyroid patient. Radiology 1985; 155:193.

109. Doppman JL, Krudy AG, Marx SJ, et al.: Aspiration of enlarged parathyroid glands for parathyroid hormone assay. Radiology 1983; 148:31.

110. Grenko RT, Anderson KM, Kauffman G, et al.: Water-clear cell adenoma of the parathyroid: A case report with immunohistochemistry and electron microscopy. Arch Pathol Lab Med 1995; 119:1072.

111. Clark OH, Gooding GA, Ljung BM: Locating a parathyroid adenoma by ultrasonography and aspiration biopsy cytology. West J Med 1981; 135:154.

112. Rastad J, Johansson H, Lindgren PG, et al.: Ultrasonic localization and cytologic identification of parathyroid tumors. World J Surg 1984; 8:501.

113. Miller DL: Pre-operative localization and interventional treatment of parathyroid tumors: When and how? World J Surg 1991; 15:706.

114. Krudy AG, Doppman JL, Marx SJ, et al.: Parathyroid aspiration directed by angiography: An alternative to venous sampling. Radiology 1984; 152:207.

115. Mincione GP, Borrelli D, Cicchi P, et al.: Fine needle aspiration cytology of parathyroid adenoma: A review of seven cases. Acta Cytol 1986; 30:65.

116. Davey DD, Glant MD, Berger EK: Parathyroid cytopathology. Diagn Cytopathol 1986; 2:76.

117. Lowhagen T, Sprenger E: Cytologic presentation of thyroid tumors in aspiration biopsy smear: A review of 60 cases. Acta Cytol 1974; 18:192.

118. Friedman M, Shimaoka K, Lopez CA, et al.: Parathyroid adenoma diagnosed as papillary carcinoma of thyroid on needle aspiration smears. Acta Cytol 1983; 27:337.

119. Guazzi A, Gabrielli M, Guadagni G: Cytologic features of a functioning parathyroid carcinoma: A case report. Acta Cytol 1982; 26:709.

120. de la Garza S, Flores de la Garza E, Hernandez-Batres F: Functional parathyroid carcinoma: Cytology, histology, and ultrastructure of a case. Diagn Cytopathol 1985; 1:232.

121. Glenthoj A, Karstrup S: Parathyroid identification by ultrasonically guided aspiration cytology: Is correct cytological identification possible? APMIS 1989; 97:497.

122. Layfield LJ: Fine needle aspiration cytology of cystic parathyroid lesions: A cytomorphologic overlap with cystic lesions of the thyroid. Acta Cytol 1991; 35:447.

123. Abati A, Skarulis MC, Shawker T, et al.: Ultrasound-guided fine-needle aspiration of parathyroid lesions: A morphological and immunocytochemical approach. Hum Pathol 1995; 26:338.

124. Solbiati L, Montali G, Croce F, et al.: Parathyroid tumors detected by fine needle aspiration biopsy under ultrasonic guidance. Radiology 1983; 148:793.

125. Kini U, Shariff S, Thomas JA: Ultrasonically guided fine needle aspiration of the parathyroid: A report of two cases. Acta Cytol 1993; 37:747.

126. Sawady J, Mendelsohn G, Sirota RL, et al.: The intrathyroidal hyperfunctioning parathyroid gland. Mod Pathol 1989; 2:652.

127. Winkler B, Gooding GA, Montgomery CK, et al.: Immunoperoxidase confirmation of parathyroid origin of ultrasound-guided fine needle aspirates of the parathyroid glands. Acta Cytol 1987; 31:40.

128. O'Connor DT, Burton D, Deftos LJ: Immunoreactive human chromogranin A in diverse polypeptide hormone producing human tumors and normal endocrine tissues. J Clin Endocrinol Metab 1983; 57:1084.

129. Silverberg SG: Imprints in the intraoperative evaluation of parathyroid disease. Arch Pathol 1975; 99:375.

130. Sulak LE, Brown RW, Butler DB: Parathyroid carcinoma with occult bone metastases diagnosed by fine needle aspiration cytology. Acta Cytol 1989; 33:645.

131. Ramos-Gabatin A, Mallette LE, Bringhurst FR, et al.: Functional mediastinal parathyroid cyst: Dynamics of parathyroid hormone secretion during cyst aspirations and surgery. Am J Med 1985; 79:633.

132. Brennan MF: Invited commentary: "Localization procedures in patients requiring reoperation for hyperparathyroidism." World J Surg 1984; 8:519.

133. Arnold A, Brown MF, Urena P, et al.: Monoclonality of parathyroid tumors in chronic renal failure and in primary parathyroid hyperplasia. J Clin Invest 1995; 95:2047.

134. Drüeke TB: The pathogenesis of parathyroid gland hyperplasia in chronic renal failure. Kidney Int 1995; 48:259.

135. Noguchi S, Motomura K, Inaji H, et al.: Clonal analysis of parathyroid adenomas by means of polymerase chain reaction. Cancer Lett 1994; 78:93.

136. Saxe AW, Baier R, Tesluk H, et al.: The role of the pathologist in the surgical treatment of hyperparathyroidism. Surg Gynecol Obstet 1985; 161:101.

137. Harrison TS, Duarte B, Reitz RE, et al.: Primary Hyperparathyroidism: Four- to eight-year postoperative follow-up demonstrating persistent functional insignificance of microscopic parathyroid hyperplasia and decreased autonomy of parathyroid hormone release. Ann Surg 1981; 194:429.

138. Attie JN, Bock G, Auguste L-J: Multiple parathyroid adenomas: Report of thirty-three cases. Surgery 1990; 108:1014.

139. Verdonk CA, Edis AJ: Parathyroid "double adenomas": Fact or fiction? Surgery 1981; 90:523.

140. Monchik JM, Farrugia R, Teplitz C, et al.: Parathyroid surgery: The role of chief cell intracellular fat staining with osmium carmine in the intraoperative management of patients with primary hyperparathyroidism. Surgery 1983; 94:877.

141. LiVolsi VA, Hamilton R: Intraoperative assessment of parathyroid gland pathology: A common view from the surgeon and the pathologist. Am J Clin Pathol 1994; 102:365.

142. Roth SI, Wang C-A, Potts JT Jr: The team approach to primary hyperparathyroidism. Hum Pathol 1975; 6:645.

143. Geelhoed GW, Silverberg SG: Intraoperative imprints for the identification of parathyroid tissue. Surgery 1984; 96:1124.

144. Ducatman BS, Wilkerson SY, Brown JA: Functioning parathyroid lipoadenoma: Report of a case diagnosed by intraoperative touch preparations. Arch Pathol Lab Med 1986; 110:645.

145. Proye CAG, Carnaille B, Bizard JP, et al.: Multiglandular disease in seemingly sporadic primary hyperparathyroidism revisited: Where are we in the early 1990s? A plea against unilateral parathyroid exploration. Surgery 1992; 112:1118.

146. Wang C-A, Castleman B, Cope O: Surgical management of hyperparathyroidism due to primary hyperplasia. Ann Surg 1982; 195:384.

147. Kasdon EJ, Cohen RB, Rosen S, et al.: Surgical pathology of hyperparathyroidism: Usefulness of fat stain and problems in interpretation. Am J Surg Pathol 1981; 5:381.

148. Ljungberg O, Tibblin S: Preoperative fat staining of frozen sections in primary hyperparathyroidism. Am J Pathol 1979; 95:633.

149. Dekker A, Watson CG, Barnes ELJ: The pathologic assessment of primary hyperparathyroidism and its impact on therapy: A prospective evaluation of 50 cases with oil-red-O stain. Ann Surg 1979; 190:671.

150. Dufour DR, Durkowski C: Sudan IV stain: Its limitations in evaluating parathyroid functional status. Arch Pathol Lab Med 1982; 106:224.

151. King DT, Hirose FM: Chief cell intracytoplasmic fat used to evaluate parathyroid disease by frozen section. Arch Pathol Lab Med 1979; 103:609.

152. Bondeson AG, Bondeson L, Ljungberg O, et al.: Fat staining in parathyroid disease: Diagnostic value and impact on surgical strategy: Clinicopathologic analysis of 191 cases. Hum Pathol 1985; 16:1255.

153. Welsh CL, Taylor GW: The density test for the intraoperative differentiation of single or multigland parathyroid disease. World J Surg 1984; 8:522.

154. Wang CA, Rieder SV: A density test for the intraoperative differentiation of parathyroid hyperplasia from neoplasia. Ann Surg 1978; 187:63.

155. Rothmund M: Invited commentary: "The density test for the intraoperative differentiation of single or multiglandular parathyroid disease." World J Surg 1984; 8:525.

156. Harlow S, Roth SI, Bauer K, et al.: Flow cytometric DNA analysis of normal and pathologic parathyroid glands. Mod Pathol 1991; 4:310.

157. Irvin GLI, Bagwell CB: Identification of histologically undetectable parathyroid hyperplasia by flow cytometry. Am J Surg 1979; 138:567.

158. Irvin GLI, Taupier M-A, Block NL, et al.: DNA patterns in parathyroid disease predict postoperative parathyroid hormone secretion. Surgery 1988; 104:1115.

159. Bowlby LS, DeBault LE, Abraham SR: Flow cytometric DNA analysis of parathyroid glands: Relationship between nuclear DNA and pathologic classifications. Am J Pathol 1987; 128:338.

160. Mallette LE: DNA quantitation in the study of parathyroid lesions: A review. Am J Clin Pathol 1992; 98:305.

161. Bondeson L, Sandelin K, Grimelius L: Histopathological variables and DNA cytometry in parathyroid carcinoma. Am J Surg Pathol 1993; 17:820.

162. Rosen IB, Musclow CE: DNA histogram of parathyroid tissue in determining extent of parathyroidectomy. Surgery 1985; 98:1024.

163. Levin KE, Chew KL, Ljung B-M, et al.: Deoxyribonucleic acid cytometry helps identify parathyroid carcinoma. J Clin Endocrinol Metab 1988; 67:779.

164. Bengtsson A, Grimelius L, Johansson H, et al.: Nuclear DNA: Content of parathyroid cells in adenomas, hyperplastic and normal glands. Acta Pathol Microbiol Scand 1977; 85:455.

165. Obara T, Fujimoto Y, Hirayama A, et al.: Flow cytometric DNA analysis of parathyroid tumors with special reference to its diagnostic and prognostic value in parathyroid carcinoma. Cancer 1990; 65:1789.

166. Hellman P, Öhrvall U, Rudberg C, et al.: Incidence, structure, and function of enlarged parathyroid glands discovered accidentally during thyroid surgery. Surgery 1993; 113:655.

167. Cope O: The study of hyperparathyroidism at the Massachusetts General Hospital. N Engl J Med 1966; 274:1174.

168. Kay S: The abnormal parathyroid. Hum Pathol 1976; 7:127.

169. Coffey RJ, Lee TC, Canary JJ: The surgical treatment of primary hyperparathyroidism: A 20-year experience. Ann Surg 1977; 185:518.

170. Paloyan E, Paloyan D, Pickleman JR: Hyperparathyroidism today. Surg Clin North Am 1973; 53:211.

171. van Heerden JA, Grant CS: Surgical treatment of primary hyperparathyroidism: An institutional perspective. World J Surg 1991; 15:688.

172. Ghandur-Mnaymneh L, Kimura N: The parathyroid adenoma: A histologic definition with a study of 172 cases of primary hyperparathyroidism. Am J Pathol 1984; 115:70.

173. Poole GV Jr, Albertson DA, Marshall RB, et al.: Oxyphil cell adenoma and hyperparathyroidism. Surgery 1982; 92:799.

174. Harness JK, Ramsburg SR, Nishiyama RH, et al.: Multiple adenomas of the parathyroids: Do they exist? Arch Surg 1979; 114:468.

175. Wang C-A, Gaz RD: Natural history of parathyroid carcinoma: Diagnosis, treatment, and results. Am J Surg 1985; 149:522.

176. van Heerden JA, Weiland LH, ReMine WH, et al.: Cancer of the parathyroid glands. Arch Surg 1979; 114:475.

177. Obara T, Fujimoto Y: Diagnosis and treatment of patients with parathyroid carcinoma: An update and review. World J Surg 1991; 15:738.

178. Chigot J-P, Menegaux F, Achrafi H: Should primary hyperparathyroidism be treated surgically in elderly patients older than 75 years? Surgery 1995; 117:397.

179. Margolis IB, Wayne R, Organ CH Jr: Parathyroid cysts: Functional and mediastinal. Surgery 1975; 77:462.

180. Spitz AF: Management of a functioning mediastinal parathyroid cyst. J Clin Endocrinol Metab 1995; 80:2866.

181. Calandra DB, Shah KH, Prinz RA, et al.: Parathyroid cysts: A report of eleven cases including two associated with hyperparathyroid crisis. Surgery 1983; 94:887.

182. Pinney SP, Daly PA: Parathyroid cyst: An uncommon cause of a palpable neck mass and hypercalcemia. West J Med 1999; 170:118.

183. Cantley LK, Ontjes DA, Cooper CW, et al.: Parathyroid hormone secretion from dispersed human hyperparathyroid cells: Increased secretion in cells from hyperplastic glands versus adenomas. J Clin Endocrinol Metab 1985; 60:1032.

184. Larsson R, Wallfelt C, Abrahamsson H, et al.: Defective regulation of the cytosolic Ca2+ activity in parathyroid cells

from patients with hyperparathyroidism. Biosci Rep 1984; 4:909.

185. Christensson T: Hyperparathyroidism and radiation therapy. Ann Intern Med 1978; 89:216.

186. Russ JE, Scanlon EF, Sener SF: Parathyroid adenomas following irradiation. Cancer 1979; 43:1078.

187. Rao SD, Frame B, Miller MJ, et al.: Hyperparathyroidism following head and neck irradiation. Arch Intern Med 1980; 140:205.

188. Beard CM, Heath HI, O'Fallon WM, et al.: Therapeutic radiation and hyperparathyroidism: A case-control study in Rochester, Minn. Arch Intern Med 1989; 149:1887.

189. Schneider AB, Gierlowski TC, Shore-Freedman E, et al.: Dose-response relationships for radiation-induced hyperparathyroidism. J Clin Endocrinol Metab 1995; 80:254.

190. Tisell LE, Carlsson S, Fjalling M, et al.: Hyperparathyroidism subsequent to neck irradiation: Risk factors. Cancer 1985; 56:1529.

191. Hedman I, Tisell LE: Associated hyperparathyroidism and nonmedullary thyroid carcinoma: The etiologic role of radiation. Surgery 1984; 95:392.

192. Paloyan E, Lawrence AM, Prinz RA, et al.: Radiation-associated hyperparathyroidism. Lancet 1977; 19:49.

193. Rosen IB, Strawbridge HG, Bain J: A case of hyperparathyroidism associated with radiation to the head and neck area. Cancer 1975; 36:1111.

194. Tisell LE, Hansson G, Lindberg S, et al.: Occurrence of previous neck radiotherapy among patients with associated nonmedullary thyroid carcinoma and parathyroid adenoma or hyperplasia. Acta Chir Scand 1978; 144:7.

195. Tisell LE, Carlsson S, Lindberg S, et al.: Autonomous hyperparathyroidism: A possible late complication of neck radiotherapy. Acta Chir Scand 1976; 142:367.

196. Tisell LE, Hansson G, Lindberg S, et al.: Hyperparathyroidism in patients treated with x-rays for tuberculous cervical adenitis. Cancer 1977; 40:846.

197. Prinz RA, Barbato AL, Braithwaite SS, et al.: Prior irradiation and the development of coexistent differentiated thyroid cancer and hyperparathyroidism. Cancer 1982; 49:874.

198. Fujiwara S, Sposto R, Shiraki M, et al.: Levels of parathyroid hormone and calcitonon in serum among atomic bomb survivors. Radiat Res 1994; 137:96.

199. Takeichi N, Dohi K, Yamamoto H, et al.: Parathyroid tumors in atomic bomb survivors in Hiroshima: Epidemiological study from registered cases at Hiroshima prefecture tumor tissue registry 1974–1987. Jpn J Cancer Res 1991; 82:875.

200. Esselstyn CB Jr, Schumacher OP, Eversman J, et al.: Hyperparathyroidism after radioactive iodine therapy for Graves' disease. Surgery 1982; 92:811.

201. Walker RP, Paloyan E: The relationship between Hashimoto's thyroiditis, thyroid neoplasia, and primary hyperparathyroidism. Otolaryngol Clin North Am 1990; 23:291.

202. Bouillon R, DeMoor P: Parathyroid function in patients with hyper- or hypothyroidism. J Clin Endocrinol Metab 1974; 38:999.

203. Lever EG: Primary hyperparathyroidism masked by hypothyroidism. Am J Med 1983; 74:144.

204. Paloyan-Walker R, Oslapsa R, Ernst K, et al.: Hyperparathyroidism induced by hypothyroidism. Laryngoscope 1993; 103:263.

205. Fialkow PJ, Jackson CE, Block MA, et al.: Multicellular origin of parathyroid "adenomas." N Engl J Med 1977; 297:696.

206. Jackson CE, Cerny JC, Block MA, et al.: Probable clonal origin of aldosteronomas versus multicellular origin of parathyroid "adenomas." Surgery 1982; 92:875.

207. Arnold A, Staunton CE, Kim HG, et al.: Monoclonality and abnormal parathyroid hormone genes in parathyroid adenomas. N Engl J Med 1988; 318:658.

208. Arnold A, Kim HG, Gaz RD, et al.: Molecular cloning and chromosomal mapping of DNA rearranged with the parathyroid hormone gene in a parathyroid adenoma. J Clin Invest 1989; 83:2034.

209. Arnold A, Kim HG: Clonal loss of one chromosome 11 in a parathyroid adenoma. J Clin Endocrinol Metab 1989; 69:496.

210. Mendelsohn G: Syndromes of multiple endocrine neoplasia and hyperplasia. In Kovacs K, Asa SL, eds.: Functional Endocrine Pathology. Boston, Blackwell Scientific Publications, 1991, p. 814.

211. Allo M, Thompson NW: Familial hyperparathyroidism caused by solitary adenomas. Surgery 1982; 92:486.

212. Mallette LE, Bilezikian JP, Ketcham AS, et al.: Parathyroid carcinoma in familial hyperparathyroidism. Am J Med 1974; 57:642.

213. Wynne AG, van Heerden J, Carney JA, et al.: Parathyroid carcinoma: Clinical and pathologic features in 43 patients. Medicine 1992; 71:197.

214. Larsson C, Skogseid B, Oberg K, et al.: Multiple endocrine neoplasia type 1 gene maps to chromosome 11 and is lost in insulinoma. Nature 1988; 332:85.

215. Byström C, Larsson C, Blomberg C, et al.: Localization of the MEN 1 gene to a small region within chromosome 11q13 by deletion mapping in tumors. Proc Natl Acad Sci U S A 1990; 87:1968.

216. Friedman E, Sakaguchi K, Bale AE, et al.: Clonality of parathyroid tumors in familial multiple endocrine neoplasia type 1. N Engl J Med 1989; 321:213.

217. Thakker RV, Bouloux P, Wooding C, et al.: Association of parathyroid tumors in multiple endocrine neoplasia type 1 with loss of alleles on chromosome 11. N Engl J Med 1989; 321:218.

218. Radford DM, Ashley SW, Wells SA, et al.: Loss of heterozygosity of markers on chromosome 11 in tumors from patients with multiple endocrine neoplasia syndrome type 1. Cancer Res 1990; 50:6529.

219. Chandrasekharappa SC, Guru SC, Manickam P, et al.: Positional cloning of the gene for multiple endocrine neoplasia-type 1. Science 1997; 276:404.

220. Knudson AGJ: Mutation and cancer: Statistical study of retinoblastoma. Proc Natl Acad Sci U S A 1971; 68:820.

221. Guru SC, Goldsmith PK, Burns AL, et al.: Menin, the product of the *MEN1* gene, is a nuclear protein. Proc Natl Acad Sci U S A 1998; 95:1630.

222. Agarwal SK, Kester MB, Debelenko LV, et al.: Germline mutations of the *MEN1* gene in familial multiple endocrine neoplasia type 1 and related states. Hum Mol Genet 1997; 6:1169.

223. Ki WF, Burgess J, Nordenskjold M, et al.: Multiple endocrine neoplasia type 1. Semin Cancer Biol 2000; 10:299.

224. Heppner C, Kester MB, Agarwal SK, et al.: Somatic mutation of the *MEN1* gene in parathyroid tumours. Nat Genet 1997; 16:375.

225. Dwight T, Twigg S, Delbridge L, et al.: Loss of heterozygosity in sporadic parathyroid tumours: Involvement of chromosome 1 and the *MEN1* gene locus in 11q13. Clin Endocrinol (Oxf) 2000; 53:85.

226. Beckers A, Abs R, Reyniers E, et al.: Variable regions of chromosome 11 loss in different pathological tissues of a patient with the multiple endocrine neoplasia type 1 syndrome. J Clin Endocrinol Metab 1994; 79:1498.

227. Tahara H, Smith AP, Gas RD, et al.: Genomic localization of novel candidate tumor suppressor gene loci in human parathyroid adenomas. Cancer Res 1996; 56:599.

228. Arnold A, Motokura T, Bloom T, et al.: *PRAD1* (cyclin D1): A parathyroid neoplasia gene on 11q13. Henry Ford Hosp Med J 1992; 40:177.

229. Arnold A: Genetic basis of endocrine disease 5: Molecular genetics of parathyroid gland neoplasia. J Clin Endocrinol Metab 1993; 77:1108.

230. Brandi ML, Aurbach GD, Fitzpatrick LA, et al.: Parathyroid mitogenic activity in plasma from patients with familial multiple endocrine neoplasia type 1. N Engl J Med 1986; 314:1287.

231. Komatsu M, Tsuchiya S, Matsuyama I, et al.: Expression of basic fibroblast growth factor in hyperplastic parathyroid glands from patients with multiple endocrine neoplasia type 1. World J Surg 1994; 18:921.

232. Gardner E, Mulligan LM, Eng C, et al.: Haplotype analysis of MEN 2 mutations. Hum Mol Genet 1994; 31:771.

233. Gardner E, Papi L, Easton DF, et al.: Genetic linkage studies map the multiple endocrine neoplasia type 2 loci to a small interval on chromosome 10q11.2. Hum Mol Genet 1993; 2:241.

234. Mole SE, Mulligan LM, Healey CS, et al.: Localization of the gene for multiple endocrine neoplasia type 2A to a 480 Kb region in chromosome band 10q11.2. Hum Mol Genet 1993; 2:247.

235. Nelkin BD, Ball DW, Baylin SB: Molecular abnormalities in tumors associated with multiple endocrine neoplasia type 2. Endocrinol Metab Clin North Am 1994; 23:187.

236. Takahashi M, Buma Y, Hiai H: Isolation of the *RET* proto-oncogene cDNA with an amino-terminal signal sequence. Oncogene 1989; 4:805.

237. Schneider R: The human Proto-oncogene *RET*: A communicative Cadherin? TIBS 1992; 17:468.

238. Jing S, Wen D, Yu Y, et al.: GDNF-induced activation of the ret protein tyrosine kinase is mediated by GDNFR-alpha, a novel receptor for GDNF. Cell 1996; 85:1113.

239. Treanor JJ, Goodman L, de Sauvage F, et al.: Characterization of a multicomponent receptor for GDNF. Nature 1996; 382:80.

240. Sanicola M, Hession C, Worley D, et al.: Glial cell line-derived neurotrophic factor-dependent RET activation can be mediated by two different cell-surface accessory proteins. Proc Natl Acad Sci U S A 1997; 94:6238.

241. Mulligan LM, Kwok JBJ, Healey CS, et al.: Germ-line mutations of the *RET* proto-oncogene in multiple endocrine neoplasia type 2A. Nature 1993; 363:458.

242. Mulligan LM, Eng C, Healey CS, et al.: Specific mutations of the *RET* proto-oncogene are related to disease phenotype in MEN 2A and FMTC. Nat Genet 1994; 670–74.

243. Mulligan L, Marsh D, Robinson B: Genotype-phenotype correlation in MEN 2: Report of the international RET mutation consortium. J Int Med 1995; 238:243.

244. Schuffenecker I, Billaud M, Calender A, et al.: *RET* proto-oncogene mutations in French MEN 2A and FMTC families. Hum Mol Genet 1994; 3:1939.

245. Mulligan LM, Ponder BAJ: Genetic basis of endocrine disease: Multiple endocrine neoplasia type 2. J Clin Endocrinol Metab 1995; 80:1989.

246. Hofstra RM, Landsvater RM, Ceccherini I, et al.: A mutation in the *RET* proto-oncogene associated with multiple endocrine neoplasia type 2B and sporadic medullary thyroid carcinoma. Nature 1994; 357:375.

247. Carlson KM, Dou S, Chi D, et al.: Single missense mutation in the tyrosine kinase catalytic domain of the *RET* proto-oncogene is associated with multiple endocrine neoplasia type 2B. Proc Natl Acad Sci U S A 1994; 91:1579.

248. Eng C, Smith DP, Mulligan LM, et al.: Point mutations within the tyrosine kinase domain of the *RET* proto-oncogene in multiple endocrine neoplasia type 2B and related sporadic tumours. Hum Mol Genet 1994; 3:237.

249. Kimura T, Yoshimoto K, Tanaka C, et al.: Obvious mRNA and protein expression but absence of mutations of the *RET* proto-oncogene in parathyroid tumors. Eur J Endocrinol 1996; 134:314.

250. Willeke F, Hauer MP, Buchick R, et al.: Multiple endocrine neoplasia type 2–associated *RET* proto-oncogene mutations do not contribute to the pathogenesis of sporadic parathyroid tumors. Surgery 1998; 124:484.

251. Szabo J, Heath B, Hill VM, et al.: Hereditary hyperparathyroidism-law tumor syndrome: The endocrine tumor gene *HRPT2* maps to chromosome 1q21-q31. Am J Hum Genet 1995; 56:944.

252. Teh BT, Farnebo F, Kristoffersson U, et al.: Autosomal-dominant primary hyperparathyroidism and jaw tumor syndrome associated with renal hamartomas and cystic kidney disease: Linkage to 1q21-q32 and loss of the wild-type allele in renal hamartomas. J Clin Endocrinol Metab 1996; 81:4204.

253. Teh BT, Farnebo F, Twigg S, et al.: Familial isolated hyperparathyroidism maps to the hyperparathyroidism–jaw tumor locus in 1q21-q32 in a subset of families. J Clin Endocrinol Metab 1998; 83:2114.

254. Hobbs MR, Pole AR, Pidwirny GN, et al.: Hyperparathyroidism–jaw tumor syndrome: The HRPT2 locus is within a 0.7-cm region on chromosome 1q. Am J Hum Genet 1999; 64:518.

255. DeLellis RA, Dayal Y, Tischler AS, et al.: Multiple endocrine neoplasia (MEN) syndromes: Cellular origins and interrelationships. Int Rev Exp Pathol 1986; 28:163.

256. Berg B, Biorklund A, Grimelius L, et al.: A new pattern of multiple endocrine adenomatosis: Chemodectoma, bronchial carcinoid, GH-producing pituitary adenoma, and hyperplasia of the parathyroid glands, and antral and duodenal gastrin cells. Acta Med Scand 1976; 200:321.

257. Hansen OP, Hansen M, Hansen HH, et al.: Multiple endocrine adenomatosis of mixed type. Acta Med Scand 1976; 200:327.

258. Rode J, Dhillon AP, Cotton PB, et al.: Carcinoid tumour of the stomach and primary hyperparathyroidism: A new association. J Clin Pathol 1987; 40:546.

259. Kassem M, Kruse TA, Wong FK, et al.: Familial isolated hyperparathyroidism as a variant of multiple endocrine neoplasia type 1 in a large Danish pedigree. J Clin Endocrinol Metab 2000; 85:165.

260. Feig DS, Gottesman IS: Familial hyperparathyroidism in association with colonic carcinoma. Cancer 1987; 60:429.

261. Cutler RE, Reiss E, Ackerman LV: Familial hyperparathyroidism: A kindred involving eleven cases, with a discussion of primary chief-cell hyperplasia. N Engl J Med 1964; 270:859.

262. Cryns VL, Thor A, Xu H-J, et al.: Loss of the retinoblastoma tumor-suppressor gene in parathyroid carcinoma. N Engl J Med 1994; 330:757.

263. Hakim JP, Levine MA: Absence of *p53* point mutations in parathyroid adenoma and carcinoma. J Clin Endocrinol Metab 1994; 78:103.

264. Cryns VL, Rubio M-P, Thor AD, et al.: *p53* abnormalities in human parathyroid carcinoma. J Clin Endocrinol Metab 1994; 78:1320.

265. Yoshimoto K, Iwahana H, Fukuda A, et al.: Role of *p53* mutations in endocrine tumorigenesis: Mutation detection by polymerase chain reaction–single strand polymorphism. Cancer Res 1992; 52:5061.

266. Levine AJ, Momand J, Finlay CA: The *p53* tumour suppressor gene. Nature 1991; 351:453.

267. Nigro JM, Baker SJ, Preisinger AC, et al.: Mutations in the *p53* gene occur in diverse human tumour types. Nature 1989; 342:705.

268. Hollstein M, Sidransky D, Vogelstein B, et al.: *p53* mutations in human cancers. Science 1991; 253:49.

269. Lloyd RV, Jin L, Qian X, et al.: Aberrant p27^{kip1} expression in endocrine and other tumors. Am J Pathol 1997; 150:401.

270. Erickson LA, Jin L, Wollan P, et al.: Parathyroid hyperplasia, adenomas, and carcinomas: Differential expression of p27^{kip1} protein. Am J Surg Pathol 1999; 23:288.

271. Golden A, Canary JJ, Kerwin DM: Concurrence of hyperplasia and neoplasia of the parathyroid glands. Am J Med 1965; 38:562.

272. Kramer WM: Association of parathyroid hyperplasia with neoplasia. Am J Clin Pathol 1970; 53:275.

273. Åkerström G, Bergström R, Grimelius L, et al.: Relation between changes in clinical and histopathological features of primary hyperparathyroidism. World J Surg 1986; 10:696.

274. Ljunghall S, Hellman P, Rastad J, et al.: Primary hyperparathyroidism: epidemiology, diagnosis and clinical picture. World J Surg 1991; 15:681.

275. Palmér M, Jakobsson S, Åkerström G, et al.: Prevalence of hypercalaemia in a health survey: A 14-year follow-up study of serum calcium values. Eur J Clin Invest 1988; 18:39.

276. Heath HI, Hodgson SF, Kennedy MA: Primary hyperparathyroidism: Incidence, morbidity, and potential economic impact in a community. N Engl J Med 1980; 302:189.

277. Shane E, Bilezikian JP: Parathyroid carcinoma: A review of 62 patients. Endocr Rev 1995; 3:218.

278. Aldinger KA, Hickey RC, Ibañez ML, et al.: Parathyroid carcinoma: A clinical study of seven cases of functioning and two cases of nonfunctioning parathyroid cancer. Cancer 1982; 49:388.

279. Sandelin K, Tullgren O, Farnebo LO: Clinical course of metastatic parathyroid cancer. World J Surg 1994; 18:594.

280. Schantz A, Castleman B: Parathyroid carcinoma: A study of 70 cases. Cancer 1973; 31:600.

281. Harrison BJ, Wheeler MH: Asymptomatic primary hyperparathyroidism. World J Surg 1991; 15:724.

282. Oertli D, Richter M, Kraenzlin M, et al.: Parathyroidectomy in primary hyperparathyroidism: Preoperative localization and

routine biopsy of unaltered glands are not necessary. Surgery 1995; 117:392.

283. Attie JN, Khan A, Rumancik WM, et al.: Preoperative localization of parathyroid adenomas. Am J Surg 1988; 156:323.

284. Thompson NW: Localization studies in patients with primary hyperparathyroidism. Br J Surg 1988; 75:97.

285. Patow CA, Norton JA, Brennan MF: Vocal cord paralysis and reoperative parathyroidectomy: A prospective study. Ann Surg 1986; 203:282.

286. Norton JA, Shawker TH, Jones BL, et al.: Intraoperative ultrasound and reoperative parathyroid surgery: An initial evaluation. World J Surg 1986; 10:631.

287. Grant CS, van Heerden JA, Charboneau JW, et al.: Clinical management of persistent and/or recurrent primary hyperparathyroidism. World J Surg 1986; 10:555.

288. Goretzki PE, Dotzenrath C, Roeher HD: Management of primary hyperparathyroidism caused by multiple gland disease. World J Surg 1991; 15:693.

289. Miller DL, Doppman JL, Shawker TH, et al.: Localization of parathyroid adenomas in patients who have undergone surgery: Part 1: Noninvasive imaging methods. Radiology 1987; 162:133.

290. Miller DL, Doppman JL, Krudy AG, et al.: Localization of parathyroid adenomas in patients who have undergone surgery: Part 2: Invasive procedures. Radiology 1987; 162:138.

291. Nilsson BE, Tisell L-E, Jansson S, et al.: Parathyroid localization by catheterization of large cervical and mediastinal veins to determine serum concentrations of intact parathyroid hormone. World J Surg 1994; 18:605.

292. Kairaluoma MV, Kellosalo J, Mäkäräinen H, et al.: Parathyroid re-exploration in patients with primary hyperparathyroidism. Ann Chir Gynaecol 1994; 83:202.

293. Schmidt N: Hyperparathyroidism: A review. Am J Surg 1980; 139:657.

294. Weber CJ, Sewell CW, McGarity WC: Persistent and recurrent sporadic primary hyperparathyroidism: Histopathology, complications, and results of reoperation. Surgery 1994; 116:991.

295. Fahey TJI, Hibbert E, Brady P, et al.: Giant double parathyroid adenoma presenting as a hypercalcaemic crisis. Aust N Z J Surg 1995; 65:292.

296. Edis AJ, Beahrs OH, van Heerden JA, et al.: "Conservative" versus "liberal" approach to parathyroid neck exploration. Surgery 1977; 82:466.

297. Purnell DC, Scholz DA, Beahrs OH: Hyperparathyroidism due to a single gland enlargement: Prospective postoperative study. Arch Surg 1977; 112:369.

298. Russell CFJ, Laird JD, Ferguson WR: Scan-directed unilateral cervical exploration for parathyroid adenoma: A legitimate approach? World J Surg 1990; 14:406.

299. Hung GU, Wu HS, Tsai SC, et al.: Recurrent hyperfunctioning parathyroid gland demonstrated on radionuclide imaging and an intraoperative gamma probe. Clin Nucl Med 2000; 25:348.

300. Rossi HL, Ali A, Prinz RA: Intraoperative sestamibi scanning in reoperative parathyroidectomy. Surgery 2000; 128:744.

301. Miccoli P, Bendinelli C, Vignali E, et al.: Endoscopic parathyroidectomy: Report of an initial experience. Surgery 1998; 124:1077.

302. Nussbaum SR, Thompson AR, Hutcheson KA, et al.: Intraoperative measurement of parathyroid hormone in the surgical management of hyperparathyroidism. Surgery 1988; 1041:121.

303. Proye CAG, Goropoulos A, Franz C, et al.: Usefulness and limits of quick intraoperative measurements of intact (1–84) parathyroid hormone in the surgical management of hyperparathyroidism: Sequential measurements in patients with multiglandular disease. Surgery 1991; 110:1035.

304. Rothmund M, Wagner PK, Schark C: Subtotal parathyroidectomy versus total parathyroidectomy and autotransplantation in secondary hyperparathyroidism: A randomized trial. World J Surg 1991; 15:745.

305. Rothmund M, Wagner PK: Assessment of parathyroid graft function after autotransplantation of fresh and cryopreserved tissue. World J Surg 1984; 8:527.

306. Wells SA Jr, Farndon JR, Dale JK, et al.: Long-term evaluation of patients with primary parathyroid hyperplasia managed by total parathyroidectomy and heterotopic autotransplantation. Ann Surg 1980; 192:451.

307. Mallette LE, Eisenberg KL, Schwaitzberg SD, et al.: Factors that influence the assessment of parathyroid graft function. Ann Surg 1984; 199:192.

308. Lundgren G, Asaba M, Magnusson G, et al.: The role of parathyroidectomy in the treatment of secondary hyperparathyroidism before and after renal transplantation. Scand J Urol Nephrol 1977; 42:149.

309. Rizzoli R, Green JI, Marx SJ: Primary hyperparathyroidism in familial multiple endocrine neoplasia type 1: Long-term follow-up of serum calcium levels after parathyroidectomy. Am J Med 1985; 78:467.

310. Levin KE, Clark OH: The reasons for failure in parathyroid operations. Arch Surg 1989; 124:911.

311. Clark OH, Duh Q-Y: Primary hyperparathyroidism: A surgical perspective. Endocrinol Metab Clin North Am 1989; 18:701.

312. Kollmorgen CF, Aust MR, Ferreiro JA, et al.: Parathyromatosis: A rare yet important cause of persistent or recurrent hyperparathyroidism. Surgery 1994; 116:111.

313. Fitko R, Roth SI, Hines JR, et al.: Parathyromatosis in hyperparathyroidism. Hum Pathol et al.: 1990; 21:234.

314. Marx SJ, Stock JL, Attie MF, et al.: Familial hypocalciuric hypercalcemia: Recognition among patients referred after unsuccessful parathyroid exploration. Ann Intern Med 1980; 92:351.

315. Ross N, Leung C-S, Kovacs K, et al.: Parathyroid nodules in a patient with chronic renal failure: Hyperplasia or neoplasia? Endocr Pathol 1993; 4:100.

316. Gogusev J, Chopard C, Duchambon P, et al.: Abnormal TGF-α expression in parathyroid gland tissue from patients with secondary hyperparathyroidism (abstract). J Am Soc Nephrol 1994; 5:879.

317. Goldsmith RS, Johnson WJ, Arnaud CD: The hyperparathyroidism of renal failure: Pathophysiology and treatment. Clin Endocrinol Metab 1974; 3:305.

318. Parfitt AM: Relation between parathyroid cell mass and plasma calcium concentration in normal and uremic subjects: A theoretical model with an analysis of the concept of autonomy, and speculations on the mechanism of parathyroid hyperplasia. Arch Intern Med 1969; 124:269.

319. Parfitt AM: Hypercalcemic hyperparathyroidism following renal transplantation: Differential diagnosis, management and implications for cell population control in the parathyroid gland. Miner Electrol Metab 1982; 9:92.

320. Szabo A, Merke J, Beier E, et al.: 1,25(OH)$_2$ Vitamin D$_3$ inhibits parathyroid cell proliferation in experimental uremia. Kidney Int 1989; 35:1049.

321. Huang Y-Y, Hsu BR-S, Huang B-Y, et al.: Value of serum alkaline phosphatase in evaluating hyperplasia of parathyroid glands in chronic hemodialysis patients. J Clin Ultrasound 1994; 22:193.

322. Vigorita VJ: The tissue pathologic features of metabolic bone disease. Orthop Clin North Am 1984; 15:613.

323. MacLean C, Brahn E: Systemic lupus erythematosus: Calciphylaxis-induced cardiomyopathy. J Rheumatol 1995; 22:177.

324. Cannella G, Bonucci E, Rolla D, et al.: Evidence of healing of secondary hyperparathyroidism in chronically hemodialyzed uremic patients treated with long-term intravenous calcitriol. Kidney Int 1994; 46:1124.

325. Hamdy NAT, Kanis JA, Beneton MNC, et al.: Effect of alfacalcidol on natural course of renal bone disease in mild-to-moderate renal failure. BMJ 1995; 310:358.

326. Kitaoka M, Fukagawa M, Ogata E, et al.: Reduction of functioning parathyroid cell mass by ethanol injection in chronic dialysis patients. Kidney Int 1994; 46:1110.

327. Ritz E: Which is the preferred treatment of advanced hyperparathyroidism in a renal patient? II. Early parathyroidectomy should be considered as the first choice. Nephrol Dial Transplant 1994; 9:1819.

328. Roth SI, Marshall RB: Pathology and ultrastructure of the human parathyroid glands in chronic renal failure. Arch Intern Med 1969; 124:397.

329. Salusky IB, Ramirez JA, Coburn JW: The renal osteodystrophies. In DeGroot LJ, ed.: Endocrinology, 3rd ed. Philadelphia, WB Saunders, 1995, p. 1151.

330. Hasleton PS, Ali HH: The parathyroid in chronic renal failure: A light and electron microscopical Study. J Pathol 1980; 132:307.

331. Krause MW, Hedinger CE: Pathologic study of parathyroid glands in tertiary hyperparathyroidism. Hum Pathol 1985; 16:772.

332. Falchetti A, Bale AE, Amorosi A, et al.: Progression of uremic hyperparathyroidism involves allelic loss on chromosome 11. J Clin Endocrinol Metab 1993; 76:139.

333. Darling GE, Marx SJ, Spiegel AM, et al.: Prospective analysis of intraoperative and postoperative urinary cyclic adenosine 3′, 5′-monophosphate levels to predict outcome of patients undergoing reoperations for primary hyperparathyroidism. Surgery 1988; 104:1128.

334. Malachi T, Zevin D, Gafter U, et al.: DNA repair and recovery of RNA synthesis in uremic patients. Kidney Int 1993; 44:385.

335. Iwamoto N, Yamazaki S, Fukuda T, et al.: Two cases of parathyroid carcinoma in patients on long-term hemodialysis. Nephron 1990; 55:429.

336. Kodama M, Ikegami M, Imanishi M, et al.: Parathyroid carcinoma in a case of chronic renal failure on dialysis. Urol Int 1989; 44:110.

337. Marx SJ, Spiegel AM, Levine MA, et al.: Familial hypocalciuric hypercalcemia: The relation to primary parathyroid hyperplasia. N Engl J Med 1982; 307:416.

338. Marx SJ, Attie MF, Levine MA, et al.: The hypocalciuric or benign variant of familial hypercalcemia: Clinical and biochemical features in fifteen kindreds. Medicine 1981; 60:397.

339. Heath HI: Familial benign hypercalcemia: From clinical description to molecular genetics. West J Med 1994; 160:554.

340. Heath HI: Familial benign (hypocalciuric) hypercalcemia: A troublesome mimic of mild primary hyperparathyroidism. Endocrinol Metab Clin North Am 1989; 18:723.

341. Marx SJ, Spiegel AM, Brown EM, et al.: Divalent cation metabolism: Familial hypocalciuric hypercalcemia versus typical primary hyperparathyroidism. Am J Med 1978; 65:235.

342. Foley TP Jr, Harrison HC, Arnaud CD, et al.: Familial benign hypercalcemia. J Pediatr 1972; 81:1060.

343. Marx SJ, Spiegel AM, Brown EM, et al.: Circulating parathyroid hormone activity: Familial hypocalciuric hypercalcemia versus typical primary hyperparathyroidism. J Clin Endocrinol Metab 1978; 47:1190.

344. Marx SJ, Attie MF, Spiegel AM, et al.: An association between neonatal severe primary hyperparathyroidism and familial hypocalciuric hypercalcemia in three kindreds. N Engl J Med 1982; 306:257.

345. Bai M, Janicic N, Trivedi S, et al.: Markedly reduced activity of mutant calcium-sensing receptor with an inserted Alu element from a kindred with familial hypocalciuric hypercalcemia and neonatal severe hyperparathyroidism. J Clin Invest 1997; 99:1917.

346. Bai M, Pearce SH, Kifor O, et al.: In vivo and in vitro characterization of neonatal hyperparathyroidism resulting from a de novo, heterozygous mutation in the Ca^{2+}-sensing receptor gene: Normal maternal calcium homeostasis as a cause of secondary hyperparathyroidism in familial benign hypocalciuric hypercalcemia. J Clin Invest 1997; 99:88.

347. Marx SJ, Spiegel AM, Sharp ME, et al.: Adenosine 3′5′-monophosphate response to parathyroid hormone: Familial hypocalciuric hypercalcemia versus typical primary hyperparathyroidism. J Clin Endocrinol Metab 1980; 50:546.

348. Heath HI, Purnell DC: Urinary cyclic 3′,5′-adenosine monophosphate responses to exogenous and endogenous parathyroid hormone in familial benign hypercalcemia and primary hyperparathyroidism. J Lab Clin Med 1980; 96:974.

349. Marx SJ, Spiegel AM, Brown EM, et al.: Family studies in patients with primary parathyroid hyperplasia. Am J Med 1977; 62:698.

350. Marx SJ, Powell D, Shimkin PM, et al.: Familial hyperparathyroidism: Mild hypercalcemia in at least nine members of a kindred. Ann Intern Med 1973; 78:371.

351. Thorgeirsson U, Costa J, Marx SJ: The parathyroid glands in familial hypocalciuric hypercalcemia. Hum Pathol 1981; 12:229.

352. Law WM Jr, Carney JA, Heath HI: Parathyroid glands in familial benign hypercalcemia (familial hypocalciuric hypercalcemia). Am J Med 1984; 76:1021.

353. Spiegel AM, Harrison HE, Marx SJ, et al.: Neonatal primary hyperparathyroidism with autosomal dominant inheritance. J Pediatr 1977; 90:269.

354. Anast CS: Disorders of calcium and phosphorus metabolism. In Taeusch TW, Ballard RA, Avery ME, eds.: Schaffer and Avery's Diseases of the Newborn, 6th ed. Philadelphia, WB Saunders, 1991, p. 927.

355. Bradford WD, Wilson JW, Gaede JT: Primary neonatal hyperparathyroidism: An unusual cause of failure to thrive. Am J Clin Pathol 1973; 59:265.

356. Thompson NW, Carpenter LC, Kessler DL, et al.: Hereditary neonatal hyperparathyroidism. Arch Surg 1978; 113:100.

357. Andersen DH, Schlesinger ER: Renal hyperparathyroidism with calcification of arteries in infancy. Am J Dis Child 1942; 63:102.

358. Marx SJ, Lasker RD, Brown EM, et al.: Secretory dysfunction in parathyroid cells from a neonate with severe primary hyperparathyroidism. J Clin Endocrinol Metab 1986; 62:445.

359. Castleman B, Roth SI: Tumors of the parathyroid glands. Atlas of Tumor Pathology, 2nd ed. Washington, D.C., Armed Forces Institute of Pathology, 1978, p. 1.

360. Wolpert HR, Vickery AL Jr, Wang C-A: Functioning oxyphil cell adenomas of the parathyroid gland: A study of 15 cases. Am J Surg Pathol 1989; 13:500.

361. Black WC, Haff RC: The surgical pathology of parathyroid chief cell hyperplasia. Am J Clin Pathol 1970; 53:565.

362. Lawrence DAS: A histological comparison of adenomatous and hyperplastic parathyroid glands. J Clin Pathol 1978; 31:626.

363. Cinti S, Colussi G, Minola E, et al.: Parathyroid glands in primary hyperparathyroidism: An ultrastructural study of 50 Cases. Hum Pathol 1986; 17:1036.

364. Block MA, Frame B, Jackson CE, et al.: Primary diffuse microscopical hyperplasia of the parathyroid glands. Arch Surg 1976; 111:348.

365. Black WCI, Utley JR: The differential diagnosis of parathyroid adenoma and chief cell hyperplasia. Am J Clin Pathol 1968; 49:761.

366. Norris EH: Primary hyperparathyroidism: Report of 5 cases that exemplify special features of this disease (infarction of parathyroid adenoma; oxyphil adenoma). Arch Pathol 1946; 42:261.

367. Williams ED: Pathology of the parathyroid glands. Clin Endocrinol Metab 1974; 32:85.

368. Rasbach DA, Monchik JM, Geelhoed GW, et al.: Solitary parathyroid microadenoma. Surgery 1984; 96:1092.

369. Redleaf MI, Walker WP, Alt LP: Parathyroid adenoma associated with a branchial cleft cyst. Arch Otolaryngol Head Neck Surg 1995; 121:113.

370. Sahin A, Robinson RA: Papillae formation in parathyroid adenoma: A source of possible diagnostic error. Arch Pathol Lab Med 1988; 112:99.

371. San Juan J, Monteagudo C, Fraker D, et al.: Significance of mitotic activity and other morphologic parameters in parathyroid adenomas and their correlation (abstract). Am J Clin Pathol 1989; 92:523.

372. Snover DC, Foucar K: Mitotic activity in benign parathyroid disease. Am J Clin Pathol 1981; 75:345.

373. Fornasier VL, Rabinovich S: A current look at hyperparathyroidism by the pathologist. Mod Med Canada. 1980; 35:29.

374. Ejerblad S, Grimelius L, Johansson H, et al.: Studies on the non-adenomatous glands in patients with a solitary parathyroid adenoma. Upsala J Med Sci 1976; 81:31.

375. Black WCI: Correlative light and electron microscopy in primary hyperparathyroidism. Arch Pathol 1969; 88:225.

376. Cinti S, Sbarbati A, Morroni M, et al.: Parathyroid glands in primary hyperparathyroidism: An ultrastructural morphometric study of 25 cases. J Pathol 1992; 167:283.

377. Ordoñez NG, Ibañez ML, Mackay B, et al.: Functioning oxyphil cell adenomas of parathyroid gland: Immunoperoxidase evidence of hormonal activity in oxyphil cells. Am J Clin Pathol 1982; 78:681.

378. Cetani F, Picone A, Cerrai P, et al.: Parathyroid expression of calcium-sensing receptor protein and in vivo parathyroid hormone-Ca^{2+} set-point in patients with primary hyperparathyroidism. J Clin Endocrinol Metab 2000; 85:4789.

379. Weber CJ, O'Dorisio TM, Howe B, et al.: Vasoactive intestinal polypeptide-, neurotensin-, substance P-, gastrin-releasing peptide-, calcitonin-, calcitonin gene-related peptide-, and so-matostatin-like immunoreactivities in human parathyroid glands. Surgery 1991; 110:1078.

380. Xu HJ, Hu SX, Benedict WF: Lack of nuclear RB protein staining in G0/middle G1 cells: Correlation to changes in total RB protein level. Oncogene 1991; 6:1139.

381. Wynford-Thomas D: p53 in tumour pathology: Can we trust immunocytochemistry? J Pathol 1992; 166:329.

382. Abbona GC, Papotti M, Gasparri G, et al.: Proliferative activity in parathyroid tumors as detected by Ki-67 immunostaining. Hum Pathol 1995; 26:135.

383. Farnebo F, Auer G, Farnebo LO, et al.: Evaluation of retinoblastoma and Ki-67 immunostaining as diagnostic markers of benign and malignant parathyroid disease. World J Surg 1999; 23:68.

384. Roth SI, Munger BL: The cytology of the adenomatous, atrophic, and hyperplastic parathyroid glands of man: A light- and electron-microscopical study. Virchows Arch 1962; 335:389.

385. Aguilar-Parada E, Gonzalez-Angulo A, del Peon L, et al.: Functioning microvillous adenoma of the parathyroid gland containing nuclear pores and annulate lamellae. Hum Pathol 1985; 16:511.

386. Bloodworth JMB: Fine Structural Pathology of the Endocrine System. In Trump BF, Jones RT, eds.: Diagnostic Electron Microscopy, vol. 3. New York, John Wiley & Sons, 1978, p. 359.

387. Nishiyama RH, Farhi D, Thompson NW: Radiation exposure and the simultaneous occurrence of primary hyperparathyroidism and thyroid nodules. Surg Clin North Am 1979; 59:65.

388. Bedetti CD, Dekker A, Watson CG: Functioning oxyphil cell adenoma of the parathyroid gland: A clinicopathologic study of ten patients with hyperparathyroidism. Hum Pathol 1984; 15:1121.

389. Christie AC: The parathyroid oxyphil cells. J Clin Pathol 1967; 20:591.

390. Arnold BM, Kovacs K, Horvath E, et al.: Functioning oxyphil cell adenoma of the parathyroid gland: Evidence for parathyroid secretory activity of oxyphil cells. J Clin Endocrinol Metab 1974; 38:458.

391. Rodriguez FH Jr, Sarma DP, Lunseth JH, et al.: Primary hyperparathyroidism due to an oxyphil cell adenoma. Am J Clin Pathol 1983; 80:878.

392. McGregor DH, Lotuaco LG, Rao MS, et al.: Functioning oxyphil adenoma of parathyroid gland: An ultrastructural and biochemical study. Am J Pathol 1978; 92:691.

393. Altenahr E, Arps H, Montz R, et al.: Quantitative ultrastructural and radioimmunologic assessment of parathyroid gland activity in primary hyperparathyroidism. Lab Invest 1979; 41:303.

394. Ober WB, Kaiser GA: Hamartoma of the parathyroid. Cancer 1958; 11:601.

395. Abul-Haj SK, Conklin H, Hewitt WC: Functioning lipoadenoma of the parathyroid gland: Report of a unique case. N Engl J Med 1962; 266:121.

396. Hargreaves HK, Wright TC Jr: A large functioning parathyroid lipoadenoma found in the posterior mediastinum. Am J Clin Pathol 1981; 76:89.

397. Daroca PJ Jr, Landau RL, Reed RJ, et al.: Functioning Lipoadenoma of the Parathyroid Gland. Arch Pathol Lab Med 1977; 101:28.

398. Geelhoed G: Parathyroid adenolipoma: Clinical and morphologic features. Surgery 1982; 92:806.

399. Legolvan DP, Moore BP, Nishiyama RH: Parathyroid hamartoma: Report of two cases and review of the literature. Am J Clin Pathol 1977; 67:31.

400. Weiland LH, Garrison RC, ReMine WH, et al.: Lipoadenoma of the parathyroid gland. Am J Surg Pathol 1978; 2:3.

401. Wolff M, Goodman EN: Functioning lipoadenoma of supernumerary parathyroid gland in the mediastinum. Head Neck Surg 1980; 2:302.

402. van Hoeven KH, Brennan MF: Lipothymoadenoma of the Parathyroid. Arch Pathol Lab Med 1993; 117:312.

403. Kovacs K, Horvath E, Murray TM: Large-cell adenoma of the parathyroid gland associated with primary hyperparathyroidism: A light and electron microscopic study. J Submicrosc Cytol 1977; 9:323.

404. Kovacs K, Horvath E, Ozawa Y, et al.: Large clear cell adenoma of the parathyroid in a patient with MEN-1 syndrome: Ultrastructural study of the tumour exhibiting unusual rER formations. Acta Biol Hung 1994; 45:275.

405. Castleman B, Mallory TB: Pathology of the Parathyroid gland in hyperparathyroidism: Study of 25 cases. Am J Pathol 1935; 11:1.

406. Levin KE, Galante M, Clark OH: Parathyroid carcinoma versus parathyroid adenoma in patients with profound hypercalcemia. Surgery 1987; 101:649.

407. Alpers CE, Clark OH: Atypical spindle cell pattern (Carcinoma?) arising in a parathyroid adenoma. Surg Pathol 1989; 2:157.

408. Murray D: The thyroid gland. In Kovacs K, Asa SL, eds.: Functional Endocrine Pathology. Boston, Blackwell Scientific Publications, 1991, p. 293.

409. Smith JF, Coombs RRH: Histological diagnosis of carcinoma of the parathyroid gland. J Clin Pathol 1984; 37:1370.

410. Haghighi P, Astarita RW, Wepsic T, et al.: Concurrent primary parathyroid hyperplasia and parathyroid carcinoma. Arch Pathol Lab Med 1983; 107:349.

411. Dinnen JS, Greenwood RH, Jones JH, et al.: Parathyroid carcinoma in familial hyperparathyroidism. J Clin Pathol 1977; 30:966.

412. Streeten EA, Weinstein LS, Norton JA, et al.: Studies in a kindred with parathyroid carcinoma. J Clin Endocrinol Metab 1992; 75:362.

413. Ireland JP, Fleming SJ, Levison DA, et al.: Parathyroid carcinoma associated with chronic renal failure and previous radiotherapy to the neck. J Clin Pathol 1985; 38:1114.

414. Kastan DJ, Kottamasu SR, Frame B, et al.: Carcinoma in a mediastinal fifth parathyroid gland. JAMA 1987; 257:1218.

415. Sandelin K, Auer G, Bondeson L, et al.: Prognostic factors in parathyroid cancer: A review of 95 cases. World J Surg 1992; 16:724.

416. Obara T, Fujimoto Y, Yamaguchi K, et al.: Parathyroid carcinoma of the oxyphil cell type: A report of two cases, light and electron microscopic study. Cancer 1985; 55:1482.

417. Jacobi JM, Lloyd HM, Smith JF: Nuclear diameter in parathyroid carcinomas. J Clin Pathol 1986; 39:1353.

418. DeLellis RA: Does the evaluation of proliferative activity predict malignancy or prognosis in endocrine tumors? Hum Pathol 1995; 26:131.

419. Saffos RO, Rhatigan RM, Urgulu S: The normal parathyroid and the borderline with early hyperplasia: A light microscopic study. Histopathology 1984; 8:407.

420. Boquist LLV: Nuclear organizer regions in normal, hyperplastic and neoplastic parathyroid glands. Virchows Archiv A Pathol Anat Histopathol. 1990; 417:237.

421. Finlay CA, Hinds PW, Tan TH, et al.: Activating mutations for transformation by p53 produce a gene product that forms an hsc70-p53 complex with an altered half-life. Mol Cell Biol 1988; 8:531.

422. Rubio MP, von Deimling A, Yandell DW, et al.: Accumulation of wild-type p53 protein in human astrocytomas. Cancer Res 1993; 53:3465.

423. Sweet JM, Gardiner GW, Horvath E, et al.: Parathyroid carcinoma with conspicuous nuclear changes: A histologic and electron microscopic study. J Submicrosc Cytol 1979; 11:495.

424. Urbanski SJ, Horvath E, Gardiner GW, et al.: Parathyroid carcinoma containing Luse bodies: A case report, including electron microscopic study. J Submicrosc Cytol 1981; 13:63.

425. Rattner DW, Marrone GC, Kasdon E, et al.: Recurrent hyperparathyroidism due to implantation of parathyroid tissue. Am J Surg 1985; 149:745.

426. Klempa I, Frei U, Röttger P, et al.: Parathyroid autografts-morphology and function: Six years experience with parathyroid autotransplantation in uremic patients. World J Surg 1984; 8:540.
427. Ordõnez NG, Samaan NA, Ibãnez ML, et al.: Immunoperoxidase study of uncommon parathyroid tumors: Report of two cases of nonfunctioning parathyroid carcinoma and one intrathyroid parathyroid tumor-producing amyloid. Am J Surg Pathol 1983; 7:535.
428. Obara T, Okamoto T, Ito Y, et al.: Surgical and medical management of patients with pulmonary metastasis from parathyroid carcinoma. Surgery 1993; 114:1040.
429. Russell CF, Grant CS, van Heerden JA: Hyperfunctioning supernumerary parathyroid glands: An occasional cause of hyperparathyroidism. Mayo Clin Proc 1982; 57:121.
430. Straus FH II, Kaplan EL, Nishiyama RH, et al.: Five cases of parathyroid lipohyperplasia. Surgery 1983; 94:901.
431. Reddick RL, Costa JC, Marx SJ: Parathyroid hyperplasia and parathyromatosis (letter). Lancet 1977; 1549.
432. Golden A, Kerwin DM: The parathyroid glands. In Bloodworth JMB Jr, ed.: Endocrine Pathology General and Surgical, 2nd ed. Baltimore/London, Williams & Wilkins, 1982, p. 205.
433. Harach HR, Jasani B: Parathyroid hyperplasia in tertiary hyperparathyroidism: A pathological and immunohistochemical reappraisal. Histopathology 1992; 21:513.
434. Ohta K, Manabe T, Katagiri M, et al.: Expression of proliferating cell nuclear antigens in parathyroid glands of renal hyperparathyroidism. World J Surg 1994; 18:625.
435. Loda M, Lipman J, Cukor B, et al.: Nodular foci in parathyroid adenomas and hyperplasias: An immunohistochemical analysis of proliferative activity. Hum Pathol 1994; 25:1050.
436. Komatsu M, Nishiyama RH, Bagwell CB: Nuclear DNA analysis of hyperplastic parathyroid glands in multiple endocrine neoplasia type 1. Arch Surg 1992; 127:1430.
437. Tominaga Y, Grimelius L, Falkmer UG, et al.: DNA ploidy pattern of parathyroid parenchymal cells in renal secondary hyperparathyroidism with relapse. Analysis Cell Pathol 1991; 3:325.
438. Albright F, Bloomberg E, Castleman B, et al.: Hyperparathyroidism due to diffuse hyperplasia of all parathyroid glands rather than adenoma of one: Clinical studies on three such cases. Arch Intern Med 1934; 54:315.
439. Tisell L-E, Hedman I, Hansson G: Clinical characteristics and surgical results in hyperparathyroidism caused by water-clear cell hyperplasia. World J Surg 1981; 5:565.
440. Miettinen M, Franssila K, Lehto V-P, et al.: Expression of intermediate filament proteins in thyroid gland and thyroid tumors. Lab Invest 1984; 50:262.
441. Hedbäck G, Odén A: Parathyroid water clear cell hyperplasia, an O-allele associated condition. Hum Genet 1994; 94:195.
442. Castleman B, Schantz A, Roth S: Parathyroid hyperplasia in primary hyperparathyroidism: A review of 85 cases. Cancer 1976; 38:1668.
443. Roth SI: The ultrastructure of primary water-clear cell hyperplasia of the parathyroid glands. Am J Pathol 1970; 61:233.
444. Dawkins RL, Tashjian AH Jr, Castleman B, et al.: Hyperparathyroidism due to clear cell hyperplasia: Serial determinations of serum ionized calcium, parathyroid hormone and calcitonin. Am J Med 1973; 54:119.
445. Schneider AB, Sherwood LM: Pathogenesis and management of hypoparathyroidism and other hypocalcemic disorders. Metabolism 1975; 24:871.
446. Eipe J, Johnson SA, Kiamko RT, et al.: Hypoparathyroidism following ^{131}I therapy for hyperthyroidism. Arch Intern Med 1968; 121:270.
447. Goldsmith RE: Hypoparathyroidism and hypothyroidism. Ann Intern Med 1971; 75:647.
448. Woodhouse NJY: Hypocalcemia and hypoparathyroidism. Clin Endocrinol Metab 1974; 3:323.
449. Burke BA, Johnson D, Gilbert EF, et al.: Thyrocalcitonin-containing cells in the DiGeorge anomaly. Hum Pathol 1987; 18:355.
450. Watanabe T, Bai M, Lane CR, et al.: Familial hypoparathyroidism: Identification of a novel gain of function mutation in transmembrane domain 5 of the calcium-sensing receptor. J Clin Endocrinol Metab 1998; 83:2497.
451. Steinberg H, Waldron BR: Idiopathic hypoparathyroidism: An analysis of fifty-two cases, including the report of a new case. Medicine 1952; 31:133.
452. Van de Casseye M, Gepts W: Primary parathyroiditis. Virchows Arch 1973; 361:257.
453. Asa SL: The pathology of autoimmune endocrine disorders. In Kovacs K, Asa SL, eds.: Functional Endocrine Pathology. Boston, Blackwell Scientific Publications, 1991, p. 961.
454. Irvine WJ: Adrenalitis, hypoparathyroidism and associated diseases. In Samter M, ed.: Immunological Diseases, 3rd ed. Boston, Little, Brown & Co, 1978, p. 1278.
455. Kopin IJ, Rosenberg IN: Idiopathic hypoparathyroidism: Report of a case with autopsy findings. Ann Intern Med 1960; 53:1238.
456. Blizzard RM, Chee D, Davis W: The incidence of parathyroid and other antibodies in the sera of patients with idiopathic hypoparathyroidism. Clin Exp Immunol 1966; 1:119.
457. Brandi ML, Aurbach GD, Fattorossi A, et al.: Antibodies cytotoxic to bovine parathyroid cells in autoimmune hypoparathyroidism. Proc Natl Acad Sci U S A 1986; 83:8366.
458. MacLaren NK, Riley WJ: Autoimmune Polyendocrinopathies. In Samter M, Talmage DW, Frank MM, et al.: eds. Immunological Diseases. 4th ed. Boston/Toronto, Little, Boston & Co, 1988, p. 1737.
459. Whyte MP, Weldon W: Idiopathic hypoparathyroidism presenting with seizures during infancy: X-linked recessive inheritance in a large Missouri kindred. J Pediatr 1981; 99:608.
460. Tolloczko T, Wozniewicz B, Sawicki A, et al.: Cultured parathyroid cell transplantation without immunosuppression in the treatment of surgical hypoparathyroidism. Transplant Proc 1994; 26:1901.
461. Albright F, Burnett CH, Smith PH, et al.: Pseudo-hypoparathyroidism: Example of "Seabright-Bantam syndrome": Report of 3 cases. Endocrinology 1942; 30:922.
462. Chase LR, Melson GL, Aurbach GD: Pseudohypoparathyroidism: Defective excretion of 3′,5′-AMP in response to parathyroid hormone. J Clin Invest 1969; 48:1832.
463. Spiegel AM, Gierschik P, Levine MA, et al.: Clinical implications of guanine nucleotide-binding proteins as receptor-effector couplers. N Engl J Med 1985; 312:26.
464. Farfel Z, Brickman AS, Kaslow HR, et al.: Defect of receptor-cyclase coupling protein in pseudohypoparathyroidism. N Engl J Med 1980; 303:237.
465. Levine MA, Downs RW Jr, Singer M, et al.: Deficient activity of guanine nucleotide regulatory protein in erythrocytes from patients with pseudohypoparathyroidism. Biochem Biophys Res Commun 1980; 94:1319.
466. Levine MA, Downs RW Jr, Moses AM, et al.: Resistance to multiple hormones in patients with pseudohypoparathyroidism: Association with deficient activity of guanine nucleotide regulatory protein. Am J Med 1983; 74:545.
467. Bastepe M, Juppner H. Pseudohypoparathyroidism: New insights into an old disease. Endocrinol Metab Clin North Am 2000; 29:569.
468. Drezner M, Neelon FA, Lebovitz HE: Pseudohypoparathyroidism type II: A possible defect in the reception of the cyclic AMP signal. N Engl J Med 1973; 289:1056.
469. Yamada K, Tamura Y, Tomioka H, et al.: Possible existence of anti-renal tubular plasma membrane autoantibody which blocked parathyroid hormone-induced phosphaturia in a patient with pseudohypoparathyroidism type II and Sjögren's syndrome. J Clin Endocrinol Metab 1984; 58:339.
470. Aurbach GD, Potts JT Jr: The parathyroids. Adv Metab Dis 1964; 14:5.
471. Kinard RE, Walton JE, Buckwalter JA: Pseudohypoparathyroidism: Report of a family with four affected sisters. Arch Intern Med 1979; 139:204.
472. Reiner L, Klayman MJ, Cohen RB: Lymphocytic infiltration of the parathyroid glands. Jewish Mem Hosp Bull. 1962; 67:103.
473. Van de Casseye M, Gepts W: Primary parathyroiditis. Virchows Arch 1973; 361:257.
474. Boyce BF, Doherty VR, Mortimer G: Hyperplastic parathyroiditis: A new autoimmune disease? J Clin Pathol 1982; 35:812.

475. Bondeson A-G, Bondeson L, Ljungberg O: Chronic parathyroiditis associated with parathyroid hyperplasia and hyperparathyroidism. Am J Surg Pathol 1984; 8:211.

476. Sinha SN, McArdle JP, Shepherd JJ: Hyperparathyroidism with chronic parathyroiditis in a multiple endocrine neoplasia patient. Aust N Z J Surg 1993; 63:981.

477. Veress B, Nordenström J: Lymphocytic infiltration and destruction of parathyroid adenomas: A possible tumour-specific autoimmune reaction in two cases of primary hyperparathyroidism. Histopathology 1994; 25:373.

478. Chetty R, Forder MD: Parathyroiditis associated with hyperparathyroidism and branchial cysts. Am J Clin Pathol 1991; 96:348.

479. Louis DN, Vickery AL Jr, Rosai J, et al.: Multiple branchial cleft-like cysts in Hashimoto's thyroiditis. Am J Surg Pathol 1989; 13:45.

480. Apel RL, Asa SL, Chalvardjian A, et al.: Intrathyroidal lymphoepithelial cysts of probable branchial origin. Hum Pathol 1994; 25:1238.

481. Fisher ER, Gruhn J: Parathyroid cysts. Cancer 1957; 10:57.

482. Wang C, Vickery AL Jr, Maloof F: Large parathyroid cysts mimicking thyroid nodules. Ann Surg 1972; 175:448.

483. Clark OH: Parathyroid cysts. Am J Surg 1978; 135:395.

484. Haid SP, Method HL, Beal JM: Parathyroid cysts: Report of two cases and a review of the literature. Arch Surg 1967; 94:421.

485. Hoehn JG, Beahrs OH, Woolner LB: Unusual surgical lesions of the parathyroid gland. Am J Surg 1969; 118:770.

486. Wick MR: Mediastinal cysts and intrathoracic thyroid tumors. Semin Diagn Pathol 1990; 7:285.

487. Ginsberg J, Young JEM, Walfish PG: Parathyroid cysts: Medical diagnosis and management. JAMA 1978; 240:1506.

488. Troster M, Chiu HF, McLarty TD: Parathyroid cysts: Report of a case with ultrastructural observations. Surgery 1978; 83:238.

489. Horwitz CA, Myers WP, Foote FW Jr: Secondary malignant tumors of the parathyroid glands: Report of two cases with associated hypoparathyroidism. Am J Med 1972; 52:797.

490. de la Monte SM, Hutchins GM, Moore GW: Endocrine organ metastases from breast carcinoma. Am J Pathol 1984; 114:131.

491. Dufour DR, Marx SJ, Spiegel AM: Parathyroid gland morphology in nonparathyroid hormone-mediated hypercalcemia. Am J Surg Pathol 1985; 94:3.

492. Hui K-S, Williams JC, Borit A, et al.: The endocrine glands in Pompe's disease: Report of two cases. Arch Pathol Lab Med 1985; 109:921.

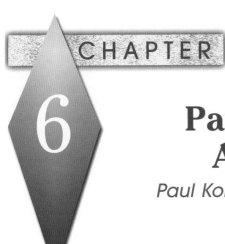

Paraganglia and the Adrenal Medulla

Paul Komminoth, Ronald R. De Krijger, and Arthur S. Tischler

HISTORICAL ASPECTS AND TERMINOLOGY

Paraganglia are dispersed neuroendocrine organs associated with the sympathetic and parasympathetic autonomic nervous system. Sympathetic paraganglia are distributed along the pre- and paravertebral sympathetic chains and follow the sympathetic innervation of the pelvic and retroperitoneal organs. Parasympathetic paraganglia are distributed along the cervical and thoracic branches of the vagus and glossopharyngeal nerves. The prototypical sympathetic paraganglion is the adrenal medulla, and the parasympathetic prototype is the carotid body. Both types of paraganglia are characterized by catecholamine- and peptide-producing secretory cells derived from the neural crest. However, differences in tissue organization and in specific secretory products suggest that these characteristic cells respond to different signals and perform varied functions in different locations.

The concept of a unified paraganglionic system was introduced by Alfred Kohn at the beginning of the 20th century.[1-3] Several investigators described histochemical reactions that functionally distinguished the adrenal medulla from the cortex. One of these reactions was the development of brown coloration in the presence of chromate salt.[4] Kohn coined the terms "chromaffin reaction" for the color change and "chromaffin cells" for the reactive cells, and described bodies of extra-adrenal chromaffin cells in the retroperitoneum. Because some cells in the carotid body exhibited a chromaffin reaction, Kohn proposed the term "paraganglia" to designate all of the tissues composed of cells analogous to neurons but not quite neuronal, including the carotid body as well as retroperitoneal chromaffin cells.

Later on, the chromaffin reaction was found to result from oxidation of stored catecholamines rather than affinity for chromium, leading to the synonym "pheochromocyte." Curiously, chromaffin cell is now the preferred term for normal adrenal medullary cells and pheochromocyte for their neoplastic counterparts. In the United States, many medical publications accepted the now widely followed suggestion by Karsner[5] that the term "pheochromocytoma" be reserved for adrenal medullary tumors and that extra-adrenal paraganglionic tumors be called "paragangliomas." However, in other literature, especially in Europe and Japan, tumors of extra-adrenal sympathetic paraganglia were referred to as "extra-adrenal pheochromocytomas" if they exhibited a positive chromaffin reaction or were associated with clinical evidence of catecholamine secretion.[6, 7] Some studies referred to all tumors of sympathetic paraganglionic cells as pheochromocytomas.[8]

Further important developments subdivided the paraganglionic system into sympathetic and parasympathetic paraganglia. These included the finding that innervation of the carotid body is primarily parasympathetic, from the glossopharyngeal nerve, and the discovery of chemoreceptor functions of the carotid bodies and similar bodies associated with the vagus nerve. The new terms "chemodecton" and "chemodectoma" were subsequently introduced for these structures and their corresponding tumors.

A persistent synonym for the parasympathetic paraganglia is "glomus." Neoplasms arising in parasympathetic paraganglia have been called "glomus tumors," often modified by specific localizations (e.g., glomus jugulare tumor).[9] This terminology is a vestige of a 19th century hypothesis that the carotid body is of vascular origin. Much confusion has resulted from its use, because it is also applied to thermoregulatory vascular structures in the skin and other locations. These structures and their corresponding tumors (vascular glomus tumors or glomangiomas) are modified arteriovenous anastomoses, unrelated to paraganglia developmentally or functionally.

Although precise terminology has been difficult to attain, we may now return to Kohn's unifying concept with a synthesis of old and new information. All paraganglionic neuroendocrine cells appear to be of neural crest origin. All produce catecholamines, detectable by methods more sensitive than the chromaffin reaction, and all express additional neuroendocrine markers. The term "paraganglion" is conceptually useful because it connotes a constellation of morphologic and functional characteristics associated with these cells and is not dependent on a single histochemical reaction. Despite the differences in the contexts in which they arise, sympathetic and parasympathetic paragangliomas strongly resemble each other microscopically and are often indistinguishable. They also exhibit a widely overlapping range of secretory products and other neuroendocrine markers, reflecting the similarities of their normal counterparts. The chromaffin reaction as a basis for diagnosis or classification should finally be considered obsolete.

EMBRYOLOGY

During embryonic development, primordia of the paraganglia are first populated by small, primitive cells morphologically similar to those that give rise to sympathetic ganglia. These cells include precursors of the neuroendocrine, neural, and glial lineages in adult paraganglia. They are readily recognized in human paraganglia at about 7 weeks' gestation and are progressively superseded by larger differentiated cells. Cytologic maturation occurs earlier in extra-adrenal paraganglia than in the adrenal medulla. Primitive cells usually disappear from these locations by week 25 of gestation, but may persist in small numbers in the adrenal medulla until after birth.[6, 10, 11]

DISTRIBUTION

Sympathetic paraganglia are associated with all parts of the peripheral sympathetic nervous system, predominantly as anatomically discrete bodies in the paraxial regions of the trunk close to the prevertebral and paravertebral sympathetic ganglia and in connective tissue in or near the walls of the pelvic organs (Fig. 6–1). In adult humans, they are especially numerous along fibers of the inferior hypogastric plexuses leading to and entering the urogenital organs, in the wall of the urinary bladder, and among the nerve fibers of the sacral plexus.[12] Sympathetic paraganglia are not generally known by individual names, and their locations are variable and not precisely defined. Exceptions are the adrenal medulla and the organs of Zuckerkandl, located at the origin of the inferior mesenteric artery. There is an inverse relationship between the volumes of adrenal and extra-adrenal paraganglionic tissue. Whereas the adrenal medulla is inconspicuous at birth and then rapidly enlarges during the first 6 months of life, the organ of Zuckerkandl reaches maturity at birth and fragments or involutes thereafter, so that by late childhood it can usually be detected only microscopically.

Parasympathetic paraganglia are almost exclusively located in the distribution of cranial and thoracic branches of the glossopharyngeal and vagus nerves (Fig. 6–2). The principal glossopharyngeal paraganglia are the tympanic paraganglia in the wall of the middle ear and the carotid bodies. Vagus nerve branches innervate the jugular paraganglia in the floor of the middle ear, superior and inferior laryngeal and subclavian paraganglia, and aorticopulmonary or cardioaortic paraganglia near the bases of the great vessels of the heart. The paraganglia of the great vessels are sometimes found within the heart in the interatrial septum.[13] In addition to the paraganglia innervated by vagus branches, intravagal paraganglia are located within or adjacent to the vagal trunk in or near the nodose and jugular ganglia.[14] With the exception of the carotid bodies, which are located just above the carotid bifurcation, parasympathetic paraganglia are highly variable in

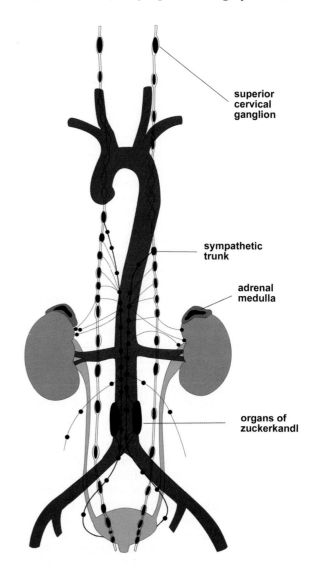

superior cervical ganglion

sympathetic trunk

adrenal medulla

organs of zuckerkandl

Figure 6–1. Anatomic distribution of sympathetic paraganglia. (Adapted from Lack E: Tumors of the adrenal gland and extra-adrenal paraganglia. In Atlas of Tumor Pathology. Armed Forces Institute of Pathology, Washington, D.C., 1997.)

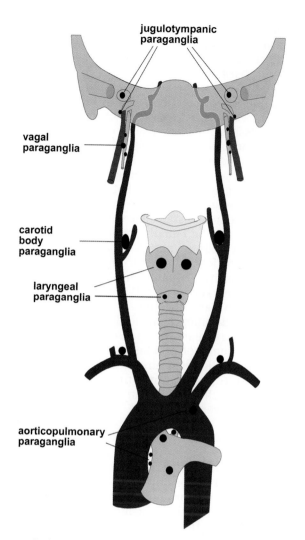

Figure 6-2. Anatomic distribution of parasympathetic paraganglia of the head and neck region. (Adapted from Lack E: Tumors of the adrenal gland and extra-adrenal paraganglia. In Atlas of Tumor Pathology. Armed Forces Institute of Pathology, Washington, D.C., 1997.)

both number and location, and their names refer to general locations rather than to specific bodies.

Paraganglia occasionally are encountered in locations outside the well-established sympathetic and parasympathetic distributions, perhaps explaining the existence of paragangliomas in unusual locations. It is possible that some of these, for example in the gallbladder, are associated with small vagus nerve branches.[15] According to scattered reports, paraganglia have been observed in various sites, including the orbit, mandible, and extremities. The validity of some of these reports, however, is questionable.

With the exception of the adrenal medulla, the organs of Zuckerkandl, and the carotid bodies, paraganglia are normally less than 1 mm in greatest dimension. The carotid bodies are the largest of the extra-adrenal paraganglia during most of one's life and vary in greatest dimension between normal adults from approximately 3 to 8 mm. The organ of Zuckerkandl at the height of development is considerably larger and may exceed 20 mm at about age 3.[16]

HISTOLOGY AND PHYSIOLOGY

Paraganglia contain two distinctive types of cells: neuroendocrine cells and Schwann cell–like glial cells. The former, initially exemplified by the chromaffin cells of the sympathetic nervous system, have been called glomus cells, type I cells, or chief cells when associated with the parasympathetic nervous system. The latter have also been called sustentacular cells, satellite cells, or type II cells.[9] In addition, there are connective tissue cells, vascular cells, and variable numbers of mast cells. Neuroendocrine cells are polyhedral cells with abundant cytoplasm and small, spherical or ovoid, pale-staining nuclei. Their chromatin is usually finely stippled and nucleoli are usually inconspicuous. However, nuclear and cellular pleomorphism and hyperchromatism may occur with advancing age, particularly in the adrenal medulla. An oncocytic variant with dense, eosinophilic cytoplasm can occur. Mitotic figures are rare. Cytoplasmic vacuolization is a common artifact of fixation and processing. Sustentacular cells have less conspicuous cytoplasm and flattened, more deeply basophilic nuclei with coarsely clumped chromatin. They may be difficult to identify in hematoxylin and eosin–stained sections but are readily identified by immunohistochemical staining for S-100 protein. Paraganglia are typically arranged with neuroendocrine cells in clusters and anastomosing cords, described as "Zellballen" by Alfred Kohn, partially or completely surrounded by sustentacular cells.[2] Sustentacular cells are present in both parasympathetic and sympathetic paraganglia, but are more numerous in the former, where they cause the Zellballen to appear more pronounced.

The characteristic ultrastructural feature of neuroendocrine cells is the presence of membrane-bound secretory granules, or "large dense-core vesicles," approximately 60–400 nm in greatest dimension. These may vary greatly in size, shape, and electron density. In addition, neuroendocrine cells sometimes contain accumulations of small synaptic-like vesicles, which may accumulate in clusters near the plasma membrane.[17] Secretory granules contain catecholamines, regulatory peptides, and a number of other constituents, including chromogranin proteins, adenosine triphosphate, peptide-processing enzymes, and dopamine β-hydroxylase.[18] Peptide growth factors such as fibroblast growth factor and transforming growth factor–β that might exert autocrine or paracrine effects may also be present.[19] The small synaptic-like vesicles probably comprise a separate compartment for regulated secretion, with substances other than those in secretory granules and without chromogranin. In addition, their membranes appear to be the principal location of synaptophysin, which, like chromogranin A, is widely used as an immunohistochemical marker for neuroendocrine cells.

The neuroendocrine cells release their secretory products by Ca^{2+}-mediated exocytosis in response to neural or chemical signals. In the adrenal medulla, secretion is triggered by splanchnic nerve endings, which synapse on chromaffin cells. Chemical signals play a more important role in extra-adrenal sympathetic paraganglia, because they are sparsely innervated.[20] Parasympathetic paraganglia appear to function as chemoreceptors, but their specific functions are not always known. The carotid and aortic bodies belong to reflex loops involving the central nervous system. Their chief cells participate in complex synaptic relationships with sensory cranial nerve endings, detecting low partial pressure of oxygen, low pH, or increased partial pressure of carbon dioxide, which may trigger respiratory and circulatory responses.[21]

The production of epinephrine is almost exclusively localized in the adrenal medulla,[22] which comprises more than 80% of human adrenal catecholamine stores.[23] In contrast, parasympathetic paraganglia produce and store little or no epinephrine, and more than 90% of their catecholamine content is norepinephrine.[24]

PATHOLOGY

The only significant pathologic changes encountered in paraganglia are neoplasia and hyperplasia. Functional differences between sympathetic and parasympathetic paraganglia are reflected in important clinicopathologic distinctions with respect to development of these lesions. First, multiple lesions within families or individuals are almost always confined to either one or the other paraganglion class. Second, although tumors arising in both classes of paraganglia produce catecholamines, large quantities of catecholamines causing clinical signs and symptoms are usually associated with tumors of sympathetic paraganglia. Tumors producing significant amounts of epinephrine are almost invariably derived from sympathetic paraganglia and most often are intra-adrenal. Third, lesions associated with prolonged hypoxia or hypercapnia are almost always parasympathetic. Fourth, sympathetic paraganglia commonly give rise to neoplasms of neuronal rather than neuroendocrine lineage, whereas tumors of parasympathetic paraganglia are almost always neuroendocrine.[25] In this chapter all tumors of sympathetic and parasympathetic paraganglia are considered paragangliomas; pheochromocytomas are paragangliomas of the adrenal medulla.

ADVANCES IN IMMUNOHISTOCHEMISTRY

Until relatively recently, the most reliable tools for diagnosis and functional assessment of paraganglionic lesions were electron microscopy and argyrophil-type silver stains to demonstrate secretory granules and fluorescence methods to demonstrate catecholamines.[26-28] The advent of many antibodies against neuroendocrine proteins and the use of heat-based antigen retrieval techniques now permits immunohistochemistry to replace these techniques for most purposes.

The neuroendocrine cells of hyperplastic and neoplastic paraganglia express many markers that are shared to varying degrees with other neural and endocrine tissues.[25] A very useful battery of functional markers consists of chromogranin A (CGA), synaptophysin, and catecholamine biosynthetic enzymes.[29] CGA is a protein of neuroendocrine secretory granules[30] and a generic marker that can usually replace electron microscopy or silver stains in the detection of normal or neoplastic neuroendocrine cells. However, it may not be demonstrable in poorly differentiated tumor cells or in cells that are degranulated as a result of low synthesis, high turnover, or low storage capacity. Synaptophysin is principally a membrane marker of small synaptic-like vesicles. Because they are located in separate secretory organelles, chromogranin and synaptophysin are complementary markers that may be differentially expressed. Immunohistochemical staining for catecholamine-synthesizing enzymes permits the pathologist to determine not only whether a tumor produced catecholamines but also what specific catecholamines were produced. They are highly specific markers that in adult humans are localized almost exclusively to paraganglia and neurons. Tyrosine hydroxylase (TH), the first enzyme in catecholamine synthesis, is found in all catecholamine-producing cells. Dopamine β-hydroxylase is found only in cells that produce norepinephrine. Phenylethanolamine N-methyltransferase (PNMT) is present only in cells that can convert norepinephrine to epinephrine.[29] It, therefore, stains almost all chromaffin cells in the adrenal medulla but only rarely normal or neoplastic extra-adrenal paraganglionic cells.

An additional very useful marker is S-100 protein, which results in intense immunoreactivity of sustentacular cells. This permits them to be identified in normal and neoplastic sympathetic and parasympathetic paraganglia despite their nondescript morphology. The same cells may, in some instances, be stained for glial fibrillary acidic protein. It is important that lymphoreticular cells expressing S-100 not be mistaken for sustentacular cells.

Paragangliomas frequently stain for neurofilament proteins but are usually negative or only focally positive for keratins.[31] Staining for cytoskeletal proteins may, therefore, be helpful in distinguishing paraganglionic tumors from carcinoids and neuroendocrine carcinomas, which frequently express both neurofilaments and cytokeratins. A notable exception to this distinction is paraganglioma of the cauda equina, which is reported to frequently be cytokeratin positive.

Rapidly advancing studies in neuroendocine cell biology have led to the discovery of many new markers that might be applied to histopathology. These include proteins such as synaptotagmin, synaptobrevin, and SNAP25, which are involved in docking and exocytosis of secretory vesicles. Because there is no shortage of highly specific markers, the pathologist should feel little compulsion to cling to relatively unspecific ones such as neuron-specific enolase. A caveat is that paraganglionic tissues may exhibit nonspecific reactivity in immunohistochemical studies, which may result in binding of normal serum to neuroendocrine cells, mast cells, and neurons.

HYPERPLASIA OF THE ADRENAL MEDULLA

Definition

Adrenal medullary hyperplasia is defined as an increase in the number and size of chromaffin cells and expansion of medullary tissue into the tail of the gland, resulting in increased gland size and weight or an increased proportion of medulla relative to cortex.[32] Adrenal medullary hyperplasia may be diffuse, nodular, or both, and the morphologic features may be symmetric or asymmetric.

Incidence and Prevalence

Adrenal medullary hyperplasia is extremely rare in the general population. The frequency is increased in association with several neurocutaneous phakomatoses. The strongest association is with multiple endocrine neoplasia (MEN) syndromes type IIA and IIB.[33, 34] Adrenal medullary hyperplasia has also been reported in some patients with von Hippel–Lindau disease[35, 36] and von Recklinghausen's disease.[32, 37] Sporadic adrenal medullary hyperplasia has been reported as a cause of hypertension in the pediatric age group, in some patients with cystic fibrosis,[32] and in association with an adrenal cortical adenoma.[38] Hyperplasia of the adrenal medulla and extra-adrenal sympathetic paraganglia also occurs in Beckwith-Wiedemann syndrome.[39]

Clinical Considerations

Adrenal medullary hyperplasia may mimic pheochromocytoma by its presentation with paroxysmal hypertension, diaphoresis, and tachycardia.[35, 40, 41] Complications include catecholamine "acute" abdomen with ileus, abdominal distention, and pain. Patients usually experience relief of signs or symptoms after surgical resection of one or both adrenal glands.[42] Catecholamine assays show episodic increases in urinary ratios of epinephrine and norepinephrine or of their metabolites in the majority of patients. Absolute increases in concentration of both norepinephrine and epinephrine may also occur. Studies of catecholamine production or content in tissue from hyperplastic adrenals have seldom been performed. The largest increases appear to be in epinephrine content in contrast to the catecholamine profile of most pheochromocytomas.[43]

Macroscopic and Microscopic Pathology

Extension of adrenal medulla into the tail and alae, which is outside the usual central portions of the head and body of the gland, should raise suspicion of diffuse hyperplasia. A definite diagnosis of diffuse adrenal medullary hyperplasia can be established only by morphometric documentation of an increase in medullary volume and weight. Cytologic changes that may accompany this increase include extreme pleomorphism, bizarre giant cells with hyperchromatic nuclei, and increased numbers of hyaline globules. Mitotic activity may also be apparent. These changes alone are not diagnostic. Medullary weight calculated for the normal adult human adrenal medulla usually is between 0.3 and 0.5 g, about 10% of the weight of the cortex.[25, 32, 44] In patients with MEN-II, synchronous or metachronous involvement of both adrenals with diffuse and superimposed nodular hyperplasia may occur (Fig. 6–3). The relationship between these two changes is highly variable, and each may be present independently. Beckwith-Wiedemann syndrome appears to be associated with an unusual type of adrenal medullary hyperplasia.[45]

Distinction Between Nodular Adrenal Medullary Hyperplasia and Pheochromocytoma

The distinction between nodular hyperplasia and pheochromocytoma is problematic. Carney et al.[44] designated nodules 1 cm or larger as pheochromocytomas and those smaller than 1 cm as "nodular adrenal medullary hyperplasia." This designation was based on an arbitrary criterion defined in the Armed Forces Institute of Pathology fascicle on adrenal neoplasms, published in 1950.[5] Clonality studies indicate that both hyperplastic nodules and

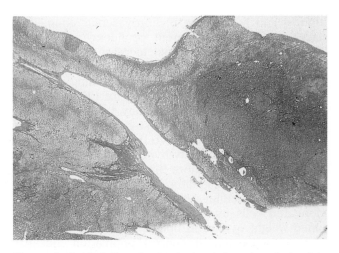

Figure 6–3. Medullary hyperplasia of the adrenal gland in a multiple endocrine neoplasia type II patient.

pheochromocytomas are often monoclonal.[46] Both lesions appear to express less PNMT than normal or diffusely hyperplastic medulla. These observations suggest that at least some lesions generally regarded as hyperplastic nodules are in fact small pheochromocytomas.

HYPERPLASIA OF EXTRA-ADRENAL PARAGANGLIA

Incidence and Prevalence

The frequency of hyperplasia in extra-adrenal paraganglia is difficult to determine because it is most often an incidental finding. Hyperplastic and neoplastic lesions of extra-adrenal sympathetic paraganglia occasionally occur with adrenal medullary lesions in patients with or without familial disorders but are quite rare. They are not a usual feature of MEN-II. Compensatory hyperplasia of the human carotid bodies occurs in response to chronic hypoxemia associated with physiologic or pathologic conditions,[47] including life at high altitude, chronic obstructive pulmonary diseases, restrictive pulmonary disease, cystic fibrosis, and cyanotic congenital heart disease.[48–50] Similar hyperplasia of vagal paraganglia sometimes accompanies chronic hypoxemia but is not as consistent as carotid body hyperplasia.[49]

Clinical Considerations

Hyperplasia of extra-adrenal paraganglia is rarely associated with clinical symptoms.

Macroscopic and Microscopic Pathology

The hyperplastic carotid body is enlarged, ovoid, often dark colored, and occasionally bilobed. Histologically, there is an increase in the number of lobules and a decrease of fibrovascular connective tissue, resulting in apparent confluence of lobules. There tends to be an equal increase in chief cells and sustentacular cells. Chief cells may show variation in size, shape, and nuclear staining intensity and diminished immunoreactivity for CGA with controls. Ultrastructurally, there may be a marked decrease in the number of dense-core neurosecretory granules. Three criteria have been proposed for the diagnosis of carotid body hyperplasia: (1) combined carotid body weight more than 300 mg; (2) mean diameter of lobules greater than 565 μm; (3) an increase of more than 47% in the differential count of elongated cells over chief cells. Individual or combined weight of carotid bodies should be correlated with an age-matched control population, because there is variation in weight and surface area with age.[49, 50]

TUMORS OF THE ADRENAL MEDULLA

Incidence and Prevalence

The annual incidence rate of sympathetic paragangliomas can be estimated to be approximately 1 per 100,000 population. Pheochromocytomas occur throughout life, with a peak between 20 and 50 years of age.[7] Familial cases are usually diagnosed before the age of 20 years, probably reflecting both earlier development and earlier detection. In adults, pheochromocytomas occur with approximately equal frequency, whereas in children about 65% occur in males.[7, 51, 52]

Clinical Considerations

Pheochromocytoma has been termed the "10% tumor": 10% bilateral, 10% extra-adrenal, 10% malignant, and about 10% occurring in childhood.[32] These conveniently remembered percentages are rough approximations. In a sporadic setting, about 95% of tumors are solitary, about 5% are bilateral, and 5% to 10% are extra-adrenal paragangliomas. In a familial setting, more than 50% of tumors are bilateral, and in the pediatric age group, which includes both familial and nonfamilial cases, there is an increased incidence of bilateral, multicentric, and extra-adrenal tumors.[53] Extra-adrenal paragangliomas are malignant considerably more often than their intra-adrenal counterparts.

Clinical presentations of patients with pheochromocytomas vary considerably. The classic diagnostic triad is paroxysmal hypertension, headache, and diaphoresis. Norepinephrine-secreting tumors reportedly are associated with sustained hypertension, whereas tumors secreting relatively large quantities of epinephrine together with norepinephrine are associated with paroxysmal or episodic hypertension. Pure epinephrine-secreting tumors have been reported to cause hypotension. Numerous other signs and symptoms attributed to catecholamine effects include anxiety, pallor and flushing, tachypnea, tremor, and cardiac arrhythmias. In some normotensive patients, the tumor, which is most frequently extra-adrenal, secretes mostly dopamine, and this profile may be associated with malignancy.[54] Some pheochromocytomas present with retroperitoneal hemorrhage.[55]

Pheochromocytoma can be localized by the use of high-resolution computed tomography or magnetic resonance imaging. On magnetic resonance imaging, pheochromocytomas usually show a very high signal intensity on T_2-weighted images.[32] Pheochromocytomas may take up iodine 131–metaiodobenzylguanidine, which appears to be correlated with the number of neurosecretory granules in the tumor cells.[32] Somatostatin scans that detect binding of labeled somatostatin to cell surface receptors have been useful in detecting small pheochromocytomas with high levels of secretory activity.[32]

Macroscopic and Microscopic Pathology

Sporadic pheochromocytomas typically present as spherical, solitary masses (Fig. 6–4). Adrenal remnants may be difficult to identify with large tumors. Most pheochromocytomas measure between 3 and 5 cm in diameter but may range between 1 and 10 cm.[32] On cross-section, the tumors are usually sharply circumscribed and may appear encapsulated.[32] However, histologically, this capsule is usually composed of a fibrous pseudocapsule or an expansion of the adrenal capsule itself. Pheochromocytomas are usually gray and firm, resembling the normal adrenal medulla (see Fig. 6–4). Areas of confluent congestion or hemorrhage may be seen within the tumor, sometimes extending into the surrounding adipose tissue or resembling a hematoma. Central degenerative changes may occur, particularly in large tumors, and may appear as zones of infarction, fibrosis, or cysts[32] (Fig. 6–5). Occasionally, pheochromocytomas have areas of calcification, which may be detected on radiographic examination. Some tumors may extend into the inferior vena cava.[25, 32]

Familial pheochromocytomas occur most frequently in the context of MEN-II but can also be seen in patients with von Recklinghausen's disease and von Hippel–Lindau disease.[33, 56–58] They are bilateral or multifocal in at least 60% to 70% of cases (Fig. 6–6) and often coexist with adrenal medullary hyperplasia, but large tumors may obliterate the

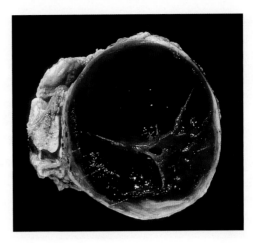

Figure 6–5. Pheochromocytoma: cystic degeneration.

non-neoplastic medulla. In MEN-II, synchronous or metachronous medullary thyroid carcinoma may occur.[59] The biologic behavior of pheochromocytomas in MEN-II varies from series to series.[60] Some suggested that these tumors are extreme examples of adrenal medullary hyperplasia.[43, 61] Malignant pheochromocytomas are rare in MEN-II and probably also in von Hippel–Lindau disease.[62–64] About 5% of pheochromocytomas are reported in association with von Recklinghausen's disease, but the percentage of such patients in whom pheochromocytomas develop is estimated to be 1% or less.[65]

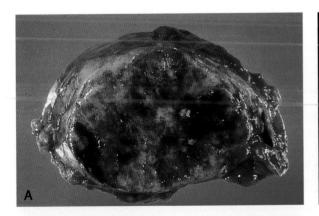

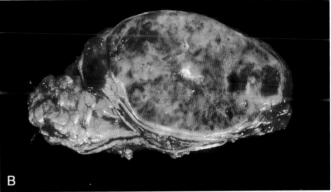

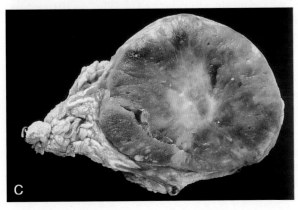

Figure 6–4. A-C, Pheochromocytoma: macroscopic aspect.

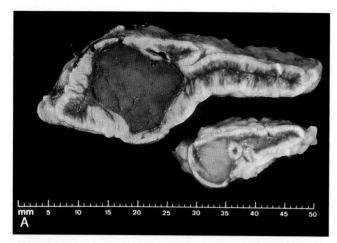

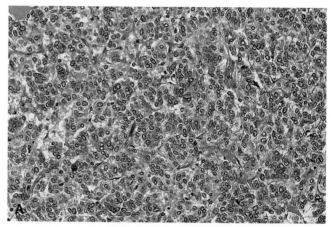

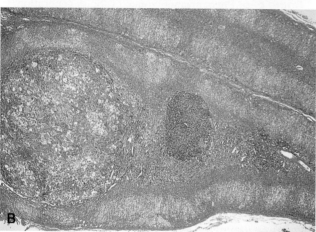

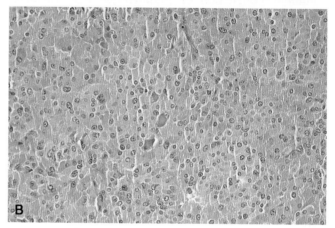

Figure 6–6. Macroscopic *(A)* and microscopic *(B)* aspects of bilateral pheochromocytoma and nodular adrenal medullary hyperplasia in a multiple endocrine neoplasia type II patient.

Figure 6–8. Pheochromocytoma: solid and diffuse pattern *(A)* and eosinophilic transformation *(B).*

Histologic patterns in pheochromocytomas include a mixture of alveolar (Zellballen) [2] and trabecular patterns (Fig. 6–7). A spindle cell pattern has been reported in about 2% of tumors but is usually not prominent throughout the tumor.[66] Some

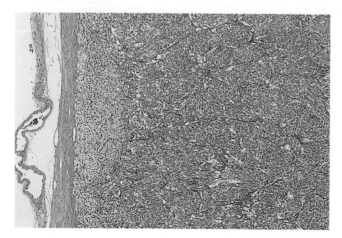

Figure 6–7. Pheochromocytoma: histologic aspect and adjacent adrenal cortex.

pheochromocytomas have areas in which the growth pattern is solid or diffuse (Fig. 6–8). Nests of tumor cells may vary considerably in size and shape, and occasional central degenerative change is seen. There is frequently peripheral intermingling of tumor cells with non-neoplastic cortical cells, without an intervening fibrous capsule. Some tumors are composed of cells that closely resemble those of the adjacent non-neoplastic medulla, whereas in others the neoplastic cells are several times the size of normal chromaffin cells, with abundant cytoplasm and vesicular nuclei with large nucleoli (Fig. 6–9). Despite these neuron-like cytologic features, the large cells contain abundant CGA (Fig. 6–10) and express PNMT and, therefore, functionally resemble chromaffin cells. However, occasional neuronal cells may be seen within a pheochromocytoma. Tumor cells are usually polygonal with sharply defined cell borders. The cytoplasm is finely granular and may be lightly eosinophilic (Fig. 6–11), amphophilic, or basophilic. Intracytoplasmic, PAS-positive, diastase-resistant hyaline globules are frequently observed (Fig. 6–12). Some cells may contain artifactual vacuoles, which resemble pseudoacini or may exhibit so-called lipid degeneration, causing them to mimic an adrenal cortical neoplasm (Fig. 6–13). Some tumor cells may exhibit oncocytic features. Tumor cell

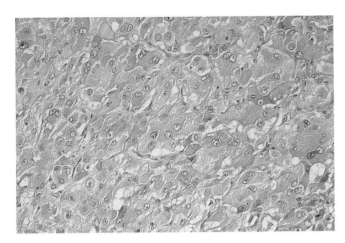

Figure 6-9. Pheochromocytoma: giant cells and prominent nucleoli.

nuclei may show cytoplasmic pseudoinclusions. Some tumors contain cells with moderate to marked nuclear enlargement and hyperchromatism, a feature that has no impact on prognosis (Fig. 6–14). Occasional mitotic figures can be identified in tumors that prove to be clinically benign. In contrast to their normal counterparts, neoplastic chromaffin cells are usually not innervated.[25, 32]

Pheochromocytomas are characteristically highly vascular neoplasms, and hemorrhage within a tumor may artifactually separate clusters of tumor cells. Some tumors may mimic angiomas or other vascular neoplasms. Areas of sclerosis may be prominent, especially in association with cystic degeneration. Amyloid has been identified in some tumors.

Pheochromocytomas are invariably positive for CGA and TH, and either of these markers should readily distinguish them from most adrenal cortical tumors and from nonendocrine tumors, including adrenal metastases. Synaptophysin is not an ideal marker for this purpose, because focal immunoreactivity for synaptophysin may be seen in normal and

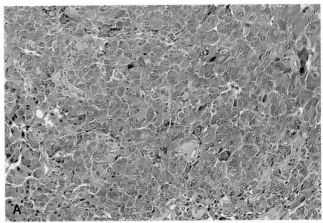

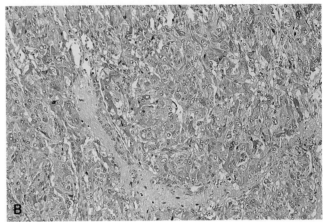

Figure 6-11. *A* and *B*, Pheochromocytoma: basophilic/amphophilic cytoplasm.

neoplastic adrenal cortex[67] (Table 6–1). A somewhat more difficult challenge is occasionally posed by adrenal cortical oncocytomas, which may strongly resemble pheochromocytomas and may show weak nonspecific reactivities in immunohistochemical studies, requiring electron microscopy.

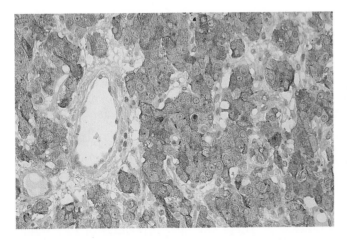

Figure 6-10. Pheochromocytoma: chromogranin A in immunohistochemistry.

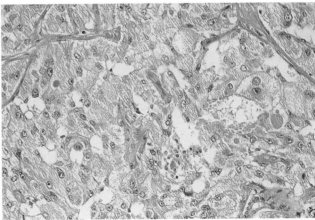

Figure 6–12. Pheochromocytoma: intracytoplasmic hyaline globules.

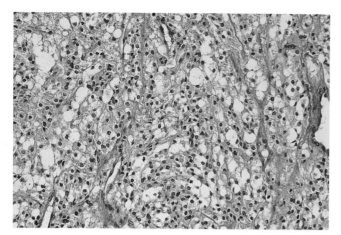

Figure 6–13. Pheochromocytoma imitating an adrenocortical tumor.

Table 6–1. Differential Diagnosis Between Adrenocortical and Medullary Tumors/Renal Carcinomas

Antigen	Adrenal Medullary Tumors (%)	Adrenocortical Tumors (%)	Renal Cell Carcinoma (%)
Pancytokeratin	0	10–36	≤100
Epithelial membrane antigen	0	0	100
Leu-M1 (CD 15)	80	0	65
Chromogranin A	95	0	
Neuron-specific enolase	95	30	
Synaptophysin	100	40–80	
D11	0	44–100	2
Polysialic acid/NCAM*	100	30	

NCAM: neural cell adhesion molecule. Adapted from Schröder S, Padberg B, Reincke M, Komminoth P: Diagnostic guidelines for adrenal gland nodules: Typing, assessment of biological potential and prognosis, molecular pathogenesis. Verh Dtsch Ges Path 1997; 81:97.

Malignancy

Pheochromocytomas metastasize in only 2%–5% of cases.[32] Up to 10% recur locally, probably as a result of small foci of local invasion, which can be found commonly in benign tumors. Malignant pheochromocytomas can metastasize widely by lymphatic or hematogenous routes (Fig. 6–15).

There are no reliable histologic criteria for predicting malignant behavior. Hyperchromatism, pleomorphism, mitoses, and vascular or capsular invasion may be observed in tumors that follow a benign course. Coarse nodularity, nests of tumor cells showing confluent necrosis, and absence of hyaline globules are features found to have a statistically significant association with malignancy.[66] Large tumor size, prominent mitoses, and extensive local or vascular invasion are worrisome findings.[68] Interestingly, malignancy in pheochromocytomas has been reported to be restricted to tumors composed of the small cells that most closely resemble chromaffin cells. The large cells with prominent nucleoli that are the major component of many pheochromocytomas may, therefore, be terminally differentiated. It has

been speculated that increased size of pheochromocytoma cells might reflect partial activation of mechanisms involved in neuronal maturation.

Studies have attempted to evaluate the malignant potential of pheochromocytomas by immunohistochemical staining for proliferation antigens and protein products of oncogenes and tumor suppressor genes (Table 6–2). In one study, benign pheochromocytomas were found to have an average of less than 10 MIB-1–labeled nuclei per 200× field in areas selected for highest labeling density, whereas metastasizing tumors had more than 20 labeled nuclei.[69] These findings have been corroborated by a study on a large series of benign and malignant pheochromocytomas, in which a high MIB–1 labeling index was significantly associated with malignancy in both uni- and multivariate analysis.[70] In another study, overexpression of p53 and immunoreactivity with bcl-2, a protein involved in blocking of apoptosis, were associated with malignant behavior of pheochromocytomas.[71] Most evidence now suggests that simple ploidy measurements are not a reliable predictor of malignancy.[72]

Molecular Pathogenesis

Molecular abnormalities in pheochromocytomas have been studied by candidate gene analysis, loss of heterozygosity of certain chromosomal regions, and, more recently, genome-wide analysis through comparative genomic hybridization (CGH). The *RET* proto-oncogene and the *VHL* tumor suppressor gene are candidate genes because pheochromocytomas occur in the multiple tumor syndromes caused by these two genes: MEN-II, and von Hippel–Lindau disease. Somatic *RET* mutations have been detected in 0%–31% of sporadic pheochromocytomas in several studies.[73–75] There was no correlation of *RET* mutations with tumor behavior.[71] Also, somatic *VHL* mutations are rare in sporadic pheochromocytomas,

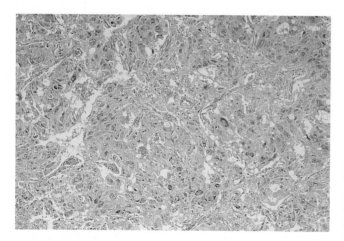

Figure 6–14. Pheochromocytoma: pleomorphic cells.

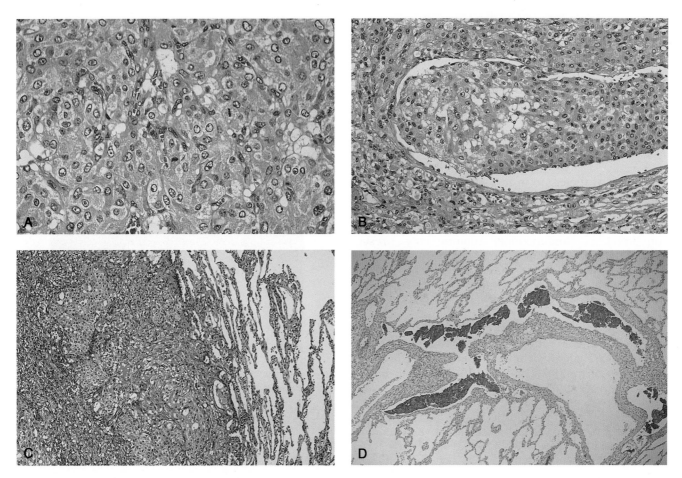

Figure 6–15. Malignant pheochromocytoma: increased mitotic rate *(A)*, vascular invasion *(B)*, pulmonary metastasis *(C)*, and lymphangiosis of the lung (chromogranin A immunohistochemistry; *D).*

although studies have demonstrated an increased frequency of mutations in malignant pheochromocytomas, with 7 of 28 tumors carrying a *VHL* missense mutation (H. Dannenberg, unpublished observations, 2000). No mutations could be detected in the c-*mos* proto-oncogene and in the p16 tumor suppressor gene.[76, 77]

Table 6–2. Criteria for Malignant Pheochromocytomas

Criteria	Benign	Suspicious for Malignancy
S-100–positive sustentacular cells	Frequent	Sparse or absent
Neuropeptide expression	Multihormonal	Sparse
DNA content	Euploid	
Weight		>200 g
Mitotic rate		Increased (>5/10 high-power fields)
Growth pattern		Small or spindle cell
Regressive changes		Frequent

Adapted from Schröder S, Padberg B, Reincke M, Komminoth P: Diagnostic guidelines for adrenal gland nodules: Typing, assessment of biological potential and prognosis, molecular pathogenesis. Verh Dtsch Ges Path 1997; 81:97.

Loss of heterozygosity studies have been performed for the detection of potential tumor suppressor genes involved in pheochromocytoma tumorigenesis. Such studies were mostly on limited numbers of benign tumors and have yielded evidence of losses on chromosomes 1p, 3p, 11p, 17p, and 22q.[78–82] With the CGH technique, the entire genome can be studied for both losses and gains of chromosomal material, allowing for the detection of tumor suppressor and oncogene loci, respectively. One study has demonstrated losses of 1p and 3q in more than half of pheochromocytomas, confirming earlier findings as well as adding a new chromosomal region of interest. In addition, a significantly higher frequency of chromosomal loss at 6q was observed in malignant compared with benign pheochromocytomas.[83]

EXTRA-ADRENAL SYMPATHETIC PARAGANGLIOMAS

Clinical Considerations

Extra-adrenal paragangliomas associated with the sympathetic nervous system occur anywhere from the upper neck to the pelvic floor (Table 6–3). More than 90% occur in the retroperitoneum, and

Table 6-3. Anatomic Distribution of Extra-Adrenal Sympathetic Paragangliomas

Type	%
Intra-abdominal	85
Superior paraaortic	45
Inferior paraaortic	30
Urinary bladder	10
Intrathoracic	12
Cervical	3

30%–50% of these are in the vicinity of the organ of Zuckerkandl.[8, 84] Between 5% and 9% are located in the thorax, and rare cases are in the neck.[85, 86] Approximately 25% to 27% of the tumors are clinically functional.[8, 87] Nonfunctional tumors may present with spinal cord compression and pain or as incidental findings. Patients may have synchronous or metachronous adrenal medullary tumors or extra-adrenal paragangliomas in other locations, whether disease is familial or not.

Despite their general similarities, extra-adrenal paragangliomas in different locations vary somewhat in terms of age distribution, gender predilection, likelihood of multicentricity, and potential to metastasize. From a clinical perspective, the most significant differences are those concerning malignancy. Extra-adrenal sympathetic paragangliomas in any location are more likely to be malignant than their intra-adrenal counterparts.[87, 88]

Intra-abdominal paragangliomas occur at all ages, but most are reported in the third to fifth decades of life, with a male predominance in some but not all series.[9, 89] In some series, up to one-third of patients are children younger than 16 years. As many as half of these children had multiple tumors. Approximately 20% to 40% of retroperitoneal paragangliomas are reported to metastasize. Most patients with metastases die of their disease, but survival for as long as 25 years has been reported[89] (Fig. 6–16).

Urinary bladder paragangliomas have been reported in patients between 11 and 78 years of age. Either there is no sex predilection or a slight female predominance. The majority of patients exhibit a clinical triad consisting of paroxysmal hypertension, gross intermittent hematuria, and micturitional "attacks" of headache, pallor, sweating, anxiety, and other catecholamine-related symptoms.[32, 90] In asymptomatic patients, the tumors are often discovered incidentally. Urinary bladder paragangliomas range in greatest dimension from 0.3 to 5.5 cm.[90] Some are circumscribed, but most grow between muscle bundles in the bladder wall. About 80% extend into the submucosa and bulge into the bladder lumen. Tumors are located in the trigone, dome, or anterior wall of the bladder.[91] Approximately 7% arise in the posterior wall and 3% in the neck. In one major series, 8% of the patients had multifocal disease. Recurrent or multifocal tumors have been reported in 18% of all cases. Metastases are reported in about 7% of patients.[90]

Intrathoracic paravertebral paragangliomas are usually located in the midthoracic region.[87] About half are associated with signs and symptoms related to catecholamine secretion. The average age at detection is 29 years and, as in paragangliomas of the retroperitoneum, two-thirds of the tumors arise in males. More than 20% of patients have multifocal disease. About 7% of patients acquire metastases.

Cervical paravertebral paragangliomas are very rare; so far, only five have been reported.[92] Some have occurred in pediatric patients in association with pheochromocytomas.[93]

Paragangliomas of the cauda equina are rare tumors that are usually located in the filum terminale.[94] The tumors are mostly intradural and rarely

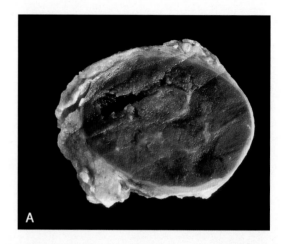

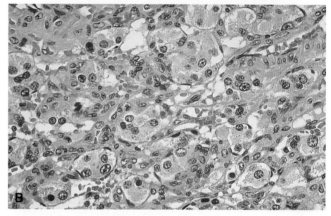

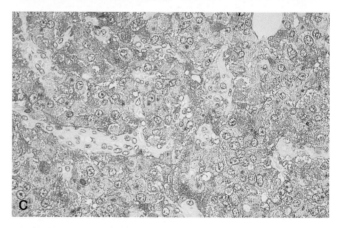

Figure 6–16. Pigmented extra-adrenal paraganglioma: macroscopic aspect (A), histology (B), and chromogranin A immunohistochemistry (C).

epidural, occur slightly more frequently in males, and exhibit similar histologic appearance as paragangliomas in other sites.[95] Typical symptoms include low back pain, neurologic deficiencies, and incontinence.

Macroscopic and Microscopic Anatomy

The most characteristic microscopic pattern is a trabecular arrangement with anastomosing cords of tumor cells. Some tumors may have a diffuse, alveolar, or admixed pattern. The morphology of adrenal and extra-adrenal tumors is usually very similar, and there is no reliable pattern to discriminate between them. Finding an attached adrenal remnant or an uninvolved adrenal may be helpful.[25]

As in the adrenal medulla, there are no reliable criteria for predicting malignancy. In a large series of pheochromocytomas and extra-adrenal sympathetic paragangliomas, a statistically significant association between malignancy and extra-adrenal location was found.[66] Indicators of malignancy that have been described in the adrenal medulla for pheochromocytomas also apply to extra-adrenal sympathetic paragangliomas. Multicentric paragangliomas, however, should not be misinterpreted as metastases of pheochromocytomas.

EXTRA-ADRENAL PARASYMPATHETIC PARAGANGLIOMAS

Clinical Considerations

Jugular and tympanic paraganglia are the most common sites of origin of parasympathetic paragangliomas in most published series (57% to 81% of tumors) followed by carotid body (8% to 36%), vagal (4% to 13%), and aortic (4% to 10%) paraganglia.[96] Paragangliomas in other locations are very rare. In two large series carotid body tumors were most common, possibly reflecting patient populations in individual institutions.[26, 97] Parasympathetic paragangliomas tend to occur most frequently in females except for familial cases, which have an equal sex distribution. Precise sex ratios vary according to tumor location and patient age.[96, 97]

In contrast to adrenal and extra-adrenal sympathetic paragangliomas, which cause catecholamine-related signs and symptoms in the majority of cases,[8, 91, 98] only about 1% of parasympathetic paragangliomas are clinically functional.[96] This contrast most likely reflects a quantitative difference in catecholamine production, because most parasympathetic paragangliomas can be shown to contain catecholamines or catecholamine-synthesizing enzymes.[25]

Carotid body paragangliomas occur in patients of all ages, the youngest reported being a 3-month-old. The most frequent age of presentation is in the fifth decade of life. Most studies show a slight female predominance.[96, 99] However, high-altitude dwellers have a 10-fold increase in tumor frequency compared with those living at sea level,[100] with a 6:1 female-male ratio. These findings suggest an increased susceptibility of females to carotid body tumors, which may be accentuated by chronic hypoxemia at high altitude.[99] Carotid body paragangliomas are bilateral in 3% to 8% of sporadic cases and up to 38% of familial cases.[96, 99, 101] Carotid body paragangliomas usually enlarge slowly; symptoms often last for several years before diagnosis. The majority of patients present with a painless neck mass, and some present with pain radiating into the head and shoulders. The tumors most commonly involve the carotid wall and displace the internal and external carotid arteries laterally.[9, 96] Most carotid body paragangliomas are 3 to 6 cm in greatest dimension, but some are larger than 20 cm.[96] The tumors are often sharply demarcated and appear to be encapsulated (Fig. 6–17). However, on histologic examination, they frequently exhibit an expansile border with a fibrous pseudocapsule. Small carotid body paragangliomas are usually not significantly adherent to the carotid artery adventitia, whereas larger tumors may surround one or both carotid arteries or the carotid bifurcation. Approximately 10% of carotid body paragangliomas are malignant.[96] Metastases are confined to regional lymph nodes in about half of these cases. Distant metastases may involve bone (28%), lung (20%), liver, and other locations. The prognosis for patients with metastases is unpredictable. Occasional tumors cause death by local infiltration.

Jugulotympanic paraganglia comprise about 20% of all tumors in the middle ear and about 66% of all benign tumors.[96] They usually occur in adult patients, with a peak incidence during the fifth decade, but have also been reported in early childhood. Similar to carotid body paragangliomas, there is a female-male ratio of 6:1, a slow growth, and a prolonged clinical course. Classic glomus tympanicum tumors produce hearing disturbances, whereas classic glomus jugulare tumors produce a jugular foramen syndrome with cranial nerve palsies.[52] More than one-third of jugulotympanic paraganglioma present as polyps in the ear channel or as retrotympanic masses. Some tumors may also grow

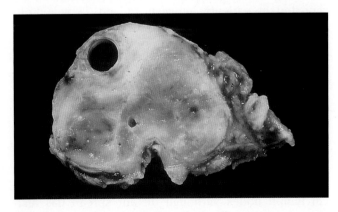

Figure 6–17. Carotid body paraganglioma: macroscopic aspect (note close proximity to carotid artery).

intracranially, where they can be confused with meningiomas, or infiltrate the internal jugular vein or dural sinuses. Microscopically, jugulotympanic paragangliomas are usually more vascular, cell nests are less uniform and smaller, and the chief cell nuclei are smaller than other paragangliomas of the head and neck region.[96] Some tumors exhibit extensive calcifications and sclerosis. Local recurrences are common and may also occur many years after initial treatment. Tumors in the jugular fossa are more difficult to remove than those in the tympanic cavity, and incomplete excision is common.[102, 103] Metastases from jugulotympanic paragangliomas occur in less than 3% of cases and are confined to cervical lymph nodes in approximately 26%. The most commonly involved sites of distant metastases are lung (44%), liver (22%), and bone (19%).

Vagal paragangliomas arise from dispersed paraganglia located in close proximity to or within the vagus nerve. They have been reported in all age groups (18 to 79 years), and the female-male ratio is similar to that of jugulotympanic paraganglioma. They usually exhibit slow growth, and approximately 83% present as painless masses in the anterolateral neck. In about 60% of cases only a pharyngeal mass is present. Cranial nerve involvement occurs in about 30% of patients, most frequently manifesting as hoarseness as a result of vagus nerve damage.[96] Gross and histologic appearance of vagal paraganglioma is similar to that of other head and neck paragangliomas. Multiple myelinized nerve bundles from the vagus nerve may be seen in the periphery of the tumor. The intraneural or paraneural presence of neoplastic chief cells does not necessarily indicate malignancy.[32] Incomplete removal has been reported in about 10% of cases treated by surgery alone, and approximately 10% metastasize, most often to regional lymph nodes and rarely to the lung (23%) or bone (9%). Local tumor infiltration into adjacent structures, including bone, is the most frequent cause of death. Reported survival of patients with metastases or locally aggressive tumors has varied between several months and 16 years.[96] Multicentric tumors occur in 15% to 20% of patients with vagal paragangliomas, of which 25% are familial.

Laryngeal paragangliomas arise from dispersed paraganglia located near the larynx. They have been reported in patients between 14 and 75 years old (mean, 47 years).[104] There is no definite sex predilection. The most common symptom is hoarseness, but rare symptoms include dyspnea, bleeding, or pain. The latter symptom is often associated with recurrent or metastatic disease.[102] The average size is 2.5 cm. Laryngeal paragangliomas usually present as red or blue-red submucosal masses and on cross-section may have a tan appearance with areas of hemorrhage. The histologic appearance is similar to that of other paragangliomas of the head and neck region. Laryngeal paragangliomas show metastases in almost 20% of cases. Most metastases are found in local lymph nodes, although distant spread has also been described. There have been no reported familial cases.[102]

Paragangliomas in Other Sites in the Head and Neck Region

Most orbital paragangliomas present with proptosis and frequently show aggressive infiltration of muscle, fatty tissue, and bone. They may extend into the cranium or the paranasal sinuses, and about 18% metastasize to regional lymph nodes. Rare paragangliomas have been reported in the nasopharynx and nasal cavity.[26, 96, 105] The tumors may show a locally aggressive behavior, but no metastases have been reported. Important differential diagnoses in these anatomic locations include neuroendocrine carcinomas and olfactory neuroblastomas.[106] Paragangliomas are occasionally found in the esophagus, trachea, and thyroid gland. At least some of the intrathyroidal tumors may be derived from laryngeal paraganglia.[96] Tumors in the parotid gland, temporalis muscle, buccal mucosa, tongue, palate, pterygopalatine fossa, and posterior and middle fossa have also been reported.[96] These lesions, like those in the orbit, are tentatively listed here as parasympathetic paragangliomas because of their location in the head and neck region. They might, however, arise from ectopic paraganglionic cells.

Aorticopulmonary and pulmonary paragangliomas are believed to arise from paraganglia near the base of the heart and great vessels, sometimes involving the heart itself.[96, 107] This category also includes intrapulmonary paragangliomas, but no lesions of the posterior mediastinum, which usually arise from the thoracic sympathetic paraganglia.[108] Most of the reported pulmonary paragangliomas were located in the vicinity of blood vessels and nerves and were often located near the pulmonary artery.[32, 104] They have been reported in all age groups (range, 6 months to 82 years; mean, 44 years). The female-male ratio is between 2 and 3:1.[96, 107] The most frequently encountered complaints are respiratory and cardiovascular symptoms, palpable masses, hypotension, and symptoms of esophageal involvement.[96, 109] About 45% of patients, however, remain asymptomatic. Aorticopulmonary paragangliomas are usually 5 to 7 cm in diameter but may range considerably in size (2 to 17 cm). They are usually sharply demarcated. Their attachment to vital structures makes complete surgical removal difficult. Histologically, these paragangliomas show the same patterns as paragangliomas from other locations. The infiltration of cardiac structures is not a reliable indicator of malignancy. Approximately 13% to 20% of tumors metastasize, a majority to distant sites.[96, 107] Approximately 10% of paragangliomas involving the great vessels are found in patients with synchronous or metachronous paragangliomas of other sites.[96, 107]

Macroscopic and Microscopic Pathology

The histologic and cytologic features of parasympathetic paragangliomas are similar to those of their sympathetic counterparts. However, a somewhat greater range of features and a more extensive differential diagnosis may pose diagnostic challenges. As in sympathetic paragangliomas, neoplastic neuroendocrine cells form nests or cords separated by fibrovascular stroma. Less common are sheets of cells and spindle cell patterns mimicking mesenchymal tumors. Different growth patterns are often admixed. Paraganglioma cells are usually cytologically similar to their normal counterparts,[2] but may be larger or smaller and may exhibit more pleomorphism. Large, bizarre, hyperchromatic cells and oncocytes are sometimes observed. Intracytoplasmic hyaline globules are rare (Fig. 6–18). Paragangliomas contain numerous small vascular channels similar to those in normal paraganglia. Some show prominent perivascular sclerosis, which may either accentuate or compress nests of tumor cells. In some cases, abundant fibrous stroma may cause isolated groups of paraganglioma cells to resemble infiltrating carcinoma. In other cases, marked dilation of the tumor vessels creates an angiomatous appearance. Perivascular rosettes of tumor cells may be observed. An abundant reticulin network usually spreads from small vessels to surround groups of tumor cells. As with tumors of the sympathetic paraganglia, there are no reliable histologic criteria for predicting malignant behavior in parasympathetic paragangliomas. Numerous mitoses, extensive vascular invasion, and central necrosis of cell nests have been associated with malignancy.

Molecular Pathogenesis

Relatively little is known about the molecular mechanisms involved in the genesis of parasympathetic paragangliomas. The oncogenes c-*myc*, *bcl-2*, and c-*jun* were found to be expressed in a proportion of carotid body paragangliomas.[110] In hereditary paragangliomas, linkage analysis and loss of heterozygosity studies indicated a gene on chromosome 11q22–q23 and 11q13,[111, 112] and a candidate gene has been identified.[113] Interestingly, those chromosomal regions have also been found to be lost in CGH analyses of sporadic paragangliomas.[83]

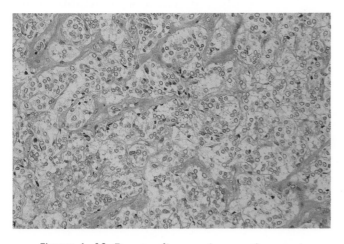

Figure 6–18. Paraganglioma: microscopic aspect.

PROLIFERATIVE LESIONS OF NEURONAL LINEAGE

Tumors of neuronal lineage (neuroblastic tumors) have traditionally been classified as neuroblastomas, ganglioneuroblastomas, or ganglioneuromas according to the degree of morphologic maturity.

Incidence and Prevalence

Neuroblastomas predominantly occur in early childhood and are the most common type of extracranial malignancy in children. They account for 15% of all neoplasms encountered in the first 4 years of life.[114] The majority of cases (90%) present before the age of 5 years.[115]

Clinical Presentation

The vast majority of neuroblastic tumors arise from the sympathetic nervous system in the adrenal medulla or sympathetic chains. Some rare tumors may develop in the bladder. More than half of the tumors occur in the abdomen or the retroperitoneum, and 30% to 40% are intra-adrenal. In contrast, ganglioneuromas are tumors of late childhood and adult life and are rare before age 3. They develop most frequently in the third decade of life. Approximately 30% to 40% of tumors are located in the mediastinum.[116–118] Ganglioneuroblastomas are both clinically and histologically intermediate. About 25% of tumors occur in patients younger than 1 year and 35% occur between 2 and 4 years. Sixty-five percent of ganglioneuroblastomas are found in extra-adrenal sites, 10% in the adrenal, and 10% in the mediastinum.

Macroscopic and Microscopic Pathology

Neuroblastomas are typically soft, gray, or white tumors with areas of hemorrhage and necrosis, and calcifications are present in 40% to 60% of cases (Fig. 6–19). Histologically, they are usually composed of small, monomorphous, hypochromatic cells with scant cytoplasm (Fig. 6–20). Areas of differentiation are characterized by larger cells with more abundant cytoplasm, vesicular nuclei, a neuropil matrix and Homer Wright rosettes.[117, 119–121] Neuroblastomas are usually glycogen poor and PAS negative and exhibit variable numbers of sustentacular or Schwann cells.[122–124] Most neuroblastomas express neuroendocrine markers (CGA, synaptophysin, neuron-specific enolase)[125] and neurofilament proteins. Distinctive ultrastructural features are axonal processes, small secretory granules and synaptic-like vesicles.[126] Neuroblastomas have been subdivided by the International Neuroblastoma Pathology Committee into undifferentiated, poorly differentiated, and differentiating. These three categories

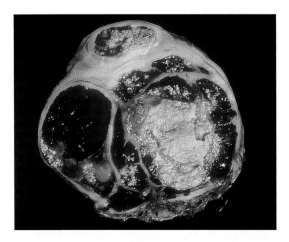

Figure 6–19. Neuroblastoma: macroscopic aspect.

have been based on the presence or absence of neuropil and on the presence of more than 5% of tumor cells with differentiation toward ganglion cells.[127]

Ganglioneuroblastomas combine both gross and microscopic features of neuroblastoma and ganglioneuroma. They are composed of mixtures of immature and mature neurons in variable amounts of stroma (Fig. 6–21). Two variants, initially described by Stout,[118] are traditionally recognized: (1) the intermixed type, in which neuroblastic cells in varying stages of maturation and ganglion cells are distributed at random in ample stroma, and the ganglioneuromatous component should at least occupy 50% of the total tumor volume; and (2) the nodular type, in which macroscopic neuroblastic nodules are seen in a tumor otherwise typical of ganglioneuroblastoma, intermixed or ganglioneuroma.[127] This last group is considered to have an unfavorable prognosis because of the presence of neuroblastic nodules, which are considered to represent aggressive malignant clones with different genetic abnormalities and biologic behavior compared with the surrounding tumor component.[127]

Ganglioneuromas are encapsulated tumors with a homogeneous-appearing gray or tan rubbery cut surface (Fig. 6–22). Histologically, they exhibit mature

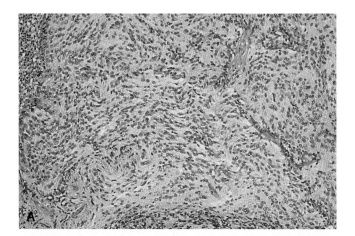

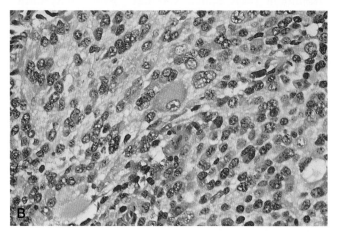

Figure 6–21. A and B, Ganglioneuroblastoma: microscopic aspect with pure neuroblastoma and mixed tumor parts.

or maturing ganglion cells in a dense stroma of Schwann cells and collagen (Fig. 6–23). Characteristically, there are no neuroblastic foci. Mitoses are usually absent. Adequate sampling is required to rule out foci of immaturity.

Immunohistochemistry

Neuroblastic tumors show immunoreactivity in a variable proportion of cases with neuron-specific

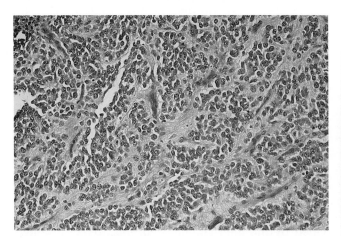

Figure 6–20. Neuroblastoma: typical histology with sheets of small "blue" cells.

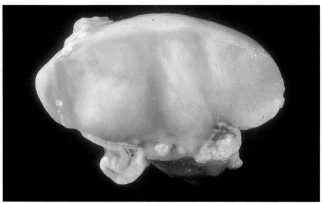

Figure 6–22. Ganglioneuroma: macroscopic aspect.

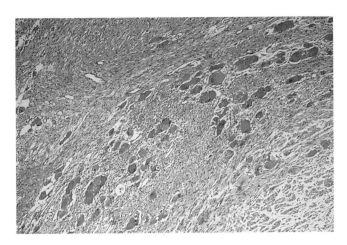

Figure 6–23. Ganglioneuroma: microscopic aspect.

enolase, chromogranin A, synaptophysin, TH, protein gene product 9.5, and NB84. In contrast, there is usually no reactivity with antibodies to actin, desmin, low-molecular-weight cytokeratin, leukocyte common antigen, and vimentin and with the CD99 antibody directed to the MIC2 gene product.[127]

Functional Activity

Catecholamines and other neuroendocrine secretory products are common in tumors of neuronal lineage, but they rarely cause typical clinical syndromes. Thus, hypertension and other catecholamine-related symptoms are only encountered in approximately 20% of patients with neuroblastomas.[128] Some patients may experience watery diarrhea as a result of vasoactive intestinal peptide (VIP) production or Cushing's syndrome.[128–130] Interestingly, VIP content appears to correlate with increasing neuronal maturation, and catecholamine-related symptoms are more frequently associated with less mature–appearing tumors. Most neuroblastomas produce dopamine or norepinephrine or both.[22] In contrast to pheochromocytomas,[22] neuroblastomas usually only contain minute amounts of catecholamines.[131] However, catecholamines and their metabolites may be detected in the urine of more than 90% of patients, most probably because of high rates of catecholamine synthesis and reduced intracellular storage.[132] A variety of neuropeptides can be found in neuroblastic tumors.[25, 133] These include VIP, somatostatin, neuropeptide Y, enkephalin, and galanin.[25] As with VIP, expression of somatostatin appears to be correlated with neuronal maturation. In contrast, neuropeptide Y is produced and secreted by a high percentage of poorly differentiated tumors.[25]

Assessment of Prognosis

Many prognostic profiles based on statistical studies have been proposed for neuroblastomas on the basis of combinations of clinical, histologic, functional, and molecular markers. Well-known prognostic factors are age at diagnosis, clinical stage, and anatomic site.[134, 135] Patients younger than 1 year with primary tumors in the mediastinum have the most favorable prognosis and patients with adrenal tumors the worst. A variety of systems for histologic classification and grading have been used.[25] The Shimada classification[136] emphasizes the improved prognosis associated with increasing numbers of S-100–reactive stromal cells.[122] Furthermore, Shimada et al. proposed the use of a mitosis/karyorrhexis index (number of mitotic and karyorrhectic nuclei per 5000 cells) as a prognostic indicator; an index above 200 imparts a poor prognosis. In the Joshi classification, the best prognosis is associated with a combination of calcification and a low mitotic rate (<10 mitoses/10 high-power fields) and the worst with absence of calcification and high mitotic rate (>10 mitoses/10 high-power fields). The outlook for tumors with calcification or a low mitotic rate is intermediate.[137] The International Neuroblastoma Pathology Committee has published a new classification, which may be regarded as an extension of the previous Shimada classification.[138] In this new classification, age, histologic subtype, and mitosis/karyorrhexis index are used as prognostic markers, whereas mitotic rate and calcification were found not to contribute to improved prognostication.

Predominance of norepinephrine or its metabolite, vanillylmandelic acid, over dopamine or its metabolite, homovanillic acid, in the urine of neuroblastoma patients is associated with a somewhat improved prognosis.[139] Among other nonhormonal circulating markers, serum ferritin has proved to be an additional prognostic marker.[25] Serum ferritin is elevated in about 40% of all neuroblastoma patients and is associated with stage III and IV disease.[140] This marker is shed by tumor cells and appears to reflect not only tumor burden but also specific metabolic characteristics, because levels are usually low in patients with stage IV-S disease. Furthermore, expression of the multidrug resistance gene product P-glycoprotein appears to correlate with tumor aggressiveness.[141] Absence of N-*myc* amplification, high levels of trkA messenger ribonucleic acid expression, absence of chromosome 1 abnormalities, and hyperdiploid/near-triploid karyotype or DNA index are favorable prognostic markers.[142] N-*myc* amplification appears to be associated with a poor prognosis for tumors at any stage, possibly because of its correlation with increased expression of the multidrug resistance gene.[143] The frequent concurrence of favorable functional and molecular markers in patients younger than 1 year has strengthened the concept that neuroblastomas of infancy are a distinct clinicopathologic entity.[144]

Molecular Pathogenesis

The most commonly encountered genetic abnormalities are loss of heterozygosity of the short arm of chromosome 1 (1p)[142, 145] and of the long arm of chromosome 14 (14q). Other reported abnormalities involve deletions at chromosome 11p, 13q, 4p, 11q, and 4q as well as extra copies of chromosome 17q.[142, 146] Trk A, the gene encoding the 140-kD high-affinity nerve growth factor receptor, is expressed in more than 90% of neuroblastomas.[142, 147] Furthermore, 25% to 30% of neuroblastomas show amplifications of the N-*myc* oncogene on chromosome 2.[142] N-*myc* amplification is correlated with deletion of chromosome 1p and other chromosomal abnormalities and with reduced trk A expression.[142]

The Phenomena of Regression and Maturation

Spontaneous regression of neuroblasts, including those from the adrenal medulla, by programmed cell death is well documented in the literature. This may be due to a lack of neurotrophic maintenance factors, such as nerve growth factors.[148, 149] These processes appear to continue until infancy, because the incidences of occult "neuroblastomas" in autopsy studies[150] or in mass population screenings for catecholamine metabolites[151] were far higher than the previously known neuroblastoma incidence. Regression of clinically apparent neuroblastomas, however, has also been reported, usually in patients younger than 1 year, with stage II or IV-S disease.[152] Although the underlying mechanisms for regression have not been fully elucidated, they appear to be associated with favorable genetic markers.[153]

Spontaneous maturation of neuroblastomas into ganglioneuromas has also been reported.[154] In fact, all ganglioneuromas are considered to have developed from neuroblastomas, in which the neuroblasts have differentiated into ganglion cells and have attracted Schwann cells by chemotactic factors.[138] Such maturation may also occur in metastases of neuroblastomas.[155] In addition, partial maturation, particularly after treatment with cytotoxic agents, is observed.[156]

Familial Tumors and Association with Other Disorders

Neuroblastomas occasionally occur in familial form, with a pattern suggestive of autosomal-dominant inheritance.[157] Some cases of neuroblastoma are associated with neurofibromatosis, Hirschsprung's disease, central hypoventilation, Beckwith-Wiedemann syndrome, nesidioblastosis, and a variety of congenital malformations.[25]

Nonhormonal Tumor–Associated Syndromes

Opsoclonus-myoclonus (ataxic eye movements and/or cerebellar ataxia) occurs in up to 2% of all neuroblastoma patients. The cause is unknown but mightbe related to immune mechanisms or toxic metabolic products. Additional neurologic syndromes associated with neuroblastic tumors include central hypoventilation (Ondine's curse)[158] and the triad of heterochromia of the iris, anisocoria, and Horner's syndrome. The latter triad occurs in up to 25% of patients with thoracic neuroblastomas involving sympathetic ganglia that affect eye development and function.

Acknowledgments

We thank P. Saremaslani, S. Muletta-Feurer, and C. Matter for excellent technical assistance, A. Vyskocil for typing the manuscript, P. U. Heitz and T. Stallmach for providing macro- and microscopic pictures, and N. Wey and I. Schmieder for photographic and computer-assisted reproductions.

References

1. Kohn A: Die chromaffinen Zellen des Sympathicus. Anat Anz 1898; 15:399.
2. Kohn A: Chromaffine Zellen; chromaffine Organe; Paraganglien. Prager Med Wochenschr 1902; 27:325.
3. Kohn A: Die Paraganglien. Arch Mikr Anat 1903; 52:262.
4. Carmichael SW: The adrenal chromaffin vesicle: An historical perspective. J Auton Nerv Syst 1983; 7:7–12.
5. Karsner H: Tumors of the Adrenal. In Atlas of Tumor Pathology. Armed Forces Institute of Pathology, Washington, D.C., 1950.
6. Coupland RE: The natural history of the chromaffin cell. Longmans Green, London, 1965.
7. Kawai K, Kimura S, Miyamoto J, et al.: A case of multiple extra-adrenal pheochromocytomas. Endocrinol Jpn 1979; 26:693.
8. Melicow MM: One hundred cases of pheochromocytoma (107 tumors) at the Columbia-Presbyterian Medical Center, 1926–1976: A clinicopathological analysis. Cancer 1977; 40:1987.
9. Glenner G, Grimley P: Tumors of the extra-adrenal paraganglion system (including chemoreceptors). In Atlas of Tumor Pathology, Second Series, Fascicle 9. Armed Forces Institute of Pathology, Washington, D.C., 1974.
10. Le Douarin NM: The Neural Crest. Cambridge University Press, Cambridge, UK, 1982.
11. Molenaar WM, Lee VM, Trojanowski JQ: Early fetal acquisition of the chromaffin and neuronal immunophenotype by human adrenal medullary cells: An immunohistological study using monoclonal antibodies to chromogranin A, synaptophysin, tyrosine hydroxylase, and neuronal cytoskeletal proteins. Exp Neurol 1990; 108:1.
12. Hervonen A, Valasti A, Partanen M: The paraganglia, a persisting endocrine system in man. Am J Anat 1976; 146:207.
13. Jacobowitz D: Histochemical studies of the relationship of chromaffin cells and adrenergic nerve fibers to the cardiac ganglia of several species. J Pharmacol Exp Ther 1967; 158:227.
14. Grillo M, Jacobs L, Comroe J: A combined fluorescence histochemical and electron microscopic method for studying special monoamine containing cells (SIF cells). J Comp Neurol 1974; 153:1.
15. Kuo T, Anderson C, Rosai J: Normal paraganglia in the human gallbladder. Arch Pathol 1974; 97:46.
16. Coupland R: Postnatal fate of the abdominal paraaortic bodies in man. J Anat 1954; 88:464.
17. Verna A: Ultrastructure of the carotid body in the mammals. Int Rev Cytol 1979; 60:271.
18. Sietzen M, Schober M, Fischer C-R, et al.: Rat adrenal medulla: Levels of chromogranins, enkephalins, dopamine beta-hydroxylase and of the amine transporter are changed by nervous activity and hypophysectomy. Neuroscience 1987; 22:131.

19. Lachmand A, Gehrke D, Krigelstein K, et al.: Trophic factors from chromaffin granules provide survival of peripheral and central nervous system neurons. Neuroscience 1994; 62:361.
20. Tischler AS, Perlman RL, Costopoulos D, et al.: Vasoactive intestinal peptide increases tyrosine hydroxylase activity in normal and neoplastic rat chromaffin cell cultures. Neurosci Lett 1985; 61:141.
21. Eyzaguirre C, Fidone S: Transduction mechanisms in carotid body: Glomus cells, putative neurotransmitters and nerve endings. Am J Physiol 1980; 239:C135.
22. Neville A: The adrenal medulla. In Symington T, ed.: Functional Pathology of the Adrenal Gland. Williams & Wilkins, Baltimore, 1969, p. 219.
23. Coupland R: The development and fate of catecholamine-secreting endocrine cells. In Parvez H, Parves S, eds.: Biogenic Amines in Development. Elsevier/North-Holland, Amsterdam, 1980, p. 3.
24. Steele R, Hinterberger H: Catecholamines and 5-hydroxytryptamine in the carotid body in vascular, respiratory and other diseases. J Lab Clin Med 1972; 80:63.
25. Tischler A: The adrenal medulla and extra-adrenal paraganglia. In Kovacs K, Asa S, eds.: Functional Endocrine Pathology, 2nd ed. Blackwell Scientific Publications, Malden, MA, 1998, p. 550.
26. Lack EE, Cubilla AL, Woodruff JM, et al.: Paragangliomas of the head and neck region: A clinical study of 69 patients. Cancer 1977; 39:397.
27. De-la-Torre JC: Standardization of the sucrose-potassium phosphate-glyoxylic acid histofluorescence method for tissue monoamines. Neurosci Lett 1980; 17:339.
28. DeLellis RA: Formaldehyde-induced fluorescence technique for the demonstration of biogenic amines in diagnostic histopathology. Cancer 1971; 28(6):1704.
29. Lloyd RV, Sisson JC, Shapiro B, et al: Immunohistochemical localization of epinephrine, norepinephrine, catecholamine-synthesizing enzymes, and chromogranin in neuroendocrine cells and tumors. Am J Pathol 1986; 125:45.
30. Heitz PU, Roth J, Zuber C, et al: Markers for neural and endocrine cells in pathology. In Gratzl M, Langley L, eds.: Markers for Neural and Endocrine Cells. Weinheim, Germany VCH, 1991, p. 203.
31. Korat O, Trojanowski J, LiVolsi V, et al.: Antigen expression in paraganglia and paragangliomas. Surg Pathol 1988; 1:33.
32. Lack E: Tumors of the adrenal gland and extra-adrenal paraganglia. In Atlas of Tumor Pathology. Armed Forces Institute of Pathology, Washington, D.C., 1997.
33. DeLellis RA: Multiple endocrine neoplasia syndromes revisited. Clinical, morphologic and molecular features. Lab Invest 1995; 72:494.
34. Komminoth P: Multiple endokrine Neoplasie Typ 1 und 2. Diagnostische Leitlinien und molekulare Pathologie 1997. Pathologe 1997; 18:286.
35. Rudy FR, Bates RD, Cimorelli AJ, et al.: Adrenal medullary hyperplasia: A clinicopathologic study of four cases. Hum Pathol 1980; 11:650.
36. Latif F, Tory K, Gnarra J, et al.: Identification of the von Hippel-Lindau disease tumor suppressor gene. Science 1993; 260:1317.
37. Ainsworth PJ, Rodenhiser DI, Costa MT: Identification and characterization of sporadic and inherited mutations in exon 31 of the neurofibromatosis (NF1) gene. Hum Genet 1993; 91:151.
38. Yoshioka M, Saito H, Kawakami Y, et al.: Adrenomedullary hyperplasia associated with cortisol producing adenoma. Endocr J 1993; 40:467.
39. Beckwith J: Macroglossia, omphalocele, adrenal cytomegaly, gigantism and hyperplastic visceromegaly. Birth Defects 1969; 5:188.
40. Streeten DH, Anderson GH Jr, Lebowitz M, et al.: Primary hyperepinephrinemia in patients without pheochromocytoma. Arch Intern Med 1990; 150:1528.
41. Qupty G, Ishay A, Peretz H, et al.: Pheochromocytoma syndrome due to unilateral adrenal medullary hyperplasia. Clin Endocrinol (Oxf) 1997; 47:613.
42. Dralle H, Schroder S, Gratz KF, et al.: Sporadic unilateral adrenomedullary hyperplasia with hypertension cured by adrenalectomy. World J Surg 1990; 14(3):308; discussion, 316.
43. DeLellis RA, Wolfe HJ, Gagel RF, et al.: Adrenal medullary hyperplasia. A morphometric analysis in patients with familial medullary thyroid carcinoma. Am J Pathol 1976; 83:177.
44. Carney JA, Sizemore GW, Sheps SG: Adrenal medullary disease in multiple endocrine neoplasia, type 2: Pheochromocytoma and its precursors. Am J Clin Pathol 1976; 66:279.
45. Drut RM, Drut R, Gilbert-Barness E, et al.: Adrenal hyperplastic nodules in Wiedemann-Beckwith syndrome. Birth Defects 1993; 29:367.
46. Diaz-Cano SJ, Blanes A: Influence of intratumour heterogeneity in the interpretation of marker results in phaeochromocytomas. J Pathol 1999; 189:627.
47. Arias-Stella J, Valcarcel J: Chief cell hyperplasia in the human carotid body at high altitudes: Physiologic and pathologic significance. Hum Pathol 1976; 7:361.
48. Heath D, Smith P, Jago R: Hyperplasia of the carotid body. J Pathol 1982; 138:115.
49. Lack EE: Hyperplasia of vagal and carotid body paraganglia in patients with chronic hypoxemia. Am J Pathol 1978; 91:497.
50. Lack EE: Carotid body hypertrophy in patients with cystic fibrosis and cyanotic congenital heart disease. Hum Pathol 1977; 8:39.
51. Remine WH, Chong GC, Van H-JA, et al.: Current management of pheochromocytoma. Bull Soc Int Chir 1975; 34:97.
52. Hume DM: Pheochromocytoma in the adult and in the child. Am J Surg 1960; 99:458.
53. Samaan NA, Hickey RC, Shutts PE: Diagnosis, localization, and management of pheochromocytoma. Pitfalls and follow-up in 41 patients. Cancer 1988; 62:2451.
54. Florkowski CM, Fairlamb DJ, Freeth MG, et al.: Raised dopamine metabolites in a case of malignant paraganglioma. Postgrad Med J 1990; 66:471.
55. Lee PH, Blute R Jr, Malhotra R: A clinically "silent" pheochromocytoma with spontaneous hemorrhage. J Urol 1987; 138:1429.
56. Greene JP, Guay AT: New perspectives in pheochromocytoma. Urol Clin North Am 1989; 16:487.
57. Xu W, Mulligan LM, Ponder MA, et al.: Loss of NF1 alleles in phaeochromocytomas from patients with type I neurofibromatosis. Genes Chromosomes Cancer 1992; 4:337.
58. Zeiger MA, Zbar B, Keiser H, et al.: Loss of heterozygosity on the short arm of chromosome 3 in sporadic, von Hippel-Lindau disease-associated, and familial pheochromocytoma. Genes Chromosomes Cancer 1995; 13:151.
59. Modigliani E, Vasen HM, Raue K, et al.: Pheochromocytoma in multiple endocrine neoplasia type 2: European study. The Euromen Study Group. J Intern Med 1995; 238:363.
60. Evans DB, Lee JE, Merrell RC, et al.: Adrenal medullary disease in multiple endocrine neoplasia type 2. Appropriate management. Endocrinol Metab Clin North Am 1994; 23:167.
61. Cho KJ, Freier DT, McCormick TL, et al.: Adrenal medullary disease in multiple endocrine neoplasia type II. AJR Am J Roentgenol 1980; 134:23.
62. Neumann HP, Berger DP, Sigmund G, et al.: Pheochromocytomas, multiple endocrine neoplasia type 2, and von Hippel-Lindau disease. N Engl J Med 1993; 329:1531. Erratum, 1994; 331:1535.
63. Cance WG, Wells SA Jr: Multiple endocrine neoplasia. Type IIa. Curr Probl Surg 1985; 22:1.
64. Chevinsky AH, Minton JP, Falko JM: Metastatic pheochromocytoma associated with multiple endocrine neoplasia syndrome type II. Arch Surg 1990; 125:935.
65. Riccardi VM: Von Recklinghausen neurofibromatosis. N Engl J Med 1981; 305:1617.
66. Linnoila RI, Keiser HR, Steinberg SM, et al.: Histopathology of benign versus malignant sympathoadrenal paragangliomas: Clinicopathologic study of 120 cases including unusual histologic features. Hum Pathol 1990; 21:1168.
67. Komminoth P, Roth J, Saremaslani P, et al.: Overlapping expression of immunohistochemical markers and synaptophysin mRNA in pheochromocytomas and adrenocortical carcinomas. Implications for the differential diagnosis of adrenal gland tumors. Lab Invest 1995; 72:424.
68. Linnoila RI, Lack EE, Steinberg SM, et al.: Decreased expression of neuropeptides in malignant paragangliomas: An immunohistochemical study. Hum Pathol 1988; 19:41.

69. Kimura N, Miura W, Noshiro T, et al.: Ki-67 is an indicator of progression in neuroendocrine tumors. Endocr Pathol 1994; 5:223.

70. Van der Harst E, Bruining H, Bonjer H, et al.: Proliferative index in phaeochromocytomas: Does it predict the occurrence of metastases? J Pathol (in press).

71. De Krijger RR, van der Harst E, van der Ham F, et al.: Prognostic value of p53, bcl-2, and c-erbB-2 protein expression in phaeochromocytomas. J Pathol 1999; 188:51.

72. Jung WH, Jung SH, Yoo CJ, et al.: Flow cytometric analysis of DNA ploidy in childhood rhabdomyosarcoma. Yonsei Med J 1994; 35:34.

73. Beldjord C, Desclaux-Arramond F, Raffin-Sanson M, et al.: The RET protooncogene in sporadic pheochromocytomas: Frequent MEN 2-like mutations and new molecular defects. J Clin Endocrinol Metab 1995; 80:2063.

74. Hofstra RM, Landsvater RM, Ceccherini I, et al.: A mutation in the RET proto-oncogene associated with multiple endocrine neoplasia type 2B and sporadic medullary thyroid carcinoma Nature 1994; 367:375.

75. Yoshimoto K, Tanaka C, Hamaguchi S, et al.: Tumor-specific mutations in the tyrosine kinase domain of the RET protooncogene in pheochromocytomas of sporadic type. Endocr J 1995; 42:265.

76. Eng C, Foster KA, Healey CS, et al.: Mutation analysis of the c-mos proto-oncogene and the endothelin-B receptor gene in medullary thyroid carcinoma and phaeochromocytoma. Br J Cancer 1996; 74:339.

77. Aguiar RC, Dahia PL, Sill H, et al.: Deletion analysis of the p16 tumour suppressor gene in phaeochromocytomas. Clin Endocrinol (Oxf) 1996; 45:93.

78. Tsutsumi M, Yokota J, Kakizoe T, et al.: Loss of heterozygosity on chromosomes 1p and 11p in sporadic pheochromocytoma. J Natl Cancer Inst 1989; 81:367.

79. Khosla S, Patel VM, Hay ID, et al.: Loss of heterozygosity suggests multiple genetic alterations in pheochromocytomas and medullary thyroid carcinomas. J Clin Invest 1991; 87:1691.

80. Moley JF, Brother MB, Fong CT, et al.: Consistent association of 1p loss of heterozygosity with pheochromocytomas from patients with multiple endocrine neoplasia type 2 syndromes. Cancer Res 1992; 52:770.

81. Vargas MP, Zhuang Z, Wang C, et al.: Loss of heterozygosity on the short arm of chromosomes 1 and 3 in sporadic pheochromocytoma and extra-adrenal paraganglioma. Hum Pathol 1997; 28:411.

82. Tanaka N, Nishisho I, Yamamoto M, et al.: Loss of heterozygosity on the long arm of chromosome 22 in pheochromocytoma. Genes Chromosomes Cancer 1992; 5:399.

83. Dannenberg H, Speel E, Zhao J, et al.: Losses of chromosome 1p and 3q are early genetic events in the development of sporadic pheochromocytomas. Am J Pathol 2000; 157:353.

84. Altergott R, Barbato A, Lawrence A, et al.: Spectrum of catecholamine-secreting tumors of the organ of Zuckerkandl. Surgery 1985; 98:1121.

85. Hervonen A, Kanerva L, Korkala O, et al.: Effects of hypoxia and glucocorticoids on the histochemically demonstrable catecholamines of the newborn rat carotid body. Acta Physiol Scand 1972; 86:109.

86. Gibbs MK, Carney JA, Hayles AB, et al.: Simultaneous adrenal and cervical pheochromocytomas in childhood. Ann Surg 1977; 185:273.

87. Gallivan MV, Chun B, Rowden G, et al.: Intrathoracic paravertebral malignant paraganglioma. Arch Pathol Lab Med 1980; 104:46.

88. Karasov RS, Sheps SG, Carney JA, et al.: Paragangliomatosis with numerous catecholamine-producing tumors. Mayo Clin Proc 1982; 57:590.

89. Lack EE, Cubilla AL, Woodruff JM, et al.: Extra-adrenal paragangliomas of the retroperitoneum: A clinicopathologic study of 12 tumors. Am J Surg Pathol 1980; 4:109.

90. Leestma JE, Price EB Jr. Paraganglioma of the urinary bladder. Cancer 1971; 28:1063.

91. Manger WM, Gifford RW: Pheochromocytoma. Springer, New York, 1977.

92. Fries JG, Chamberlin JA: Extra-adrenal pheochromocytoma: Literature review and report of a cervical pheochromocytoma. Surgery 1968; 63:268.

93. Cone TE Jr: Recurrent pheochromocytoma: Report of a case in a previously treated child. Pediatrics 1958; 21:994.

94. Hirose T, Sano T, Mori K, et al.: Paraganglioma of the cauda equina: An ultrastructural and immunohistochemical study of two cases. Ultrastruct Pathol 1988; 12:235.

95. Sonneland PR, Scheithauer BW, LeChago J, et al.: Paraganglioma of the cauda equina region. Clinicopathologic study of 31 cases with special reference to immunocytology and ultrastructure. Cancer 1986; 58:1720.

96. Zak FG, Lawson W: The Paraganglionic Chemoreceptor System. Physiology, Pathology and Clinical Medicine. Springer, New York, 1983.

97. McCaffrey TV, Meyer FB, Michels VV, et al.: Familial paragangliomas of the head and neck. Arch Otolaryngol Head Neck Surg 1994; 120:1211.

98. Scalafani LM, Woodruff JM, Brennan MF: Extra-adrenal retroperitoneal paragangliomas: Natural history and response to treatment. Surgery 1990; 108:1124.

99. Parry DM, Li FP, Strong LC, et al.: Carotid body tumors in humans: Genetics and epidemiology. J Natl Cancer Inst 1982; 68:573.

100. Saldana MJ, Salem LE, Travezan R: High altitude hypoxia and chemodectomas. Hum Pathol 1973; 4:251.

101. Zollinger R, Hedinger C: Pheochromocytoma and sympathetic paragangliomas. Schweiz Med Wochenschr 1983; 113:1057.

102. Ali S, Aird DW, Bihari J: Pain-inducing laryngeal paragangliomas (non-chromaffin). J Laryngol Otol 1983; 97:181.

103. Gnepp DR, Ferlito A, Hyams V: Primary anaplastic small cell (oat cell) carcinoma of the larynx. Review of the literature and report of 18 cases. Cancer 1983; 51:1731.

104. Blessing MH, Hora B: Glomera in der Lunge des Menschen. Z Zellforsch 1968; 87:562.

105. Himelfarb MZ, Ostrzega NL, Samuel J, et al.: Paraganglioma of the nasal cavity. Laryngoscope 1983; 93:350.

106. Kameya T, Shimosato Y, Adachi I, et al.: Neuroendocrine carcinoma of the paranasal sinus: A morphological and endocrinological study. Cancer 1980; 45:330.

107. Johnson TL, Shapiro B, Beierwaltes WH, et al.: Cardiac paragangliomas. A clinicopathologic and immunohistochemical study of four cases. Am J Surg Pathol 1985; 9:827.

108. Singh G, Lee RE, Brooks DH: Primary pulmonary paraganglioma: Report of a case and review of the literature. Cancer 1977; 40:2286.

109. DeLellis RA, Tischler AS, Lee AK, et al.: Leu-enkephalin-like immunoreactivity in proliferative lesions of the human adrenal medulla and extra-adrenal paraganglia. Am J Surg Pathol 1983; 7:29.

110. Wang DG, Barros D'Sa AA, Johnston CF, et al.: Oncogene expression in carotid body tumors. Cancer 1996; 77:2581.

111. Heutink P, van Schothorst EM, van der Mey AG, et al.: Further localization of the gene for hereditary paragangliomas and evidence for linkage in unrelated families. Eur J Hum Genet 1994; 2:148.

112. Devilee P, van SE, Bardoel AF, et al.: Allelotype of head and neck paragangliomas: Allelic imbalance is confined to the long arm of chromosome 11, the site of the predisposing locus PGL. Genes Chromosomes Cancer 1994; 11:71.

113. Baysal BE, Ferrell RE, Willett-Brozick JE, et al.: Mutations in SDHD, a mitochondrial complex II gene, in hereditary paraganglioma. Science 2000; 287:848.

114. Ross JA, Severson RK, Pollock BH, et al.: Childhood cancer in the United States. A geographical analysis of cases from the Pediatric Cooperative Clinical Trials groups. Cancer 1996; 77:201.

115. Monforte-Munoz H, Kawakami T, Stram D, et al.: Neuroblastoma in children over 5 years of age: Recognition of a rare and aggressive subset with "unconventional" morphology. Mod Pathol 1997; 10:4P.

116. Enzinger FM, Weiss SW: Soft Tissue Tumors, 3rd ed. CV Mosby, St. Louis, MO, 1995.

117. Stowens D: Neuroblastoma and related tumors. Arch Pathol 1959; 63:451.

118. Stout AP: Ganglioneuroma of the sympathetic nervous system. Surg Gynecol Obstet 1947; 84:101.

119. Beckwith JB, Martin RF: Observations on the histopathology of neuroblastomas. J Pediatr Surg 1968; 3:106.

120. Makinen J: Microscopic patterns as a guide to prognosis of neuroblastoma in childhood. Cancer 1972; 29:1637.

121. Hughes M, Marsden HB, Palmer MK: Histologic patterns of neuroblastoma related to prognosis and clinical staging. Cancer 1974; 34:1706.

122. Shimada H, Aoyama C, Chiba T, et al.: Prognostic subgroups for undifferentiated neuroblastoma: Immunohistochemical study with anti-S-100 protein antibody. Hum Pathol 1985; 16:471.

123. Katsetos CD, Karkavelas G, Frankfurter A, et al.: The stromal Schwann cell during maturation of peripheral neuroblastomas. Immunohistochemical observations with antibodies to the neuronal class III beta-tubulin isotype (beta III) and S-100 protein. Clin Neuropathol 1994; 13:171.

124. Ambros IM, Zellner A, Roald B, et al.: Role of ploidy, chromosome 1p, and Schwann cells in the maturation of neuroblastoma. N Engl J Med 1996; 334:1505.

125. Molenaar WM, Baker DL, Pleasure D, et al.: The neuroendocrine and neural profiles of neuroblastomas, ganglioneuroblastomas, and ganglioneuromas. Am J Pathol 1990; 136:375.

126. Taxy JB: Electron microscopy in the diagnosis of neuroblastoma. Arch Pathol Lab Med 1980; 104:355.

127. Shimada H, Ambros IM, Dehner LP, et al.: Terminology and morphologic criteria of neuroblastic tumors: Recommendations by the International Neuroblastoma Pathology Committee. Cancer 1999; 86:349.

128. Weinblatt ME, Heisel MA, Siegel SE: Hypertension in children with neurogenic tumors. Pediatrics 1983; 71:947.

129. Mendelsohn G, Eggleston JC, Olson JL, et al.: Vasoactive intestinal peptide and its relationship to ganglion cell differentiation in neuroblastic tumors. Lab Invest 1979; 41:144.

130. Normann T, Havnen J, Mjolnerod O: Cushing's syndrome in an infant associated with neuroblastoma in two ectopic adrenal glands. J Pediatr Surg 1971; 6(2):169.

131. Hortnagl H, Winkler H, Asamer H, et al.: Storage of catecholamines in neuroblastoma and ganglioneuroma. A biochemical, immunologic, and morphologic study. Lab Invest 1972; 27:613.

132. Lopes-Ibor B, Schwartz AD: Neuroblastoma. Pediatr Clin North Am 1985; 32:755.

133. Qualman SJ, O'Dorisio MS, Fleshman DJ, et al.: Neuroblastoma. Correlation of neuropeptide expression in tumor tissue with other prognostic factors. Cancer 1992; 70:2005.

134. Evans AE, D'Angio GJ, Koop CE: Diagnosis and treatment of neuroblastoma. Pediatr Clin North Am 1976; 23:161.

135. Jaffe N: Neuroblastoma: Review of the literature and an examination of factors contributing to its enigmatic character. Cancer Treat Rev 1976; 3:61.

136. Shimada H, Chatten J, Newton WA Jr, et al.: Histopathologic prognostic factors in neuroblastic tumors: Definition of subtypes of ganglioneuroblastoma and an age-linked classification of neuroblastomas. J Natl Cancer Inst 1984; 73:405.

137. Joshi VV, Silverman JF: Pathology of neuroblastic tumors. Semin Diagn Pathol 1994; 11:107.

138. Shimada H, Ambros IM, Dehner LP, et al.: The International Neuroblastoma Pathology Classification (the Shimada system). Cancer 1999; 86:364.

139. Gitlow SE, Dziedzic LB, Strauss L, et al.: Biochemical and histologic determinants in the prognosis of neuroblastoma. Cancer 1973; 32:898.

140. Evans AE, D'Angio GJ, Propert K, et al.: Prognostic factor in neuroblastoma. Cancer 1987; 59:1853.

141. Brodeur GM, Pritchard J, Berthold F, et al.: Revisions of the international criteria for neuroblastoma diagnosis, staging, and response to treatment. J Clin Oncol 1993; 11:1466.

142. Brodeur GM: Molecular pathology of human neuroblastomas. Semin Diagn Pathol 1994; 11:118.

143. Norris MD, Bordow SB, Marshall GM, et al.: Expression of the gene for multidrug-resistance-associated protein and outcome in patients with neuroblastoma. N Engl J Med 1996; 334:231.

144. Woods WG, Lemieux B, Tuchman M: Neuroblastoma represents distinct clinical-biologic entities: A review and perspective from the Quebec Neuroblastoma Screening Project. Pediatrics 1992; 89:114.

145. Kaneko Y, Kanda N, Maseki N, et al.: Different karyotypic patterns in early and advanced stage neuroblastomas. Cancer Res 1987; 47:311.

146. Caron H, van Sluis P, de Kraker J, Bokkerink J, et al.: Allelic loss of chromosome 1p as a predictor of unfavorable outcome in patients with neuroblastoma. N Engl J Med 1996; 334:225.

147. Nakagawara A, Arima N-M, Scavarda NJ, et al.: Association between high levels of expression of the TRK gene and favorable outcome in human neuroblastoma. N Engl J Med 1993; 328:847.

148. Oppenheim R: Naturally occurring cell death during neural development. Trends Neurosci 1985; 487.

149. Levi-Montalcini R, Angeletti P: Nerve growth factor. Physiol Rev 1968; 48:534.

150. Beckwith J, Perrin R: In-situ neuroblastoma: Its contribution to the natural history of neural crest tumors. Am J Pathol 1963; 43:1089.

151. Bessho F, Hashizume K, Nakajo T, et al.: Mass screening in Japan increased the detection of infants with neuroblastoma without a decrease in cases in older children. J Pediatr 1991; 119:237.

152. Haas D, Ablin AR, Miller C, et al.: Complete pathologic maturation and regression of stage IVS neuroblastoma without treatment. Cancer 1988; 62:818.

153. Ambros PF, Ambros IM, Strehl S, et al.: Regression and progression in neuroblastoma. Does genetics predict tumour behaviour? Eur J Cancer 1995; 31A:510.

154. Cushing H, Wolbach S: Transformation of malignant paravertebral sympathicoblastoma into benign ganglioneuroma. Am J Pathol 1927; 3:203.

155. Matthay KK, Sather HN, Seeger RC, et al.: Excellent outcome of stage II neuroblastoma is independent of residual disease and radiation therapy. J Clin Oncol 1989; 7:236.

156. McLaughlin JE, Urich H: Maturing neuroblastoma and ganglioneuroblastoma: A study of four cases with long survival. J Pathol 1977; 121:19.

157. Robertson CM, Tyrrell JC, Pritchard J: Familial neural crest tumours. Eur J Pediatr 1991; 150:789.

158. Bower RJ, Adkins JC: Ondine's curse and neurocristopathy. Clin Pediatr (Phila) 1980; 19:665.

CHAPTER

7

The Adrenal Cortex

Anne Marie McNicol

Although Eustachius first illustrated the adrenal glands in 1563, their physiologic importance was not appreciated until 1855, when Addison described the effects of their destruction.[1] The outer cortex and central medulla have functional interactions, but these are as yet poorly understood and the pathologic features of each are therefore considered separately. Diseases of the adrenal cortex are rare but important because they cause significant morbidity because of the crucial roles of glucocorticoids, mineralocorticoids, and androgens in homeostasis. It is important for the pathologist to have some understanding of normal structure and function for the proper interpretation of pathologic states.

NORMAL ADRENAL CORTEX

Development

The adrenal cortex develops from mesoderm adjacent to the dorsal celomic epithelium beside the urogenital ridge.[2] The detailed control of its development is beyond the scope of this chapter, but transcription factors such as steroidogenic factor-1 (SF-1/Ad4BP)[3] and a nuclear hormone receptor *DAX-1*[4] appear to have important roles. The cortex first appears at the 7- to 8-mm stage and is recognizable as a mass of immature cells by 10–15 mm. At 20–25 mm, early evidence of definitive and fetal zones is seen, and by 50 mm, these are obvious. The inner fetal (or provisional) zone accounts for about 80% of the fetal cortex, with the narrower definitive (or adult) zone lying under the capsule. The zones seem to develop independently, as both show significant levels of proliferation.[5] The fetal zone is composed of large eosinophilic granular cells, whereas the cells of the definitive zone are smaller, with a higher nuclear-to-cytoplasmic ratio (Fig. 7–1). After birth the fetal zone regresses, possibly by apoptosis,[5] and the definitive zone grows and migrates inward to form the adult cortex. In stillbirths, microcystic structures may be seen in the definitive zone, but whether this is a normal variant or a response to stress[6] is unclear. Vacuolar change in the outer cortex in erythroblastosis fetalis[7] may also be related to hypoxia and stress.

At birth, the combined gland weight is between 6 g[8] and 10 g.[9] Regression of the fetal zone causes a fall to 4 g or 5 g by 2 weeks,[8] and little further change occurs over the first 2 years, after which the glands grow to reach adult weight by 15–20 years. Some claim that adult zonation develops by 2 years of age; others report that it is not seen until 8–9 years and is not complete until about 18 years.[10]

Gross Anatomy

The glands sit in the retroperitoneal tissues at the upper poles of the kidneys. The right is pyramidal in shape, lying behind the right lobe of the liver and inferior vena cava and in front of the diaphragm and right kidney. The left is crescentic and lies behind the omentum and stomach. Its lower pole may be separated from these organs by the pancreas and splenic artery. There is a groove on the anterior surface of each, where the adrenal vein emerges. The normal adult gland weighs about 4 g at surgery[11] or in cases of sudden death[12] but can range 2–6 g. The cortex comprises about 90% of the total weight.[12] The average weight of 6 g in hospital autopsy studies is thought to be the result of stimulation by adrenocorticotropic hormone (ACTH) in the stress of terminal illness.[11] The glands are divided into head, body, and tail from inferomedial to superolateral aspects, with alae lying laterally. The medulla is present only in the head and body and focally in the alae, the corticomedullary ratio ranging from 5:1 in the head to 15:1 in the body.[13, 14] The boundary between cortex and medulla is irregular, with considerable admixture in some areas. There is also a cuff of cortical tissue that invaginates into the medulla around the central vein.

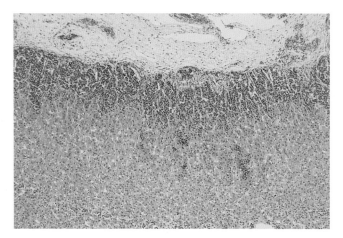

Figure 7-1. This is a section through the human fetal adrenal showing the inner fetal zone comprising large eosinophilic cells and the outher definitive zone made up of smaller cells lying below the capsule.

Microscopic Anatomy

The adult cortex is divided into three zones, each with characteristic histologic features (Fig. 7–2). The zona glomerulosa consists of discontinuous subcapsular aggregates of small angular cells with a high nuclear-to-cytoplasmic ratio and little lipid storage. The major part is the zona fasciculata, with large, clear, lipid-laden cells arranged in columns extending from the glomerulosa or capsule to the inner zona reticularis. The cells of the zona reticularis are eosinophilic, with little lipid storage (compact cells), and many contain lipofuscin. These are arranged in cords around a network of vascular sinusoids.

Immunohistochemistry

Immunopositivity for low-molecular-weight cytokeratins in the normal cortex is consistent with glandular differentiation, and occasional cells also express vimentin.[15, 16] Zonal differences in the expression of steroidogenic enzymes help explain the functional zonation.[17-21] Surprisingly, immunopositivity has been detected for neuroendocrine markers, including neuron-specific enolase, synaptophysin, and CD56 (neural cell adhesion molecule).[22, 23] Class II major histocompatibility antigens are expressed, mainly in the zona reticularis.[24-26] The transmembrane efflux pump, P-glycoprotein, has a potential role in steroid transport.[27, 28] The function of inhibin-α, expressed primarily in the zona reticularis,[29-31] is unknown. Parathyroid hormone–related peptide[32] may influence steroidogenesis by altering transmembrane calcium fluxes.[33] Immunoreactivity with antibody melan-A (clone A103), which recognizes a melanoma-associated protein, most probably reflects a cross-reaction.[34] Blood vessels may be outlined by staining of endothelium for CD34[33, 35] or by binding to the lectin *Ulex europaeus*.[36] PGP9.5 identifies

nerves.[37] Type IV collagen shows the distribution of basement membrane.[38]

Ultrastructure

The ultrastructural features have been documented in detail,[39, 40] but this technique is not commonly used in diagnostic practice. In the zona glomerulosa, smooth endoplasmic reticulum is scant, as are lysosomes and lipid. Mitochondria are plentiful and are elongated with small lamellar cristae, and the Golgi apparatus is more prominent than in the other zones. In the zona fasciculata,

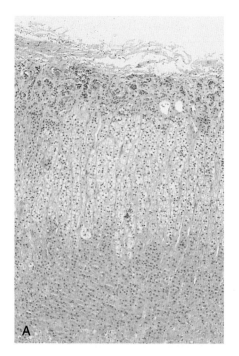

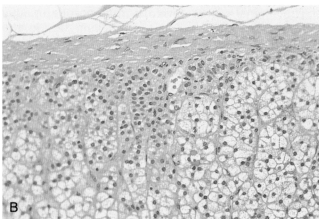

Figure 7-2. The adult cortex comprises the outer zona glomerulosa (ZG); the zona fasciculata (ZF), consisting of cords of lipid-laden cells; and the inner zona reticularis (ZR), made up of eosinophilic compact cells, some of which may contain lipofuscin. The ZF and ZR can be identified in *A,* and *B* shows the focal subcapsular distribution of the ZG.

mitochondria are ovoid or spherical with tubular and vesicular cristae, and smooth endoplasmic reticulum is often prominent. Lipid droplets are plentiful. In the zona reticularis, the cells contain large numbers of tubulovesicular mitochondria, lysosomes and lipofuscin are common, and rough endoplasmic reticulum is prominent. Cells with mixed features are found at the zonal junctions.[39-41]

Vasculature

The adrenal glands are highly vascular, supplied by 50–60 small arteries derived from the inferior phrenic artery, aorta, and renal artery that pierce the capsule and form an extensive subcapsular plexus. This gives rise to a complex intra-adrenal system comprising spiral arterioles opening into a capillary plexus in the zona glomerulosa; sinusoids traversing the zona fasciculata and forming a network in the zona reticularis; and arteriovenous loops that dip into the cortex, then turn back and drain into veins near their site of origin. Medullary sinusoids drain into venous channels that leave the gland through a single central vein emerging from the hilum. These veins have a pronounced longitudinal muscle coat, arranged concentrically in the extraglandular and immediate intraglandular portions of the vein but in an eccentric fashion within the gland[13] (Fig. 7–3). These complex arrangements may regulate function by altering blood flow. The veins are more constant than the arteries and are more useful in identifying atrophic glands, which may be difficult to find at autopsy. The right adrenal vein is less than 5 mm long and joins the vena cava between the renal vein and the inferior right hepatic vein. The left adrenal vein is longer and joins the left renal vein about 30 mm from its junction with the inferior vena cava. It may join the left inferior phrenic vein before entering the renal vein. Lymphatic vessels are readily visible only as a subcapsular plexus.[42] They emerge to form larger channels, which drain into para-aortic and celiac lymph nodes.

Innervation

Sympathetic preganglionic cholinergic neurons[43] reach the gland through the splanchnic nerves. Postganglionic fibers arise within sympathetic nerves, in the celiac or superior mesenteric plexuses, or within the gland itself. Most fibers traverse the cortex to synapse on chromaffin cells, directly regulating catecholamine release.[44] However, a cortical plexus also exists[37, 45] that includes catecholaminergic,[46] acetylcholinesterase-positive,[46] and peptidergic fibers.[47] These are now thought to regulate not only blood flow[48] but also cortical function and growth.[49, 50]

Regulation of Adrenal Growth

There are two theories, based mostly on animal studies, as to how adrenal cell mass is maintained. The migration theory proposes that proliferation occurs at the junction of the zona glomerulosa and zona fasciculata, with cells differentiating into the zona glomerulosa, then migrating in a centripetal manner into the zona fasciculata and zona reticularis before programmed cell death.[51, 52] The zonal theory suggests that each zone proliferates to maintain itself.[51, 53-55] Apoptosis appears to take place in the zona reticularis.[56] It is probable that both mechanisms are involved, with the balance changing in different situations.

The factors regulating growth are not fully understood. Hypophysectomy and exogenous glucocorticoids result in atrophy, implicating pituitary factors, most likely derived from cells that produce ACTH. ACTH induces hypertrophy of fasciculata and reticularis cells in vivo,[57, 58] followed by increased mitotic activity.[59, 60] However, ACTH is not directly mitogenic in vitro,[61] so this may reflect interaction with growth factors or facilitation of their access by alterations in blood flow.[62] Peptides from the N-terminal region of the ACTH precursor, proopiomelanocortin, may stimulate hypertrophy and hyperplasia.[60] Other factors implicated are vasopressin[63] and angiotensin II[64, 65] (particularly with respect to the glomerulosa), basic fibroblast growth factor,[66, 67] and cytokines including interleukin-1.[68] The roles of insulin-like growth factors I and II (IGFI and IGFII)[69, 70] and epidermal growth factor[71-73] may differ in adult and fetal glands. Transforming growth factor-β (TGF-β)[74] and activin[75] may have an inhibitory role in the fetal gland.

Steroidogenesis and Steroid Metabolism

The adrenal cortex synthesizes three main groups of steroids: glucocorticoids, mineralocorticoids, and androgens. All are derived from cholesterol

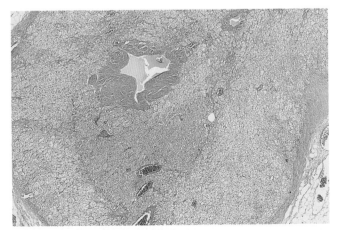

Figure 7–3. The asymmetric muscle bundles that characterize the intraglandular portion of the central vein are clearly shown. The physiologic relevance is unclear, but there may be a role in regulating blood flow.

Cholesterol

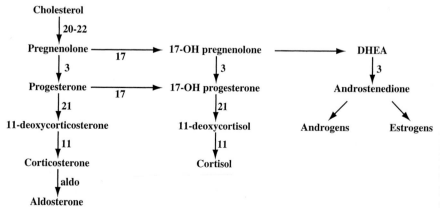

Figure 7-4. All steroids are derived from cholesterol, based on the cyclopentanophenanthrene ring. The carbon atoms have a specific numbering sequence. Different steroids are characterized by the substitution of various chemical groups at specific carbon atoms. These are designated α if lying above the ring and β if below. Double bonds are identified by Δ. Examples are shown in Table 7-1.

Table 7-1. Steroid Nomenclature

Systematic Name	Trivial Name
4-Pregn-11β,21-diol-3,18,20-trione	Aldosterone
4-Androsten-3,17-dione	Androstenedione
4-Pregnen-11β,7α,21-triol-3,20-dione	Cortisol
5-Androsten-3β-ol-17-one	Dehydroepiandrosterone
4-Pregnen-21-ol-3,20-dione	Deoxycorticosterone
5-Pregnen-3β-ol-20-one	Pregnenolone
4-Pregn-3,20-dione	Progesterone
1,3,5(10)-Estratrien-3,17β-diol	Estradiol
4-Androsten-17β-ol-3-one	Testosterone

(Fig. 7-4). About 80% of adrenal cholesterol comes from plasma low-density lipoproteins (LDL)[76] internalized by specific LDL receptors[77] and stored as cholesterol esters. Free cholesterol is generated by the action of cholesterol ester hydrolase. The remainder is synthesized de novo from acetyl coenzyme A.[76] Cholesterol is transported to the inner mitochondrial membrane by the steroid acute response (StAR) protein.[78] The biosynthetic pathways are shown in Figure 7-5 and are discussed elsewhere.[79, 80] They involve the catalytic action of four of the family of cytochrome P-450 enzymes, mainly with hydroxylase activities, and of a 3β-hydroxysteroid dehydrogenase. Steroids are known by trivial and by systematic names. The latter are based on their specific structure, indicating the type of substitution, the carbon atom on which it has taken place, and whether it projects above (α) or below

(β) the nucleus. The symbol Δ indicates a double bond. Examples of these two systems are shown in Table 7-1.

The pattern of steroid production differs among the zones because of differential expression of specific enzymes and response to a variety of regulatory factors. The zona glomerulosa is the source of aldosterone, the main mineralocorticoid, and the absence of immunoreactivity for P-450$_{17\alpha}$ in this zone[21] is in keeping with its inability to divert precursors into the cortisol and sex steroid pathways. The preferential expression of aldosterone synthase (CYPBII)[81] permits the production of aldosterone. Both zona fasciculata and zona reticularis express the complement of enzymes necessary for the synthesis of glucocorticoids and androgens.[17-21, 82] However, biochemical[83] and immunohistochemical[84] evidence suggests that major androgen production is confined to the zona reticularis because most secreted androgen is dehydroepiandrosterone (DHEA) sulfate, and sulfotransferase is present only in that zone.

Cortisol production is mainly controlled by the hypothalamic-pituitary-adrenal (HPA) axis (Fig. 7-6). ACTH from the anterior pituitary binds to a specific membrane receptor[85] and activates the cyclic adenosine monophosphate pathway,[86] which regulates the expression of all the steroid hydroxylase genes.[87]

Adrenal Steroidogenesis

Cholesterol
↓ 20-22
Pregnenolone ——17——→ 17-OH pregnenolone ——————→ DHEA
↓ 3 ↓ 3 ↓ 3
Progesterone ——17——→ 17-OH progesterone   Androstenedione
↓ 21 ↓ 21   ↙   ↘
11-deoxycorticosterone   11-deoxycortisol   Androgens   Estrogens
↓ 11 ↓ 11
Corticosterone   Cortisol
↓ aldo
Aldosterone

Figure 7-5. Pathways of adrenal steroidogenesis. The main steroids produced in the human gland are mineralocorticoids (aldosterone), glucocorticoids (cortisol), and sex steroids. Each is produced via a defined pathway within the gland, involving the action of specific enzymes. The enzymes involved are **20-22**, 20-22 desmolase; **3**, 3β-hydroxysteroid dehydrogenase; **21**, 21-hydroxylase, P-450$_{c21}$; **11**, 11β-hydroxylase, P-450$_{11\beta}$; **aldo**, aldosterone synthase, P-450$_{aldo}$; **17**, 17α-hydroxylase, P-450$_{17\alpha}$. **DHEA** is dehydroepiandrosterone.

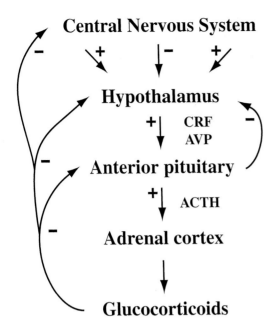

Figure 7–6. Synthesis of glucocorticoids is under the control of the hypothalamic-pituitary-adrenal (HPA) axis. The hypothalamus receives both stimulatory and inhibitory inputs from the central nervous system. It releases corticotropin-releasing hormone (CRH) and arginine vasopressin (AVP) that act together to stimulate the secretion of adrenocorticotropic hormone (ACTH) from the anterior pituitary. This stimulates the adrenal cortex to produce cortisol. There is negative feedback at a number of levels by both cortisol and ACTH.

Other factors, including calcium, chloride ions, and arachidonic acid metabolites, may also be involved.[86] ACTH secretion is controlled by corticotropin-releasing factor and vasopressin from the hypothalamus, and glucocorticoids exert negative feedback at pituitary, hypothalamic, and central loci.[88] ACTH and cortisol show a circadian rhythm of secretion, with a peak in early morning and a low in the evening.[79] The renin-angiotensin system is the major element in the production of aldosterone. Angiotensinogen, produced in the liver, is cleaved to angiotensin I (AI) by renin, secreted by the kidney, and then to AII by angiotensin-converting enzyme. Further cleavage occurs to AIII. AII and AIII bind to specific membrane receptors, effecting their actions via G proteins and the phosphoinositide-Ca^{2+} signaling pathway.[89] ACTH also controls androgen secretion, but there is probably also a specific androgen-stimulating factor, yet to be identified, because adrenal androgen levels may rise (e.g., at adrenarche) without a change in ACTH secretion.[90]

A number of other factors also play roles in steroidogenesis. IGFI and IGFII have been shown to stimulate both cortisol and DHEA secretion.[91] Vasopressin may also play a stimulatory role,[92] whereas TGF-β may be inhibitory.[93, 94] Catecholamines, probably derived from both nerves and medullary cells,[95, 96] may also exert effects.

The majority of steroids in plasma are bound to proteins. These are either high-affinity, low-capacity specific binding proteins, such as corticosteroid-binding protein, which bind cortisol and aldosterone, or proteins such as albumin, which bind at a higher capacity but with low affinity.[97] Inactivation occurs mainly in the liver, and the products are excreted in the urine, largely as glucuronides. Not all conversion results in inactivation, some active steroids being generated. Steroid metabolism also takes place in kidney, muscle, and connective tissue, and this peripheral metabolism may play an important role in regulating specific tissue responses.[98]

Steroid Action

Steroids interact with intracellular receptor proteins belonging to the superfamily that includes thyroid hormone, vitamin D, and retinoic acid receptors.[99] Binding of the appropriate ligand activates the receptor and permits binding to DNA, thus regulating the transcription of a variety of genes.[100] Glucocorticoid receptors are present in most cells, permitting them to exert wide-ranging effects. They promote gluconeogenesis and oppose the action of insulin. Protein synthesis is inhibited, and catabolism is stimulated, with the release of glucogenic amino acids. Lipolysis is increased. Glucocorticoids are immunosuppressive, reducing the number of circulating lymphocytes, both by redistribution within tissues and inhibition of proliferative and activation-related responses. Their anti-inflammatory properties are linked to inhibition of the phagocytic and bactericidal properties of macro-phages and neutrophil polymorphs. Healing is slowed because of suppression of fibroblast function. Effects on bone formation and calcium metabolism favor the development of osteopenia, and growth may be affected. Significant central effects can induce behavioral changes. Aldosterone plays a major role in regulating plasma volume and potassium balance by increasing renal tubular secretion of potassium and reabsorption of sodium and chloride. Adrenal androgens have weak androgenic effects but are converted peripherally to testosterone. Most estrogenic effects are the result of peripheral conversion of androstenedione.

DEVELOPMENTAL AND CONGENITAL ABNORMALITIES

Cortical Tissue in Extra-adrenal Locations

Small capsular extrusions are extremely common (Fig. 7–7), and are probably best regarded as a variant of normal. They consist only of cortex, often with cells of all three types arranged in a centripetal manner. They may appear to be continuous with, or apparently separate from, the cortex. Accessory

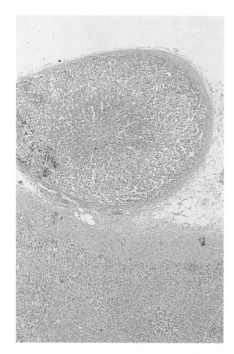

Figure 7–7. Small extracapsular extrusions are common. These should be interpreted as a variant of normal.

adrenal tissue is found within the upper abdomen and in the pathways of gonadal descent. Some rests consist of cortex and medulla, others of cortical tissue alone. The most common site is around the celiac axis.[101] They may also be found in the kidney, liver, broad ligament, ovary,[102] spermatic cord, testis,[103, 104] and hernial sacs.[105] There have been rare reports at places more difficult to explain embryologically: placenta,[106] gallbladder,[107] lung,[108, 109] and intracranial sites.[110] The whole adrenal gland may occasionally fuse with the liver[111] or the kidney,[112, 113] both organs sharing a common capsule, referred to as adrenal-hepatic or adrenal-renal heterotopia. Rare midline fusion of both glands is always associated with multiple congenital abnormalities.[114] Malposition is unusual, even in the presence of renal agenesis. Absence, even unilateral, is rare.

Congenital Adrenal Cytomegaly

Cytomegaly of the fetal cortex is found incidentally in 3%–6.5% of stillbirths or neonatal deaths.[115, 116] The cells may reach 150 μm in diameter, usually lie in nodules or wedges surrounded by normal cells, and can show DNA polyploidy.[117] The significance is unclear.

Adrenal cytomegaly is also found in a high proportion of infants with the rare Beckwith-Wiedemann syndrome, characterized by exomphalos, macroglossia, and gigantism. It is usually sporadic but may occur as an autosomal-dominant trait with incomplete penetrance.[118] The adrenal glands are usually enlarged, with severe cytomegaly, and macrocysts may

develop,[119, 120] although children who survive may show involution with a reduction in cytomegaly. Adrenocortical carcinoma is more common than in the normal population.[121]

Wolman's disease,[122] which results from deficiency of a lysosomal lipase activity, affects a variety of organs and is usually fatal in the first 6 months. Cholesterol esters and triglycerides accumulate, causing cellular damage and calcification, particularly in the inner zones. Adrenal enlargement has also been noted in Niemann-Pick disease.[123, 124]

Congenital Adrenal Hypoplasia

This rare condition causes weight loss, dehydration, vomiting, and salt loss; it can be fatal if unrecognized. The adrenals are small and difficult to find at autopsy. The condition may be a primary abnormality in adrenocortical development or secondary to other abnormalities of the HPA. Primary disease shows an X-linked pattern of inheritance and is the result of mutations or deletion in the *DAX-1* gene on Xp21,[4, 125] important in the development of steroidogenic tissues. Hypogonadotropic hypogonadism often coexists.[4, 125, 126] Patients with deletions may have familial associations with glycerol kinase deficiency[127, 128] and Duchenne's muscular dystrophy,[129] the genes for which are contiguous at this locus.

Anencephaly is the most common cause of congenital adrenal hypoplasia because of the lack of ACTH. The anterior pituitary is usually present but is small. The adrenal glands are normal up to the 20th week of pregnancy, but they become hypoplastic, typically weighing about 0.5–1 g at birth.[130] The fetal zone fails to develop normally and makes up only 20% of the gland, compared with 80% in normal infants.[131] Cytomegaly is occasionally seen.[132] Isolated deficiency of ACTH has also been reported,[133] and congenital adrenal insufficiency may occur in association with other defects of the brain.[134] These result in similar changes in the adrenal glands.

Familial Glucocorticoid or Aldosterone Insufficiency

Familial glucorticoid deficiency is a rare condition that affects both sexes and is characterized by very low cortisol levels, relatively normal levels of mineralocorticoids, and very high levels of ACTH.[135, 136] Patients develop hypoglycemia, muscle weakness, and hyperpigmentation, usually before the age of 2 years. Where this occurs in isolation, mutations have been identified in the ACTH receptor.[137, 138] There is also a variant associated with alacrima and achalasia,[135, 138, 139] but its basis is not known. The adrenal glands are small, with a normal zona glomerulosa, but there is significant atrophy of the zona fasciculata and zona reticularis.[140] The pathologic features of isolated aldosterone deficiency[141, 142] have not been documented.

Adrenoleukodystrophy (Addison-Schilder Disease)

Adrenoleukodystrophy is an X-linked peroxisomal disorder in which there is accumulation of saturated very-long-chain fatty acids (VLCFA) in the white matter of the brain and in the adrenal cortex as a result of a reduced capacity for beta oxidation.[143] Progressive demyelination and adrenal insufficiency develop, the extent of involvement of each tissue defining a number of phenotypes. The gene involved on Xq28 encodes a peroxisomal membrane protein of unknown function with homology to the adenosine triphosphate–binding cassette (ABC) transmembrane transporter superfamily.[144] More than 100 different mutations have been identified. About 50% are missense, but deletions and insertions are also found,[145, 146] with no correlation between genotype and phenotype.

Because the adrenals undergo gradual atrophy with progression of the disease, they vary in size at autopsy. The zona glomerulosa is often normal, but the zona fasciculata contains nests of degenerate ballooned cells. Even on light microscopy, striations are visible in the cytoplasm of some cells, and the rest have a granular appearance. Ultrastructural examination reveals a characteristic proliferation of smooth endoplasmic reticulum and accumulation of lamellae of lipid and crystalloid clefts, thought to be the deposits of VLCFAs. Similar appearances may be seen in Leydig cells, microglia, and Schwann cells. As the disease progresses, the nests of degenerate cells enlarge to affect the entire adrenal cortex. In the later stages, the adrenals can resemble those in autoimmune Addison's disease as the characteristic cells may degenerate and disappear. The principal distinguishing feature in such cases is the absence of lymphocytic infiltrate. Recent evidence suggests that this may be the cause of a significant proportion of clinical Addison's disease in young men, where adrenal antibodies are not detected.[147]

Neonatal adrenoleukodystrophy is part of a continuum with infantile Refsum's disease and Zellweger's (cerebro-hepato-renal) syndrome, in which mutations in genes encoding peroxins result in abnormal assembly of peroxisomes. Striated cells containing lamellar-lipid profiles have been described in the inner zona fasciculata and zona reticularis in seven of the eight reported cases.[148]

Congenital Adrenal Hyperplasia

Congenital adrenal hyperplasia (CAH) is a group of diseases inherited in an autosomal-recessive fashion, involving impairment of enzymatic function in the steroidogenic pathways. Low levels of cortisol reduce steroid negative feedback to the pituitary and hypothalamus and result in excessive secretion of ACTH. The increased stimulation of the adrenals causes the glands to become hyperplastic. With each enzyme, there is a characteristic pattern of steroid secretion and clinical findings,[149] which can be useful in pinpointing the defective gene.

21-Hydroxylase deficiency is the commonest form, accounting for more than 90% of cases. Precursor steroids are diverted into pathways of androgen synthesis. In the classic form, which presents at birth, there are varying degrees of masculinization of the external genitalia in female infants. The internal genitalia are normal because the development of a male phenotype is dependent not only on testosterone but also on an inhibitory anti-müllerian hormone secreted by the Sertoli cells of the testis. In boys there is no genital ambiguity, but they may later develop precocious puberty. Both sexes show rapid growth and early closure of epiphyses. In 65%–75% of cases there is also a defect in aldosterone synthesis, resulting in hyponatremia and hyperkalemia (salt wasting), with hypovolemia and shock. The nonclassic form is linked to less severe impairment of enzyme activity and may be asymptomatic or cause milder symptoms of androgen excess.

The gene encoding P-450$_{c21}$ *(CYP21)* is located on the short arm of chromosome 6 in the human major histocompatibility complex (MHC).[150] It lies close to a pseudogene with 98% homology *(CYP21P)*.[151] The mutations in CAH are the result of recombinations between the two, resulting in deletions or transfer of sequences from the pseudogene. However, genotype may not always be linked to phenotype.[152] The global incidence of the classic disease is 1 in 15,000 live births, but in some groups the incidence is much higher, e.g., 1 in 27 in Ashkenazic Jews and 1 in 40 in Hispanics.[149] The nonclassic form is the most common autosomal-recessive condition known, occuring in around 1 in 100 of the general population.[153]

Impairment of activity of *11β-hydroxylase deficiency* is the second most common form of CAH, comprising 5%–8% of all cases. In the classic form, androgens are increased, and there is accumulation of deoxycorticosterone (DOC). The signs of hyperandrogenism are therefore accompanied by hypertension. Numerous mutations have been identified in the gene encoding the 11β-hydroxylase enzyme (CYP11B1),[149] including frameshift, missense, and premature terminations. A mild late-onset form has also been identified.[154]

Deficiency of *17α-hydroxylase* is an unusual cause of CAH, responsible for about 1% of cases. The gene involved *(CYP17)* lies on chromosome 10, and a variety of mutations have been identified.[155] In the adrenal the synthesis of both cortisol and androgen is impaired, and gonadal steroidogenesis is also affected. The external genitalia are female in both sexes. Genetic females have normal internal genitalia. In genetic males the testes may be found at any point in the path of descent. Raised levels of DOC cause hypertension. Corticosterone excess achieves reasonable levels of glucocorticoid action.

The rare *3β-hydroxysteroid dehydrogenase (3βHSD) deficiency* also affects both adrenal and gonadal steroidogenesis. Mutations have been identified in the type II 3βHSD gene, which is predominantly expressed in adrenal glands and gonads.[156, 157] Males are incompletely masculinized owing to lack of testicular androgens. Females show some virilization, usually only clitoral enlargement, because of the high levels of DHEA. Some patients show salt wasting. Again, nonclassic disease has been reported with mild virilization in females. Glomerulosal function may be normal in some cases.[158]

Adrenal Pathology in CAH

Descriptions have been based mainly on autopsy studies, principally in cases of 21-hydroxylase deficiency. In untreated patients, the glands are grossly enlarged, the average weight of a single gland being 15 g in children (normal 1.5–3 g) and up to 30–35 g in adults.[159] They have a characteristic cerebriform appearance (Fig. 7–8), and in most cases the cut surface of the cortex is red-brown. Compact cells extend almost to the glomerulosa, with only a small number of peripheral lipid-laden cells; the appearances resemble those seen in ectopic ACTH syndrome. The zona glomerulosa is hyperplastic only if aldosterone synthesis is also impaired. Any accessory adrenal tissue is also hyperplastic. Adrenal nodules are said to be more common in both homozygous and heterozygous patients.[160] Adenoma[161] and carcinoma[162] have been reported, suggesting that continued hyperstimulation may play some role in neoplastic transformation. Myelolipomas are also described.[163, 164]

Males with CAH can develop testicular swelling if steroid replacement is inadequate. This is best demonstrated by ultrasonography because it picks up even small lesions.[165, 166] The lesions are usually bilateral, and many are palpable, measuring more than than 20 mm in diameter.[167] They are multilobated, with a brown cut surface. The histologic appearance resembles that of Leydig cells arranged in sheets or alveolar structures, but Reinke's crystalloids are absent. Whether this is a neoplastic or hyperplastic process is unclear. Most lesions regress to some extent with adequate steroid replacement, suggesting dependency on ACTH.[168] Their origin is also a matter of debate, with adrenal rests, Leydig cells, or testicular stroma proposed.

Congenital lipoid hyperplasia is a rare cause of CAH that was thought to be due to side-chain cleavage (cholesterol desmolase) deficiency. It has now been shown that it is the result of mutations in the gene encoding StAR protein,[169] which transports cholesterol to the mitochondrion. Because this is a critical early step in steroidogenesis, production of all adrenal and gonadal steroids is affected. Many cases are fatal. Males who survive are incompletely masculinized. The extremely high levels of ACTH and related peptides may result in pigmentation. The defect adequately explains the histologic appearance of this disease, in which there is significant accumulation of lipid in the cortex.

ADRENAL CORTICAL HYPERFUNCTION

The Adrenal Response to Stress

Chronic stress causes an increase in secretion of ACTH and thus stimulation of the adrenal cortex, with a shift in steroidogenesis to favor glucocorticoid production.[148] Adrenal weight increases with enlargement of the zona fasciculata and zona reticularis. Hypertrophy, hyperplasia, and a reduction in apoptosis probably all contribute.[55, 170] Lipid depletion of the zona fasciculata (Fig. 7–9) develops in a centripetal manner, the cells coming to resemble the compact cells of the zona reticularis. This change tends to be focal in the adult but is more diffuse in children. Degenerative changes may occur in the outer zona

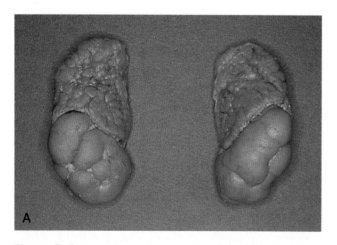
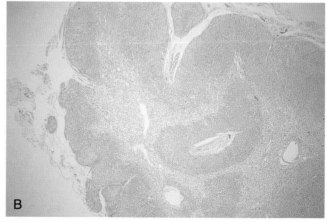

Figure 7–8. In congenital adrenal hyperplasia, there is massive enlargement of the glands, giving rise to the characteristic cerebriform appearance of the hyperplastic cortex *(A)*. This is reflected in the histologic appearance *(B)*, accompanied by a significant centripetal extension of compact cells. (Courtesy of Professor P.J. Berry, Bristol, UK.)

Figure 7–9. Lipid depletion of the cortex. This gland shows loss of lipid stores from the zona fasciculata, with compact cells extending almost to the capsule. This occurs when the adrenal gland is subject to increased stimulation by ACTH in situations of stress.

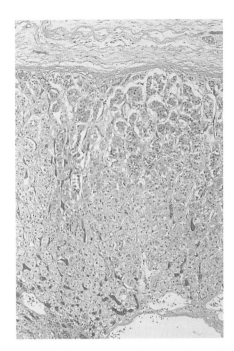

Figure 7–10. Lipid reversion of the cortex. In patients who survive severe stress, lipid reaccumulates first in the inner layers of the cortex, the outer zona fasciculata. The zone of lipid depletion in the outer zona fasciculata should not be misinterpreted as a hyperplastic zona glomerulosa.

fasciculata with the solid cords converted into tubular structures.[171] Lipid reversion[172] is characterized by the presence of lipid in the outer zona fasciculata and its abundance in its inner part (Fig. 7–10), and it is thought to reflect reaccumulation of lipid following stress; but why it happens in a centripetal manner is unclear. Care should be taken not to misinterpret the compact cells of the outer zone as a hyperplastic zona glomerulosa.

Chronic Hypersecretion of Steroids

Three clinical syndromes are associated with hypersecretion of adrenal steroids; Cushing's syndrome (hypercortisolism), Conn's syndrome (primary hyperaldosteronism), and adrenogenital syndrome (excess androgens or estrogens).

Cushing's Syndrome (Glucocorticoid Excess)

The clinical features of Cushing's syndrome are well known (Fig. 7–11). There is centripetal obesity, moon face and plethora, a buffalo hump, bruising, abdominal striae, and proximal muscle wasting. Wound healing is delayed. Osteoporosis leads to back pain and vertebral compression fracture.

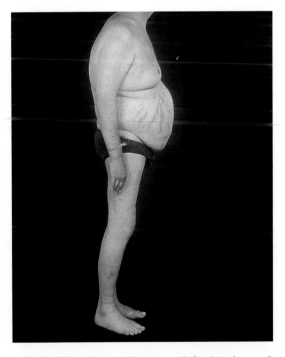

Figure 7–11. The clinical features of Cushing's syndrome are well recognized. Note the centripetal distribution of fat, the relative wasting of limbs, and the abdominal striae. (Courtesy of Professor J.M.C. Connell, Glasgow, UK.)

Increased secretion of cortisol precursors with mineralocorticoid effects (e.g., DOC) frequently causes hypertension. The anti-insulin effects of glucocorticoids lead to hyperglycemia and glycosuria with frank diabetes mellitus in 10%–15% of cases. Increased susceptibility to infection reflects interactions with the immune system. Psychiatric symptoms are common, particularly depression. Virilization may occur if there is also increased sec-retion of androgens (mixed Cushing's syndrome).

In adults, the majority of cases are the result of excessive secretion of ACTH from the pituitary gland (Cushing's disease). In some cases, ACTH is derived from an extrapituitary tumor (ectopic ACTH syndrome). Alternatively, there is autonomous secretion of cortisol from an adrenal tumor. This is the most common cause in young children. Rarer causes include primary pigmented adrenocortical nodular dysplasia.[173, 174] There have been a few reports of highly unusual patients in whom cortisol excess is induced by eating, the adrenal showing an aberrant response to gastric inhibitory polypeptide.[175, 176] An iatrogenic form may result from excessive therapeutic administration of steroids.

Cushing's disease accounts for roughly two-thirds of cases; it is three times more common in women than in men, with a peak in the third and fourth decades. Circulating ACTH levels are usually only mildly raised with loss of circadian rhythm. High-dose dexamethasone suppresses ACTH and cortisol secretion. Of all patients, 80%–90% have a corticotroph adenoma of the pituitary gland; removal often results in cure.[177, 178] It is now less common to have surgical resection specimens of the adrenals in these cases. A minority has corticotroph hyperplasia, or the pituitary may appear normal,[179] perhaps reflecting primary hypothalamic or central dysfunction. These patients may proceed to adrenal surgery.

The adrenals most commonly show bilateral diffuse cortical hyperplasia (Fig. 7–12), with each gland weighing 6–12 g.[41] They can often be visualized on scanning. The cortex is broadened, and it may be possible with the naked eye to distinguish the red-brown zona reticularis in the inner third to half from the outer yellow zona fasciculata. Histologic examination confirms the relative predominance of the zona reticularis. The bigger the gland, the easier it is to define these changes. Microscopic nodules are not uncommon, usually in the outer zona fasciculata. Of all patients, 10%–20% have bilateral nodular (or macronodular) hyperplasia (Fig. 7–13). This diagnosis used to be restricted to glands with nodules visible to the naked eye.[180] It now tends to be employed when nodules are visualized on computed tomography,[181] which can usually show those with a diameter of 6 mm or more. In many instances, the nodules are large, measuring up to ≥2.5 cm. These glands often weigh up to 30 g and may show significant disparity between the two sides. The cut surface of the nodules is yellow, with variable foci of brown-red. This is reflected in histology, with lipid-laden zona fasciculata–like cells predominant and only scattered groups of compact cells. The intervening cortex is similar to the diffusely hyperplastic gland, and the nodules are usually seen to merge with it. Lipomatous or myelolipomatous change may be seen. It is probable that diffuse and nodular hyperplasia are a continuum,[182] with nodules developing in long-standing disease.[183] The relationship with macronodular hyperplasia with marked enlargement (see below) is unclear. The emergence of adrenal autonomy[184, 185] suggests that neoplastic transformation can occur in a background of hyperplasia. A single case of adrenal carcinoma in a patient with Cushing's disease has been reported.[186]

The ultrastructural features of the hyperplastic gland include an increase in smooth endoplasmic reticulum, greater numbers of cristae, and an increase in matrix density in mitochondria,[40, 187] consistent with enhanced steroidogenesis.

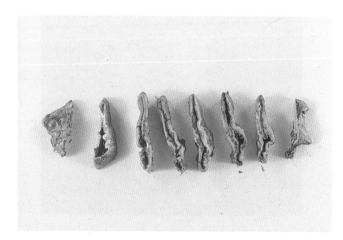

Figure 7–12. In pituitary-dependent Cushing's syndrome (Cushing's disease), the majority of patients have diffuse hyperplasia of the cortex, with moderate enlargement of the gland.

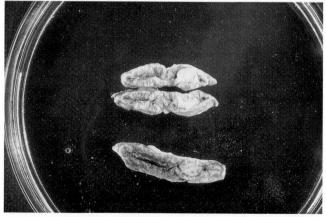

Figure 7–13. A minority of patients with Cushing's disease have nodular hyperplasia as shown here, the gland containing cortical nodules visible to the naked eye on a background of hyperplasia.

Ectopic ACTH syndrome accounts for 15% of cases of Cushing's syndrome. It occurs more commonly in males and is most frequently seen in association with bronchial carcinoid and small-cell lung carcinoma (SCLC), these tumors accounting for about half of cases.[188] ACTH secretion also occurs from 35% of thymic carcinoids,[189, 190] more rarely from islet cell tumors of pancreas, medullary carcinoma of thyroid, or pheochromocytoma,[191] and occasionally from tumors at other sites such as the ovary.[192] Ectopic secretion of corticotropin-releasing factor, either alone[193] or along with ACTH,[194, 195] may give a similar clinical picture and can be accompanied by pituitary corticotroph hyperplasia.[193] The characteristic clinical syndrome may not develop in patients with SCLC because of the other effects of the tumor. Classically, plasma ACTH levels are significantly elevated, as are levels of ACTH precursors, and they are not usually suppressed by dexamethasone. However, it may be difficult in some cases to distinguish this from pituitary-dependent disease, and the source of ectopic secretion may take some time to reveal itself.[196] The presence of hypokalemia is suggestive of the diagnosis.

The adrenals show marked bilateral symmetric enlargement, weighing on average 15–16 g each and not infrequently more than 20 g. On section, the cortex is prominent and diffusely brown. Well-defined nodules are uncommon. Histologically, compact cells extend up to or close to the capsule. Mitotic figures may occasionally be found, and cellular and nuclear pleomorphism is common. Metastases may be found in the gland, particularly in patients with bronchial carcinoma. Ultrastructural examination[197] showed massive increase in smooth endoplasmic reticulum, enlargement and pleomorphism of mitochondria, and a preponderance of vesicular cristae.

Of adults with Cushing's syndrome, 15%–20% have an *adrenal tumor*.[198] Because a general account of adrenal cortical tumors follows in the next section, only a brief comment on Cushing's-associated tumors is included here. They are most common in the fourth and fifth decades. The proportion of benign to malignant has been reported as 1:1 to 2:1,[199–201] the disparity perhaps reflecting the difficulty in making the histologic distinction between the two. In contrast, more than half of children with the disease have a tumor, and the majority are malignant.[198] Females are affected four times as often as males at all ages. Adenomas usually weigh less than 50 g and appear encapsulated (Fig. 7–14), but they can weigh more than 100 g.[202] The cut surface is yellow with focal small brown areas. Histology shows mainly lipid-laden fasciculata-like cells arranged in cords and alveolar structures with foci of compact cells (Fig. 7–15). The compact cells may contain lipofuscin, which helps account for the brown foci. If present in large amounts, lipofuscin may produce a black adenoma. The nuclei are usually rather bland, but occasional cellular and nuclear pleomorphism may occur. Mitoses are almost never seen. Occasional cases of bilateral adenoma have been

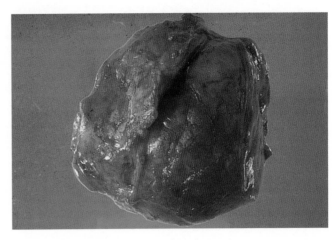

Figure 7–14. This is an adrenal adenoma from a patient with Cushing's syndrome, showing the atrophic normal cortex stretched over the surface on the top left. The excessive secretion of cortisol by the tumor causes increased negative feedback and inhibits the secretion of ACTH by the pituitary gland. This leads to atrophy of the adjacent normal cortex and of the contralateral gland.

reported,[203] but it might be difficult to differentiate this from an adenoma arising on a background of nodular glands. Carcinomas show features similar to those in other syndromes. Coexistent virilization is more common.

Because the high levels of cortisol suppress ACTH secretion from the pituitary, the adjacent cortex and the contralateral gland are atrophic (see Fig. 7–14). They show thickening of the capsule and a reduction in width of the cortex that consists of only clear cells and zona glomerulosa (see Fig. 7–15). The latter may appear more prominent than in the normal gland because of the relative loss of the other two zones.

A rare variant is *macronodular hyperplasia without ACTH hypersecretion*.[204–206] The glands are markedly enlarged and distorted. The nodules are composed mainly of lipid-laden cells that appear inefficient in steroidogenesis,[204, 207] with weak signal for steroidogenic enzymes and poorly developed smooth endoplasmic reticulum. The intervening cortex can be difficult to recognize but has been reported atrophic.[204] Whether this represents a primary adrenocortical abnormality or a response to an as yet unidentified stimulus is unknown.

Primary pigmented nodular adrenocortical disease[173, 208, 209] is a rare familial condition of children and young adults. Patients present with the typical features of Cushing's syndrome, but the osteopenia is more severe than in other variants.[210] Both adrenal glands consist of multiple nodules (Fig. 7–16), usually 1–3 mm in diameter, although nodules up to 1.8 cm have been reported.[209] The combined weights range 4–21g.[211] On cross-section, the nodules appear dark brown to black and rarely yellow.[212] As in black adenomas, the pigment is probably a combination of lipofuscin and

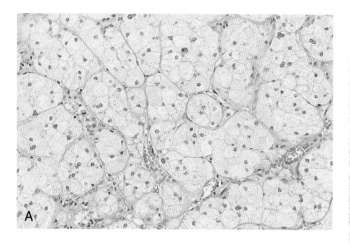

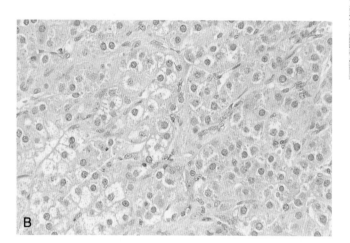

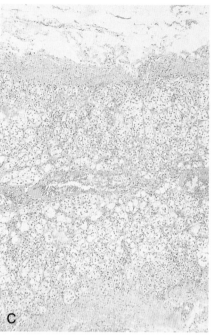

Figure 7–15. Adrenocortical adenoma in Cushing's syndrome. The tumor consists mainly of lipid-laden cells arranged in an organized alveolar pattern *(A)*, with focal groups of compact cells, some of which contain lipofuscin *(B)*. There is little evidence of pleomorphism, and mitotic activity is not identified. The adjacent atrophic cortex is narrowed and comprises only lipid-laden cells *(C)*.

neuromelanin. Focal lipomatous or myelolipomatous change may been seen as well as lymphoid infiltration in some cases.[124, 210] The intervening cortex may be difficult to identify. It consists of small regular cells with clear cytoplasm, consistent with functional suppression. Plasma ACTH levels

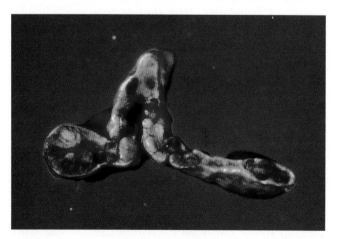

Figure 7–16. Primary pigmented nodular disease. This adrenal gland shows the typical pattern, consisting of multiple nodules, dark brown to black in color. (Courtesy of Dr. R.J.M. Croughs, Utrecht, Netherlands.)

are low,[213] indicating adrenal autonomy. The pathogenesis is unknown, but a link with chromosome 16 has been proposed.[207] The identification of circulating adrenal growth-stimulating immunoglobulins raised the possibility of an autoimmune mechanism,[214, 215] but the supporting evidence is weak. The condition may be part of the Carney complex, in association with myxomas, spotty skin pigmentation, schwannomas, and tumors of the pituitary, testis, andthyroid.[216–218] This is transmitted as an autosomal-dominant trait, but there may be more than one gene involved, as linkage to chromosome 2 has been reported in some families[219] and to chromosome 17 in others.[220]

Conn's Syndrome (Aldosterone Excess)

This rare cause of hypertension accounts for less than 1% of patients attending clinics. High aldosterone levels are coupled with low renin levels and hypokalemia. Patients complain of muscle weakness, fatigue, and polyuria. Periodic paralysis may occur, and there is an increased risk of cardiac arrhythmias. In the past, about two-thirds of patients were

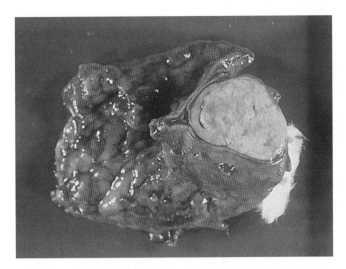

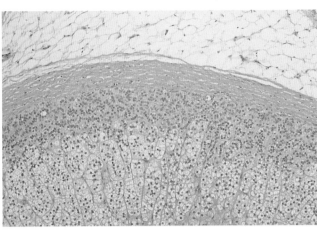

Figure 7–17. This adrenal from a patient with Conn's syndrome contains a small circumscribed adrenal adenoma, deep yellow in color. Note that the normal gland is of normal size, as ACTH secretion is normal.

Figure 7–19. Hyperplasia of zona glomerulosa (ZG) in Conn's syndrome. In contrast to the focal distribution in the normal gland, the ZG extends around the whole circumference of the gland and lies several layers deep.

reported to have a single adrenal adenoma.[221] Unilateral adrenalectomy is usually curative in these cases if the condition is recognized before the vascular changes of hypertension develop. Bilateral adenomas have been recorded.[222, 223] The tumors are usually small, often less than 2 cm in diameter,[224, 225] and half weigh less than 4 g.[226] Women are more commonly affected than men, with the peak incidence rate in the third to fifth decades.[227] The cut surface has a characteristic golden-yellow color (Fig. 7–17), deeper than most Cushing's adenomas. Histologic examination reveals a variety of cell types (Fig. 7–18). Most resemble the zona fasciculata, with a minority having features of glomerulosal cells. Hybrid cells show features of both, containing lipid but having a higher nuclear-to-cytoplasmic ratio than that for fasciculata-like cells. Compact cells are also found. Ultrastructural examination confirms the range of cell types.[228]

Focal nuclear pleomorphism is not uncommon. Very occasional black adenomas have been reported.[229] Carcinomas are extremely rare.[230, 231] As in Cushing's disease, micronodules are not uncommon in the paratumoral gland. The adjacent zona glomerulosa may be normal in distribution, and immunoreactivity for steroidogenic enzymes suggests that it is not fully suppressed.[10] In some cases, the ipsilateral zona glomerulosa appears hyperplastic (Fig. 7–19), but whether this relates to the pathogenesis of the adenoma or indicates effects of treatment is not clear. Where spironolactone has been given as treatment, small globular intracellular bodies known as spironolactone bodies[232] may be seen in the zona glomerulosa and outer zona fasciculata (Fig. 7–20) and, in some instances, in tumor cells. These are up to 20 μm in diameter and stain positively with periodic acid–Schiff and often have a whorled appearance

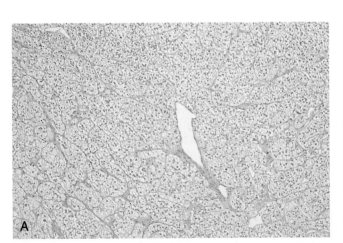

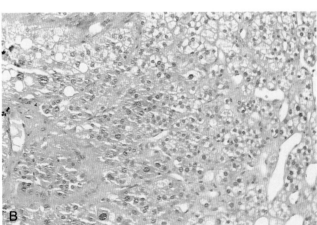

Figure 7–18. Adrenal cortical adenoma from a patient with Conn's syndrome. The majority of cells resemble the zona fasciculata *(A)*. Focally, there is some variation *(B)*, with subpopulations reminiscent of compact cells (mid to lower left), and others show features midway between the glomerulosa and fasciculata, so-called hybrid cells (right of field).

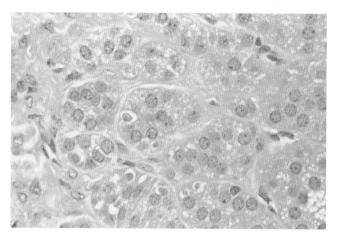

Figure 7–20. When spironolactone is given as treatment in Conn's syndrome, whorled globular inclusion bodies can be found in glomerulosal cells in the para-adenomatous gland and sometimes in the tumor.

and a halo around them. Ultrastructural analysis shows lamellar myelin bodies, probably derived from smooth endoplasmic reticulum.[233]

Initially, hyperplasia of the zona glomerulosa, so-called "idiopathic hyperaldosteronism," was reported only in a minority of cases, more commonly in older patients, with no sex difference in incidence rate.[234] However, it is probably more common than that, accounting for 45% of cases at the Mayo Clinic between 1978 and 1987, compared with 26% before 1970.[225] It may be associated with the milder forms of primary hyperaldosteronism that are now recognized. Adrenocortical nodules may also be found in these cases, possibly as a result of hypertensive arteriopathic change.[235] Hyperplasia of the outer zona fasciculata is found infrequently.[10] Unless nodules are present, glands with glomerulosal hyperplasia may be of normal weight because the zone comprises such a small fraction of the total. Instead of the normal focal distribution of the zona glomerulosa, it usually forms a continuous band in the subcapsular region and may extend in places into the zona fasciculata.

A further rare variant is glucocorticoid-suppressible hyperaldosteronism, in which aldosterone may be derived from the outer zona fasciculata.[236] This is inherited in an autosomal-dominant manner because of the formation of a chimeric gene. Unequal crossover results in a protein formed from the ACTH-dependent part of 11β-hydroxylase (CYP11B1) and the functional part of aldosterone synthase (CYP11B2).[237, 238] Little is known of the pathology of such cases, but hyperplasia of both zona glomerulosa and outer zona fasciculata has been described.[239]

Adrenogenital Syndrome (Sex Steroid Excess)

Excessive secretion of sex steroids causes virilization, feminization, or precocious puberty, depending on the steroids secreted and the age and sex of the patient. The pathologic features of CAH have already been discussed. Adrenocortical tumors may also produce sex steroids, either as the predominant hormone or, more commonly, in combination with cortisol (mixed Cushing's syndrome). Androgen secretion is the usual pattern, with DHEA and DHEA sulfate more common than testosterone.[240] Of all cases, 80% are diagnosed in females and the majority in children.[241] Prepubertal girls develop clitoral hypertrophy and secondary male sex characteristics, whereas boys undergo precocious puberty. Both show accelerated growth with early closure of epiphyses. Amenorrhea, hirsutism, and virilization occur in adult women. Suppression of the pituitary-gonadal axis by the high level of androgens results in testicular atrophy. The apparent excess of these tumors in women may be due to the fact that they appear nonfunctional in men and present only if there are general features of malignancy. Estrogen-secreting tumors most frequently cause feminization in men between the ages of 20 and 50 years, with gynecomastia, loss of secondary sex characteristics, testicular atrophy, and loss of libido.[242] They are also an occasional cause of precocious puberty in girls. In rare instances, they appear to respond to gonadotropins,[243, 244] and it is unclear whether these tumors arise from the adrenal cortex or from heterotopic gonadal steroid-producing cells.

A higher proportion of this subgroup is malignant, particularly in feminizing cases. The usual criteria must be applied to distinguish benign and malignant potential, but there are certain caveats. Tumor weights are extremely variable, and even benign tumors may be very large. Also, compact cells are more common in androgen-secreting adenomas than in other subtypes.

ADRENAL CORTICAL TUMORS: GENERAL CONSIDERATIONS

Incidental Adrenal Cortical Nodules

Adrenal cortical nodules are not uncommon at autopsy. Solitary lesions are present in 1.5%–29% of unselected cases,[211] and these are often classified as adenomas. Careful examination reveals that in most cases, however, nodules are multiple and bilateral.[235] Most of these are small, and it is unusual to find more than one or two large nodules in any individual. They are more common in older patients and in those with hypertension or diabetes mellitus.[235, 245] They range in size from microscopic foci (Fig. 7–21) to 2–3 cm in diameter, and large nodules may cause disparity in the weight between the glands. The cut surface is yellow, often with focal brown areas. Although they appear circumscribed, they have no true capsule, and at microscopic level they merge with the cells of the normal gland. Micronodules are most often found in the outer fasciculata, and larger

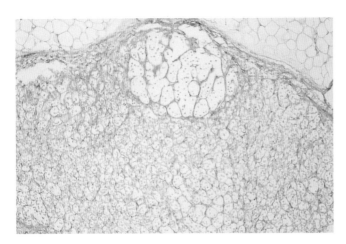

Figure 7-21. Adrenal cortex immunostained for type IV collagen to demonstrate the basement membrane. This shows a microscopic adrenocortical nodule sited in the outer zona fasciculata. These nodules are not uncommon in adrenal glands from older patients or those with vascular disease.

lesions occupy the greater proportion of the cortex. They also develop in the cortical cuff around the central vein.

Most are composed of hypertrophied lipid-laden cells, even when the adjacent cortex shows signs of lipid depletion, although compact cells may occasionally predominate. There is no pleomorphism or mitotic activity. Myelolipomatous change and osseous metaplasia are occasionally seen.[235] Dobbie[235] proposed that they represent compensatory hyperplasia following local ischemic damage and atrophy. He found that they were more common in glands showing hyalinization and luminal occlusion of capsular vessels. Others have debated this[246] on the grounds that vascular changes may be identified in glands without nodules and that abnormal vessels may be found within nodules themselves.

These nodules are now more often identified in life when the abdomen is scanned for other reasons, up to 1% of abdominal CT scans revealing a lesion of 1 cm or more in diameter.[247] Not surprisingly, they are more common in older patients, with a prevalence of about 7% in patients older than 70 years of age.[248] The average size is about 2.5 cm, but with increasingly sensitive techniques smaller lesions may be detected. They pose clinical problems. How can they be distinguished from other lesions, such as metastases? Enhanced scanning techniques have helped[249] (Fig. 7–22), but cytologic examination may be required for confirmation. If they are cortical, do they need to be removed? Most are not associated with hormonal dysfunction, although some patients have low levels of autonomous cortisol secretion: subclinical Cushing's syndrome.[250, 251] Malignant po-

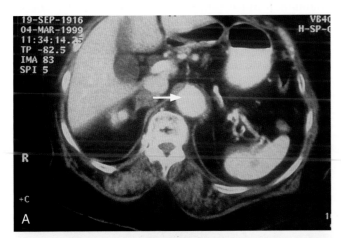

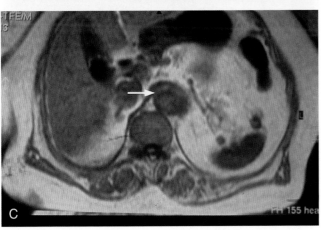

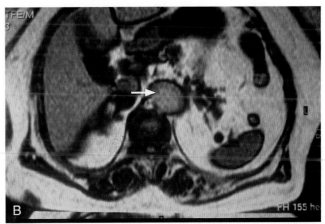

Figure 7-22. Incidental macronodules of 1 cm or more in diameter are found in up to 1% of patients undergoing abdominal CT scans. They must be distinguished from other disorders (for example, metastasis). A 58-year-old woman with carcinoma of the colon was found to have a nodule in the left adrenal gland on CT scan *(A)*. Further investigation was undertaken using chemical-shift MRI. This technique is able to distinguish adrenal adenomas and nodules with a high lipid content from other lesions. The in-phase image *(B)* shows the signal intensity of the lesion. The out-of-phase image *(C)* shows a loss of signal intensity ("blackening" of the lesion). This change is based on a high lipid content, defining the lesion as an adrenal adenoma rather than a metastasis. (Courtesy of Dr. F.W. Poon, Glasgow, UK.)

tential would also warrant surgery but, as discussed below, this is difficult to assess. At present, treatment is rather arbitrarily based on size (larger lesions are more likely to be malignant), but cut-off points between 3 cm[252] and 6 cm[253] have been proposed. Even with larger lesions, most are likely to pose no risk. It has been estimated that 60 lesions ≥6 cm would have to be removed to find one carcinoma.[254]

Adrenal Cortical Adenomas

The real incidence of adrenal adenomas is almost certainly underestimated because a firm diagnosis is made with confidence only when there is clinical evidence of autonomous hormone secretion. Women are more frequently affected. The tumors are usually unilateral and solitary, involving both glands equally, although occasional cases of bilateral adenoma have been reported.[203, 222, 223] They may show true encapsulation or the presence of a pseudocapsule. The cut surface is in general yellow with focal brown pigmentation, probably a combination of lipofuscin and neuromelanin.[255] In some cases—so-called black adenomas[256, 257]—this is pronounced. Micronodules may be seen in the para-adenomatous gland.

Adrenal Cortical Carcinoma

Adrenal cortical carcinoma is a rare but highly aggressive tumor, accounting for 0.05%[258, 259] to 0.2%[260] of all malignancies, with an incidence of between 0.5 and 2 per million.[261-263] The bulk of evidence suggests that they occur more commonly in women.[264] There is a bimodal age distribution, with a peak in early childhood and a second peak in the fifth to seventh decades.[265-267] The prognosis is very poor, with a 67%–94% mortality rate.[260, 268-271] The median or mean survival interval from diagnosis lies between 4 and 30 months.[260, 271-275] Many tumors are locally invasive, and 15%[276]–67%[273] have metastasized at the time of initial presentation. The most common sites of metastasis are liver, lung, retroperitoneum, and lymph nodes.[277]

Functioning tumors may present with signs of hormone excess and comprise 24%–74%,[264] the difference probably reflecting variances in the level of investigation of steroid hormone secretion. Cushing's syndrome is the most common clinical presentation, often accompanied by androgen excess (mixed Cushing's syndrome). Virilization may be the sole presenting feature, but feminizing tumors are rare. Mineralocorticoid excess is usually associated with secretion of DOC,[278, 279] whereas hyperaldosteronism is almost never found.[272, 278] Other presenting symptoms include abdominal or loin pain, fullness, and sometimes fever. Weight loss may be less marked than in other malignancies, possibly because of the anabolic effects of androgens. In recurrent or metastatic disease, the clinical syndrome is usually the same as that of the primary tumor, although conversion from virilization to feminization has been reported.[280]

Most tumors respond poorly to treatment. Complete surgical excision is the mainstay of cure, but that may not be possible. The tumors are extremely resistant to chemotherapy, which may be explained in part by the expression of P-glycoprotein[281-283] and glutathione-S-transferases,[284-286] which play roles in various types of drug resistance. Mitotane (o'p'-DDD, a derivative of DDT) has a nonspecific adrenolytic effect and may be of use in controlling the disease in some cases.[263, 287]

Most adrenal cortical carcinomas weigh more than 100 g[41, 288] and some weigh as much as 5 kg. However, tumors weighing less than 50 g have behaved in a malignant fashion.[283, 289] A range of 3–40 cm diameter has been reported.[290] Grossly, they may appear encapsulated or may be obviously adherent to surrounding structures. The normal adrenal gland is often not easily identified. Lobulation is common (Fig. 7–23), with fibrous tissue separating the tumor nodules. The cut surface is fleshy, with variable coloration ranging from pink-brown to yellow. Hemorrhage and necrosis are often seen (Fig. 7–24), and there may be cystic change. In occasional cases, there is gross evidence of vascular invasion.[291]

The architectural features are less ordered than in adenomas. A trabecular arrangement is commonly seen, with wide cords of cells separated by vascular channels. Diffuse patterns of growth are also found (Fig. 7–25), and alveolar patterns are uncommon. The architecture may be fairly constant or may show marked variation. Compact cells are more frequent than in adenomas, and they often predominate. Nuclear hyperchromatism and pleomorphism

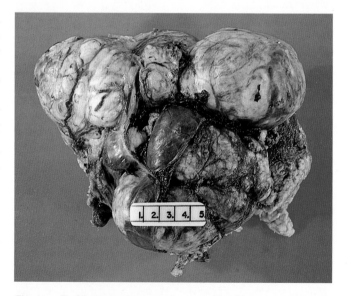

Figure 7–23. This large adrenocortical carcinoma presented with upper abdominal pain. It shows an obvious lobular pattern of growth (scale in centimeters).

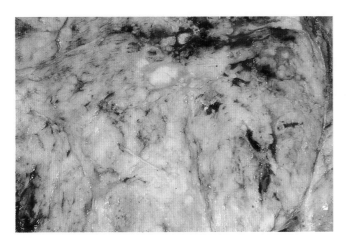

Figure 7-24. The cut surface of the tumor shows obvious areas of hemorrhage and necrosis.

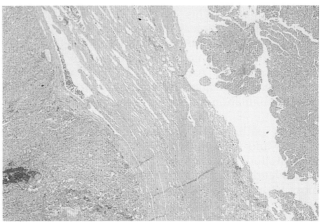

Figure 7-27. Adrenal cortical carcinoma. This tumor shows the presence of broad fibrous bands.

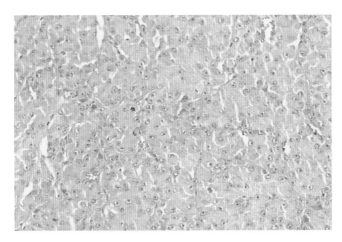

Figure 7-25. Adrenal cortical carcinoma. This tumor consists mainly of compact cells showing a diffuse pattern of growth. Mitotic figures are present.

are seen (Fig. 7-26), sometimes with multinucleated giant cells. Many of the cells have vesicular nuclei with prominent nuclear membranes and conspicuous nucleoli. Mitotic activity is often seen, sometimes with atypical forms. Oncocytic change has been described.[292] A single case of adenosquamous carcinoma in the absence of an obvious other primary site has been documented.[293] Confluent necrosis is common, and broad fibrous bands are present in a significant proportion of cases (Fig. 7-27). Vascular invasion of sinusoidal and venous channels may be identified (Fig. 7-28). Capsular invasion may be more difficult to identify, partly because of necrosis and fibrosis. Metastases and invasion of surrounding organs provide unequivocal evidence of malignant behavior.

Diagnosis of Malignancy

In most cases the diagnosis of carcinoma can be made without difficulty, but the pathologist must assess the risk of malignant potential in all adrenal

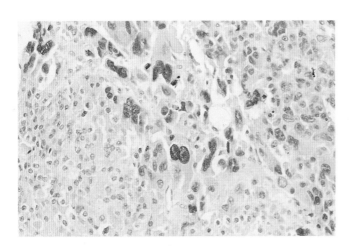

Figure 7-26. Adrenal cortical carcinoma. There is significant nuclear pleomorphism in this case.

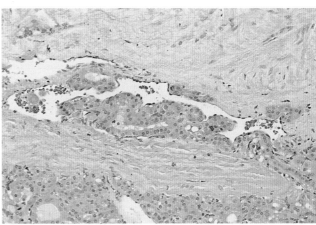

Figure 7-28. Adrenal cortical carcinoma. Obvious vascular invasion is seen.

cortical tumors. This is best done by taking an overview of all clinical, biochemical, and histologic findings. Patients who present with virilization, feminization, or large nonfunctional tumors are more likely to have a carcinoma. Elevated urinary 17-oxosteroids and failure of the tumor to respond to ACTH stimulation in vivo are also suspicious features.[266]

Often, pathologists are not given the appropriate clinical information and must rely on morphologic criteria alone for diagnosis. Important features have been identified by examining differences between tumors with known benign and malignant outcome. In addition to weight, assessment is based on the following: extensive necrosis; broad fibrous bands; capsular, venous, and sinusoidal invasion; architectural features (organized or diffuse); the proportion of clear cells; nuclear pleomorphism; mitotic activity; and the presence of atypical mitoses. Two types of analysis have been proposed. In the first,[266, 294] features are given a numerical weighted risk value, and the diagnosis of malignancy is based on summation. In the approach of Hough et al[266] weighting is given to clinical and biochemical features also. The system proposed by Weiss et al[275, 295] is easier to apply in everyday diagnostic practice. It is based on the assessment of the features outlined above, apart from the broad fibrous bands. There is a cutoff point of 25% for the proportion of clear cells, and of 6 in 50 high-power (×400) fields for mitotic activity. The presence of three of the nine features indicates malignant potential. All three systems have value, but not all will give the same answer in an individual case. In difficult cases, all clinical and histologic information should be taken into account, but in a few instances, a diagnosis of indeterminate or "borderline" tumor may have to be made.

Assessment of Prognosis

A staging system for adrenal cortical carcinoma[296] is shown in Table 7–2. It is clear that most patients have advanced disease at the time of diagnosis.[276, 297] Some researchers would combine stages I and II,[297, 298] as these patients have a similar prognosis after complete surgical excision.[299] It is unclear whether histologic grade correlates with outcome, although there is some evidence to support this.[300] High mitotic activity is associated with more aggressive behavior.[294, 295] Tumors with a mitotic rate greater than 20 per 50 high-power fields show a shorter disease-free interval.[295] This has been confirmed using the Ki-67 index as a measure of proliferation, with a cutoff of 3%.[301] However, there appears to be no correlation with overall survival. Antibodies to proliferating cell nuclear antigen should not be used to assess proliferation[302–304] in diagnostic practice.

Additional Studies

Immunocytochemistry. The main diagnostic problems may be in differentiating adrenal cortical carcinoma from hepatocellular carcinoma, renal cell carcinoma and, occasionally, pheochromocytoma. Specific identification of a tumor as of adrenal cortical origin is difficult. Antibody D11 has been reported useful.[305] Immunopositivity for inhibin-α[29, 30, 306] (Fig. 7–29) and immunoreactivity with melan-A clone A103[34] may help. Expression of steroidogenic enzymes[17–21] can also be helpful, but antibodies are not freely available, and the enzymes may not be expressed in nonfunctional tumors. Adrenal cortical tumors show little if any positivity for cytokeratins, particularly in the absence of enzyme pretreatment.[15, 16, 307, 308] Vimentin positivity is found in up to 100% of some series.[15, 307] These tumors are immunonegative for epithelial membrane antigen (EMA).[305] Renal carcinoma usually shows positivity for both EMA and cytokeratins.[308] Hepatocellular carcinoma may be immunopositive for α-fetoprotein, α-antitrypsin, or carcinoembryonic antigen (CEA).

Table 7–2. Staging of Adrenal Cortical Tumors	
Stage	
I	T1 N0 M0
II	T2 N0 M0
III	T1 or T2 N1 M0 T3 N0 M0
IV	Any T or N, M1 T3 N1 T4
Criteria	
T1	Tumor ≤5 cm, no invasion
T2	Tumor >5 cm, no invasion
T3	Tumor of any size, locally invasive but not involving adjacent organs
T4	Tumor of any size with invasion of adjacent organs
N0	Negative regional nodes
N1	Positive regional nodes
M0	No distant metastases
M1	Distant metastases

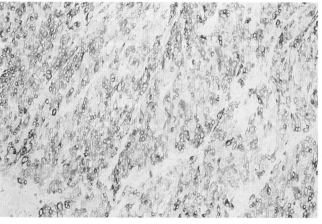

Figure 7–29. Adrenal cortical carcinoma. Immunostaining for inhibin-α shows widespread positivity. This can be useful in the differential diagnosis.

Occasionally, one needs to distinguish a cortical carcinoma from a pheochromocytoma. Immunopositivity of cortical carcinomas for general neuroendocrine markers including neuron-specific enolase (NSE) and synaptophysin may cause difficulty, but chromogranin staining is negative.[22, 23, 309]

Studies have demonstrated positivity for the transcription factor SF-1/Ad4BP[310] and the nuclear receptor DAX-1,[311] both of which are important in cortical development and steroidogenesis. Whether they are of any diagnostic relevance is unknown.

Ultrastructural Features. Adenomas often resemble normal glands,[39, 40, 312] with characteristic mitochondria, abundant smooth endoplasmic reticulum, and rough endoplasmic reticulum arranged in parallel arrays. Some, however, show changes in the distribution of organelles and mitochondrial changes with inclusion bodies and loss of cristae. These alterations are more marked in malignant tumors, and loss of basement membrane may be seen. However, there are often sufficiently characteristic mitochondrial features to allow a positive diagnosis of adrenal cortical tumor. The presence of neuroendocrine granules is of uncertain significance.

Tumor Ploidy. Initial studies appeared to indicate that the majority of adrenal cortical carcinomas were aneuploid and that adenomas were diploid.[313, 314] However, it is now clear that the extent of overlap is too great to make it a useful investigation for diagnosing malignancy in an individual case.[315, 316] There is no direct correlation between DNA content and survival.[315–317]

Other Studies. Conflicting data also exist on the usefulness of counting nucleolar organizer regions as identified by silver staining (AgNORs).[318–320] Patterns of lectin binding are unhelpful both in diagnosis and in prognosis.[321]

Adrenal Cortical Tumors at Other Sites

Benign and malignant tumors may occur wherever ectopic adrenal tissue is found. They are reported most commonly in the liver, kidney, and gonads.[322–326] In the gonads, they may be difficult to characterize as adrenal in origin because of the similarities to gonadal steroidogenic cells. The testicular lesions occurring in males with adrenogenital syndrome were discussed earlier.

PATHOGENESIS OF ADRENAL CORTICAL TUMORS

The molecular pathogenesis of adrenal cortical tumors is still poorly understood. Clonality studies based on X chromosome inactivation[327] have shown that, although all carcinomas are monoclonal, adenomas may show monoclonal, polyclonal, or intermediate patterns.[328] This might suggest that adenomas arise by two different pathways, some from a single cell and others by clonal expansion of a population with a growth advantage within a polyclonal proliferation. Whether the polyclonal proliferation is truly neoplastic is unclear.

Detection of cytogenetic abnormalities has been hampered by the difficulties in culturing these tumors, and there is evidence that culture may select unrepresentative subpopulations of tumor cells.[329] However, allelic loss on chromosomes 11p, 13q, and 17p in carcinomas[330, 331] suggests involved genes at these loci. New techniques provide more opportunity of detecting changes. Comparative genomic hybridization indicates widespread chromosomal gains and losses in carcinomas with few changes in adenomas.[332] An interphase cytogenetic study[333] suggests that changes in chromosomes 3, 9, and X are early events and that there is increasing chromosomal instability with tumor progression. Loss of heterozygosity has been shown at 2p16 and at 11q13.[334]

A number of oncogenes and tumor suppressor genes have been investigated. Adrenal cortical carcinoma occurs more commonly in Li-Fraumeni syndrome,[335] associated with germline mutations in the *p53* gene.[336] Abnormal expression of p53 protein and *p53* mutations in a majority of sporadic adrenal cortical carcinomas with rare changes in adenoma[337–339] would support a role in tumor progression, although there appears to be no prognostic correlation.[339] The high incidence of mutations in exon 4, which is not a known hot spot, in cases from Taiwan[340] has not been confirmed in a series of white patients.[341] This may reflect ethnic differences. Adrenal cortical tumors also form part of the disease spectrum of multiple endocrine neoplasia (MEN) type 1. However, although there is frequent loss of 11q13 where the *MEN-1* gene is located,[334] there is no evidence for gene mutation in sporadic tumors.[342, 343] There may be another tumor suppressor gene nearby. Preliminary data indicate that p16[344, 345] and retinoblastoma protein[344] may play a role, particularly in carcinoma. Inactivation of both alleles has been demonstrated in adrenocortical tumors in two patients with adenomatous polyposis coli, but the mechanism does not seem important in sporadic tumors.[346, 347]

Conflicting data exist on the *RAS* family of proto-oncogenes. Whereas two studies have shown no involvement,[338, 348] others report 12.5% of tumors with mutations in *N-ras* but none in *Ki-ras* or *Ha-ras*[349] and 46% of cases with mutations in *Ki-ras,* but none in *Ha-ras.*[350] Expression of c-myc protein may vary with tumor type, but it does not seem to be involved in neoplastic transformation.[351]

Familial tumors also occur in Beckwith-Wiedemann syndrome, associated with dysregulation of a group of growth-controlling genes on 11p15.5,[352] including paternal disomy of the *IGF-II* gene. Rearrangement at this locus and overexpression of *IGF-II* have been reported in sporadic cases.[353, 354] Other growth factors that may be involved are TGF-α, epidermal growth factor receptor[71, 355] *IGF-I* and its binding proteins and receptors,[353, 356, 357] and the activin and inhibin subgroups of the TGF-β superfamily.[29, 30, 358]

Constitutive activation of functional signaling pathways by mutation has been implicated in tumorigenesis in other endocrine glands, including pituitary[359] and thyroid.[360] There is no current evidence that this is important in the adrenal cortex. No mutations have been shown in either the ACTH[361, 362] or AII type 1 receptors[363] in cortical tumors. Mutation in the α subunit of the stimulatory G protein is extremely rare in sporadic tumors,[364] but it plays a role in some cortical tumors in McCune-Albright syndrome.[365] Likewise, an early report of mutation in the inhibitory subunit, $\alpha_i 2$,[366] has not been substantiated.[364, 367] Immortalization of cells by the action of the protein/RNA telomerase complex, not normally expressed in differentiated cells, may also play a role in tumorigenesis. Published data to date on expression in adrenal cortical tumors are equivocal.[368–370] The role of apoptosis has been poorly investigated. A single study showed no difference in apoptotic index between benign and malignant tumors,[371] and BCL2 protein, which has a critical role in the process, has been reported as detectable[372] or undetectable[301] by immunohistochemistry.

OTHER TUMORS

An unusual tumor is the adrenal oncocytoma[373, 374] (Fig. 7–30). This resembles oncocytic lesions at other sites, showing accumulation of mitochondria. It is assumed to be of adrenal origin, although no specific features have been documented. It has generally behaved in a benign fashion, although uncertain malignant potential and carcinoma have been described.[292, 373]

Mesenchymal tumors are rare. Hemangiomas are usually chance findings at autopsy but may present clinically if large or if calcification is identified on abdominal radiograph.[375–377] Primary angiosarcoma[378, 379] and lymphangiomas[246, 380, 381] have been described. Leiomyomas and leiomyosarcomas[382–384] presumably arise from vascular smooth muscle. They seem to occur more commonly in patients with AIDS,[385–389] and Epstein-Barr virus infection has been implicated.[384] Carcinosarcoma,[390–392] neural tumors including schwannomas and neurofibromas,[264] adenomatoid tumor,[393, 394] and xanthofibroma[395] have also been described.

Other *steroid-producing tumors* include granulosa/theca cell tumor,[396] Leydig cell adenoma,[397–399] and a testosterone-secreting adrenal ganglioneuroma containing Leydig cells.[400] A highly unusual virilizing neoplasm in an infant, consisting of immature epithelial and mesenchymal cells with slit-like spaces, is named adrenocortical blastoma.[401]

At autopsy, there are *metastases* to the adrenals in up to 27% of patients dying of cancer,[402] and 41% of these have bilateral involvement.[403] Certain tumors

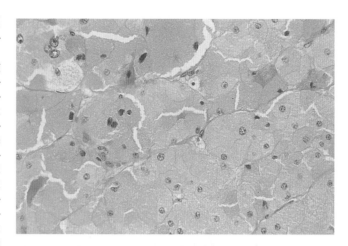

Figure 7–30. Adrenal oncocytoma. This was an intra-adrenal tumor composed of large eosinophilic cells arranged in a diffuse pattern. There were no features to suggest malignancy.

show a higher incidence rate: around 30%–40% in breast[404] and lung cancer.[403] Melanomas commonly metastasize to the adrenal,[405, 406] presumably because of a favorable growth environment in the medulla. Occasionally, the metastasis is to an adrenal cortical tumor.[407, 408] Metastatic tumor is usually asymptomatic, but adrenal insufficiency has been reported in 19%–33% of patients with computed tomography evidence of bilateral adrenal involvement. The nature of the infiltrating lesion is usually apparent. Difficulty may be encountered with metastatic hepatocellular carcinoma or renal cell carcinoma that may mimic adrenal cortical tumors.

Involvement by *lymphoma* is uncommon apart from Burkitt's lymphoma.[409] Both T- and B-cell tumors have been reported, and infiltration is usually asymptomatic, but hypoadrenalism can occur.[410, 411] These tumors should be characterized in the usual fashion.

TUMOR-LIKE LESIONS

Myelolipoma is a benign lesion consisting of an admixture of mature adipose tissue and hemopoietic cells (Fig. 7–31). Occasional examples have been reported in heterotopic adrenal[412, 413] and in other extra-adrenal sites, such as the presacral area[414, 415] and in the liver.[416] Image-guided fine-needle aspiration cytology may be of use in confirming the diagnosis at these unusual sites. Microscopic lesions are present in up to 0.4% of autopsies,[417] more commonly in cortical hyperplasia, nodules, and adenomas than in normal cortex. Diagnosis is usually made when a patient is between 40 and 70 years and rarely younger than 30 years of age.[418, 419] These lesions are usually single, unencapsulated, and less than 4 cm in diameter. Occasional patients have multiple and/or bilateral lesions, and the lesions

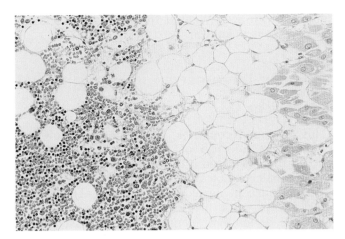

Figure 7–31. Adrenal myelolipoma. This lesion consists of an admixture of mature adipose tissue and hemopoietic cells. Hemosiderin-laden macrophages are found in this case. Adrenal cortical cells are seen to the right of the field. Similar changes may be seen focally in adrenal cortical nodules and adenomas.

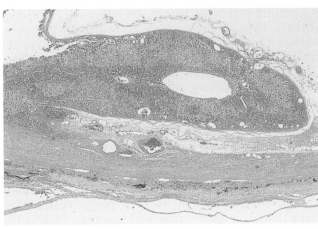

Figure 7–32. Adrenal pseudocyst. This lesion presented with upper abdominal pain. The cyst had a fibrous wall and no obvious lining. As illustrated, the cyst wall appeared to abut cortical tissue. (Courtesy of Dr. K. McLaren, Edinburgh, UK.)

may reach a very large size.[164] Like nodules and adenomas, they appear on scans.[420] Most are asymptomatic, but larger lesions may present clinically because of abdominal discomfort. The cut surface is yellow with red or pink areas. Histology shows variable combinations of fat and hemopoietic tissue of normal appearance in which all elements can be identified. Cortical cells may be interspersed. A few lesions show osseous metaplasia. Their origin is not clear, but stromal metaplasia has been suggested.[419]

Ovarian thecal metaplasia is the name given to wedge-shaped microscopic nodules of stellate spindle cells closely resembling ovarian stroma found in the adrenals of about 4% of postmenopausal women. Some of the nodules may show hyalinization. Lesions are usually but not always solitary.[421] Similar foci have been documented, although rarely, in men.[422]

Adrenal cysts are rare lesions; there are fewer than 500 cases reported in the literature.[423, 424] Most are small and are incidental findings at autopsy, but they are now more commonly visualized on scanning. Occasional large lesions may be found.[425–427] They are heterogeneous in origin. Endothelial cysts are the most common (45%) and are mainly lymphangiomatous.[428] Pseudocysts (39%) are heterogeneous in origin and are the most common to present clinically (Fig. 7–32). They have fibrous walls, usually with no obvious lining, although adrenal cortical cells may be scattered within the fibrous tissue, and there is often calcification. The contents consist of organizing thrombus and blood-stained fluid. The cysts may be derived from cortical nodules or tumors by hemorrhage or degeneration, or they may have a vascular origin.[429, 430] Epithelial cysts account for 9% and are either degenerate neoplasms or, rarely, retention or embryonal cysts. Mesothelial

origin has been reported in a few cases.[431, 432] In some countries, parasitic cysts are more common, accounting for 7% overall. These are usually due to echinococcal[433, 434] infection.

CHRONIC ADRENAL CORTICAL INSUFFICIENCY

This is often a disease of insidious onset, with general weakness, lethargy, anorexia, nausea, weight loss, abdominal pain, and other gastrointestinal symptoms. Patients may also have postural dizziness, hypotension, and hypoglycemic attacks. Most eventually show pigmentation of skin and mucous membranes because of increased pituitary secretion of ACTH and related peptides with melanocyte-stimulating activity. Psychiatric symptoms include depression and frank psychosis. A prevalence of 20 to 60 per million has been reported in Europe and North America, but the true figure may be higher.[435] It occurs mainly in women, with the onset between 30 and 40 years of age. The most frequent cause in developed countries is autoimmune adrenalitis, but tuberculosis remains the major cause in developing countries. Other infections may occasionally be involved. Involvement of the gland by amyloidosis, hemochromatosis, and secondary tumor rarely results in clinical impairment.[410, 436, 437]

Autoimmune Adrenalitis

This is one of the organ-specific autoimmune diseases. It may occur in isolation, but about 50% of patients also have other autoimmune diseases. Two variants of polyglandular autoimmune syndromes have been described.[438] Type 1 is the rarer;

it comprises at least two of the following: Addison's disease, hypoparathyroidism, and chronic mucocutaneous candidiasis. There may also be hypogonadism, alopecia, pernicious anemia, and hepatitis. The term autoimmune polyendocrinopathy-candidiasis-ectodermal dystrophy (APECED) has been applied.[439] It is associated with mutations in the APECED or AIRE (autoimmune regulator) gene on chromosome 21q22.3, which encodes a putative transcription factor.[440-443] This variant typically occurs in children or young adults. Type 2 is seen in adults. Adrenalitis is associated with autoimmune thyroid disease and/or insulin-dependent diabetes mellitus.[440] It is thought to be a polygenic disorder with dominant inheritance and linkage to HLA-DR3. The majority of patients have autoantibodies to adrenal antigens, including the enzyme $P450_{c21}$ (70%–80% of cases).[444, 445] Antibodies to $P450_{scc}$ and $P-450_{c17\alpha}$ are more commonly seen in polyglandular disease.[446, 447]

The adrenals show a chronic inflammatory infiltrate in the cortex with destruction of cortical cells, which may be due to both cell- and antibody-mediated immune mechanisms.[448] Surviving cortical cells strongly express class II MHC molecules, most likely as a result of the inflammatory process[26] rather than the cause.[449] The end result of this destructive process is cortical atrophy. Unless there is some precipitating factor, cortical failure does not usually occur until about 90% of the cortex is destroyed. At autopsy the glands weigh only 1.2–2.5 g and consist eventually of only medulla and a thickened fibrous capsule (Fig. 7–33). Some investigators have reported complete loss of the gland, but this is most likely due to the inability to locate the tiny medulla in perirenal fat.

Focal lymphocytic infiltration, mainly T cells,[450] can be found in adrenal glands of patients with no evidence of clinical dysfunction[451] and appears to increase with age. Whether this represents subclinical disease is unknown.

Infectious Diseases

Tuberculosis

In developed countries, tuberculosis is now less common as a cause of Addison's disease, but it should be considered if the adrenals are enlarged or there is calcification on scanning.[452, 453] It is still the leading cause in developing countries. There is almost always a past history of tuberculosis. However, although about 50% of patients with disseminated tuberculosis have adrenal lesions, fewer than 2% have adrenal insufficiency.[454] The glands are usually enlarged and replaced by fibrocaseous tissue. Both medulla and cortex are involved, showing caseous necrosis, with a chronic inflammatory infiltrate and Langhan-type giant cells (Fig. 7–34), although full-blown epithelioid granulomas are less common than in other sites, suggesting that glucocorticoids may inhibit their formation. Special stains for acid/alcohol-fast bacilli or polymerase chain reaction may demonstrate the presence of mycobacteria.

Other Bacterial Infections

Other bacterial infections are rare, and most occur in children. They often follow adrenal hemorrhage, with unilateral adrenal abscess formation.[455-457] Spread is probably hematogenous, and *Escherichia coli,* group B streptococci, and *Bacteroides* are most commonly involved.[457] Local spread may involve the kidney or spleen.[458, 459] Abscesses are rare in adults but may be a rare complication of fine-needle aspiration.[460] Syphilis may occasionally cause adrenal

Figure 7–33. Autoimmune Addison's disease. The figure shows the remnants of an adrenal gland composed of the central medulla surrounded by inflamed fibrous tissue. The adrenal cortex has been largely destroyed by the inflammatory process.

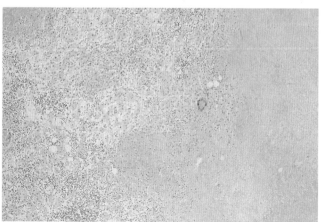

Figure 7–34. Addison's disease caused by tuberculosis. There is granulomatous inflammation of the cortex with a Langhan-type giant cell seen in the center of the field and caseous necrosis to the right.

insufficiency, with extensive fibrosis, and gumma formation.[454] Malakoplakia has been reported.[461]

Fungal Infections

Histoplasmosis involves the adrenals in about 80% of cases, with Addison's disease reported in 7%.[462] The adrenals show gross enlargement with caseation. South American[463] and North American[464] blastomycosis, cryptococcosis,[458, 465] coccidioidomycosis,[466] and paracoccidioidomycosis[467, 468] can also cause hypoadrenalism.

Viral Infections

Viral infections are uncommon and usually affect immunocompromised patients, including neonates and those with acquired immunodeficiency syndrome (AIDS; see below). Herpesviruses[469] have been implicated, and neonatal infection with echovirus types 11 and 12 can result in adrenal hemorrhage.[470, 471]

Secondary Cortical Insufficiency

Reduced ACTH secretion as a result of pituitary or hypothalamic disease, exogenous glucocorticoids, or autonomous cortisol production by an adrenal tumor causes cortical atrophy. The glands each weigh less than 2.5 g. The capsule is thickened, and the cortex is reduced in width. The zona glomerulosa is normal and may appear prominent because of the loss of zona fasciculata and reticularis, which consist of only a narrow band of lipid-laden cells. The medulla is normal.

ACUTE ADRENAL INSUFFICIENCY

The increased demands of an infective illness or trauma in a patient with subclinical chronic insufficiency may precipitate an acute episode. The withdrawal of therapeutic steroids can have similar effects. Abdominal symptoms, hypotension, and collapse are the predominant clinical features.

Waterhouse-Friderichsen syndrome is associated most often with meningococcal septicemia in children[472] but also occurs with pneumococcal, staphylococcal, or *Haemophilus influenzae* septicemia; rarely with *Pseudomonas aeruginosa*[473] or *Klebsiella oxytoca*.[474] The vascular collapse is believed to be the result of endotoxemia and disseminated intravascular coagulation rather than adrenal cortical insufficiency, although mineralocorticoid deficiency may contribute to the hypotension. Neonatal infection with echovirus types 11 or 12 can give rise to a similar syndrome.[470, 471]

Adrenal cortical hemorrhage can also occur with anticoagulant therapy or coagulopathies,[475, 476] rarely

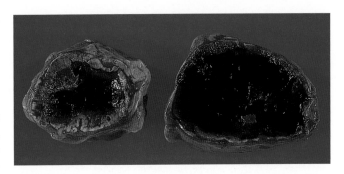

Figure 7–35. Waterhouse-Friderichsen syndrome. There is hemorrhage into both adrenal glands in this patient, who died of septicemia.

as the result of adrenal embolus or adrenal vein thrombosis following trauma.[477, 478] Fatal adrenal hemorrhage has also followed vapor inhalation.[479] Antemortem hypotension may result in minor adrenal hemorrhage confined to the corticomedullary junction.[480] The adrenals may be of normal size but show congestion or hemorrhage, or they may be enlarged (Fig. 7–35). In some cases the hemorrhage extends into the retroperitoneal tissues.

Acquired Immunodeficiency Syndrome

Patients infected with the human immunodeficiency virus without AIDS show evidence of mild abnormalities in the HPA axis.[481–483] Adrenal insufficiency has been reported in AIDS,[484–486] although others have questioned this.[487] The pathologic features of the adrenals in AIDS have not been fully documented.[488, 489] Most show lipid depletion, consistent with stress. Cytomegalovirus infection is common[490, 491] and is usually associated with adrenal hemorrhage and necrosis. Because less than 50% of the gland is usually involved, the necrosis itself is unlikely to result in cortical insufficiency. *Cryptococcus* and *Mycobacterium avium-intracellulare* are identified less commonly. Involvement by Kaposi's sarcoma is seen.[488]

INVOLVEMENT IN SYSTEMIC DISEASES

Small amounts of amyloid may be detected in most cases of systemic amyloidosis, but it is rarely symptomatic.[454] Diffuse involvement is said to be more common in secondary amyloidosis (AA type), with deposition in vessel walls in primary amyloidosis. Stainable iron is often found in the zona glomerulosa in hemochromatosis and hemosiderosis (Fig. 7–36), but it does not affect function.

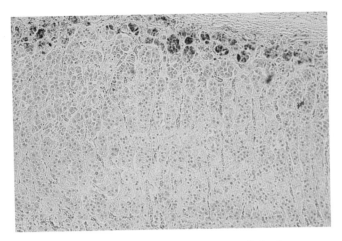

Figure 7-36. In hemochromatosis, intracellular iron accumulates mainly in the zona glomerulosa (Perl's stain).

Effects of Drugs and Other Chemicals on the Adrenal Cortex

A number of drugs may have functional and/or structural effects on the adrenal cortex. Inhibition of cortisol synthesis is reported with metyrapone,[492] the antifungal agent ketoconazole,[493] the anesthetic etomidate,[494] the antiepileptic aminoglutethimide,[495] and suramin, an antiparasitic agent.[496] These are sometimes now used therapeutically for their anti-adrenal effects. Other drugs induce hepatic enzymes responsible for steroid metabolism, and thus increase turnover. These include the antiepileptic phenytoin, rifampicin, and barbiturates.[497] The effects are not usually sufficient to cause hypoadrenalism per se, but they may precipitate it in patients with reduced cortical reserve. Paraquat poisoning may result in extensive adrenocortical necrosis.[497]

References

1. Addison T: On the constitutional and local effects of disease of the suprarenal capsules. 1855. In a collection of the published writings of Thomas Addison, MD, physician to Guy's Hospital, London. New Sydenham Society, London, 1868. Medical Classics 1937; 2:244.
2. Crowder RE: Development of the adrenal gland in man with special reference to origin and ultimate locations of cell types and evidence in favour of cell migration theory. Contrib Embryol 1975; 36:193.
3. Morohashi K: The ontogenesis of the steroidogenic tissues. Genes Cells 1997; 2:95.
4. Burris TP, Guo W, McCabe ER: The gene responsible for adrenal hypoplasia congenita, DAX-1, encodes a nuclear hormone receptor that defines a new class within the superfamily. Recent Prog Horm Res 1996; 51:241.
5. Spencer SJ, Mesiano S, Lee JY, et al.: Proliferation and apoptosis in the human adrenal cortex during the fetal and perinatal periods: Implications for growth and remodeling. J Clin Endocrinol Metab 1999; 84:1110.
6. Oppenheimer EH: Cyst formation in the outer adrenal cortex: Studies in the human fetus and newborn. Arch Pathol 1969; 87:653.
7. Bartman J, Driscoll SG: Fetal adrenal cortex in erythroblastosis fetalis. Arch Pathol 1969; 87:343.
8. Tahka A: On the weight and structure of the adrenal glands and the factors affecting them in children of 0–2 years. Acta Pediatrica 1951; 40:4.
9. Stoner HB, Whiteley HJ, Emery JL: Effect of systemic disease on adrenal cortex of children. J Pathol Bacteriol 1953; 66:171.
10. Sasano N, Sasano H: The adrenal cortex. In Kovacs K, Asa SL, eds.: Functional Endocrine Pathology. Blackwell Scientific Publications, Boston, 1990, p. 546.
11. Studzinski GP, Hay DCF, Symington T: Observations on the weight of the human adrenal gland and the effect of preparations of corticotropin of different purity on the weight and morphology of the human adrenal gland. J Clin Endocrinol Metab 1963; 23:248.
12. Quinan C, Berger AA: Observations on human adrenals with especial reference to the relative weight of the normal medulla. Ann Int Med 1933; 6:1180.
13. Dobbie JW, Symington T: The human adrenal gland with special reference to the vasculature. J Endocrinol 1966; 34:479.
14. De Lellis RA, Wolfe HJ, Gagel RF, et al.: Adrenal medullary hyperplasia: A morphometric analysis in patients with familial medullary thyroid carcinoma. Am J Pathol 1976; 83:177.
15. Cote RJ, Cordon-Cardo C, Reuter VE, et al.: Immunopathology of adrenal and renal cortical tumors: Coordinated change in antigen expression is associated with neoplastic conversion in the adrenal cortex. Am J Pathol 1990; 136:1077.
16. Henzen-Logmans SC, Stel HV, van Muijen GN, et al.: Expression of intermediate filament proteins in adrenal cortex and related tumours. Histopathology 1988; 12:359.
17. Sasano H, Mason JI, Sasano N, et al.: Immunolocalization of 3 beta-hydroxysteroid dehydrogenase in human adrenal cortex and in its disorders. Endocr Pathol 1990; 1:94.
18. Sasano H, Okamoto M, Sasano N: Immunohistochemical study of cytochrome P-450 11 beta-hydroxylase in human adrenal cortex with mineralo- and glucocorticoid excess. Virchows Arch A Pathol Anat Histopathol 1988; 413:313.
19. Sasano H, Sasano N, Okamoto M: Immunohistochemical demonstration of cholesterol side-chain cleavage cytochrome P-450 in bovine and human adrenals. Pathol Res Pract 1989; 184:337.
20. Sasano H, White PC, New MI, et al.: Immunohistochemical localization of cytochrome P-450C21 in human adrenal cortex and its relation to endocrine function. Hum Pathol 1988; 19:181.
21. Sasano H, Mason JI, Sasano N: Immunohistochemical study of cytochrome P-45017 alpha in human adrenocortical disorders. Hum Pathol 1989; 20:113.
22. Erhart-Bornstein M, Hilbers U: Neuroendocrine properties of adrenocortical cells. Horm Metab Res 1998; 30:436.
23. Haak HR, Fleuren GJ: Neuroendocrine differentiation of adrenocortical tumors. Cancer 1995; 75:860.
24. Khoury EL, Greenspan JS, Greenspan FS: Adrenocortical cells of the zona reticularis normally express HLA-DR antigenic determinants. Am J Pathol 1987; 127:580.
25. Khoury EL, Berline JW: HLA-DR expression by adrenocortical cells of the zona reticularis: Structural and allotypic characterization. Tissue Antigens 1988; 31:191.
26. Jackson R, McNicol AM, Farquharson M, et al.: Class II MHC expression in normal adrenal cortex and cortical cells in autoimmune Addison's disease. J Pathol 1988; 155:113.
27. Gros P, Croop J, Housman D: Mammalian multidrug resistance gene: Complete cDNA sequence indicates strong homology to bacterial transport proteins. Cell 1986; 47:371.
28. Yang CP, de Pinho SG, Greenberger LM, et al.: Progesterone interacts with P-glycoprotein in multidrug-resistant cells and in endometrium of gravid uterus. J Biol Chem 1989; 264:782.
29. McCluggage WG, Burton J, Maxwell P, et al.: Immunohistochemical staining of normal, hyperplastic, and neoplastic adrenal cortex with a monoclonal antibody against alpha inhibin. J Clin Pathol 1998; 51:114.
30. Munro LM, Kennedy A, McNicol AM: The expression of inhibin/activin subunits in the human adrenal cortex and its tumours. J Endocrinol 1999; 161:341.
31. Spencer SJ, Rabinovici J, Mesiano S, et al.: Activin and inhibin in the human adrenal gland: Regulation and differential effects in fetal and adult cells. J Clin Invest 1992; 90:142.

32. Asa SL, Henderson J, Goltzman D, et al.: Parathyroid hormone-like peptide in normal and neoplastic human endocrine tissues. J Clin Endocrinol Metab 1990; 71:1112.

33. Kojima I, Lippes H, Kojima K, et al.: Aldosterone secretion: Effect of phorbol ester and A23187. Biochem Biophys Res Commun 1983; 116:555.

34. Busam KJ, Iversen K, Coplan KA, et al.: Immunoreactivity for A103, an antibody to melan-A (Mart-1), in adrenocortical and other steroid tumors. Am J Surg Pathol 1998; 22:57.

35. Magennis DP, McNicol AM: Vascular patterns in the normal and pathological human adrenal cortex. Virchows Arch 1998; 433:69.

36. Gonzalez-Campora R, Montero C, Martin-Lacave I, et al.: Demonstration of vascular endothelium in thyroid carcinomas using Ulex europaeus I agglutinin. Histopathology 1986; 10:261.

37. McNicol AM, Richmond J, Charlton BG: A study of general innervation of the human adrenal cortex using PGP 9.5 immunohistochemistry. Acta Anat 1994; 151:120.

38. Kendall CH, Sanderson PR, Cope J, et al.: Follicular thyroid tumours: A study of laminin and type IV collagen in basement membrane and endothelium. J Clin Pathol 1985; 38:1100.

39. Tannenbaum M: Ultrastructural pathology of the adrenal cortex. Pathol Annu 1973; 8:109.

40. Mackay AM: Atlas of human adrenal cortex ultrastructure. In Symington T, ed.: Functional Pathology of the Human Adrenal Gland. Churchill Livingstone, Edinburgh, 1969, p. 346.

41. Neville AM, O'Hare MJ: The Human Adrenal Cortex: Pathology and Biology—An Integrated Approach. Springer-Verlag, Berlin, 1982.

42. Merklin RJ: Suprarenal gland lymphatic drainage. Am J Anat 1966; 119:359.

43. Moskowitz MS: Diseases of the autonomic nervous system. Clin Endocrinol Metab 1977; 6:745.

44. Neville A: The adrenal medulla. In Symington T, ed.: Functional Pathology of the Human Adrenal Gland. Churchill Livingstone, Edinburgh, 1969, p. 217.

45. Mikhail Y, Amin F: Intrinsic innervation of the human adrenal gland. Acta Anat 1969; 72:25.

46. Charlton BG, Nkomazana OF, McGadey J, et al.: A preliminary study of acetylcholinesterase-positive innervation in the human adrenal cortex. J Anat 1991; 176:99.

47. Heym C, Braun B, Shuyi Y, et al.: Immunohistochemical correlation of human adrenal nerve fibers and thoracic dorsal root neurons with special reference to substance P. Histochem Cell Biol 1995; 104:233.

48. Engeland WC, Lilly MP, Gann DS: Sympathetic adrenal denervation decreases adrenal blood flow without altering the cortisol response to hemorrhage. Endocrinology 1985; 117:1000.

49. Kleitman N, Holzwarth MA: Compensatory adrenal cortical growth is inhibited by sympathectomy. Am J Physiol 1985; 248:E261.

50. Dorovni-Zis K, Zis AP: Innervation of the zona fasciculata of the human adrenal cortex: A light and electron microscopic study. J Neural Transm 1991; 84:75.

51. McNicol AM, Duffy AE: A study of cell migration in the adrenal cortex of the rat using bromodeoxyuridine. Cell Tissue Kinet 1987; 20:519.

52. Wright NA, Voncina D, Morley AR: An attempt to demonstrate cell migration from the zona glomerulosa in the prepubertal male rat adrenal cortex. J Endocrinol 1973; 59:451.

53. Race CJ, Green RF: Studies on zonation and regeneration of the adrenal cortex of the rat. Am Med Assoc Arch Pathol 1955; 59:59.

54. McEwan PE, Lindop GB, Kenyon CJ: In vivo studies of the control of DNA synthesis in the rat adrenal cortex and medulla. Endocr Res 1995; 21:91.

55. Carr I: The human adrenal cortex at the time of death. J Pathol Bacteriol 1959; 78:533.

56. Wyllie AH, Kerr JF, Macaskill IA, et al.: Adrenocortical cell deletion: The role of ACTH. J Pathol 1973; 111:85.

57. Nickerson PA: Quantitative study on the effect of an ACTH-producing pituitary tumor on the ultrastructure of the mouse adrenal gland. Am J Pathol 1975; 80:295.

58. Nussdorfer GG, Mazzocchi G, Rebonato LZ: Long term trophic effect of ACTH on rat adrenocortical cells. Z Zellforsch Mikrosk Anat 1971; 115:30.

59. Malendowicz LK: Correlated stereological and functional studies on the long-term effect of ACTH on rat adrenal cortex. Folia Histochem Cytobiol 1986; 24:203.

60. Estivariz FE, Iturriza FC, Hope J, et al.: Stimulation of adrenal mitogenesis by N-terminal proopiocortin peptide. Nature 1982; 297:419.

61. Hornsby PJ: Regulation of adrenocortical cell proliferation in culture. Endocr Res 1984; 10:259.

62. Vinson GP, Pudney JA, Whitehouse BJ: The mammalian adrenal circulation and the relationship between adrenal blood flow and steroidogenesis. J Endocrinol 1985; 105:285.

63. Payet N, Deziel Y, Lehoux JG. Vasopressin: A potent growth factor in adrenal glomerulosa cells in culture. J Steroid Biochem 1984; 20:449.

64. McEwan PE, Lindop GB, Kenyon CJ: Control of cell proliferation in the rat adrenal gland in vivo by the renin-angiotensin system. Am J Physiol 1996; 271:E192.

65. Gill GN, Ill CR, Simonian MH: Angiotensin stimulation of bovine adrenocortical cell growth. Proc Natl Acad Sci U S A 1977; 74:5569.

66. Gospodarowicz D, Hadley HH: Stimulation of division of Y1 adrenal cells by growth factor isolated from bovine pituitary glands. Endocrinology 1975; 97:102.

67. Feige JJ, Baird A: Growth factor regulation of adrenal cortex growth and function. Prog Growth Factor Res 1991; 3:103.

68. Nussdorfer GG, Mazzocchi G: Immune-endocrine interactions in the mammalian adrenal gland: Facts and hypotheses. Int Rev Cytol 1998; 183:143.

69. Naaman E, Chatelain P, Saez JM, et al.: In vitro effect of insulin and insulin-like growth factor I on cell multiplication and adrenocorticotropin responsiveness of fetal adrenal cells. Biol Reprod 1989; 40:570.

70. van Dijk JP, Tanswell AK, Challis JRG: Insulin-like growth factor (IGF)-II and insulin, but not IGF-I, are mitogenic for fetal rat adrenal cells in vitro. J Endocrinol 1988; 119:509.

71. Sasano H, Suzuki T, Shizawa S, et al.: Transforming growth factor alpha, epidermal growth factor, and epidermal growth factor receptor expression in normal and diseased human adrenal cortex by immunohistochemistry and in situ hybridization. Mod Pathol 1994; 7:741.

72. Mesiano S, Jaffe RB: Role of growth factors in the developmental regulation of the human fetal adrenal cortex. Steroids 1997; 62:62.

73. McAllister JM, Hornsby PJ: Improved clonal and nonclonal growth of human, rat and bovine adrenocortical cells in culture. In Vitro Cell Dev Biol 1987; 23:677.

74. Riopel L, Branchaud CL, Godyer CG, et al.: Growth-inhibitory effects of TGF-beta on human fetal adrenal cells in primary monolayer culture. J Cell Physiol 1989; 140:233.

75. Spencer SJ, Rabinovici J, Jaffe RB: Human recombinant activin-A inhibits proliferation of human fetal adrenal cells in vitro. J Clin Endocrinol Metab 1990; 71:1678.

76. Gwynne JT, Strauss JF: The role of lipoprotein in steroidogenesis and cholesterol metabolism in steroidogenic glands. Endocr Rev 1982; 3:299.

77. Brown MS, Kovanen PT, Goldstein JL: Receptor mediated uptake of lipoprotein-cholesterol and its utilization for steroid synthesis in the adrenal cortex. Recent Prog Horm Res 1979; 35:215.

78. Kallen CB, Arakane F, Christenson LK, et al.: Unveiling the mechanism of action and regulation of the steroidogenic acute regulatory protein. Mol Cell Endocrinol 1998; 145:39.

79. Orth DN, Kovacs WJ, DeBold CR: The adrenal cortex. In Wilson JD, Foster DW, eds.: Williams Textbook of Endocrinology, 8th ed. WB Saunders, Philadelphia, 1992, p. 489.

80. Fraser R: Biosynthesis of adrenocortical steroids. In James VHT, ed.: The Adrenal Gland, 2nd ed. Raven Press, New York, 1992, p. 117.

81. Rainey WE: Adrenal zonation: Clues from 11beta-hydroxylase and aldosterone synthase. Mol Cell Endocrinol 1999; 151:151.

82. Sasano H, Sasano N, Okamoto M, et al.: Immunohistochemical demonstration of adrenodoxin reductase in bovine and human adrenals. Pathol Res Pract 1989; 184:473.

83. Cameron EHD, Jones T, Jones D, et al.: Further studies on the relationship between C-19 and C-21 steroid synthesis. J Endocrinol 1969; 45:215.

84. Kennerson AR, McDonald DA, Adams JB: Dehydroepiandrosterone sulfotransferase localization in human adrenal glands: A light and electron microscopic study. J Clin Endocrinol Metab 1983; 56:786.

85. Penhoat A, Jaillard C, Saez JM: Identification and characterization of corticotropin receptors in bovine and human adrenals. J Steroid Biochem Mol Biol 1993; 44:21.

86. Cooke BA: Signal transduction involving cyclic AMP–dependent and cyclic AMP–independent mechanisms in the control of steroidogenesis. Mol Cell Endocrinol 1999; 151:25.

87. Waterman MR, Bischof LJ: Mechanisms of ACTH (cAMP)–dependent transcription of adrenal steroid hydroxylases. Endocr Res 1996; 22:615.

88. Keller-Wood ME, Dallman MF: Corticosteroid inhibition of ACTH secretion. Endocr Rev 1984; 5:1.

89. Tian Y, Baukal AJ, Sandberg K, et al.: Properties of AT1a and AT1b angiotensin receptors expressed in adrenocortical Y-1 cells. Am J Physiol 1996; 270:E831.

90. Parker LN: Adrenarche. Endocrinol Metab Clin North Am 1991; 20:71.

91. Fottner C, Engelhardt D, Weber MM: Regulation of steroidogenesis by insulin-like growth factors (IGFs) in adult human adrenocortical cells: IGF-I and, more potently, IGF-II preferentially enhance androgen biosynthesis through interaction with the IGF-I receptor and IGF-binding proteins. J Endocrinol 1998; 158:409.

92. Gallo-Payet N, Guillon G: Regulation of adrenocortical function by vasopressin. Horm Metab Res 1998; 30:360.

93. Lebrethon MC, Jaillard C, Naville D, et al.: Effects of transforming growth factor-beta 1 on human adrenocortical fasciculata-reticularis cell-differentiated functions. J Clin Endocrinol Metab 1994; 79:1033.

94. Rainey WE, Naville D, Saez JM, et al.: Transforming growth factor-beta inhibits steroid 17 alpha-hydroxylase cytochrome P-450 expression in ovine adrenocortical cells. Endocrinology 1990; 127:1910.

95. Ehrhart-Bornstein M, Bornstein SR, Gonzalez-Hernandez J, et al.: Sympathoadrenal regulation of adrenocortical steroidogenesis. Endocr Res 1995; 21:13.

96. Haidan A, Bornstein SR, Glasow A, et al.: Basal steroidogenic activity of adrenocortical cells is increased 10-fold by coculture with chromaffin cells. Endocrinology 1998; 139:772.

97. Rosner W. The function of corticosteroid-binding globulin and sex hormone–binding globulin: Recent advances. Endocr Rev 1990; 11:80.

98. Edwards CR, Benediktsson R, Lindsay RS, et al.: 11 Beta-hydroxysteroid dehydrogenases: Key enzymes in determining tissue-specific glucocorticoid effects. Steroids 1996; 61:263.

99. Carson-Jurica MA, Schrader WT, O'Malley BW: Steroid receptor family: Structure and functions. Endocr Rev 1990; 11:201.

100. King RJB: Effects of steroid hormones and related compounds on gene transcription. Clin Endocrinol 1992; 36:1.

101. Graham LS: Celiac accessory adrenal glands. Cancer 1953; 6:149.

102. Nelson AA: Accessory adrenal cortical tissue. Arch Pathol 1939; 27:955.

103. Mares AJ, Shkolnik A, Sacks M: Aberrant (ectopic) adrenocortical tissue along the spermatic cord. J Pediatr Surg 1980; 15:289.

104. Dahl EV, Bahn RC: Aberrant adrenal cortical tissue near the testis in human infants. Am J Pathol 1962; 40:587.

105. MacLennan A: On the presence of adrenal rests in hernial sac walls. Surg Gynecol Obstet 1919; 29:387.

106. Qureshi F, Jacques SM: Adrenocortical heterotopia in the placenta. Pediatr Pathol Lab Med 1995; 15:51.

107. Busuttil A: Ectopic adrenal within the gall-bladder wall. J Pathol 1974; 113:231.

108. Bozic C: Ectopic fetal adrenal cortex in the lung of a newborn. Virchows Arch (Pathol Anat) 1974; 363:371.

109. Armin A, Castelli M: Congenital adrenal tissue in the lung with adrenal cytomegaly: Case report and review of the literature. Am J Clin Pathol 1984; 82:225.

110. Wiener MF, Dallgaard SA: Intracranial adrenal gland: A case report. Arch Pathol 1959; 67:228.

111. Dolan MF, Janovski NA: Adreno-hepatic union. Arch Pathol 1968; 86:22.

112. Culp OS: Adrenal heterotopia: A survey of the literature and report of a case. J Urol 1939; 41:303.

113. O'Crowley CR, Martland HS. Adrenal heterotopia, rests and the so-called Grawitz tumor. J Urol 1943; 50:756.

114. D'Cruz C, Huff D, deSa D, et al.: Fused adrenals in the Cornelia de Lange syndrome. Lab Invest 1987; 56:IP.

115. Bech K: Cytomegaly of the foetal adrenal cortex. Acta Pathol Microbiol Scand (A) 1971; 79:279.

116. Craig JM, Landing BH: Anaplastic cells of fetal adrenal cortex. Am J Clin Pathol 1951; 21:940.

117. Favara BE, Steele A, Grant JH, et al.: Adrenal cytomegaly: Quantitative assessment by image analysis. Pediatr Pathol 1991; 11:521.

118. Pettenati MJ, Haines JL, Higgins RR, et al.: Wiedemann-Beckwith syndrome: Presentation of clinical and cytogenetic data on 22 new cases and review of the literature. Hum Genet 1986; 74:143.

119. McCauley RG, Beckwith JB, Elias ER, et al.: Benign hemorrhagic adrenocortical macrocysts in Beckwith-Wiedemann syndrome. AJR Am J Roentgenol 1991; 157:549.

120. Akata D, Haliloglu M, Ozmen MN, et al.: Bilateral cystic adrenal masses in the neonate associated with the incomplete form of Beckwith-Wiedemann syndrome. Pediatr Radiol 1997; 27:1.

121. Wiedemann HR: Tumors and hemihypertrophy associated with Wiedemann-Beckwith syndrome. Eur J Pediatr 1983; 141:129.

122. Wolman M, Sterk VV, Gratl S, et al.: Primary familial xanthomatosis with involvement and calcification of the adrenal. Pediatrics 1961; 28:742.

123. Elleder M, Smid F: Adrenal changes in Niemann-Pick disease: Differences between sphingomyelinase deficiency and type C. Acta Histochem 1985; 76:163.

124. Crocker AC, Farber S: Niemann-Pick disease: A review of eighteen patients. Medicine 1958; 37:1.

125. Zanaria E, Muscatelli F, Bardoni B, et al.: An unusual member of the nuclear hormone receptor superfamily responsible for X-linked adrenal hypoplasia congenita. Nature 1994; 372:635.

126. Golden MP, Lippe BM, Kaplan SA: Congenital adrenal hypoplasia and hypogonadotropic hypogonadism. Am J Dis Child 1977; 131:1117.

127. Guggenheim MA, McCabe ERB, Roig M, et al.: Glycerol kinase deficiency with neuromuscular, skeletal and adrenal abnormalities. Ann Neurol 1980; 7:441.

128. Wise JE, Matalon R, Morgan AM, et al.: Phenotypic features of patients with congenital adrenal hypoplasia and glycerol kinase deficiency. Am J Dis Child 1987; 141:744.

129. Peter M, Viemann M, Partsch CJ, et al.: Congenital adrenal hypoplasia: Clinical spectrum, experience with hormonal diagnosis, and report on new point mutations of the DAX-1 gene. J Clin Endocrinol Metab 1998; 83:2666.

130. Benirschke K. Adrenals in anencephaly and hydrocephaly. Obstet Gynecol 1956; 8:412.

131. van Hale HM, Turkel SB: Neuroblastoma and adrenal morphologic features in anencephalic infants. Arch Pathol 1979; 103:119.

132. Aterman K, Kerenyi N, Lee M: Adrenal cytomegaly. Virchows Arch (Pathol Anat) 1972; 355:105.

133. de Luis DA, Aller R, Romero E: Isolated ACTH deficiency. Horm Res 1998; 49:247.

134. Aimone V, Campagnoli C: Severe adrenal hypoplasia in a live-born normocephalic infant with neurohypophyseal aplasia. Am J Obstet Gynecol 1970; 107:327.

135. Geffner ME, Lippe BM, Kaplan SA, et al.: Selective ACTH insensitivity, achalasia and alacrima: A multisystem disorder presenting in childhood. Pediatr Res 1983; 17:532.

136. Shephard TH, Landing BH, Mason DG: Familial Addison's disease: Case report of two sisters with corticoid deficiency unassociated with hypoaldosteronism. Am J Dis Child 1959; 97:154.

137. Slavotinek AM, Hurst JA, Dunger D, et al.: ACTH receptor mutation in a girl with familial glucocorticoid deficiency. Clin Genet 1998; 53:57.

138. Tsigos C, Arai K, Latronico AC, et al.: A novel mutation of the adrenocorticotropin receptor (ACTH-R) gene in a family with the syndrome of isolated glucocorticoid deficiency, but no ACTH-R abnormalities in two families with the triple A syndrome. J Clin Endocrinol Metab 1995; 80:2186.

139. Heinrichs C, Tsigos C, Deschepper J, et al.: Familial adrenocorticotropin unresponsiveness associated with alacrima and achalasia: Biochemical and molecular studies in two siblings with clinical heterogeneity. Eur J Pediatr 1995; 154:191.

140. Kelch RP, Kaplan SL, Biglieri EG, et al.: Hereditary adrenal cortical unresponsiveness to ACTH. J Pediatr 1972; 81:726.

141. Hudson JB, Chobanian AV, Relman AS: Hypoaldosteronism: A clinical study of a patient with an isolated adrenal mineralocorticoid deficiency, resulting in hyperkalemia and Stokes-Adams attacks. N Engl J Med 1957; 257:529.

142. White PC: Abnormalities of aldosterone synthesis and action in children. Curr Opin Pediatr 1997; 9:424.

143. Smith KD, Kemp S, Braiterman LT, et al.: X-linked adrenoleukodystrophy: Genes, mutations, and phenotypes. Neurochem Res 1999; 24:521.

144. Savary S, Troffer-Charlier N, Gyapay G, et al.: Chromosomal localization of the adrenoleukodystrophy-related gene in man and mice. Eur J Hum Genet 1997; 5:99.

145. Krasemann EW, Meier V, Korenke GC, et al.: Identification of mutations in the ALD-gene of 20 families with adrenoleukodystrophy/adrenomyeloneuropathy. Hum Genet 1996; 97:194.

146. Dodd A, Rowland SA, Hawkes SL, et al.: Mutations in the adrenoleukodystrophy gene. Hum Mutat 1997; 9:500.

147. Laureti S, Casucci G, Santeusanio F, et al.: X-linked adrenoleukodystrophy is a frequent cause of idiopathic Addison's disease in young adult male patients. J Clin Endocrinol Metab 1996; 81:470.

148. Goldfischer S, Powers JM, Johnson AB, et al.: Striated adrenocortical cells in cerebro-hepato-renal (Zellweger) syndrome. Virchows Arch (Pathol Anat) 1983; 401:355.

149. New MI: Diagnosis and management of congenital adrenal hyperplasia. Annu Rev Med 1998; 49:311.

150. Dupont B, Oberfield SE, Smithwick EM, et al.: Close genetic linkage between HLA and congenital adrenal hyperplasia (21-hydroxylase deficiency). Lancet 1977; 1309.

151. White PC, New MI, Dupont B: Structure of the human steroid 21-hydroxylase genes. Proc Natl Acad Sci U S A 1986; 83:5111.

152. Wilson RC, Mercado AB, Cheng KC, et al.: Steroid 21-hydroxylase deficiency: Genotype may not predict phenotype. J Clin Endocrinol Metab 1995; 80:2322.

153. Speiser PW, Dupont B, Rubinstein P, et al.: High frequency of nonclassical steroid 21-hydroxylase deficiency. Am J Hum Genet 1985; 37:650.

154. Newmark S, Dluhy RG, Williams GH, et al.: Partial 11- and 21-hydroxylase deficiencies in hirsute women. Am J Obstet Gynecol 1977; 127:594.

155. New MI, Crawford C, Wilson RC: Genetic disorders of the adrenal steroidogenic enzymes. In Emery AEH, Rimoin D, eds.: Principles and Practice of Medical Genetics, 3rd ed. Churchill Livingstone, New York, 1996, p. 1441.

156. Rheaume E, Simard J, Morel Y, et al.: Congenital adrenal hyperplasia due to point mutations in the type II 3 beta-hydroxysteroid dehydrogenase gene. Nat Genet 1992; 1:239.

157. Simard J, Rheaume E, Sanchez R, et al.: Molecular basis of congenital adrenal hyperplasia due to 3 beta-hydroxysteroid dehydrogenase deficiency. Mol Endocrinol 1993; 7:716.

158. Pang S, Levine LS, Stoner E, et al.: Nonsalt-losing congenital adrenal hyperplasia due to 3 beta-hydroxysteroid dehydrogenase deficiency with normal glomerulosa function. J Clin Endocrinol Metab 1983; 56:808.

159. Lack EE, Kosakewich HP: Embryology, developmental anatomy, and selected aspects of non-neoplastic pathology. In Lack EE, ed.: Pathology of the Adrenal Glands. Churchill Livingstone, New York, 1990, p. 1.

160. Jaresch S, Kornely E, Kley HK, et al.: Adrenal incidentaloma and patients with homozygous or heterozygous congenital adrenal hyperplasia. J Clin Endocrinol Metab 1992; 74:685.

161. Pang S, Becksen D, Cotelingham J, et al.: Adrenocortical tumor in a patient with congenital adrenal hyperplasia due to a 21-hydroxylase deficiency. Pediatrics 1981; 68:242.

162. Hamwi GJ, Serbin RA, Kruger FA: Does adrenocortical hyperplasia result in adrenocortical carcinoma? N Engl J Med 1957; 257:1153.

163. Condom E, Villabona CM, Gomez JM, et al.: Adrenal myelolipoma in a woman with congenital 17-hydroxylase deficiency. Arch Pathol Lab Med 1985; 109:1116.

164. Boudreaux D, Waisman J, Skinner DG, et al.: Giant adrenal myelolipoma and testicular interstitial cell tumor in a man with congenital 21-hydroxylase deficiency. Am J Surg Pathol 1979; 3:109.

165. Avila NA, Shawker TS, Jones JV, et al.: Testicular adrenal rest tissue in congenital adrenal hyperplasia: Serial sonographic and clinical findings. Am J Roentgenol 1999; 172:1235.

166. Willi U, Atares M, Prader A, et al.: Testicular adrenal-like tissue (TALT) in congenital adrenal hyperplasia: Detection by ultrasonography. Pediatr Radiol 1991; 21:284.

167. Rutgers JL, Young RH, Scully RE: The testicular "tumor" of the adrenogenital syndrome: A report of six cases and review of the literature on testicular masses in patients with adrenocortical disorders. Am J Surg Pathol 1988; 12:503.

168. Kirkland RT, Kirkland JL, Keenan BS, et al.: Bilateral testicular tumors in congenital adrenal hyperplasia. J Clin Endocrinol Metab 1977; 44:369.

169. Caron KM, Soo SC, Parker KL: Targeted disruption of StAR provides novel insights into congenital adrenal hyperplasia. Endocr Res 1998; 24:827.

170. Willenberg HS, Bornstein SR, Dumser T, et al.: Morphological changes in adrenals from victims of suicide in relation to altered apoptosis. Endocr Res 1998; 24:963.

171. Rich AR: A peculiar type of adrenal cortical damage associated with acute infections and its possible relation to circulatory collapse. Bull Johns Hopkins Hosp 1944; 74:1.

172. Sarason EL: Adrenal cortex in systemic disease: A morphological study. Arch Int Med 1943; 71:702.

173. Meador CK, Bowdoin B, Owen WC Jr., et al.: Primary adrenocortical nodular dysplasia: A rare cause of Cushing's syndrome. J Clin Endocrinol Metab 1967; 27:1255.

174. Chute AL, Robinson CG, Donohue WC: Cushing's syndrome in children. J Pediatr 1949; 34:20.

175. Lacroix A, Bolte E, Tremblay J, et al.: Gastric inhibitory polypeptide-dependent cortisol hypersecretion: A new cause of Cushing's syndrome. N Engl J Med 1992; 327:974.

176. Lebrethon MC, Avallet O, Reznik Y, et al.: Food-dependent Cushing's syndrome: Characterization and functional role of gastric inhibitory polypeptide receptor in the adrenals of three patients. J Clin Endocrinol Metab 1998; 83:4514.

177. Nakane T, Kuwayama A, Watanabe M, et al.: Long-term results of transsphenoidal adenomectomy in patients with Cushing's disease. Neurosurgery 1987; 21:218.

178. Tyrrell JB, Brooks RM, Fitzgerald PA, et al.: Cushing's disease: Selective transsphenoidal resection of pituitary microadenomas. N Engl J Med 1978; 298:753.

179. McNicol AM. Patterns of corticotropic cells in the adult human pituitary in Cushing's disease. Diagn Histopathol 1981; 4:335–341.

180. Neville AM, Symington T: The pathology of the adrenal gland in Cushing's syndrome. J Pathol Bacteriol 1967; 93:19.

181. Doppman JL, Miller DL, Dwyer AJ, et al.: Macronodular adrenocortical hyperplasia in long-standing Cushing's disease. Radiology 1988; 166:347.

182. Neville AM: The nodular adrenal. Invest Cell Pathol 1978; 1:99.

183. Smals AGH, Pieters G, van Haelst VJG, et al.: Macronodular adrenocortical hyperplasia in long-standing Cushing's disease. J Clin Endocrinol Metab 1984; 58:25.

184. Sturrock ND, Morgan L, Jeffcoate WJ: Autonomous nodular hyperplasia of the adrenal cortex: Tertiary hypercortisolism? Clin Endocrinol (Oxf) 1995; 43:753.

185. Choi Y, Werk EE Jr., Sholiton LJ: Cushing's syndrome with dual pituitary-adrenal control. Arch Intern Med 1970; 125:1045.

186. Anderson DC, Child DF, Sutcliffe CH, et al.: Cushing's syndrome, nodular adrenal hyperplasia and virilizing carcinoma. Clin Endocrinol 1978; 9:1.

187. Hashida Y, Kenny FM, Yunis EJ: Ultrastructure of the adrenal cortex in Cushing's disease in children. Hum Pathol 1970; 1:595.

188. Jey RK, van Heerden JA, Carpenter PC, et al.: Ectopic ACTH syndrome: Diagnostic and therapeutic aspects. Am J Surg 1985; 149:276.

189. Singer W, Kovacs K, Ryan N, et al.: Ectopic ACTH syndrome: Clinicopathological correlations. J Clin Pathol 1978; 31:591.

190. Wick MR, Rosai J: Neuroendocrine neoplasms of the thymus. Pathol Res Pract 1988; 183:188.

191. Howlett TA, Drury PL, Perry L, et al.: Diagnosis and management of ACTH-dependent Cushing's syndrome: Comparison of the features in ectopic and pituitary ACTH production. Clin Endocrinol 1986; 24:699.

192. Ball SG, Davison JM, Burt AD, et al.: Cushing's syndrome secondary to ectopic ACTH secretion from a primary ovarian carcinoma. Clin Endocrinol (Oxf) 1996; 45:775.

193. Carey RM, Varma SK, Drake CR Jr., et al.: Ectopic secretion of corticotropin-releasing factor as a cause of Cushing's syndrome: A clinical, morphologic, and biochemical study. N Engl J Med 1984; 311:13.

194. Schteingart DE, Lloyd RV, Akil H, et al.: Cushing's syndrome secondary to ectopic corticotropin-releasing hormone adrenocorticotropin secretion. J Clin Endocrinol Metab 1986; 63:770.

195. Zarate A, Kovacs K, Flores M, et al.: ACTH and CRF-producing bronchial carcinoid associated with Cushing's syndrome. Clin Endocrinol (Oxf) 1986; 24:523.

196. Findling JW, Tyrrell JB: Occult ectopic secretion of corticotropin. Arch Intern Med 1986; 146:929.

197. Kovacs K, Horvath E, Singer W, et al.: Fine structure of adrenal cortex in ectopic ACTH syndrome. Endokrinologie 1977; 69:94.

198. Neville AM, Mackay AM: The structure of the human adrenal cortex in health and disease. Clin Endocrinol Metab 1972; 1:361.

199. Gold EM: The Cushing syndromes: Changing views of diagnosis and treatment. Ann Intern Med 1979; 90:829.

200. Heinbecker P, O'Neal LW, Ackerman LV: Functioning and nonfunctioning adrenal cortical tumors. Surg Gynecol Obstet 1957; 105:21.

201. Orth DN, Liddle GW: Results of treatment in 108 patients with Cushing's syndrome. N Engl J Med 1971; 285:243.

202. Bertagna X, Orth DN: Clinical and laboratory findings and results of therapy in 58 patients with adrenocortical tumors admitted to a single medical center (1951 to 1978). Am J Med 1981; 71:855.

203. Aiba M, Kawakami M, Ito Y, et al.: Bilateral adrenocortical adenomas causing Cushing's syndrome: Report of two cases with enzyme histochemical and ultrastructural studies and a review of the literature. Arch Pathol Lab Med 1992; 116:146.

204. Aiba M, Hirayama A, Iri H, et al.: Adrenocorticotropic hormone-independent bilateral adrenocortical macronodular hyperplasia as a distinct subtype of Cushing's syndrome: Enzyme histochemical and ultrastructural study of four cases with a review of the literature. Am J Clin Pathol 1991; 96:334.

205. Doppman JL, Nieman LK, Travis WD, et al.: CT and MR imaging of massive macronodular adrenocortical disease: A rare cause of autonomous primary adrenal hypercorticism. J Comput Assist Tomogr 1991; 15:773.

206. Swain JM, Grant CS, Schlinkert RT, et al.: Corticotropin-independent macronodular adrenal hyperplasia: A clinicopathologic correlation. Arch Surg 1998; 133:541.

207. Sasano H, Suzuki T, Nagura H: ACTH-independent macronodular adrenocortical hyperplasia: Immunohistochemical and in situ hybridization studies of steroidogenic enzymes. Mod Pathol 1994; 7:215.

208. Schweizer-Cagianut M, Froesch ER, Hedinger EC: Familial Cushing's syndrome with primary adrenocortical microadenomatosis (primary adrenocortical nodular dysplasia). Acta Endocrinol 1980; 94:529.

209. Shenoy BV, Carpenter PC, Carney JA: Bilateral primary pigmented nodular adrenocortical disease: Rare cause of the Cushing syndrome. Am J Surg Pathol 1984; 8:335.

210. Ruder HJ, Loriaux DL, Lipsett MB: Severe osteopenia in young adults associated with Cushing's syndrome due to micronodular adrenal disease. J Clin Endocrinol 1974; 39:1138.

211. Lack EE, Travis WD, Oertel JE: Adrenal cortical nodules, hyperplasia and hyperfunction. In Lack EE, ed. Pathology of the Adrenal Gland. Churchill Livingstone, New York, 1990, p. 75.

212. Larsen JL, Cathey WJ, Odell WD: Primary adrenocortical nodular dysplasia, a distinct subtype of Cushing's syndrome. Case report and review of the literature. Am J Med 1986; 80:976.

213. Degennes J-L, Garnier H, Calmette M, et al.: Etude clinique, biologique et histologique d'un cas exemplaire de polymicroadenomatose corticosurrenale. Ann Endocrinol (Paris) 1970; 31:1022.

214. Tieding van Berkhout F, Croughs RJM, Kater L, et al.: Familial Cushing's syndrome due to nodular adrenocortical dysplasia: A putative receptor-antibody disease? Clin Endocrinol 1986; 24:299.

215. Cartensen H, Krabbe S, Wulffraat NM, et al.: Autoimmune involvement in Cushing syndrome due to primary adrenocortical nodular dysplasia. Eur J Pediatr 1989; 149:84.

216. Schweizer-Cagianut M, Salomon F, Hedinger EC: Primary adrenocortical nodular dysplasia with Cushing's syndrome and cardiac myxomas. Virchows Arch (Pathol Anat) 1982; 397:183.

217. Danoff A, Jormark S, Lorber D, et al.: Adrenocortical nodular dysplasia, cardiac myxomas, lentigines and spindle cell tumors. Arch Intern Med 1987; 147:443.

218. Carney JA, Gordon H, Carpenter PC, et al.: The complex of myxomas, spotty pigmentation, and endocrine overactivity. Medicine (Baltimore) 1985; 64:270.

219. Stratakis CA, Carney JA, Lin JP, et al.: Carney complex, a familial multiple neoplasia and lentiginosis syndrome: Analysis of 11 kindreds and linkage to the short arm of chromosome 2. J Clin Invest 1996; 97:699.

220. Casey M, Mah C, Merliss AD, et al.: Identification of a novel genetic locus for familial cardiac myxomas and Carney complex. Circulation 1998; 98:2560.

221. Conn JW: Primary aldosteronism, a new clinical entity. J Lab Clin Med 1955; 45:6.

222. Favre L, Jacot-des-Combes E, Morel P, et al.: Primary aldosteronism with bilateral adrenal adenomas. Virchows Arch A (Pathol Anat) 1980; 388:229.

223. Watanabe N, Tsunoda K, Sasano H, et al.: Bilateral aldosterone-producing adenomas in two patients diagnosed by immunohistochemical analysis of steroidogenic enzymes. Tohoku J Exp Med 1996; 179:123.

224. Dunnick NR, Leight GS Jr., Roubidoux MA, et al.: CT in the diagnosis of primary aldosteronism: Sensitivity in 29 patients. Am J Roentgenol 1993; 160:321.

225. Young WF Jr., Hogan MJ, Klee GG, et al.: Primary aldosteronism: Diagnosis and treatment. Mayo Clin Proc 1990; 65:96.

226. Neville AM, Symington T: Pathology of primary hyperaldosteronism. Cancer 1966; 19:1854.

227. Melby JC: Diagnosis of hyperaldosteronism. Endocrinol Metab Clin North Am 1991; 20:247.

228. Eto T, Kumamoto K, Kawasaki T, et al.: Ultrastructural types of cell in adrenal cortical adenoma with primary aldosteronism. J Pathol 1979; 128:1.

229. Caplan RH, Virata RL: Functional black adenoma of the adrenal cortex: A rare cause of primary aldosteronism. Am J Clin Pathol 1974; 62:97.

230. Telner AH: Adrenal cortical carcinoma: An unusual cause of hyperaldosteronism. Can Med Assoc J 1983; 129:731.

231. Weingartner K, Gerharz EW, Bittinger A, et al.: Isolated clinical syndrome of primary aldosteronism in a patient with adrenocortical carcinoma: Case report and review of the literature. Urol Int 1995; 55:232.

232. Davis DA, Medline NM: Spironolactone (Aldactone) bodies: Concentric lamellar formations in the adrenal cortices of

patients treated with spironolactone. Am J Clin Pathol 1970; 54:22.

233. Jenis EH, Hertzog RW: Effect of spironolactone on the zona glomerulosa of the adrenal cortex: Light and electron microscopy. Arch Pathol 1969; 88:530.

234. Ferris JB, Brown JJ, Fraser R, et al.: Hypertension with aldosterone excess and low plasma renin: Preoperative distinction between patients with and without adrenocortical tumour. Lancet 1970; 2:995.

235. Dobbie JW: Adrenocortical nodular hyperplasia: The aging adrenal. J Pathol 1969; 99:1.

236. Connell JM, Kenyon CJ, Corrie JE, et al.: Dexamethasone-suppressible hyperaldosteronism: Adrenal transition cell hyperplasia. Hypertension 1986; 8:669.

237. Connell JM, Inglis GC, Fraser R, et al.: Dexamethasone-suppressible hyperaldosteronism: Clinical, biochemical and genetic relations. J Hum Hypertens 1995; 9:505.

238. Miyahara K, Kawamoto T, Mitsuchi Y, et al.: The chimeric gene linked to glucocorticoid-suppressible hyperaldosteronism encodes a fused P-450 protein possessing aldosterone synthase activity. Biochem Biophys Res Commun 1992; 189:885.

239. Sasano H, Ojima M, Fukuchi S, et al.: An endocrine-pathological spectrum of non-neoplastic hyperaldosteronism with suppressed plasma renin activity. Lab Invest 1988; 58:81A.

240. Gabrilove JL, Seeman AT, Sabet R, et al.: Virilizing adrenal adenoma with studies on the steroid content of the adrenal venous effluent and a review of the literature. Endocr Rev 1981; 2:462.

241. Mendonca BB, Lucon AM, Menezes CA, et al.: Clinical, hormonal and pathological findings in a comparative study of adrenocortical neoplasms in childhood and adulthood. J Urol 1995; 154:2004.

242. Gabrilove JL, Sharma DC, Wotiz HH, et al.: Feminizing adrenocortical tumours in the male: A review of 52 cases including a case report. Medicine (Baltimore) 1965; 44:37.

243. Givens JR, Andersen RN, Wiser WL, et al.: A gonadotrophin-responsive adrenocortical adenoma. J Clin Endocrinol Metab 1974; 38:126.

244. Werk EE, Sholiton LJ, Kalejs L. Testosterone secreting adrenal adenoma under gonadotropin control. N Engl J Med 1973; 289:767.

245. Hedeland H, Ostberg G, Hökfelt B: On the prevalence of adrenocortical adenomas in autopsy material in relation to hypertension and diabetes. Acta Med Scand 1968; 184:211.

246. Page DL, DeLellis RA, Hough AJ: Tumors of the adrenal. Fascicle 23. Atlas of Tumor Pathology. Armed Forces Institute of Pathology, Washington, DC. 1985.

247. Mitnick JS, Bosniak MA, Megibow AJ, et al.: Non-functioning adrenal adenomas discovered incidentally on computed tomography. Radiology 1983; 148:495.

248. Kloos RT, Gross MD, Francis IR, et al.: Incidentally discovered adrenal masses. Endocrine Rev 1995; 16:460.

249. Bilbey JH, McLoughlin RF, Kurkjian PS, et al.: MR imaging of adrenal masses: Value of chemical-shift imaging for distinguishing adenomas from other tumors. Am J Radiol 1995; 164:637.

250. Reincke M, Nieke J, Krestin GP, et al.: Preclinical Cushing's syndrome in adrenal incidentalomas: Comparison with adrenal Cushing's syndrome. J Clin Endocrinol Metab 1992; 75:826.

251. Herrera MF, Grant CS, van Heerden JA, et al.: Incidentally discovered adrenal tumors: An institutional perspective. Surgery 1991; 110:1014.

252. Carpenter PC: Cushing's syndrome: Update of diagnosis and management. Mayo Clin Proc 1986; 61:49.

253. Thompson NW, Cheung PSY: Diagnosis and treatment of functioning and non-functioning adrenocortical neoplasms including incidentalomas. Surg Clin North Am 1987; 67:423.

254. Copeland PM: The incidentally discovered adrenal mass. Ann Surg 1984; 199:116.

255. Damron TA, Schelper RL, Sorensen L: Cytochemical demonstration of neuromelanin in black pigmented adrenal nodules. Am J Clin Pathol 1987; 87:334.

256. Macadam RF: Black adenomas of the human adrenal cortex. Cancer 1971; 27:116.

257. Visser HKA, Boejinga JK, Meer CVD: A functioning black adenoma of the adrenal cortex: A clinicopathological entity. J Clin Pathol 1974; 27:955.

258. Ibanez ML: The pathology of adrenal cortical carcinomas: Study of 22 cases. In Endocrine and Nonendocrine Hormone-Producing Tumors. Year Book Medical Publishers, Chicago, 1971, p. 231.

259. Macfarlane DA: Cancer of the adrenal cortex. Ann R Coll Surg Engl 1958; 23:155.

260. Hutter AMJ, Kayhoe DE: Adrenal cortical carcinoma. Am J Med 1966; 41:572.

261. Correa P, Chen VW: Endocrine gland cancer. Cancer 1995; 75:338.

262. Brennan MF: Adrenocortical carcinoma. Cancer J Clin 1987; 37:348.

263. Lubitz JA, Freeman L, Okun R: Mitotane use in inoperable adrenal cortical carcinoma. JAMA 1973; 223:1109.

264. Lack EE: Tumors of the Adrenal Gland and Extra-adrenal Paraganglia, 3rd series. Armed Forces Institute of Pathology, Washington, DC, 1997.

265. Javadpour N, Woltering EA, Brennan MF: Adrenal neoplasms. Cur Prob Surg 1980; 17:3.

266. Hough AJ, Hollifield JW, Page DL, et al.: Prognostic factors in adrenal cortical tumours. Am J Clin Pathol 1979; 72:390.

267. Wooten MD, King DK: Adrenal cortical carcinoma: Epidemiology and treatment with mitotane and a review of the literature. Cancer 1993; 72:3145.

268. Hajjar RA, Hickey RC, Samafin NA: Adrenal cortical carcinoma. Cancer 1975; 35:549.

269. Harrison JH, Mahoney EM, Bennet AH: Tumors of the adrenal cortex. Cancer 1973; 32:1227.

270. Huvos AG, Hajdu SI, Brasfield RD, et al.: Adrenal cortical carcinoma. Cancer 1970; 25:354.

271. King DR, Lack EE: Adrenal cortical carcinoma: A clinical and pathologic study of 49 cases. Cancer 1979; 44:2399.

272. Didolkar MS, Bescher RA, Elias EG, et al.: Natural history of adrenal cortical carcinoma: A clinicopathologic study of 42 patients. Cancer 1981; 47:2153.

273. Hogan TF, Gilchrist KW, Westring DW, et al.: A clinical and pathological study of adrenocortical carcinoma: Therapeutic implications. Cancer 1980; 45:2880.

274. Nader S, Hickey RC, Sellin RV, et al.: Adrenal cortical carcinoma: A study of 77 cases. Cancer 1983; 52:707.

275. Weiss LM: Comparable histologic study of 43 metastasizing and nonmetastasizing adrenocortical tumors. Am J Surg Pathol 1984; 8:163.

276. Cohn K, Gottesman L, Brennan MF: Adrenocortical carcinoma. Surgery 1986; 100:1170.

277. Lack EE, Travis WD, Oertel JE: Adrenal cortical neoplasms. In Lack EE, ed.: Pathology of the Adrenal Glands. New York, Churchill Livingstone, 1990, p. 115.

278. Kelly WF, O'Hare MJ, Loizou S, et al.: Hypermineralocorticism without excessive aldosterone secretion: An adrenal carcinoma producing deoxycorticosterone. Clin Endocrinol (Oxf) 1982; 17:353.

279. Powell-Jackson JD, Calin A, Fraser R, et al.: Excess deoxycorticosterone secretion from adrenocortical carcinoma. Br Med J 1974; 2:32.

280. Halmi KA, Lascari AD: Conversion of virilization to feminization in a young girl with adrenal cortical carcinoma. Cancer 1971; 27:931.

281. Haak HR, van Seters AP, Moolenaar AJ, et al.: Expression of P-glycoprotein in relation to clinical manifestation, treatment and prognosis of adrenocortical cancer. Eur J Cancer 1993; 7:1036.

282. Flynn SD, Murren JR, Kirby WM, et al.: P-glycoprotein expression and multidrug resistance in adrenocortical carcinoma. Surgery 1992; 112:981.

283. McNicol AM: The human adrenal gland: Aspects of structure, function and pathology. In James VHT, ed: The Adrenal Gland, 2nd ed. Raven Press Ltd, New York, 1992, p. 1.

284. Sundberg AG, Nilsson R, Appelkvist EL, et al.: Immunohistochemical localization of alpha and pi class glutathione transferases in normal human tissues. Pharmacol Toxicol 1993; 72:321.

285. Papadopoulos D, Seidegard J, Rydstrom J: Metabolism of xenobiotics in the human adrenal gland. Cancer Lett 1984; 22:23.

286. Campbell JA, Bass NM, Kirsch RE: Immunohistological localization of ligandin in human tissues. Cancer 1980; 45:503.
287. Haak HR, Hermans J, van de Velde CJ, et al.: Optimal treatment of adrenocortical carcinoma with mitotane: Results in a consecutive series of 96 patients. Br J Cancer 1994; 69:947.
288. Tang CK, Gray GF: Adrenocortical neoplasms: Prognosis and morphology. Urology 1975; 5:691.
289. Gandour MJ, Grizzle WE: A small adrenocortical carcinoma with aggressive behavior: An evaluation of criteria for malignancy. Arch Pathol Lab Med 1986; 110:1076.
290. Lewinsky BS, Grigor KM, Symington T, et al.: The clinical and pathologic features of "non-hormonal" adrenocortical tumors: Report of twenty new cases and review of the literature. Cancer 1974; 33:778.
291. Symington T, ed.: Functional Pathology of the Adrenal Gland. Churchill Livingstone, Edinburgh, 1969.
292. El Naggar AK, Evans DB, Mackay B: Oncocytic adrenal cortical carcinoma. Ultrastruct Pathol 1991; 15:549.
293. Drachenberg CB, Lee HK, Gann DS, et al.: Adrenal cortical carcinoma with adenosquamous differentiation: Report of a case with immunohistochemical and ultrastructural studies. Arch Pathol Lab Med 1995; 119:260.
294. Van Slooten H, Schaberg A, Smeenk D, et al.: Morphologic characteristics of benign and malignant adrenocortical tumors. Cancer 1985; 55:766.
295. Weiss LM, Medeiros LJ, Vickery AL Jr.: Pathologic features of prognostic significance in adrenocortical carcinoma. Am J Surg Pathol 1989; 13:202.
296. Henley DJ, van Heerden JA, Grant CS, et al.: Adrenal cortical carcinoma: A continuing challenge. Surgery 1983; 94:926.
297. Bodie B, Novick AC, Pontes JE, et al.: The Cleveland Clinic experience with adrenal cortical carcinoma. J Urol 1989; 141:257.
298. Luton JP, Cerdas S, Billaud L, et al.: Clinical features of adrenocortical carcinoma, prognostic factors, and the effect of mitotane therapy. N Engl J Med 1990; 372:1195.
299. Medeiros LJ, Weiss LM: New developments in the pathologic diagnosis of adrenal cortical neoplasms. Am J Clin Pathol 1992; 97:73.
300. Zografos GC, Driscoll D, Karakousis C, et al.: Staging and grading in the survival of adrenal carcinomas. Eur J Surg Oncol 1994; 20:449.
301. McNicol AM, Struthers AJ, Nolan CE, et al.: Proliferation in adrenocortical tumors: Correlation with clinical outcome and p53 status. Endocr Pathol 1997; 8:29.
302. Edgren M, Eriksson B, Wilander E, et al.: Biological characteristics of adrenocortical carcinoma: A study of p53, IGF, EGF-r, Ki-67 and PCNA in 17 adrenocortical carcinomas. Anticancer Res 1997; 17:1303.
303. Goldblum JR, Shannon R, Kaldjian EP, et al.: Immunohistochemical assessment of proliferative activity in adrenocortical neoplasms. Mod Pathol 1993; 6:663.
304. Bergada I, Venara M, Maglio S, et al.: Functional adrenal cortical tumors in pediatric patients: A clinicopathologic and immunohistochemical study of a long-term follow-up series. Cancer 1996; 77:771.
305. Schroder S, Padberg BC, Achilles E, et al.: Immunocytochemistry in adrenocortical tumours: A clinicomorphological study of 72 neoplasms. Virchows Arch A Pathol Anat Histopathol 1992; 420:65.
306. Fetsch PA, Powers CN, Zakowski MF, et al.: Anti-alpha-inhibin: Marker of choice for the consistent distinction between adrenocortical carcinoma and renal cell carcinoma in fine-needle aspiration. Cancer 1999; 87:168.
307. Miettinen M, Lehto VP, Virtanen I: Immunofluorescence microscopic evaluation of the intermediate filament expression of the adrenal cortex and medulla and their tumors. Am J Pathol 1985; 118:360.
308. Wick MR, Cherwitz DL, McGlennen RC, et al.: Adrenocortical carcinoma: An immunohistochemical comparison with renal cell carcinoma. Am J Pathol 1986; 122:343.
309. Miettinen M: Neuroendocrine differentiation in adrenocortical carcinoma: New immunohistochemical findings supported by electron microscopy. Lab Invest 1992; 66:169.
310. Sasano H, Shizawa S, Suzuki T, et al.: Ad4BP in the human adrenal cortex and its disorders. J Clin Endocrinol Metab 1995; 80:2378.
311. Reincke M, Beuschlein F, Lalli E, et al.: DAX-1 expression in human adrenocortical neoplasms: Implications for steroidogenesis. J Clin Endocrinol Metab 1998; 83:2597.
312. Mackay B, el-Naggar A, Ordonez NG: Ultrastructure of adrenal cortical carcinoma. Ultrastruct Pathol 1994; 18:181.
313. Klein FA, Kay S, Ratliff JE, et al.: Flow cytometric determinations of ploidy and proliferation patterns of adrenal neoplasms: An adjunct to histological classification. J Urol 1985; 134:862.
314. Bowlby LS, DeBault LE, Abraham SR: Flow cytometric analysis of adrenal cortical tumor DNA: Relationship between cellular DNA and histopathologic classification. Cancer 1986; 58:1499.
315. Haak HR, Cornelisse CJ, Hermans J, et al.: Nuclear DNA content and morphological characteristics in the prognosis of adrenocortical carcinoma. Br J Cancer 1993; 68:151.
316. Cibas ES, Medeiros LJ, Weinberg DS, et al.: Cellular DNA profiles of benign and malignant adrenocortical tumors. Am J Surg Pathol 1990; 14:948.
317. Pignatelli D, Leitao D, Maia M, et al.: DNA quantification and ploidy patterns in human adrenocortical neoplasms. Endocr Res 1998; 24:869.
318. Kida Y, Takano Y, Okudaira M: Argyrophilic nucleolar organizer regions in human adrenocortical neoplasms. J Cancer Res Clin Oncol 1992; 119:49.
319. Oz B, Dervisoglu S, Dervisoglu M, et al.: Silver binding nucleolar organizer regions in adrenocortical neoplasia. Cytopathology 1992; 3:93.
320. Sasano H, Saito Y, Sato I, et al.: Nucleolar organizer regions in human adrenocortical disorders. Mod Pathol 1990; 3:591.
321. Sasano H, Nose M, Sasano N: Lectin histochemistry of adrenocortical hyperplasia and neoplasms with emphasis on carcinoma. Arch Pathol Lab Med 1989; 113:68.
322. Nguyen GK, Vriend R, Ronaghan D, et al.: Heterotopic adrenocortical oncocytoma: A case report with light and electron microscopic studies. Cancer 1992; 70:2681.
323. Adashi EY, Rosenwaks A, Lee PA, et al.: Endocrine features of an adrenal-like tumor of the ovary. J Clin Endocrinol Metab 1979; 48:241.
324. Hamwi GJ, Gwinup G, Mostow JH, et al.: Activation of testicular adrenal rest tissue by prolonged excessive ACTH production. J Clin Endocrinol Metab 1963; 23:861.
325. Strauch GO, Vinnick L: Persistent Cushing's syndrome apparently cured by ectopic adrenalectomy. JAMA 1972; 221:183.
326. Uehling DT: Adrenal rest tumors of the testis: A case report of fertility following treatment. Fertil Steril 1978; 29:583.
327. Vogelstein B, Fearon ER, Hamilton SR, et al.: Clonal analysis using recombinant DNA probes from the X-chromosome. Cancer Res 1987; 47:4806.
328. Gicquel C, Leblond-Francillard M, Bertagna X, et al.: Clonal analysis of human adrenocortical carcinomas and secreting adenomas. Clin Endocrinol (Oxf) 1994; 40:465.
329. Rosenberg C, Della-Rosa VA, Latronico AC, et al.: Selection of adrenal tumor cells in culture demonstrated by interphase cytogenetics. Cancer Genet Cytogenet 1995; 79:36.
330. Henry I, Grandjouan S, Couillin P, et al.: Tumor-specific loss of 11p 15.5 alleles in del 11 p13 Wilms tumor and in familial adrenocortical carcinoma. Proc Natl Acad Sci U S A 1989; 86:3247.
331. Yano T, Linehan M, Anglard P, et al.: Genetic changes in adrenocortical carcinoma. J Natl Cancer Inst 1989; 81:518.
332. Kjellman M, Kallioniemi OP, Karhu R, et al.: Genetic aberrations in adrenocortical tumors detected using comparative genomic hybridization correlate with tumor size and malignancy. Cancer Res 1996; 56:4219.
333. Russell AJ, Sibbald J, Haak H, et al.: Increasing genome instability in adrenocortical carcinoma progression with involvement of chromosomes 3, 9 and X at the adenoma stage. Br J Cancer 1999; 81:684.
334. Kjellman M, Roshani L, Teh BT, et al.: Genotyping of adrenocortical tumors: Very frequent deletions of the MEN1 locus in 11q13 and of a 1-centimorgan region in 2p16. J Clin Endocrinol Metab 1999; 84:730.

335. Li FP, Fraumeni JF: Soft tissue sarcomas, breast cancer, and other neoplasms: A familial syndrome? Ann Intern Med 1969; 71:747.

336. Srivastava S, Zou Z, Pirollo K, et al.: Germline transmission of a mutated p53 gene in a cancer-prone family with Li-Fraumeni syndrome. Nature 1990; 348:747.

337. Reincke M, Karl M, Travis WH, et al.: p53 mutations in human adrenocortical neoplasms: Immunohistochemical and molecular studies. J Clin Endocrinol Metab 1994; 78:790.

338. Ohgaki H, Kleihues P, Heitz PU: p53 mutations in sporadic adrenocortical tumors. Int J Cancer 1993; 54:408.

339. McNicol AM, Nolan CE, Struthers AJ, et al.: Expression of p53 in adrenocortical tumours: Clinicopathological correlations. J Pathol 1997; 181:146.

340. Lin SR, Lee YJ, Tsai JH: Mutations of the p53 gene in human functional adrenal neoplasms. J Clin Endocrinol Metab 1994; 78:483.

341. Reincke M, Wachenfeld C, Mora P, et al.: p53 mutations in adrenal tumors: Caucasian patients do not show the exon 4 "hot spot" found in Taiwan. J Clin Endocrinol Metab 1996; 81:3636.

342. Gortz B, Roth J, Speel EJ, et al.: MEN1 gene mutation analysis of sporadic adrenocortical lesions. Int J Cancer 1999; 80:373.

343. Heppner C, Reincke M, Agarwal SK, et al.: MEN1 gene analysis in sporadic adrenocortical neoplasms. J Clin Endocrinol Metab 1999; 84:216.

344. Fogt F, Vargas MP, Zhuang Z, et al.: Utilization of molecular genetics in the differentiation between adrenal cortical adenomas and carcinomas. Hum Pathol 1998; 29:518.

345. Pilon C, Pistorello M, Moscon A, et al.: Inactivation of the p16 tumor suppressor gene in adrenocortical tumors. J Clin Endocrinol Metab 1999; 84:2776.

346. Seki M, Tanaka K, Kikuchi-Yanoshita R, et al.: Loss of normal allele of the APC gene in an adrenocortical carcinoma from a patient with familial adenomatous polyposis. Hum Genet 1992; 89:298.

347. Wakatsuki S, Sasano H, Matsui T, et al.: Adrenocortical tumor in a patient with familial adenomatous polyposis: A case associated with a complete inactivating mutation of the APC gene and unusual histological features. Hum Pathol 1998; 29:302.

348. Moul JW, Bishoff JT, Theune SM, et al.: Absent ras gene mutations in human adrenal cortical neoplasms and pheochromocytomas. J Urol 1993; 149:1389.

349. Yashiro T, Hara H, Fulton NC, et al.: Point mutations of ras genes in human adrenal cortical tumors: Absence in adrenocortical hyperplasia. World J Surg 1994; 18:455.

350. Lin SR, Tsai JH, Yang YC, et al.: Mutations of K-ras oncogene in human adrenal tumours in Taiwan. Br J Cancer 1998; 77:1060.

351. Liu J, Voutilainen R, Kahri AI, et al.: Expression patterns of the c-myc gene in adrenocortical tumors and pheochromocytomas. J Endocrinol 1997; 152:175.

352. Li M, Squire JA, Weksberg R: Molecular genetics of Wiedemann-Beckwith syndrome. Am J Med Genet 1998; 79:253.

353. Ilvesmaki V, Kahri AI, Miettinen PJ, et al.: Insulin-like growth factors (IGFs) and their receptors in adrenal tumors: high IGF-II expression in functional adrenocortical carcinomas. J Clin Endocrinol Metab 1993; 77:852.

354. Gicquel C, Bertagna X, Schneid H, et al.: Rearrangements at the 11p15 locus and overexpression of insulin-like growth factor-II gene in sporadic adrenocortical tumors. J Clin Endocrinol Metab 1994; 78:1444.

355. Balnave SE, Longman CA, Hamilton FA, et al.: Epidermal growth factor receptor and transforming growth factor alpha immunoreactivity in adrenocortical tumours. J Pathol 1992; 167:130A.

356. Weber MM, Auernhammer CJ, Kiess W, et al.: Insulin-like growth factor receptors in normal and tumorous adult human adrenocortical glands. Eur J Endocrinol 1997; 136:296.

357. Ilvesmaki V, Liu J, Heikkila P, et al.: Expression of insulin-like growth factor binding protein 1-6 genes in adrenocortical tumors and pheochromocytomas. Horm Metab Res 1998; 30:619.

358. Pelkey TJ, Frierson HF Jr., Mills SE, et al.: The alpha subunit of inhibin in adrenal cortical neoplasia. Mod Pathol 1998; 11:516.

359. Spada A, Lania A, Ballare E: G protein abnormalities in pituitary adenomas. Mol Cell Endocrinol 1998; 142:1.

360. Derwahl M, Manole D, Sobke A, et al.: Pathogenesis of toxic thyroid adenomas and nodules: Relevance of activating mutations in the TSH-receptor and Gs-alpha gene, the possible role of iodine deficiency and secondary and TSH-independent molecular mechanisms. Exp Clin Endocrinol Diabetes 1998; 106:S6.

361. Light K, Jenkins PJ, Weber A, et al.: Are activating mutations of the adrenocorticotropin receptor involved in adrenal cortical neoplasia? Life Sciences 1995; 56:1523.

362. Latronico AC, Reincke M, Mendonca BB, et al.: No evidence for oncogenic mutations in the adrenocorticotropin receptor gene in human adrenocortical neoplasms. J Clin Endocrinol Metab 1995; 80:875.

363. Sachse R, Shao X-J, Rico A, et al.: Absence of angiotensin II type 1 receptor gene mutations in human adrenal tumors. Eur J Endocrinol 1997; 137:262.

364. Reincke M, Karl M, Travis W, et al.: No evidence for oncogenic mutations in guanine nucleotide-binding proteins of human adrenocortical neoplasms. J Clin Endocrinol Metab 1993; 77:1419.

365. Weinstein LS, Shenker A, Gejman PV, et al.: Activating mutations of the stimulatory G protein in the McCune-Albright syndrome. N Engl J Med 1991; 325:1688.

366. Lyons J, Landis CA, Harsh G, et al.: Two G protein oncogenes in human endocrine tumors. Science 1990; 249:655.

367. Gicquel C, Dib A, Bertagna X, et al.: Oncogenic mutations of alpha-Gi2 protein are not determinant for human adrenocortical tumourigenesis. Eur J Endocrinol 1995; 133:166.

368. Hirano Y, Fujita K, Suzuki K, et al.: Telomerase activity as an indicator of potentially malignant adrenal tumors. Cancer 1998; 83:772.

369. Teng L, Tucker O, Malchoff C, et al.: Telomerase activity in the differentiation of benign and malignant adrenal tumors. Surgery 1998; 124:1123.

370. Bamberger CM, Else T, Bamberger AM, et al.: Telomerase activity in benign and malignant adrenal tumors. Exp Clin Endocrinol Diabetes 1999; 107:272.

371. Sasano H, Imatani A, Shizawa S, et al.: Cell proliferation and apoptosis in normal and pathologic human adrenal. Mod Pathol 1995; 8:11.

372. Fogt F, Vortmeyer AO, Poremba C, et al.: bcl-2 expression in normal adrenal glands and in adrenal neoplasms. Mod Pathol 1998; 11:716.

373. Lin BT, Bonsib SM, Mierau GW, et al.: Oncocytic adrenocortical neoplasms: A report of seven cases and review of the literature. Am J Surg Pathol 1998; 22:603.

374. Sasano H, Suzuki T, Sano T, et al.: Adrenocortical oncocytoma: A true nonfunctioning adrenocortical tumor. Am J Surg Pathol 1991; 15:949.

375. Rothberg M, Bastidas J, Mattey WE, et al.: Adrenal hemangiomas: Angiographic appearance of a rare tumor. Radiology 1978; 126:341.

376. Plaut A: Hemangiomas and related lesions of the adrenal gland. Virchows Arch (Pathol Anat) 1962; 335:345.

377. Proye C, Jafari Manjili M, Combemale F, et al.: Experience gained from operation of 103 adrenal incidentalomas. Langenbecks Arch Surg 1998; 383:330.

378. Kareti LR, Katlein S, Siew S, et al.: Angiosarcoma of the adrenal gland. Arch Pathol Lab Med 1988; 112:1163.

379. Fiordelise S, Zangrandi A, Tronci A, et al.: Angiosarcoma of the adrenal gland: Case report. Arch Ital Urol Nefrol Androl 1992; 64:341.

380. Mortele KJ, Hoier MR, Mergo PJ, et al.: Bilateral adrenal cystic lymphangiomas in nevoid basal cell carcinoma (Gorlin-Goltz) syndrome: US, CT, and MR findings. J Comput Assist Tomogr 1999; 23:562.

381. Hoeffel CC, Kamoun J, Aubert JP, et al.: Bilateral cystic lymphangioma of the adrenal gland. South Med J 1999; 92:424.

382. Choi SH, Liu K: Leiomyosarcoma of the adrenal gland and its angiographic features: A case report. J Surg Oncol 1981; 16:145.

383. Lack EE, Graham CW, Azumi N, et al.: Primary leiomyosarcoma of adrenal gland: Case report with immunohistochemical and ultrastructural study. Am J Surg Pathol 1991; 15:899.

384. Zetler PJ, Filipenko JD, Bilbey JH, et al.: Primary adrenal leiomyosarcoma in a man with acquired immunodeficiency syndrome (AIDS): Further evidence for an increase in smooth muscle tumors related to Epstein-Barr infection in AIDS. Arch Pathol Lab Med 1995; 119:1164.

385. Rosenfeld DL, Girgis WS, Underberg-Davis SJ: Bilateral smooth-muscle tumors of the adrenals in a child with AIDS. Pediatr Radiol 1999; 29:376.

386. Parola P, Petit N, Azzedine A, et al.: Symptomatic leiomyoma of the adrenal gland in a woman with AIDS. AIDS 1996; 10:340.

387. Jimenez-Heffernan JA, Hardisson D, Palacios J, et al.: Adrenal gland leiomyoma in a child with acquired immunodeficiency syndrome. Pediatr Pathol Lab Med 1995; 15:923.

388. Dahan H, Beges C, Weiss L, et al.: Leiomyoma of the adrenal gland in a patient with AIDS. Abdominal Imaging 1994; 19:259.

389. Radin DR, Kiyabu M: Multiple smooth-muscle tumors of the colon and adrenal gland in an adult with AIDS. AJR Am J Roentgenol 1992; 159:545.

390. Decorato JW, Gruber H, Petti M, et al.: Adrenal carcinosarcoma. J Surg Oncol 1990; 45:134.

391. Barksdale SK, Marincola FM, Jaffe G: Carcinosarcoma of the adrenal cortex presenting with mineralocorticoid excess. Am J Surg Pathol 1993; 17:941.

392. Fischler DF, Nunez C, Levin HS, et al.: Adrenal carcinosarcoma presenting in a woman with clinical signs of virilization: A case report with immunohistochemical and ultrastructural findings. Am J Surg Pathol 1992; 16:626.

393. Travis WD, Lack EE, Azumi N, et al.: Adenomatoid tumor of the adrenal gland with ultrastructural and immunohistochemical demonstration of a mesothelial origin. Arch Pathol Lab Med 1990; 114:722.

394. Simpson PR: Adenomatoid tumor of the adrenal gland. Arch Pathol Lab Med 1990; 114:722.

395. Nakada T, Sasagawa I, Yamaguchi T, et al.: Xanthofibroma of the adrenal gland. Int Urol Nephrol 1992; 24:337.

396. Orselli RC, Bassler TJ: Theca granulosa cell tumor arising in adrenal. Cancer 1973; 31:474.

397. Vasiloff J, Chideckel EW, Boyd CB, et al.: Testosterone-secreting adrenal adenoma containing crystalloids characteristic of Leydig cells. Am J Med 1985; 79:772.

398. Trost BN, Koenig MP, Zimmerman A, et al.: Virilization of a postmenopausal woman by a testosterone-secreting Leydig cell–type adrenal adenoma. Acta Endocrinol 1981; 98:274.

399. Pollock WJ, McConnell CF, Hilton C, et al.: Virilizing Leydig cell adenoma of adrenal gland. Am J Surg Pathol 1986; 10:816.

400. Aguirre P, Scully RE: Testosterone-secreting adrenal ganglioneuroma containing Leydig cells. Am J Surg Pathol 1983; 7:699.

401. Molberg K, Vuitch F, Stewart D, et al.: Adrenocortical blastoma. Hum Pathol 1992; 23:1187.

402. Abrams HL, Spiro R, Goldstein N: Metastases in carcinoma. Cancer 1950; 3:74.

403. Sahagian-Edwards A, Holland JF: Metastatic carcinoma to the adrenal glands with cortical hypofunction. Cancer 1954; 7:1242.

404. Cho SY, Choi HY: Causes of death and metastatic patterns in patients with mammary cancer. Am J Clin Pathol 1980; 73:232.

405. Saboorian MH, Katz RL, Charnsangavej C: Fine needle aspiration cytology of primary and metastatic lesions of the adrenal gland: A series of 188 biopsies with radiologic correlation. Acta Cytol 1995; 39:843.

406. Das Gupta T, Brasfield R: Metastatic melanoma: A clinicopathological study. Cancer 1964; 17:1323.

407. Moriya T, Manabe T, Yamashita K, et al.: Lung cancer metastasis to adrenocortical adenomas: A chance occurrence or a predilected phenomenon? Arch Pathol Lab Med 1988; 112:286.

408. McMahon RF: Tumour to tumour metastasis: Bladder carcinoma metastasising to an adrenocortical adenoma. Br J Urol 1991; 67:216.

409. Ejeckam GC, Attah Ed B: Pattern of secondary adrenal tumors in Ibadan, Nigeria. Int Surg 1975; 60:368.

410. Pimentel M, Johnston JB, Allan DR, et al.: Primary adrenal lymphoma associated with adrenal insufficiency: A distinct clinical entity. Leuk Lymphoma 1997; 24:363.

411. Pool MO, Janssen MJ, van der Valk P, et al.: Adrenocortical insufficiency: A rare presentation of non-Hodgkin's lymphoma. J Intern Med 1991; 229:377.

412. Damjanov I, Katz SM, Catalano E, et al.: Myelolipoma in a heterotopic adrenal gland: Light and electron microscopic findings. Cancer 1979; 44:1350.

413. Stein SH, Latour F, Frost SS: Myelolipoma arising from ectopic adrenal cortex: Case report and review of the literature. Am J Gastroenterol 1986; 81:999.

414. Del Gaudio A, Solidaro G: Myelolipoma of the adrenal gland: Report of two cases and a review of the literature. Surgery 1986; 99:293.

415. Hunter SB, Schemankewitz EH, Patterson C, et al.: Extra-adrenal myelolipoma: A report of two cases. Am J Clin Pathol 1992; 97:402.

416. Nishizaki T, Kanematsu T, Matsumata T, et al.: Myelolipoma of the liver: A case report. Cancer 1989; 63:930.

417. Olsson CA, Krane RJ, Klugo RC, et al.: Adrenal myelolipoma. Surgery 1973; 73:665.

418. Plaut A: Myelolipoma in the adrenal cortex (myeloadipose structures). Am J Pathol 1958; 34:487.

419. Dieckman K, Hamm B, Pickartz H, et al.: Adrenal myelolipoma: Clinical, radiologic, and histologic features. Urology 1987; 29:1.

420. Musante F, Derchi LE, Bazzocchi M, et al.: MR imaging of adrenal myelolipomas. J Comput Assist Tomogr 1991; 15:111.

421. Fidler WJ: Ovarian thecal metaplasia in adrenal glands. Am J Clin Pathol 1977; 67:318.

422. Romberger CF, Wong TW: Thecal metaplasia in the adrenal gland of a man with acquired bilateral testicular atrophy. Arch Pathol Lab Med 1989; 113:1071.

423. Foster DG: Adrenal cysts. Arch Surg 1966; 92:131.

424. Incze JS, Lui PS, Merriam JC, et al.: Morphology and pathogenesis of adrenal cysts. Am J Pathol 1979; 95:423.

425. Tagge DU, Baron PL: Giant adrenal cyst: Management and review of the literature. Am Surg 1997; 63:744.

426. Ulusoy E, Adsan O, Guner E, et al.: Giant adrenal cyst: Preoperative diagnosis and management. Urol Int 1997; 58:186.

427. Sahu KK, Pai RR, Raghuveer CV: Giant adrenal cysts. Indian J Pathol Microbiol 1994; 37:S12.

428. Gaffey MJ, Mills SE, Fechner RE, et al.: Vascular adrenal cysts: A clinicopathologic and immunohistochemical study of endothelial and hemorrhagic (pseudocystic) variants. Am J Surg Pathol 1989; 13:740.

429. Medeiros LJ, Lewandrowski KB, Vickery AL Jr.: Adrenal pseudocyst: A clinical and pathologic study of eight cases. Hum Pathol 1989; 20:660.

430. Torres C, Ro JY, Batt MA, et al.: Vascular adrenal cysts: A clinicopathologic and immunohistochemical study of six cases and a review of the literature. Mod Pathol 1997; 10:530.

431. Medeiros LJ, Weiss LM, Vickery AL Jr.: Epithelial-lined (true) cyst of the adrenal gland: A case report. Hum Pathol 1989; 20:491.

432. Fukushima N, Oonishi T, Yamaguchi K, et al.: Mesothelial cyst of the adrenal gland. Pathol Int 1995; 45:156.

433. Schoretsanitis G, de Bree E, Melissas J, et al.: Primary hydatid cyst of the adrenal gland. Scand J Urol Nephrol 1998; 32:51.

434. Fitzgerald EJ: Hydatid disease of the adrenal gland. Ir J Med Sci 1987; 156:366.

435. Kong MF, Jeffcoate W: Eighty-six cases of Addison's disease. Clin Endocrinol (Oxf) 1994; 41:757.

436. Dobnig H, Silly H, Ohlinger W, et al.: Successful treatment of primary adrenal insufficiency due to malignant non-Hodgkin's lymphoma. Clin Invest 1992; 70:938.

437. Navarro M, Felip E, Garcia L, et al.: Addison's disease secondary to prostatic carcinoma: A case report. Tumori 1990; 76:611.

438. Neufeld M, MacLaren NK, Blizzard RM: Two types of autoimmune Addison's disease associated with different polyglandular autoimmune (PGA) syndromes. Medicine 1981; 60:355.

439. Ahonen P: Autoimmune polyendocrinopathy-candidosis-ectodermal dystrophy (APECED): Autosomal recessive inheritance. Clin Genet 1985; 27:535.

440. Obermayer-Straub P, Manns MP: Autoimmune polyglandular syndromes. Baillieres Clin Gastroenterol 1998; 12:293.

441. Bjorses P, Aaltonen J, Vikman A, et al.: Genetic homogeneity of autoimmune polyglandular disease type I. Am J Hum Genet 1996; 59:879.

442. Wang CY, Davoodi-Semiromi A, Huang W, et al.: Characterization of mutations in patients with autoimmune polyglandular syndrome type 1 (APS1). Hum Genet 1998; 103:681.

443. Gibson TJ, Ramu C, Gemund C, et al.: The APECED polyglandular autoimmune syndrome protein, AIRE-1, contains the SAND domain and is probably a transcription factor. Trends Biochem Sci 1998; 23:242.

444. Betterle C, Volpato M, Pedini B, et al.: Adrenal-cortex autoantibodies and steroid-producing cell autoantibodies in patients with Addison's disease: Comparison of immunofluorescence and immunoprecipitation assays. J Clin Endocrinol Metab 1999; 84:618.

445. Soderbergh A, Winqvist O, Norheim I, et al.: Adrenal autoantibodies and organ-specific autoimmunity in patients with Addison's disease. Clin Endocrinol (Oxf) 1996; 45:453.

446. Seissler J, Schott M, Steinbrenner H, et al.: Autoantibodies to adrenal cytochrome P450 antigens in isolated Addison's disease and autoimmune polyendocrine syndrome type II. Exp Clin Endocrinol Diabetes 1999; 107:208.

447. Uibo R, Aavik E, Peterson P, et al.: Autoantibodies to cytochrome P450 enzymes P450scc, P450c17, and P450c21 in autoimmune polyglandular disease types I and II and in isolated Addison's disease. J Clin Endocrinol Metab 1994; 78:323.

448. Weetman AP: Autoimmunity to steroid-producing cells and familial polyendocrine autoimmunity. Baillieres Clin Endocrinol Metab 1995; 9:157.

449. Bottazzo GF, Pujol-Borrell R, Hanafusa T, et al.: Role of aberrant HLA-DR expression and antigen presentation in induction of endocrine autoimmunity. Lancet 1983; 2:1115.

450. Hayashi Y, Hiyoshi T, Takemura T, et al.: Focal lymphocytic infiltration in the adrenal cortex of the elderly: Immunohistological analysis of infiltrating lymphocytes. Clin Exp Immunol 1989; 77:101.

451. Petri M, Nerup J: Addison's adrenalitis. Acta Pathol Microbiol Scand 1971; 79:381.

452. Johnson TL: Tuberculous Addison's disease. Postgrad Med 1991; 90:139.

453. Efremidis SC, Harsoulis F, Douma S, et al.: Adrenal insufficiency with enlarged adrenals. Abdom Imaging 1996; 21:168.

454. Guttman PH: Addison's disease: A statistical analysis of 566 cases and a study of the pathology. Arch Pathol 1930; 10:742.

455. Steffens J, Zaubitzer T, Kirsch W, et al.: Neonatal adrenal abscesses. Eur Urol 1997; 31:347.

456. Rajani K, Shapiro SR, Goetzman BW: Adrenal abscess: Complication of supportive therapy of adrenal hemorrhage in the newborn. J Pediatr Surg 1980; 15:676.

457. Atkinson GO, Kodroff MB, Gay BB, et al.: Adrenal abscess in the neonate. Radiology 1985; 155:101.

458. Shah B, Taylor HC, Pillay I, et al.: Adrenal insufficiency due to cryptococcosis. JAMA 1986; 256:3247.

459. O'Brien WM, Choyke PL, Copeland J, et al.: Computed tomography of adrenal abscess. J Comput Assist Tomogr 1987; 11:550.

460. Masmiquel L, Hernandez-Pascual C, Simo R, et al.: Adrenal abscess as a complication of adrenal fine-needle biopsy. Am J Med 1993; 95:244.

461. Benjamin E, Fox H: Malakoplakia of the adrenal gland. J Clin Pathol 1981; 34:606.

462. Goodwin RA, Shapiro JL, Thurman GH, et al.: Disseminated histoplasmosis: Clinical and pathologic correlations. Medicine 1980; 59:1.

463. Osa SR, Peterson RE, Roberts RB: Recovery of adrenal reserve following treatment of disseminated South American blastomycosis. Am J Med 1981; 71:298.

464. Abernathy RS, Melby JC: Addison's disease in North American blastomycosis. N Engl J Med 1962; 266:552.

465. Walker BF, Gunthel CJ, Bryan JA, et al.: Disseminated cryptococcosis in an apparently normal host presenting as primary adrenal insufficiency: Diagnosis by fine needle aspiration. Am J Med 1989; 86:715.

466. Maloney PJ: Addison's disease due to chronic disseminated coccidioidomycosis. Arch Intern Med 1952; 90:869.

467. Faical S, Borri ML, Hauache OM, et al.: Addison's disease caused by *Paracoccidioides brasiliensis:* Diagnosis by needle aspiration biopsy of the adrenal gland. AJR Am J Roentgenol 1996; 166:461.

468. Do Valle AC, Guimaraes MR, Cuba J, et al.: Recovery of adrenal function after treatment of paracoccidioidomycosis. Am J Trop Med Hyg 1993; 48:626.

469. Haas GM: Hepato-adrenal necrosis with intranuclear inclusion bodies: Report of a case. Am J Pathol 1935; 11:127.

470. Mostoufizadeh M, Lack EE, Gang DL, et al.: Postmortem manifestations of echovirus 11 sepsis in five newborn infants. Hum Pathol 1983; 14:818.

471. Speer ME, Yawn DH: Fatal hepatoadrenal necrosis in the neonate associated with echovirus types 11 and 12 presenting as a surgical emergency. J Pediatr Surg 1984; 19:591.

472. Migeon CJ, Kenny FM, Hung W, et al.: Study of adrenal function in children with meningitis. Pediatrics 1967; 40:163.

473. Margaretten W, Nakai H, Landing BH: Septicemic adrenal hemorrhage. Am J Dis Child 1963; 105:346.

474. Hori K, Yasoshima H, Yamada A, et al.: Adrenal hemorrhage associated with *Klebsiella oxytoca* bacteremia. Intern Med 1998; 37:990.

475. McCroskey RD, Phillips A, Mott F, et al.: Antiphospholipid antibodies and adrenal hemorrhage. Am J Hematol 1991; 36:60.

476. Wong R, Topliss DJ, Metz GL, et al.: Postoperative primary adrenal failure from bilateral hemorrhagic adrenal infarction associated with coagulation factor XI deficiency. J Endocrinol Invest 1993; 16:61.

477. Xarli VP, Steele AA, Davis PJ, et al.: Adrenal hemorrhage in the adult. Medicine (Baltimore) 1978; 57:211.

478. Ikekpeazzu N, Bonadies JA, Sreenivas VI: Acute bilateral adrenal hemorrhage secondary to rough truck ride. J Emerg Med 1996; 14:15.

479. Kamijo Y, Soma K, Hasegawa I, et al.: Fatal bilateral adrenal hemorrhage following acute toluene poisoning: A case report. J Toxicol Clin Toxicol 1998; 36:365.

480. Kuhajda F, Hutchins GM: Adrenal cortico-medullary junction necrosis: A morphologic marker for hypotension. Am Heart J 1979; 98:294.

481. Verges B, Chavanet P, Desgres J, et al.: Adrenal function in HIV infected patients. Acta Endocrinol (Copenh) 1989; 121:633.

482. Raffi F, Brisseau JM, Planchon B, et al.: Endocrine function in 98 HIV-infected patients: A prospective study. AIDS 1991; 5:729.

483. Opocher G, Mantero F: Adrenal complications of HIV infection. Baillieres Clin Endocrinol Metab 1994; 8:769.

484. Freda PU, Wardlaw SL, Brudney K, et al.: Primary adrenal insufficiency in patients with the acquired immunodeficiency syndrome: A report of five cases. J Clin Endocrinol Metab 1994; 79:1540.

485. Geusau A, Stingl G: Primary adrenal insufficiency in two patients with the acquired immunodeficiency syndrome associated with disseminated cytomegaloviral infection. Wien Klin Wochenschr 1997; 109:845.

486. Piedrola G, Casado JL, Lopez E, et al.: Clinical features of adrenal insufficiency in patients with acquired immunodeficiency syndrome. Clin Endocrinol (Oxf) 1996; 45:97.

487. Hawken MP, Ojoo JC, Morris JS, et al.: No increased prevalence of adrenocortical insufficiency in human immunodeficiency

virus–associated tuberculosis. Tuberc Lung Dis 1996; 77:444.

488. Reichert CM, O'Leary TJ, Levens DL, et al.: Autopsy pathology in the acquired immune deficiency syndrome. Am J Pathol 1983; 112:357.

489. Glasgow BJ, Steinsapir KD, Anders K, et al.: Adrenal pathology in the acquired immune deficiency syndrome. Am J Clin Pathol 1985; 84:594.

490. Guarda LA, Luna MA, Smith LJR, et al.: Acquired immune deficiency syndrome: Postmortem findings. Am J Clin Pathol 1984; 81:549.

491. Klatt EC: Adrenal findings with CMV infection in AIDS. Am J Clin Pathol 1990; 94:368.

492. Liddle GW, Island D, Lance EM, et al.: Alterations of adrenal steroid patterns in man resulting from treatment with a chemical inhibitor of 11beta-hydroxylation. J Clin Endocrinol Metab 1958; 18:906.

493. Sonino N: The use of ketoconazole as an inhibitor of steroid production. N Engl J Med 1987; 317:812.

494. Wagner RL, White PF, Kan PB, et al.: Inhibition of adrenal steroidogenesis by the anesthetic etomidate. N Engl J Med 1984; 310:1415.

495. Fishman LM, Liddle GW, Island DP, et al.: Effects of aminoglutethimide on adrenal function in man. J Clin Endocrinol Metab 1967; 27:481.

496. Stein CA, Saville W, Yarchoan R, et al.: Suramin and function of the adrenal cortex. Ann Intern Med 1986; 104:286.

497. Elias AN, Gwinup G: Effects of some clinically encountered drugs on steroid synthesis and degradation. Metabolism 1980; 29:582.

CHAPTER 8

Endocrine Pancreas

Irina Lubensky

INTRODUCTION

Both exocrine and endocrine pancreatic tissue originate from the ductular system, which arises from the foregut during embryogenesis.[1] Therefore, endocrine cells of the pancreas develop from the endoderm rather than from the neural crest. The support for the origin of the pancreatic endocrine cells and tumors from the pluripotent stem cell in the ductular epithelium rather than from the islets of Langerhans comes from the evaluation of proliferative conditions of endocrine pancreas, multiple endocrine neoplasia type I (MEN1) pancreata, and sporadic endocrine tumors.[2] In nesidioblastosis of infancy, budding off of endocrine cells from ductular epithelium can be observed. In focal adenomatosis or in insulinomas in infancy, an intimate contact of the endocrine cell clusters or endocrine tumors with ductules is often seen.[3] The hallmark of pancreatic disease in MEN1 is the multifocal, multicellular ductuloinsular proliferation and multiple microadenomas. Focal proliferation of ductules and endocrine tissue is often associated with sporadic pancreatic endocrine tumors, and ductular cells are frequently seen inside these tumors. Evaluation of these lesions for the genes and other factors involved in human pancreatic endocrine tumorigenesis and progression is necessary to confirm the origin of the endocrine cells and tumors of the pancreas from the ductular epithelium.

Pancreatic endocrine tumors are relatively rare; however, it is important to distinguish them from the more common neoplasms of the exocrine pancreas. Pancreatic endocrine tumors frequently produce characteristic clinical syndromes and are slowly progressive. Clinicopathologic correlation is important in diagnosis and surgical and medical management of these tumors. Clinical, radiologic, and morphologic features of pancreatic common and uncommon endocrine tumors and tumor-like lesions of the pancreas are summarized in this chapter. Molecular genetic alterations in pancreatic endocrine tu-

mors and current approach to their therapy are also discussed.

NORMAL ENDOCRINE PANCREAS

Development

The pancreas develops from the dorsal and right ventral primordia, which first appear during the 5th week of gestation at the level of the distal foregut and fuse at 7 weeks.[4, 5] The primitive pancreas at this stage consists of small unbranched tubules of undifferentiated epithelial cells surrounded by loose connective tissue.[6] Endocrine cells appear during the 8th week as scattered cells at the base of the tubules. A, B, and D cells appear at the same time, and pancreatic polypeptide (PP) cells follow a few days later. Clusters of epithelial cells bud off from the tubules as terminal buds or paratubular buds at 10–13 weeks. In some paratubular buds, cells develop secretory endocrine granules and form primitive islets, which are later penetrated by a capillary bed. The other paratubular buds and all the terminal buds become primitive acini formed by large cells abundant in glycogen, basophilic cytoplasm, and a few zymogen granules. Cells located at the center of some acini (centroacinar cells) remain small and glycogen-rich with clear cytoplasm without secretory granules. The common embryologic origin of early islets, acini, and centroacinar cells from primitive ductules is important and may explain the presence of ductular cells inside pancreatic endocrine tumors and pancreatic disorder of nesidioblastosis and MEN1.

A, B, D, and PP islet cells are actively formed along the intralobular and intercalated ductules during gestation and up to the early postnatal period.[7] Islet cells stop to form in lobar or main ducts. A few "primary" islet cells originating from such ducts may remain in interlobular connective tissue until the 5th month, when they degenerate and disappear.[4] Three

205

types of islets form in the fetal pancreas: the "mantle" islets, composed of multiple layers of A and D cells around a compact central nucleus of B cells; the "bipolar" islets, with non-B and B cells clustering at opposite poles of the islet; and the PP-rich islets located at the posteroinferior part of the head (ventral pouch origin), characterized by irregular size and shape and by columnar cells arranged in trabecular architecture.

Endocrine Pancreas of Newborns and Infants

The pancreas of the newborn differs from the adult pancreas. The newborn pancreas has prominent lobules separated by thick connective tissue septa. The stroma comprises about 28% of pancreatic volume in newborns[8] and only 10% in adults. The islet volume in newborns is about 10% of the total pancreatic tissue, compared with 1%–2% in the adult pancreas. The total islet weight is estimated at 0.3 g, and the maximum islet diameter ranges from 85 to 210 μm. In addition to the well-formed islets located in the central part of the lobules, numerous endocrine cells are scattered as clusters and single cells in the exocrine tissue and are most prominent at the periphery of the lobules. These scattered endocrine cells account for a considerable proportion of the total endocrine tissue in the newborn pancreas, whereas they constitute less than 10% of the endocrine component in the adult pancreas.

The larger islets in the newborn pancreas are similar to the regular islets in the adult pancreas and have a ribbon-lobular appearance. Such islets are composed of centrally located B cells surrounded by A and D cells at the islet periphery or along the capillaries. The smaller compact islets and cell clusters are associated with intralobular ductules. Only rare mantle and bipolar islets characteristic of the fetal pancreas are present in the newborn.

Similar to the adult pancreas, irregular trabecular PP-rich islets are located in the posteroinferior head in the newborn. Budding-off endocrine cells from the interlobular and main duct epithelium are rare.

During early postnatal life, the exocrine pancreas rapidly expands, leading to the decrease of the volume density of the endocrine and stromal elements. In infants up to 6 months of age, the endocrine component constitutes only 5%–7% of the exocrine tissue. The number of small endocrine cellular clusters and scattered single endocrine cells decreases significantly. Furthermore, the budding of the endocrine cells from ductular epithelium stops nearly completely.[8]

Endocrine Pancreas of Adults

Ninety percent of all pancreatic endocrine cells in the adult pancreas are located in the islets of Langerhans (Fig. 8–1A), whereas fewer than 10% are distributed singly or in clusters among ductal cells or paraductular acinar cells.[9, 10] Extrainsular endocrine cells are usually PP and glucagon cells, which may be found in the small ducts (see Fig. 8–1B). A few enterochromaffin or serotonin cells are present in the epithelium of large ducts.[11]

The pancreatic islets were first recognized in 1869 by Paul Langerhans (1849–1888), a Berlin-based pathologist.[12, 13] The islets consist of aggregates of lightly staining endocrine cells well demarcated from the surrounding exocrine tissue (Fig. 8–2A). They are embedded in reticulin and collagen fibers and lack a true capsule. Two types of islets are recognized based on their architecture and location: ordinary, or regular, islets and PP-rich, or irregular, islets (see Fig. 8–2B).

According to morphometric studies, ordinary or regular islets are evenly distributed in the anterior part of the head, body, and tail of the pancreas. They are round to ovoid in shape, with cells

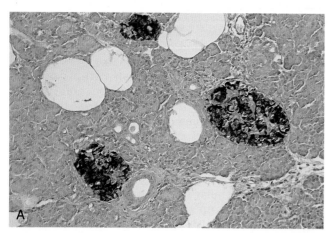
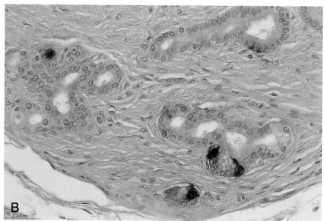

Figure 8–1. Endocrine cell distribution in adult pancreas. *A,* 90% of all pancreatic endocrine cells are located in the islets of Langerhans, 75 to 225 μm in size (insulin immunostain, ×200); *B,* Extrainsular endocrine cells, usually PP and glucagon cells, are found in the small ducts (PP immunostain ×400).

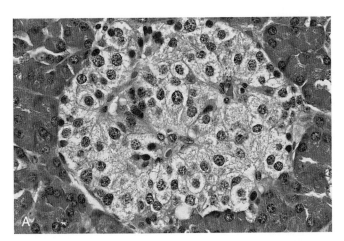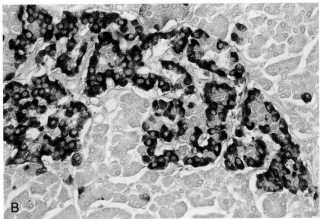

Figure 8-2. Islets of Langerhans of adult pancreas. *A,* Ordinary type islet, rich in B cells, is characterized by regular contour and compact shape (H&E ×630); *B,* Irregular type islet, rich in PP cells, is characterized by irregular contour and trabecular architecture (chromogranin A, ×400).

arranged into partly delineated ribbons or lobules (see Fig. 8-2A). The diameter of ordinary islets ranges from 75 to 225 μm.

PP-rich, irregular islets are large, are 400–500 μm in diameter, and have trabecular structure (see Fig. 8-2B). Therefore, they may be mistaken for hyperplastic islets. Irregular islets are located in the posterior part of the pancreatic head and derive embryologically from the ventral premordium.

The islets are penetrated by a system of anastomosing sinusoids. The capillaries are lined by endocrine cells, which are in contact with blood vessels.[14] The innervation of the islets derives from both sympathetic and parasympathetic nerve fibers, which are closely associated with the blood vessels. In addition, peptidergic fibers originating from the intrinsic autonomic system ganglia act as neuroregulators of local control of the endocrine function of the pancreas.[15]

Each islet of Langerhans is composed of approximately 1000 endocrine cells filled with characteristic secretory granules. Four major cell types are recognized in the islets: glucagon-producing A (alpha) cells, insulin-producing B (beta) cells, somatostatin-producing D (delta) cells, and pancreatic polypeptide-producing PP cells (Table 8-1) (Fig. 8-3).

A cells constitute 15%–20% of total endocrine mass and contain characteristic 180–300-nm secretory granules with a centrally or eccentrically located, round, highly electron-dense core and a pale peripheral mantle (see Table 8-1). Glucagon, glucagon-37, and the major proglucagon fragment (MPGF) are stored in the core, whereas chromogranins and glicentin-related pancreatic peptide (GRPP) are stored in the pale mantle.[16, 17] Immunohistochemical stain using specific C-terminal glucagon sera demonstrates A cells in the tissue (see Fig. 8-3A).

B cells are the most numerous types of islet cells and form 60%–70% of total endocrine mass (see Table 8-1). B cells synthesize, store, and secrete insulin. The secretory granules of B cells measure about 225–375 nm and contain either a crystalline or compact, finely granular core. Crystalline granules contain insulin, whereas compact granules contain proinsulin and are considered immature.[18] B cell granules also contain chromogranin A[19] and islet amyloid polypeptide (IAPP).[20] Positive immunohistochemical stains for both insulin (see Fig. 8-3B) and

Table 8-1. Characteristics of Islet Cells

Cell Type	Hormone	Granule Morphology	Percent of Total Endocrine Cells
A cell	Glucagon	180–300-nm granules with round, electron-dense core and pale peripheral mantle	15–20
B cell	Insulin	225–375-nm granules with crystalline or compact granular core and pale peripheral mantle	60–70
D cell	Somatostatin	170–220-nm granules with moderate and uniform cores, tight limiting membrane	5–10
PP cell	Pancreatic polypeptide	138–208-nm granules of variable shape, density, and structure	15–20

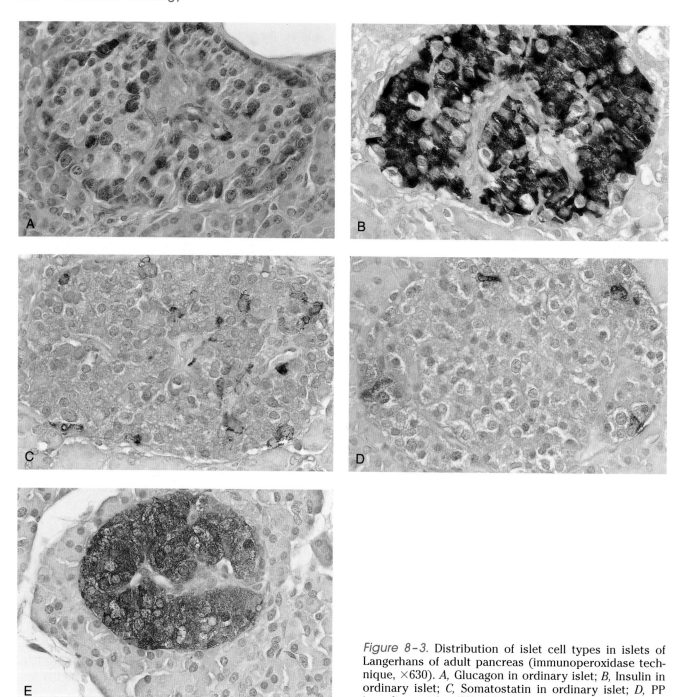

Figure 8-3. Distribution of islet cell types in islets of Langerhans of adult pancreas (immunoperoxidase technique, ×630). *A,* Glucagon in ordinary islet; *B,* Insulin in ordinary islet; *C,* Somatostatin in ordinary islet; *D,* PP in ordinary islet (2%–5%); *E,* PP in irregular islet (70%).

proinsulin provide direct evidence of the presence of insulin in the B cells.

D cells constitute 5%–10% of endocrine cells in the islets. The majority of D cells are located in the periphery of the islet, and some are scattered among the B-cell clusters in the center (see Table 8–1, Fig. 8–3C). Somatostatin is stored in 170–220-nm secretory granules with moderate and uniform cores. D cells contain short processes in contact with adjacent endocrine cells and long processes in contact with intrainsular capillaries.[14] Somatostatin secreted by D cells modulates insulin and glucagon release from the B and A cells by both paracrine

and endocrine mechanisms.[14] D cells stain positively with somatostatin immunohistochemical stain (see Fig. 8–3C) and alcoholic silver solutions but do not react with Grimelius silver stain.

PP cells constitute up to 70% of islet cells in the irregular islets of the posterior pancreatic head and only 2%–5% of endocrine cells in the rest of the islets (see Table 8–1 and Fig. 8–3D–E). Overall, PP cells form 15%–20% of total endocrine mass. PP cells of the ventrally derived posterior pancreatic head are large, 208 nm in size, and contain granules of variable shape, density, and structure.[21] PP cells of the dorsally derived pancreas demonstrate small, round granules, 138 nm in diameter, with a fairly dense core closely surrounded by a membrane. All PP cells contain pancreatic polypeptide and stain positively on PP immunohistochemistry stain (see Fig. 8–3D–E).

TUMORS OF THE ENDOCRINE PANCREAS

General Characteristics

Pancreatic endocrine tumors are benign or malignant epithelial neoplasms that show evidence of endocrine cell differentiation. They are relatively uncommon and represent 1%–2% of all pancreatic tumors.[2] The annual incidence of clinically relevant endocrine tumors reported in surgical series is 1 per 2 million people.[2] The incidence of 1 to 5 per year per million population for all pancreatic endocrine tumors was reported in Northern Ireland.[22] In the United States, the incidence is estimated at less than 1 per 100,000 people.[23] The relative frequency of pancreatic endocrine tumors has been estimated: 30% for insulinoma, 16%–30% for gastrinoma, 10% for vasoactive intestinal polypeptide-secreting tumor (VIPoma), 5%–6% for glucagonoma, 25%–36% for nonfunctioning tumor, and 0%–3% for tumor with ectopic hormone production. In autopsy series, incidental nonfunctioning endocrine tumors were reported in 0.4%–1.6% of random pancreatic sections and in 10% of systematically examined pancreata.[24, 25]

Nichols published the first description of a pancreatic "islet cell adenoma" in 1902[26]; a year later,

Fabozzi reported a malignant counterpart as an "islet cell carcinoma."[27] The hormonal activity of such lesions was noted in 1927 by Wilder et al. who recorded hyperinsulinism associated with a pancreatic endocrine carcinoma.[28] Subsequently in 1955, Zollinger and Ellison described the causal association of an ulcerogenic syndrome with pancreatic endocrine tumors, leading to the recognition of gastrin as a product of the endocrine pancreatic tumor.[29]

Different nomenclatures have been used for tumors of the endocrine pancreas. The term "islet cell tumor," which is still widely used, is misleading because tumors like gastrinoma and VIPoma produce hormones not normally present in the endocrine cells of the human adult pancreas. Furthermore, it is now believed that endocrine tumors arise from pluripotent stem cells or committed endocrine precursors in the wall of the pancreatic ducts rather than from the cells of the islets of Langerhans.[30-32] Other terms previously used are "carcinoid-islet cell tumor," because of the histologic resemblance to the intestinal carcinoids,[33] and "APUDoma," reflecting once-popular theory of a common embryologic origin from cells of the amine precursor uptake and decarboxylation system.[34]

The preferred term is "pancreatic endocrine tumor,"[31, 35] which combines histologic, immunohistochemical, ultrastructural, and/or clinical features of endocrine differentiation. However, many of the endocrine tumors that occur in the pancreas can occur at other sites (Tables 8–2 and 8–3). The term "endocrine tumor" is preferable to "adenoma" because a benign clinical course cannot be predicted

Table 8-2. Classification of Pancreatic Endocrine Tumors Based on Hormone Production

Major Hormone	Clinical Syndrome	Tumor Location	Percent Malignant
Insulin	Hypoglycemia	Pancreas (>99%)	<10
Glucagon	Glucagonoma syndrome	Pancreas (100%)	50–80
Somatostatin	Somatostatinoma syndrome	Pancreas (55%) Duodenum/ Jejunum (44%)	>70
Gastrin	Zollinger-Ellison syndrome	Duodenum (70%) Pancreas (25%) Other sites (5%)	60–90
Vasoactive intestinal peptide	Verner-Morrison syndrome or WDHA (pancreatic cholera)	Pancreas (90%) Other sites (10%)	40–80
ACTH, CRH	Cushing's syndrome	Pancreas (10%) Other sites (90%)	>88
GHRH, GH	Acromegaly	Pancreas (30%) Lung (54%) Other sites (20%)	>60
Serotonin	Carcinoid syndrome	Pancreas (<1% of all carcinoids)	68–88
PTHrP, PTH	Hypercalcemia	Pancreas (rare cause of hypercalcemia)	84
Pancreatic polypeptide; various hormones	Nonfunctioning	Pancreas (100%)	>60

WDHA: watery diarrhea, hypokalemia, achlorhydria; ACTH, adrenocorticotropic hormone; CRH: corticotropin-releasing hormone; GHRH: growth hormone-releasing hormone; GH: growth hormone, PTHrP: parathyroid hormone-related peptide; PTH: parathyroid hormone.

Table 8–3. Pancreatic Endocrine Tumors (PET) in Hereditary Syndromes

Syndrome	Location of the Gene (gene product)	Frequency of PET
Multiple endocrine neoplasia type 1	11q13 (610–amino acid protein, *MENIN*)	80%–100% pancreas (nonfunctioning> gastrinoma > insulinoma)
Von Hippel-Lindau disease	3p25.5 (213–amino acid protein)	12%–17% (almost always nonfunctioning)
Von Recklinghausen's disease (neurofibromatosis 1)	17q11.2 (2485–amino acid protein, neurofibromin)	6% pancreatic somatostatinoma

with certainty. If the tumor is known to be clinically malignant, then the term "pancreatic endocrine carcinoma" may be used. The ultimate classification into prognostic groups (benign versus malignant) is the most difficult aspect of pancreatic endocrine tumor pathology. Classic morphologic features of malignancy are unreliable in predicting the biologic behavior of these tumors. The only reliable criterion of malignancy is infiltration of adjacent organs and/or metastases to regional lymph nodes and distant organs.

Pancreatic endocrine tumors occur sporadically or as a part of hereditary syndromes. Sporadic pancreatic endocrine tumors are solitary, whereas pancreatic tumors in patients with hereditary syndromes

such as MEN1 (prevalence of 82%–100%)[36-39] and von Hippel-Lindau (VHL) disease (prevalence of 12%–17%) are frequently multiple[40-43] (see Table 8–3). The mean reported age at presentation for sporadic tumors is 58 (age range is 12–78 years).[35] Tumors associated with hereditary syndromes occur in younger patients (mean age 35 in VHL disease), and most are detected during radiologic screening.[42, 43]

Pancreatic endocrine tumors can be classified morphologically according to their histologic, immunohistochemical, and ultrastructural characteristics. The tumors may show trabecular (gyriform), solid (medullary, diffuse), or acinar (duct-like) architectural growth patterns (Fig. 8–4).[35, 44] Although these patterns may suggest the endocrine nature of

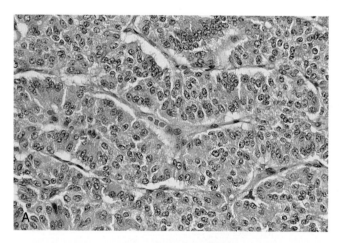

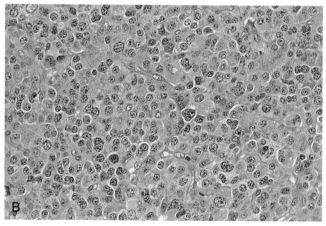

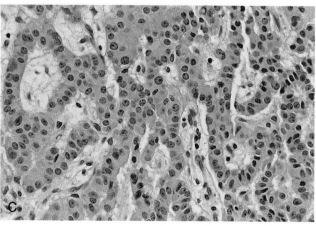

Figure 8–4. Architectural patterns of pancreatic endocrine tumors (H&E, ×400). *A,* Trabecular; *B,* Solid; *C,* Acinar.

the tumors, there is no reliable relationship between architectural pattern and cell type, hormone production, or biologic behavior. Immunohistochemical and molecular analyses allow subclassification by hormone production in many cases but are less helpful in tumors demonstrating multiple hormones. Ultrastructural assessment of tumor morphology may indicate the cell type in well-differentiated tumors; however, the presence of atypical granules in other tumors may prevent accurate ultrastructural classification.[44] Therefore, classification of tumors according to morphologic characteristics, including all recognized cell types identified by immunohistochemistry and/or electron microscopy, is not practical.

At present, the most practical classification of pancreatic endocrine tumors is their functional subclassification by the type of clinical syndrome[35, 44] (see Table 8–2). Pancreatic endocrine tumors are subdivided into functioning, or hormonally active, tumors that induce clinical symptoms by inappropriate hormone secretion, and nonfunctioning, or hormonally inactive (silent), tumors. Because both functioning and nonfunctioning endocrine tumors may stain with one or several peptide hormones by immunohistochemistry, but the clinical picture is usually dominated by the effects of one hormone, the classification of functioning tumors should be based on the hormone giving rise to the clinical syndrome. The majority of clinically relevant pancreatic endocrine tumors are functioning and include insulinoma, gastrinoma, glucagonoma, somatostatinoma, and VIPoma. Nonfunctioning tumors are reported at 15%–35% of surgical cases and usually present with symptoms of an expanding mass.[45] It has been observed that all pancreatic endocrine tumors, with or without associated hyperfunctional syndrome, that are composed of cells that are normally found in pancreatic islets and that produce hormones like insulin, glucagon, somatostatin, and PP, have much lower malignancy rates (1%–20%) than those producing "gut" hormones, like gastrin, VIP, and neurotensin (60%–80%),[2, 35, 46, 47] or "ectopic" hormones, such as adrenocorticotropic hormone, vasopressin, or parathyroid hormone (90%–100%).[35, 48]

The practical value of the new approach to classification of pancreatic endocrine tumors in particular and tumors of the "diffuse endocrine system" in general proposed in World Health Organization (WHO) publication *Histological Typing of Endocrine Tumors*[49] remains to be determined. The classification subdivides pancreatic endocrine lesions into five categories: (1) well-differentiated endocrine tumor, (2) well-differentiated endocrine carcinoma, (3) poorly differentiated endocrine carcinoma, (4) mixed exocrine-endocrine tumor, and (5) tumor-like lesions. The tumor classification proposed by the WHO Committee is based largely on the microscopic characteristics of the tumor integrated with hormonally characterized cell types detectable in the tumor and by recognition of related hyperfunctional syndromes at the clinical level.[49] However, the histopathologic criteria for malignancy in pancreatic

endocrine tumors are unreliable, and the hyperfunctional syndromes associated with the various tumors are often more predictive of the tumor's natural history than are the purely morphologic findings or tumor size.[50, 51] For example, a gastrin-producing tumor may have a high metastatic potential even when it is small (<2 cm) and has no histologic atypia or local invasion. Therefore, the distinction between a well-differentiated endocrine tumor and a well-differentiated endocrine carcinoma in the WHO classification may be difficult. The categories of the poorly differentiated endocrine carcinoma, mixed exocrine endocrine tumor, and tumor-like lesions of the pancreas are important and are considered in this chapter.

Recent studies demonstrate that plasma chromogranin A, a protein produced by neuroendocrine cells, is elevated in about 60% of both functioning and nonfunctioning pancreatic endocrine tumors as well as carcinoid tumors.[52, 53] Measurement of plasma chromogranin A level may be an important nonimaging method for diagnosis of nonfunctioning endocrine tumors that do not secrete detectable levels of specific hormones. Chromogranin A level is elevated in patients with advanced disease and liver metastasis in all endocrine tumor types. Patients with gastrinoma, however, have high chromogranin A values even in the absence of liver metastasis.[54, 55] In an individual patient, measurement of chromogranin A levels could be useful in assessment of tumor progression, relapse, and tumor burden.[52, 53, 55] However, the course of disease in patients with functioning endocrine tumors is best monitored by measuring the specific hormone secreted by the tumor.[55] There is no correlation between chromogranin A or specific hormone secretion and malignancy in any given pancreatic endocrine tumor.

Functioning Pancreatic Endocrine Tumors Associated with Hormone Excess Syndromes

More than 75% of patients with pancreatic endocrine tumors have clinical evidence of hormone hypersecretion that results in characteristic clinical syndromes (see Table 8–2). The diagnosis may be suspected on clinical grounds, but tissue confirmation is essential.

Insulin-Producing Tumors. Insulinomas are the most common pancreatic endocrine tumors[47] (Fig. 8–5A). Ninety percent of insulinomas are benign.[56] The clinical hallmarks of the tumor are hypoglycemia (less than 40 mg/dL) and inappropriate plasma insulin levels occurring after periods of fasting. Because insulin is secreted intermittently and unpredictably, the diagnosis may be difficult. Patients experience headaches, weakness, dizziness, dysarthria, incoherence, convulsion, and coma because of the deleterious effect of hypoglycemia on brain function. Owing to central nervous system manifestations, insulin-producing tumors may simulate epilepsy, brain tumors, or psychiatric disorders.[56]

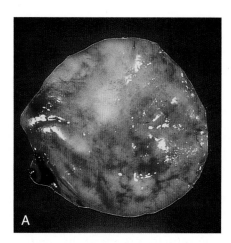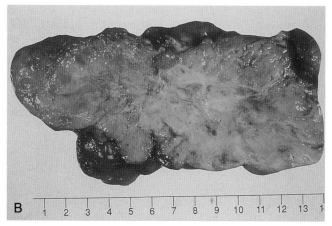

Figure 8–5. Gross pathology of pancreatic endocrine tumors. *A,* Insulinoma, 2.3 cm (enucleated); *B,* Glucagonoma, 14 cm (distal pancreatectomy). (Courtesy of Dr. Ernest Lack, Washington Hospital Center, Washington, D.C.)

Glucagon-Producing Tumors. Tumors secreting glucagon may produce the "glucagonoma syndrome," which is characterized by necrolytic migratory erythema, glossitis, cheilitis, nail dystrophy, glucose intolerance, anemia, hypoaminoacidemia, weight loss, depression, and deep venous thrombosis.[57] There is a close correlation between tumor size and clinical symptoms and malignancy. Glucagonomas usually become symptomatic after they become large (mean diameter >5 cm) and produce high levels of glucagon[58, 59] (see Fig. 8–5B). Sixty to eighty percent of large glucagonomas are malignant.[56] Because these tumors are initially asymptomatic or the symptoms are unrecognized for a long time, the diagnosis may be delayed for many years (up to 15 years).[60]

Somatostatin-Producing Tumors. "Somatostatinoma syndrome" is rare and is characterized by diabetes mellitus, cholelithiasis, steatorrhea, and hypochlorhydria.[61, 62] The majority of pancreatic endocrine tumors associated with this syndrome were reported to be malignant, with metastasis to the liver at the time of presentation.[63, 64] The diagnosis is frequently delayed because the early symptoms of dyspepsia, cholelithiasis, and mild diabetes are common and nonspecific. Not all patients with somatostatinomas present with the syndrome.[65] These clinical differences may be attributed to the level and molecular form of the secreted somatostatin and/or other hormones released by the tumor.[65] Duodenal somatostatinomas do not induce the classic somatostatinoma syndrome and usually present with symptoms related to their location (jaundice, pancreatitis, right upper quadrant pain). The diagnosis of somatostatinoma is suspected on clinical grounds and is usually proven by hypersomatostatinemia (10 to 100 times the normal level). However, normal basal somatostatin plasma levels do not exclude the diagnosis of a somatostatin-producing tumor; provocative testing with tolbutamide may be required to demonstrate somatostatin secretion by the tumor.[66]

Gastrin-Producing Tumors. Gastrinoma is an enteropancreatic endocrine tumor of high malignant potential (60%–90% are metastatic at the time of diagnosis) that follows an indolent clinical course (Fig. 8–6). The tumor cells release gastrin into the blood stream, causing Zollinger-Ellison syndrome (ZES). Gastrin is not present in islets of the normal adult pancreas, but it is produced by fetal islets prior to the onset of synthesis of other pancreatic hormones and may have an important trophic role.[67]

The tumor may occur in sporadic and familial forms. Twenty to twenty-five percent of ZES cases are associated with familial MEN1 (ZES-MEN1). Sporadic gastrinomas are solitary, whereas MEN1 associated gastrinomas are commonly multiple, extrapancreatic (the duodenum is the most common site), and small (see Fig. 8–6). The preoperative localization of gastrin-producing tumors is challenging.[68, 69] Tumor localization studies demonstrate that ultrasonography, computed tomography (CT) scanning, and angiography localize only 20%, 30%, and 50% of primary gastrinomas, respectively. Exploratory laparotomy with intraoperative ultrasonography, transduodenal endoscopic illumination, duodenotomy, and surgical resection of the tumor are currently recommended for patients with sporadic ZES without MEN1.

The diagnosis of ZES is usually established clinically and then confirmed by demonstration of the specific tumor type (gastrin-positive endocrine tumor) in the pathology specimen. Clinical diagnosis of ZES is based on the finding of concurrent hypergastrinemia (increased serum gastrin produced by the tumor) and hyperchlorhydria (increased gastric acid secretion by hyperplastic parietal cells secondary to the trophic action of gastrin) in patients with ulcer disease.[70] Because ZES symptoms overlap with those of much more common peptic ulcer disease, the diagnosis of gastrinoma (ZES) may be delayed for many years. Multiple ulcers and unusual (low duodenal and intestinal) location; resistance to medical therapy; frequent and early recurrence;

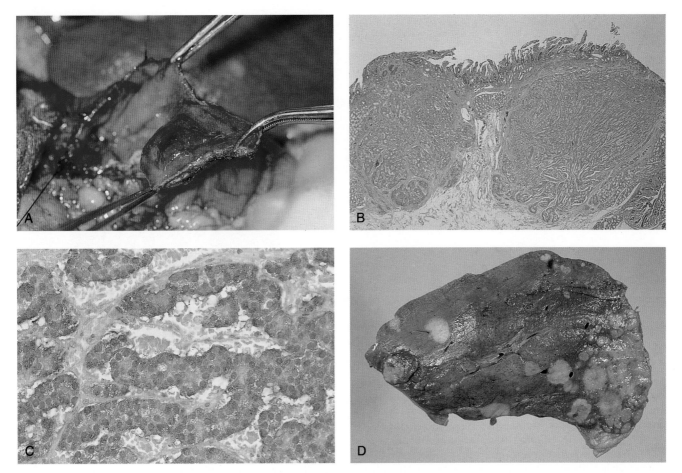

Figure 8–6. Gastrin-producing tumors causing Zollinger-Ellison syndrome. *A*, Sporadic solitary duodenal gastrinoma, 1 cm in size (intraoperative photograph); *B*, Multiple microgastrinomas in duodenum of a patient with MEN1 (H&E, ×25); *C*, Gastrin-producing pancreatic endocrine tumor (gastrin immunostain, ×400); *D*, Metastatic gastrinoma in the liver (autopsy).

prolonged, unexplained diarrhea or steatorrhea; enlarged gastric or duodenal folds; and negative test results for *Helicobacter pylori* raise a suspicion for ZES. The diagnosis is established by positive results with two or more of the following: elevated fasting serum level of gastrin (>100 ng/L), abnormal secretin stimulation test (increment in fasting serum level of gastrin >200 ng/L after intravenous secretin), and an elevated basal level of gastric acid output (>10 mEq/hr).

Gastrinomas may cause severe hypergastrinimia and be malignant even when less than 0.5 cm in diameter. The prognosis of gastrinoma is directly related to the spread of the tumor. Patients with liver metastases (see Fig. 8–6D) have only a 20%–30% chance of surviving for 5 years, whereas patients without liver metastases have an excellent long-term prognosis (>90% 5-year survival rate).[70]

The excess gastrin produced by gastrinoma has trophic effects on a variety of cells of the stomach. These long-term effects include hypertrophy of oxyntic mucosa, hyperplasia of parietal cells (Fig. 8–7A) and hyperplasia of the enterochromaffin-like (ECL) cells (see Fig. 8–7B). Simple, linear,

micronodular and adenomatoid hyperplasias of the histamine-producing ECL cells in the stomach have been described.[71, 72] Gastric ECL cell carcinoids are seen in more than 13% of patients with ZES-MEN1.[73]

Treatment of patients with ZES is also directed at reducing gastric acid hypersecretion, the first and the most severe clinical manifestation of the disease. Total gastrectomy or vagotomy was used in the past to control hyperchlorhydria but is presently not recommended routinely.[74] Over the past 15 years, due to advent of highly potent antisecretory agents, gastric acid output can be effectively suppressed by therapeutic methods. Introduction of histamine H_2-antagonists and especially the proton pump inhibitor omeprazole significantly decreased the early mortality of patients due to complications of ulcer disease. With the increased ability to control hyperchlorhydria, the progression of gastrinoma and metastases are becoming the primary factor in long-term survival of patients with ZES.[75]

Vasoactive Intestinal Peptide–Producing Tumors. Tumors secreting vasoactive intestinal peptide (VIP) produce Verner-Morrison or WDHA (watery diarrhea, hypokalemia, achlorhydria) syndrome. Other

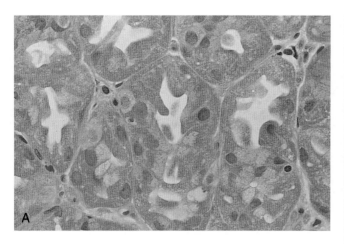
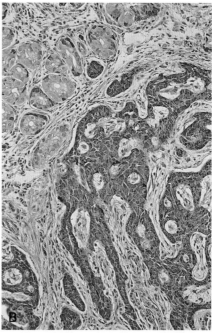

Figure 8–7. Stomach pathology in Zollinger-Ellison syndrome. *A,* Parietal cell hyperplasia (H&E, ×400); *B,* Gastric ECL cell carcinoid and ECL cell hyperplasia (Grimelius silver stain, ×200).

peptides such as PP, secretin, neurotensin, prostaglandins, calcitonin, peptide histidine is oleucine, and peptide histidine methionine (PHM) have been implicated in the pathophysiology of this syndrome.[76–79] A VIP plasma level should be measured in all patients with severe secretory diarrhea. In patients with VIPoma, the VIP levels are usually above 60 pmol/L. High PHM levels in plasma may facilitate the diagnosis. Although cases of VIPomas associated with MEN1 have been reported,[46, 78, 80] most VIP-producing tumors are sporadic.[66] Sporadic tumors are usually large and solitary. Up to 80% of VIPomas are reported to be metastatic at the time of diagnosis.[66]

Functioning Pancreatic Endocrine Tumors Associated with Uncommon Hormone Excess Syndromes

Other syndromes due to ectopic hormone production have been reported in association with pancreatic endocrine tumors (see Table 8–2). The syndromes include Cushing's syndrome (adrenocorticotropic hormone [ACTH][81, 82]), corticotropin-releasing hormone,[83] acromegaly (growth hormone–releasing hormone),[84] growth hormone,[85] carcinoid syndrome (serotonin),[86] and hypercalcemia (parathyroid hormone [PTH] and PTH related peptide [PTHrP][87, 88]). Other hormones secreted ectopically by pancreatic endocrine tumors include vasopressin, norepinephrine, substance P, calcitonin, and neurokinin.[44] Tumors secreting ectopic hormones are more often malignant as compared with other hormone-secreting pancreatic tumors.[89] ACTH-secreting pancreatic tumors correspond to about 10% of ectopic Cushing's syndrome cases and

occur predominantly in women (64% of cases).[81] Eighty-eight percent of these tumors are metastatic to lymph nodes, liver and, often, kidney, thyroid, and bone.[81] In some cases the same tumor produces both Cushing's syndrome and ZES, and both ACTH and gastrin immunoreactive cells are documented in the tumor. This association occurs in 5% of ZES cases and 14% of Cushing's cases because of pancreatic tumor and carries a worse prognosis.[81, 89]

Pancreatic endocrine tumors causing the carcinoid syndrome are extremely rare. They are usually large, and 68%–88% are malignant.[90, 91] Diarrhea; cutaneous flushing; hypotension; and endocardial, mesenteric, and retroperitoneal fibrosis are components of the carcinoid syndrome. The syndrome is due to a variety of substances released by the tumor such as serotonin, kallikreins, substance P, and other tachykinins and prostaglandins.

Pancreatic endocrine tumors causing hypercalcemia are almost all malignant and large (>5 cm).[92] Serum PTH is usually not elevated. PTHrP is produced in normal pancreatic islets[93] and is commonly detected in pancreatic endocrine tumors.[93] When the serum level of PTHrP is elevated in isolation, it does not lead to hypercalcemia. Additional tumor-derived factors may be necessary to cause hypercalcemia.[88]

Nonfunctioning Tumors (Including PP-Cell Tumors)

Fifteen to thirty-five percent of all pancreatic endocrine tumors are clinically silent or nonfunctioning.[94] These tumors may be found incidentally during radiologic imaging for other reasons or they may be present with nonspecific symptoms.

Symptoms include abdominal pain, abdominal mass, gastrointestinal bleeding, weight loss, or jaundice. Nonfunctioning tumors that produce local symptoms are more often malignant than those found incidentally.[58] Survival rates do not differ significantly between patients with functioning and nonfunctioning tumors when patients are matched for age, sex, and extent of disease.[95] The most important indicator of prognosis and survival is the extent of disease at the time of presentation.[95, 96] In nonfunctioning and functioning malignant endocrine tumors, regional lymph node involvement frequently occurs and does not imply that a tumor is incurable.[44, 97] Liver metastases indicate a more biologically aggressive tumor; however, some patients with liver involvement live for many years.[96–98]

PP-Cell Tumors. Plasma levels of PP are frequently elevated in patients with functional and nonfunctional endocrine tumors of the pancreas.[99] Approximately 45% of all pancreatic endocrine tumors contain PP,[99, 100] and elevated plasma PP level alone is not a useful marker. In fact, large tumors producing extremely high levels of serum PP have been reported, and the tumors were clinically nonfunctioning.[101] No distinctive clinical syndrome associated with PP-producing tumors has been described.[2, 66] Some patients with elevated PP levels have been reported with symptoms of watery diarrhea, weight loss, gastrointestinal bleeding, epigastric pain, and chronic duodenal ulcers.[76, 77, 102] However, these clinical symptoms can be attributed to the production of VIP, somatostatin, and other hormones by plurihormonal pancreatic endocrine tumors.[66] Most clinically silent and functional small tumors (<2 cm) are benign. Tumors reported to have metastases have a mean size of 6.3–8.1 cm.[102]

Multiple nonfunctioning endocrine tumors are the most common tumors found in the pancreas of patients with MEN1[37, 39, 70] (see Table 8–3). von Hippel–Lindau–associated pancreatic endocrine tumors are almost always nonfunctioning.[42, 43] Sporadic and hereditary nonfunctioning tumors usually contain several hormones by immunohistochemistry.[37, 39, 42, 94] The lack of clinical symptoms may be the result of the production of small amount of hormones, secretion of biologically inactive forms, or production of hormones not causing recognizable symptoms (PP, neurotensin, cacitonin, bombesin).[2, 44]

Pancreatic Endocrine Tumors in Heredity Syndromes

MEN1

MEN1 is a familial disorder inherited as an autosomal-dominant trait in which tumors occur in at least two of the following organs: parathyroid (88%–97%), endocrine pancreas and duodenum (81%–100%, including gastrinomas in 54% and insulinomas in 21%–24%), and pituitary (21%–65%). The MEN1 tumor suppressor gene was identified in 1997.[103] The gene plays a causative role in the development of MEN1 tumors and a subset of sporadic counterpart tumors.[103–106]

Multiple nonfunctioning microadenomas (<0.5 cm) are the predominant lesions in the pancreas (Fig. 8–8A and 8–8B). They have trabecular or mixed solid-trabecular growth pattern with or without interspersed dense stroma.[107] The cells in microadenoma show immunoreactivity for one or several hormones and frequently stain for glucagon, PP, and/or insulin by immunohistochemistry.[107, 108] Gastrinoma is the most common functioning enteropancreatic tumor in MEN1 (see Fig. 8–6B). It may be an initial manifestation of the syndrome in up to one-third of familial ZES cases.[109] Therefore, it is currently recommended to evaluate all ZES patients for medical and family history of the endocrine neoplasms and to assess parathyroid function (serum calcium and plasma parathormone levels), pituitary function (prolactin levels and magnetic resonance imaging [MRI] of sella turcia), and adrenal status (24-hour urinary cortisol). It is important to distinguish patients with familial ZES-MEN1 from patients with sporadic ZES because of the differences in natural history of ZES, need for family screening, difficulty in controlling acid hypersecretion, potential for developing gastric carcinoid tumors, and need for exploratory laparotomy for cure. Gastrinomas in ZES-MEN1 are multiple, are located in the duodenum (most common site) and pancreas, and are associated with metastases in 60%–90% of cases. Because gastrinomas are small and multiple, they are hard to localize preoperatively and intraoperatively. Therefore, it is difficult to achieve a long-term biochemical cure, and the usefulness of surgery has not been established for patients with ZES-MEN1.

Other hyperfunctional syndromes of pancreatic origin reported in MEN1 patients are the result of insulinoma, VIPoma, glucagonoma, and growth hormone–releasing factor. Hyperinsulinism has been diagnosed in 21%–24% of MEN1 patients. Excision of a single insulinoma did not result in a long-term cure in 42% of MEN1 patients with hyperinsulinism most likely due to multifocality of insulin-producing lesions.

Nesidioblastosis-like lesions are common in MEN1 pancreata (see Fig. 8–8C). Such lesions most likely represent proliferations of endocrine cells from stem cells when small endocrine nests bud off the ducts and ductules. Endocrine dysplasia is found in MEN1 pancreata. It is defined by an endocrine cell growth less than 0.5 mm in size, which deviates from the normal architecture of the islets by having a trabecular growth pattern, abnormal prevalence of one of the four islet cell types, and mild cellular atypia (see Fig. 8–8D). Both dysplastic and nesidioblastosis-like lesions are nonfunctioning.

Gastric tumors of ECL cells—carcinoids (ECLomas)—are reported in about 13% of patients with ZES-MEN1 (see Fig. 8–7B). Molecular genetic studies demonstrate a causative role of the *MEN1* gene in tumorigenesis of ZES-MEN1 gastric carcinoids.[110]

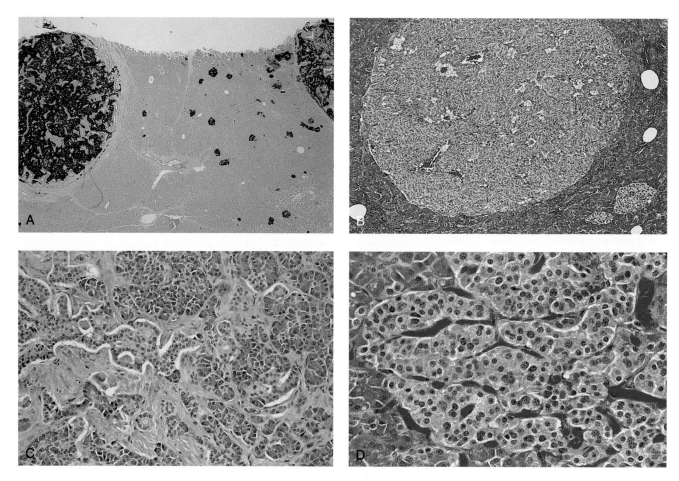

Figure 8–8. Pancreatic pathology in MEN1. *A,* Multiple microadenomas (Insulin, ×25); *B,* Microadenoma (H&E, ×100); *C,* Nesidioblastosis and dysplasia (H&E, ×200); *D,* Endocrine dysplasia (H&E, ×400).

Gastric carcinoids associated with MEN1 are nonfunctioning. Microscopically, carcinoids are mucosal-submucosal tumors composed of endocrine cells arranged in a trabecular, acinar, or solid pattern. ECL cell hyperplasia may be seen in gastric mucosa adjacent to the tumor (see Fig. 8–7B).

ECL-omas are histologically similar to other endocrine tumors of the gastrointestinal tract and cannot be distinguished from gastrinomas on hematoxylin and eosin–stained slides. Silver stains (Sevier-Munger and Grimelius) may be helpful in determining the ECL cell origin of carcinoids. Gastric carcinoids stain positively with panendocrine immunohistochemical stains for chromogranin A and synaptophysin but, unlike gastrinomas, stain negatively for gastrin. Unlike gastrinomas, gastric argyrophil carcinoids in ZES-MEN1 patients usually pursue a benign clinical course.[71, 111] Although a 12% prevalence of metastatic spread to a local perigastric lymph node in ZES-MEN1–associated gastric carcinoids was reported by Rindi et al., no carcinoid-related death was observed among the six patients after 6.7 years of follow-up.[111]

VHL Disease

VHL disease is an autosomal-dominant disorder in which affected individuals develop multiple neoplasms in target organs. The neoplasms include hemangioblastomas of the central nervous system, retinal hemangiomas, renal cell carcinomas, pheochromocytomas, and cysts of the kidneys and epididymis.[112] The most common manifestations of pancreatic VHL disease are benign cysts and microcystic (serous) adenomas that occur in 35%–75% of patients.[113]

Multiple pancreatic endocrine tumors are reported in 12%–17% of VHL patients.[40–43] Loss of the wild-type allele of the VHL tumor suppressor gene was documented in VHL-associated pancreatic endocrine tumors, providing direct molecular evidence for a role of the gene in their tumorigenesis.[42]

Almost all tumors are clinically nonfunctioning and are usually found incidentally or during screening for VHL disease. The tumors are located anywhere in the pancreas, are well circumscribed, and vary in size from 0.4 to 8 cm (median 2 cm)

(Fig. 8–9A–B). They demonstrate tan, red-brown, and gray or yellow color. Invasion of adjacent organs is not usually observed.

Morphologically, the tumors are characterized by solid, trabecular, and/or glandular architecture and prominent stromal collagen bands. Interestingly, 60% of the tumors reveal clear cell cytology at least focally (see Fig. 8–9C). Focal cytologic atypia are occasionally present (see Fig. 8–9D). The tumors are positive for panendocrine immunohistochemistry markers (chromogranin A and/or synaptophysin). Immunohistochemistry stains demonstrate focal positivity for pancreatic polypeptide, somatostatin, insulin, and/or glucagon in 35% of tumors, whereas no immunostaining for pancreatic and gastrointestinal hormones is observed in 65% of tumors.[42] Dense core neurosecretory granules are evident by electron microscopic examination, and the clear cells additionally reveal abundant intracytoplasmic lipid (see Fig. 8–9E).[42] Although usually well circumscribed and confined to the pancreas,

VHL-associated endocrine tumors can metastasize. The median primary tumor diameter in patients with metastases was 5 cm compared with a median primary tumor diameter of 2 cm for patients without evidence of metastatic disease. Therefore, the size of the primary VHL-associated pancreatic endocrine tumor appears to be related to the risk of metastatic disease.[43]

It is important to recognize several differences between pancreatic pathology of MEN1 and VHL patients. First, although multiple pancreatic endocrine tumors occur in both syndromes, they are much more frequent in MEN1 (82%–100%) than in VHL (12%–17%) patients (see Table 8–1).[37, 42, 108] Second, hormonally functioning tumors are extremely rare in VHL disease[42] but relatively common in MEN1.[37] Finally, pancreatic resection specimens in MEN1 patients demonstrate multiple microadenomas and nesidioblastosis in 30% of cases.[108] In contrast, VHL patients usually have a mean of two pancreatic endocrine tumors. Although scattered islets and duc-

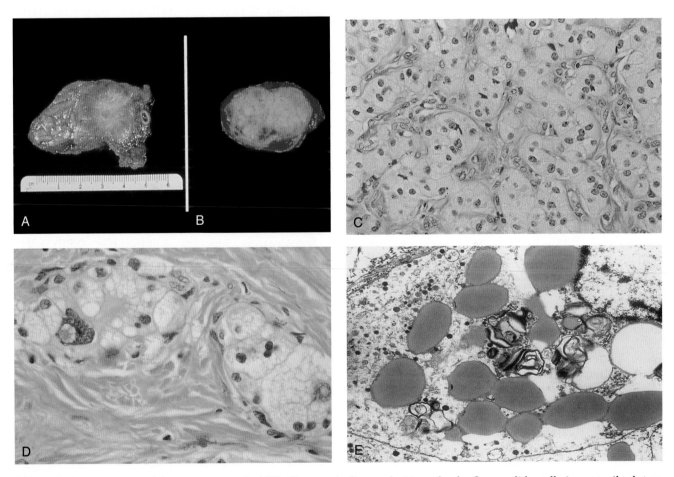

Figure 8–9. Pancreatic endocrine tumors in VHL disease. *A,* Gross photograph of a 3-cm solid, well-circumscribed, tan-gray tumor (partial pancreatectomy); *B,* Gross photograph of a 1-cm tumor with prominent yellow color secondary to abundant lipid content (enucleation); *C,* Endocrine tumor with solid architecture, small vessels, and cells with prominent clear cytoplasm (H&E, ×400); *D,* Tumor cells with clear cytoplasm and focal nuclear atypia surrounded by stromal collagen bands (H&E, ×630); *E,* Electron micrograph of a "clear" cell from a tumor showing prominent lipid globules and myelin figures as well as small dense core granules (magnification ×8900).

tules were frequent within VHL-associated tumors, nesidioblastosis and/or lesions smaller than 0.4 cm in size are not observed in the adjacent pancreas. Multiple cysts and microcystic adenomas common in VHL pancreata are not seen in MEN1 cases.

von Recklinghausen's Disease (Neurofibromatosis 1)

Patients with von Recklinghausen's disease (neurofibromatosis 1) develop duodenal somatostatinomas; only rarely do they develop pancreatic somatostatinomas (6%; see Table 8–3).[114] Many of these tumors stain immunohistologically for somatostatin but do not produce clinical "somatostatinoma syndrome" and, therefore, strictly speaking, are nonfunctioning. The histology and clinical behavior of somatostatinomas in von Recklinghausen's disease are similar to those of sporadic somatostatinomas. Pancreatic and duodenal somatostatinomas show similar morphologic features, except for psammoma bodies that are more frequently seen in duodenal tumors. In contrast to its duodenal counterpart, the pancreatic somatostatinoma is more often associated with a recognizable "somatostatinoma syndrome" and with demonstrable liver or lymph node metastases at the time of operation.

PREOPERATIVE AND INTRAOPERATIVE LOCALIZATION OF PANCREATIC ENDOCRINE TUMORS

Radiology

Pancreatic endocrine tumors of a large size can be localized with standard noninvasive radiologic techniques such as CT scans and transcutaneous ultrasonography. Small tumors, in contrast, frequently require specialized localization techniques for diagnosis. Sporadic and MEN1-associated gastrinomas are frequently small and located in the wall of the duodenum or other extrapancreatic location.[115] Both noninvasive and invasive radiology techniques are used to localize small tumors. In more than 20% of patients with sporadic gastrinomas and in even more patients with MEN1-associated gastrinomas, preoperative localization of the tumors is unsuccessful. Insulinomas are detected successfully in more than 90% of patients.

Noninvasive Studies. Ultrasonography is a noninvasive and relatively inexpensive procedure with highly variable sensitivity.[116] The value of preoperative ultrasound localization of pancreatic endocrine tumors is controversial.[69, 117–120]

CT scanning is the most commonly used initial localization procedure. Intravenous contrast-enhanced thin sections are especially useful.[116] Primary pancreatic endocrine tumor localization rates range from 56% to 96%[96, 108] (Fig. 8–10A). Tumors smaller than 1 cm in size usually cannot be visualized. CT scanning has 70%–100% sensitivity in identification of liver metastases.[69, 98, 121] (see Fig. 8–10B).

MRI is more expensive and less sensitive than CT scanning for identifying pancreatic endocrine tumors.[121]

Invasive Studies. Arteriography with selective injection into branches of the celiac and superior mesenteric arteries supplying the pancreas is a sensitive technique for localization of small, highly vascular endocrine tumors and liver metastases[69, 121] (see Fig. 8–10C).[69, 121]

Selective portal venous sampling has been used when arteriography and noninvasive studies failed to localize a tumor.[115, 119] Catheterization of the splenic and superior mesenteric veins is performed under fluoroscopic guidance after intrahepatic branches of the portal vein are cannulated.[121] Hormone concentrations are measured in blood samples obtained from veins draining different regions of the pancreas. Peptide concentration gradient proximal and distal to the suspected mass is established. Selective venous sampling is highly sensitive for preoperative tumor localization, but it is expensive, invasive, and technically difficult.[119–121] Hormone assays on portal venous blood can be used intraoperatively to confirm complete removal of tumors.

Selective arterial stimulation testing has been used for detection of small insulin- and gastrin-producing tumors. Stimulating agents are sequentially injected into arteries supplying different regions of the pancreas and hormone concentrations are then measured in the cannulated hepatic vein.[121]

Intraoperative ultrasonography is highly sensitive and reveals small tumors as focal areas of decreased echogenicity in the more echogenic pancreas.[115, 122–124] This technique also demonstrates the relationship of tumors to pancreatic ducts, common bile duct, and vessels, which is important in local tumor resection.

Somatostatin receptor scintigraphy (SRS) using gamma scanners is performed preoperatively to localize pancreatic endocrine tumors.[125] The somatostatin analog octreotide, labeled with radioactive iodine (^{123}I) or indium (^{111}In), binds to tissues that express somatostatin receptors. Pancreatic endocrine tumors and carcinoids possess high densities of somatostatin receptors.[70, 126, 127] Using [^{111}In-DTPA-DPhe^1] octreotide for scintigraphy, SRS has proved to be the most sensitive modality for imaging pancreatic endocrine tumors[70, 126] (see Fig. 8–10D). Furthermore, SRS may be useful in differentiating pancreatic endocrine tumors from adenocarcinoma of the pancreas.[128] Sixty-five percent of patients with suspected pancreatic endocrine tumors in the study showed positive SRS localization, whereas no patient with pancreatic adenocarcinoma did.[128] However, the results of SRS should be interpreted carefully within the clinical context of the patient. A prospective study[129] showed that 12% of SRS localizations for pancreatic endocrine tumors could be false positive if interpreted without the clinical context. If interpreted within the clinical context, the

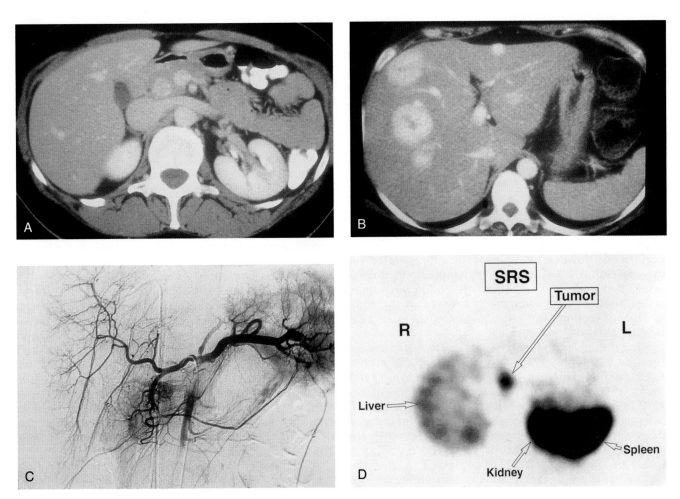

Figure 8–10. Preoperative localization of pancreatic endocrine tumors. *A,* CT scan with contrast demonstrates a tumor in the head of the pancreas; *B,* CT scan with contrast shows multiple tumor metastases in the liver; *C,* Arteriogram of pancreatic insulinoma; *D,* SRS + scan of a 2-cm gastrin-producing tumor in the head of the pancreas. (*A–C,* Courtesy of Dr. Steven K. Libutti, Surgery Branch, National Cancer Institute; *D,* Courtesy of Dr. Robert T. Jensen, Digestive Diseases Branch, National Institute of Diabetes, Digestive and Kidney Diseases, National Institutes of Health, Bethesda, MD.)

SRS false-positive results cause a change in clinical management in only 3% of cases.[129]

Fine-Needle Aspiration Biopsy

The diagnosis of an endocrine tumor or endocrine tumor metastasis can be suspected on cytologic examination of the fine needle aspirate from a pancreatic mass or liver, respectively.[130, 131] Fine-needle aspiration may provide a preoperative diagnosis. It has also been used intraoperatively to evaluate whether small (0.3 cm in diameter) indurated areas in the pancreas represent endocrine tumors.[132] The aspirates are frequently cellular and contain loosely cohesive cells and cell aggregates (Fig. 8–11). The cells are usually monotonous and have eccentric, round, and uniform nuclei with delicate nuclear membranes, a small nucleolus, and finely granular chromatin. The cells have scanty, poorly defined, nonvacuolated cytoplasm. Some cells may have a plasmacytoid appearance, and occasional large

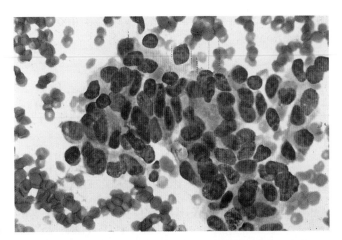

Figure 8–11. Fine-needle aspiration biopsy of a pancreatic endocrine tumor. Tumor cells with eccentric, uniform nuclei and finely granular chromatin. The cells have scanty, nonvacuolated cytoplasm. Some cells may have plasmacytoid appearance, and occasional large atypical cells may be found. (Courtesy of Cytology Section, Laboratory of Pathology, National Cancer Institute, National Institutes of Health, Bethesda, MD.)

atypical cells may be found. Application of panendocrine immunohistochemistry stains to cytologic material is useful in differential diagnosis of nonendocrine pancreatic lesions. Immunohistochemical characterization of a tumor's hormone content, ultrastructural features of endocrine differentiation, and somatostatin receptor status for therapeutic guidelines may also be obtained from cytologic material.[121]

Frozen Section

Intraoperative frozen section assessment of pancreatic endocrine tumors is of limited value because of enzymatic tissue damage if an incisional biopsy is performed. However, it is useful if applied after tumor resection or evaluation of lymph node metastases. If diagnosis of a pancreatic endocrine tumor rather than an adenocarcinoma is made at the time of frozen section, the extent of surgical resection may be altered.[44]

Tumor enucleation and partial pancreatic resection are commonly used for endocrine tumors confined to the pancreas. On the rare occasion, the frozen section may reveal invasion into adjacent organs and confirm the malignant nature of the tumor. Documentation of tumor lymph node metastasis does not contraindicate removal of a pancreatic endocrine tumor,[97] whereas presence of metastases from an adenocarcinoma will prevent aggressive surgery. It is important to distinguish endocrine tumors from well-differentiated adenocarcinomas and acinar carcinomas on frozen section. Touch preparation of the fresh tumor made at the time of frozen section is very useful in visualizing characteristic features of the endocrine tumor. Noncohesive cell groups with round, uniform nuclei and inconspicuous nucleoli and scanty, poorly defined eosinophilic cytoplasm are readily seen on the touch preparations.

MORPHOLOGY OF PANCREATIC ENDOCRINE TUMORS

Gross Appearance and Location

Pancreatic endocrine tumors are usually fairly well circumscribed and may be encapsulated. The tumors occur throughout the pancreas. The predominant distribution of tumor subtypes may or may not reflect the distribution of the corresponding islet cell types throughout the pancreas.[133] Thus, 75% of insulin- and glucagon-secreting tumors are located in the body and tail of the pancreas, whereas 75% of PP-producing tumors are found in the head of the pancreas, reflecting the corresponding islet cell distribution.[133] However, somatostatinomas are commonly found in the head of the pancreas, even though somatostatin-producing D cells are evenly distributed throughout the pancreas.[13] Seventy-five percent of pancreatic gastrinomas are found in the head, yet there are no gastrin-secreting cells in the adult pancreas.

The size of pancreatic endocrine tumors varies. Functioning tumors that produce marked symptoms are usually smaller (0.5–4 cm) than tumors producing nonspecific symptoms or nonfunctioning tumors (>5 cm).[96] Insulinomas and gastrinomas are frequently small (0.5–2 cm in diameter).[115] (see Figs. 8–5A and 8–6A).

Sporadic pancreatic endocrine tumors are usually solitary. Pancreatic endocrine tumors in MEN1 and VHL syndromes are typically multiple, and many are small or microscopic in size[37, 42] (see Fig. 8–8A). If more than one tumor is present in the pancreas, the hereditary syndrome should be suspected.

Extrapancreatic insulin- and glucagon-secreting tumors are very rare, whereas extrapancreatic gastrin- and somatostatin-secreting tumors are more frequent.[65, 68] In fact, both somatostatin- and gastrin-producing tumors occur more commonly in the duodenum than in the pancreas (see Tables 8–2 and 8–3 and Fig. 8–6A–B). Gastrinomas may be located anywhere in the "gastrinoma triangle," defined by the anatomic junctions of cystic and common bile ducts superiorly, second and third portion of the duodenum inferiorly, and neck and body of the pancreas medially.[134] Somatostatin-producing tumor can occur in the small intestine, thyroid, lung, kidney, and hypothalamus.[65, 135, 136]

The gross appearance of pancreatic endocrine tumors varies, based on the degree of vascularity and the amount of stroma. Many tumors are soft and red or yellow-tan (see Fig. 8–5). Other tumors have marked fibrosis and are firm and gray or white. Insulin-secreting tumors are frequently firm and sclerotic due to amyloid stroma.

Histology

The histology of pancreatic endocrine tumors is similar to the histology of intestinal and other endocrine tumors. Several architectural patterns are recognized: (1) trabecular (gyriform), (2) acinar (rosette-like perivascular, glandular, alveolar or duct-like), and (3) solid (medullary or diffuse) patterns[35] (see Fig. 8–4). The sheets or nests of cells may be separated by strands of fibrous tissue or closely packed with a thin vascular stroma (Fig. 8–12A–B). Frequently, cells are arranged around blood vessels or spaces with eosinophilic material. The growth pattern in the tumors varies extensively, and various architectural patterns may be found in different areas of the same tumor. Although architectural patterns suggest the endocrine nature of the tumors, there is no reliable relationship between architectural pattern and cell type, hormone production, or biologic behavior. Therefore, architecture and histology of pancreatic endocrine tumor are unreliable parameters for precise diagnosis of tumor type or malignancy.

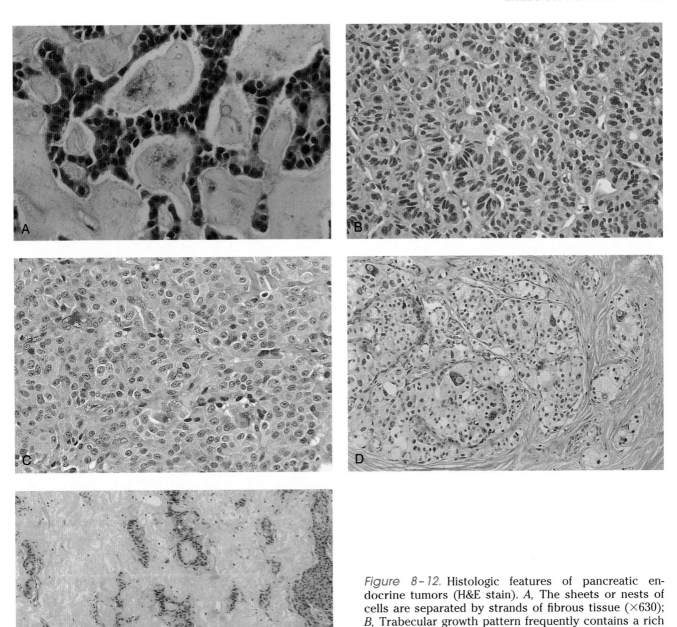

Figure 8-12. Histologic features of pancreatic endocrine tumors (H&E stain). *A,* The sheets or nests of cells are separated by strands of fibrous tissue (×630); *B,* Trabecular growth pattern frequently contains a rich capillary network and elongated neuroendocrine cells (×400); *C,* The tumor cells are in general uniform in size and shape, round and polygonal (×400); *D,* Fibrous bands, scattered pleomorphic cells (×200); *E,* Amyloid in the stroma is seen in about 50% of insulinomas (×200).

The tumor cells are generally uniform in size and shape. They may be round, polygonal, or elongated (see Fig. 8–12). The cytoplasmic border is usually well defined. The cytoplasm is generally slightly eosinophilic but may be strongly eosinophilic or clear. The nuclei are uniform and nucleoli range from inconspicuous to prominent. The "salt and pepper" chromatin pattern is seen in some tumors but not in others. Pleomorphic large cells may be scattered throughout the tumor[31] (see Fig. 8–12D). Mitoses are generally rare.[31] The presence of pleomorphism and mitoses has no prognostic significance.

Pancreatic endocrine tumors frequently contain a rich capillary network and variable amount of stroma. Hyalinization of the tumor stroma is common and sometimes extensive (see Fig. 8–12A and D). Amyloid may be present and is chemically different from AL or AA amyloid. It is composed of a 37-amino-acid peptide IAPP (islet amyloid peptide) that shows 50% homology with calcitonin gene-related peptide.[137] IAPP is co-stored with insulin in B-cell secretory granules.[138] Amyloid in the stroma is seen in about 50% of insulinomas (see Fig. 8–12E) but is rare in other pancreatic endocrine tumors.[139]

A number of histologic features have been described rarely in pancreatic endocrine tumors. Large globules that stain with periodic acid–Schiff stain may be present in the tumor cell cytoplasm or within the stroma. These globules may stain with antibodies to α-antitrypsin.[140] Mucin droplets are occasionally seen in the duct-like structures.[141] Tumor cells may have clear cytoplasm secondary to the presence of glycogen and/or lipid.[42, 142] Clear cytoplasm is commonly seen in VHL-associated pancreatic endocrine tumors[42] (see Fig. 8–9). Pancreatic endocrine tumors composed of oncocytic cells with abundant, finely granular eosinophilic cytoplasm with numerous mitochondria have been described.[143] Dystrophic calcifications and psammoma bodies may be present in the tumor. Psammoma bodies have been reported predominantly in pancreatic insulinomas and duodenal somatostatinomas.[44, 65]

Immunohistochemistry

Pancreatic endocrine tumors are epithelial neoplasms that stain positively with cytokeratin immunohistochemistry stains (Fig. 8–13A). Their endocrine phenotype is confirmed with general markers of endocrine differentiation (pan-endocrine markers). Neuron-specific enolase (NSE) is a sensitive but nonspecific pan-endocrine marker. NSE is a glycolitic enzyme that localizes a soluble cytoplasmic antigen in all pancreatic endocrine tumors and shows a diffuse, homogenous, cytoplasmic staining pattern[144–146] (see Fig. 8–13B). Synaptophysin is an endocrine marker that is as sensitive as NSE but is more specific for identification of pancreatic endocrine tumors.[147, 148] Synaptophysin is an acidic glycoprotein isolated from the neuronal presynaptic vesicles. It demonstrates a uniform, delicate granular staining pattern marking all tumors regardless of their hormone content or biologic behavior[148] (see Fig. 8–13C). Synaptophysin has been recommended as a marker of choice for the broad categorization of pancreatic tumors as endocrine in nature.[148] Chromogranins are far more specific but not as sensitive for detecting the endocrine nature of pancreatic endocrine tumors.

Chromogranin A is an acidic glycoprotein isolated from chromaffin granules.[146, 149] Chromogranin A gives an irregular, coarsely granular staining pattern[145, 146] (see Fig. 8–13D). It is the major chromogranin of the pancreatic islets where it is present only in a subset of cells such as A cells and PP cells and is not

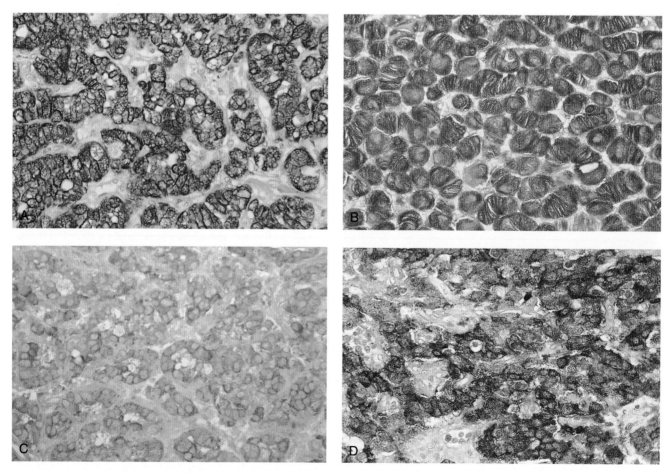

Figure 8–13. Immunohistochemistry staining of pancreatic endocrine tumors with cytokeratin and pan-endocrine markers (×400). *A,* Cytokeratin AE1/AE3; *B,* NSE; *C,* Synaptophysin; *D,* Chromogranin A.

expressed strongly by B and D cells.[145, 146] Only those tumors with certain hormonal products are positive for chromogranin A, and many tumors, such as insulin-containing lesions, may be negative.

Pan-endocrine markers that are used less commonly to demonstrate the endocrine nature of a pancreatic endocrine neoplasm include Leu-7, PGP 9.5, and HISL-19.[146, 149] Leu-7 is a monoclonal antibody raised against a human T-cell leukemia cell line that also has been shown to react with myelin-associated glycoproteins and matrix components of endocrine secretory granules.[150] Leu-7 is less specific than synaptophysin and less sensitive than chromogranin A in detecting endocrine differentiation. PGP 9.5 (protein gene product) is a cytoplasmic protein of unknown function isolated from the brain[151] and found in pancreatic endocrine tumors of all types.[146] It is not a specific marker for endocrine cells. HISL-19 is a monoclonal antibody made by immunizing mice with human cadaveric islet cells.[152] It reacts with antigens in secretory granules and labels Golgi's complexes.[146, 152] HISL-19 may give a positive reaction and be useful in tumors with sparse secretory granules.[122] HISL-19 reacts most strongly with benign glucagon- and PP-secreting tumors and less strongly with insulin-secreting and malignant neoplasms.[146, 152] Like chromogranin A, HISL-19 is a specific but not sensitive indicator of endocrine differentiation.

Immunohistochemical assessment of the hormone profile of a tumor is important in classification of pancreatic endocrine neoplasms. In the majority of cases, the predominant hormone detected by immunohistochemistry correlates with the clinical symptoms and biochemical blood profile (Fig. 8–14A). In some cases, however, discrepancies may occur. In sparsely granulated insulin-producing tumors with rapid secretion rates and classic clinical manifestations, the tumors may not store the hormone product in sufficient amounts to be visualized by immunohistochemistry. In such cases, in situ hybridization technique or electron microscopy are useful for clarifying structure-function correlation.[62, 153, 154] Immunohistochemical assessment of the hormone profile of a tumor provides prognostic information and may determine a chemical marker for postoperative monitoring of tumor progression.[31, 46] Immunohistochemical detection of

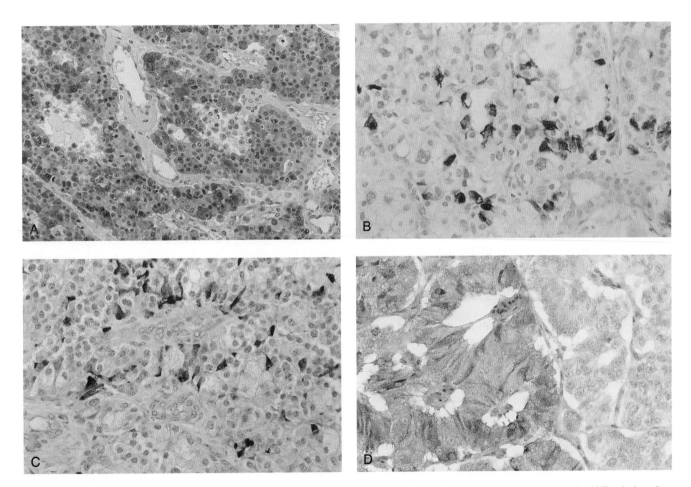

Figure 8–14. Immunohistochemistry of pancreatic endocrine tumors with hormone-specific markers (×400). *A,* Insulin-immunoreactive cells in insulin-producing tumor; *B,* Focal insulin-immunoreactive cells in nonfunctioning tumor; *C,* Focal somatostatin-immunoreactive cells in nonfunctioning tumor; *D,* PP-immunoreactive tumor cells are found as a minor component in up to 47% of pancreatic endocrine tumors.

hormone production is particularly helpful in tumors unassociated with clinical manifestations of the hormone. These tumors are frequently not suspected to be endocrine in nature, and preoperative blood hormone levels are not measured.[31]

Immunohistochemistry analysis of pancreatic endocrine tumors has revealed that many tumors produce, although not necessarily secrete, more than one hormone and may be termed "plurihormonal tumors" (see Fig. 8–14B–C). It is thought that multipotential stem cells exist and are capable of differentiating into each of the cell types normally present in the islets. The distribution of hormone-producing cells is irregular and may vary from one area of the tumor to another. Furthermore, multiple tumors may each produce a different hormone or several hormones. PP-immunoreactive tumor cells are found as a minor component in up to 47% of pancreatic endocrine tumors.[102] (see Fig. 8–14D). Clinically nonfunctional pancreatic tumors in MEN1 and VHL patients are commonly plurihormonal by immunohistochemistry.[37, 42]

In Situ Hybridization

Hormone mRNA detection by in situ hybridization can be used to identify hormone expression at the cellular level in the rare tumors in which immunohistochemistry fails.[155] This approach may help to correlate clinical signs of hormone hyperfunction or increased hormone blood levels and the precise source in primary pancreatic tumors, tumor recurrences, metastases, or extrapancreatic tumors.

Electron Microscopy

Ultrastructural analysis of pancreatic endocrine tumors is mainly useful in establishing the endocrine nature of the neoplasm and allowing further structure-function correlation in tumors with typical secretory granules. In well-differentiated pancreatic endocrine tumors, secretory granules have the characteristic structure of granules found in normal endocrine cells (Fig. 8–15A–C). However, frequently there is heterogenei0ty of granule structure within tumors, and atypical granules may be present that cannot be defined[2] (see Fig. 8–15D). In some tumors, heterogeneity of granule morphology is attributed to the plurihormonal nature of the tumors. The size, shape, and electron density of secretory granules may change according to the functional activity and cellular maturation.[65] Variable structure of the granules may also reflect the storage of prohormones or other molecular species of the peptides in the tumor cells.[59, 65, 156] Therefore, ultrastructure of secretory granules cannot be used as the only criterion of tumor cell differentiation.[13, 60] Because electron microscopy is often not iagnostic,immunohistochemical analysis of the tumors is faster and more reliable.

Ultrastructural analysis may be useful in highly hormonally active pancreatic endocrine tumors. The presence of cells with abundant rough endoplasmic reticulum and Golgi's complexes may be characteristic of such tumors. These tumors may be sparsely granulated if they are actively and rapidly secreting their product. These electron microscopic features may explain apparent discrepancies between immunohistochemistry results and clinical symptoms.[154]

Electron microscopic immunohistochemistry is useful for localization of hormones within individual tumor cells. Double immunogold staining of tumors may show co-localization of peptide hormones within single secretory granules of uniform tumor cells. In a polymorphous tumor cell population, the staining may show different hormones in different cells.

Assessment of Malignancy

Pancreatic endocrine tumors are slow-growing neoplasms, and it is difficult to predict whether an individual tumor will behave in a clinically benign or aggressive manner. Invasion into adjacent organs and/or metastases are the only absolute criteria of malignancy.

Histologic criteria such as nuclear pleomorphism and mitotic activity are unreliable for distinguishing benign from malignant pancreatic endocrine tumors.[31, 46, 157] The significance of perineural, lymphatic, and vascular invasion is being debated and has not been proved (Fig. 8–16). Some authors believe that vascular invasion per se does not indicate malignancy; they advocate closer surveillance of patients with pancreatic tumors that show vascular invasion.[58] Other authors suggest that vascular invasion is one of the few reliable signs of metastatic potential.[68] Perineural and vascular invasion are frequently not seen in primary pancreatic endocrine tumors with documented metastases.[58] Malignant pancreatic endocrine tumors most commonly metastasize to regional lymph nodes and the liver, but they may spread to bone and other distant organs. The rare poorly differentiated pancreatic endocrine tumors demonstrate malignant cytology and frequently show invasion of adjacent organs.

Hormonal subtyping of pancreatic tumors may provide a better prognostic value than histologic features. It has been observed that all pancreatic endocrine tumors, with or without associated hyperfunctional syndrome, that are composed of cells normally found in pancreatic islets and that produce hormones like insulin, glucagon, somatostatin, and PP have much lower malignancy rates (10%–20%) than those producing "gut" hormones such as gastrin, VIP, and neurotensin (60%–80%)[2, 35, 46, 47] or "ectopic" hormones such as ACTH, vasopressin, or parathyroid hormone (90%–100%)[48] (see Table 8–2).

Tumor size is an unreliable criterion of malignancy in many functioning pancreatic endocrine tumors but may be of value in nonfunctioning

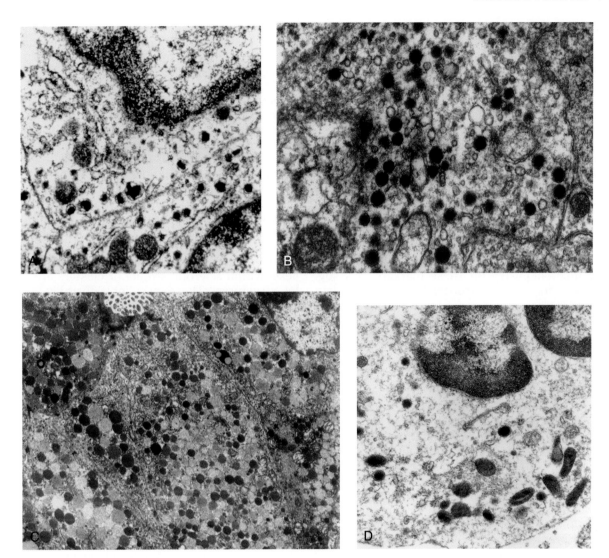

Figure 8-15. Electron microscopy of pancreatic endocrine tumors. *A,* B-cell granules with crystalline or compact granular core and pale peripheral mantle in insulinoma; *B,* A-cell granules with round, electron-dense core and pale peripheral mantle in glucagonoma; *C,* D-cell granules with moderate and uniform cores and tight limiting membrane in somatostatinoma; *D,* Atypical granules in a pancreatic endocrine tumor. (Courtesy of Dr. Maria Tsokos, Laboratory of Pathology, National Cancer Institute, National Institutes of Health, Bethesda, MD.)

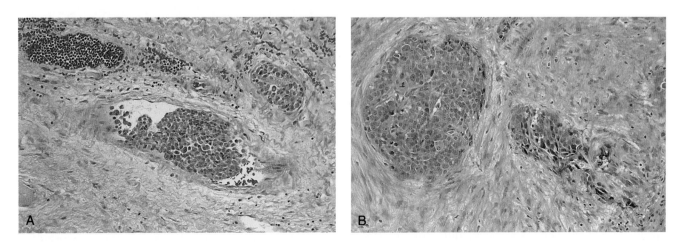

Figure 8-16. Nonfunctioning pancreatic endocrine tumor showing *(A)* vascular and *(B)* capsular invasion (H&E, ×200). The definitive diagnosis of malignancy in this tumor was established by the presence of liver metastases.

sporadic tumors and nonfunctioning tumors associated with MEN1 and VHL. For example, many gastrinomas are small (0.5–2 cm in diameter), yet they are frequently metastatic at the time of diagnosis. Although usually well circumscribed and confined to the pancreas, VHL-associated nonfunctioning pancreatic endocrine tumors can metastasize. The median primary tumor diameter in VHL patients with metastases is 5 cm compared with a median primary tumor diameter of 2 cm for patients without evidence of metastatic disease. Therefore, the size of the primary VHL pancreatic tumors appears to be related to the risk of metastatic disease.[42, 43]

Elevated serum levels of the human chorionic gonadotropin (hCG) and its alpha and beta subunits have been initially suggested as markers of malignancy in pancreatic endocrine tumors.[158, 159] Immunohistochemistry for these markers was suggested for diagnostic purposes.[159–161] These data are contradictory,[162] and most investigators believe that alpha-hCG is frequently localized in tumors with benign behavior.[146]

Ploidy analysis and determinations of S-phase fractions have not proved helpful in distinguishing benign from malignant endocrine tumors.[163, 164] Proliferation marker studies have also showed contradictory results. Although mitotic counts are unreliable,[165] it has been suggested that immunohistochemical positivity for proliferating cell nuclear antigen (PCNA) may predict malignant behavior.[165] Tumors with >5% PCNA-positive cells were more likely to have extrapancreatic spread.[165] The Ki-67 proliferative rate index is thought to be more reliable than PCNA in separating benign from malignant nonfunctioning tumors,[50] but it is not clear if it is helpful in predicting behavior of functioning pancreatic tumors. The proportion of AgNOR-rich cells may predict prognosis of insulinomas but is less reliable for evaluation of gastrinomas.[166]

In summary, although various techniques and markers have been suggested to predict malignant behavior, no reproducible, convenient, and reliable methods are currently available. The multiparametric approach, including size, angio/neuroinvasion, proliferative rate, and the presence or absence of hyperfunctional syndrome, has been suggested for identifying tumors at higher risk of recurrence or metastasis.[2] However, because each of these parameters is unreliable, using a combination of them will not accurately predict prognosis in many tumors.

Differential Diagnosis

The most important differential diagnosis in a patient presenting with a solid tumor in the pancreas is between pancreatic adenocarcinoma and endocrine tumor. Natural history, prognosis, and surgical management are very different in these diseases. Clinical and radiologic data obtained before surgery should be confirmed by pathologic evaluation of the tumor intraoperatively. Other pancreatic neoplasms included in differential diagnosis of endocrine tumor are solid-cystic (papillary-cystic) tumors of adolescent and young females and acinar cell carcinoma of the pancreas.[44] Pancreatic poorly differentiated endocrine carcinoma and mixed exocrine-endocrine tumor of the pancreas should be distinguished from the well-differentiated endocrine tumors. Because many nonfunctioning pancreatic endocrine tumors in VHL patients share the clear cell histology with other tumors of the syndrome, careful consideration should be given to differential diagnosis between primary endocrine tumor and metastatic renal cell carcinoma and microcystic adenoma of the pancreas.[42] In chronic pancreatitis and other disorders associated with chronic duct obstruction and fibrosis, endocrine cells may proliferate and form nests within sclerotic stroma or clusters around ductal structures. These nesidioblastosis-like proliferations can mimic invasive endocrine tumors.

UNCOMMON TUMORS AND TUMOR-LIKE LESIONS OF THE PANCREAS

Poorly Differentiated Endocrine Carcinoma

Poorly differentiated endocrine carcinoma is defined as an epithelial tumor showing highly atypical, small-to-intermediate cells with high nucleocytoplasmic ratio and a poorly granular or agranular cytoplasm. The cells form large, poorly defined solid aggregates, often with central necrosis (Fig. 8–17). Poorly differentiated (small-cell) endocrine carcinomas were previously classified as exocrine tumors.[167, 168] Recent studies have demonstrated a variable degree of reactivity for hormones or endocrine markers and ultrastructural features of

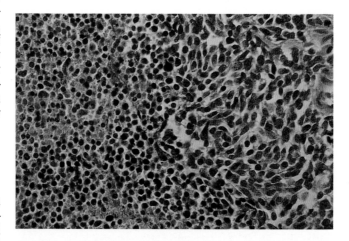

Figure 8–17. Poorly differentiated (small-cell) endocrine carcinoma of the pancreas. The tumor shows solid-diffuse architectural pattern, poorly differentiated fusiform cells, and focal early necrosis (H&E, ×400).

scattered abortive endocrine differentiation in these tumors. Furthermore, the tumors lack reactivity for markers of exocrine differentiation.[169] These neoplasms make up about 2%–3% of pancreatic endocrine tumors in surgical series.[2] The structure and natural history of pancreatic poorly differentiated (small-cell) endocrine carcinomas closely resemble those of pulmonary and extrapulmonary small-to-intermediate-cell carcinomas. They are highly invasive tumors, frequently associated with distant metastases to the liver and extra-abdominal sites. Large areas of tumor necrosis, 10 or more mitoses per 10 high-power fields, and 10% or more Ki-67 positive cells are commonly found. The diagnosis of small-cell carcinoma of the pancreas should be made after the possibility of metastasis from other sites, especially from the lung, is excluded.[170] The differential diagnosis also includes non-Hodgkin's lymphoma and pancreatic adenocarcinoma. Because almost all cases of pancreatic poorly differentiated (small-cell) endocrine carcinoma present with advanced stage of disease in which the tumor resection is impossible, the prognosis is poor. When patients with small-cell tumors received supportive treatment only, their survival time was 1–2 months; in patients with intermediate-cell tumors, the survival period was 6–12 months.[171, 172] Chemotherapy with etoposide and cis-platinum has been shown to prolong survival up to 50 months in some patients.[173, 174]

Mixed Exocrine-Endocrine Tumor of the Pancreas

Mixed exocrine-endocrine tumor of the pancreas is defined as an epithelial tumor with a prevalently exocrine growth pattern and an endocrine component. Endocrine component forms at least one-third of the tumor cell population. These rare tumors demonstrate an intimate admixture of exocrine and endocrine elements[175–177] supporting a close histogenetic origin for the two functional components of the pancreas. The biologic behavior of a mixed exocrine-endocrine tumor is dictated by the exocrine component, which may be solid-pseudopapillary, acinar, or ductal. In the case of solid-pseudopapillary and acinar exocrine components, the endocrine component is frequently composed of endocrine cell types found in normal islets, whereas in the case of ductal-endocrine carcinoma, both islet-type and gut-type (serotonin, gastrin) endocrine cells may be present. Immunohistochemistry confirms the mixture of endocrine and exocrine components. The endocrine cell population stains positively for chromogranin, NSE, and hormone markers, whereas the exocrine component is negative for endocrine markers and stains positively for CEA, for carbohydrate antigen (CA19-9), and for cytokeratins.[176, 178] Electron microscopy may also be helpful in demonstrating exocrine and endocrine features of the tumors.

Tumor-Like Lesions of the Pancreas

Islet hyperplasia is defined as an increase of pancreatic islet mass resulting from an increase of islet size, number, or both (Fig. 8–18). It has been reported rarely in adult patients with hyperinsulinism in the absence of insulinoma[179] or with α_1-antitrypsin deficiency.[180] In newborns, it has been described in association with maternal diabetes, erythroblastosis fetalis, hereditary tyrosinemia, and Beckwith-Wiedemann syndrome.[181–183] Abnormalities of islet size and number are subtle and may be difficult to document.

Nesidioblastosis is a hyperfunctional disorder of insulin-producing cells characterized by hypertrophic B cells within enlarged or normal-appearing islets, small scattered endocrine cell clusters, and ductuloinsular complexes (Fig. 8–19). It most likely represents a proliferation of endocrine cells from

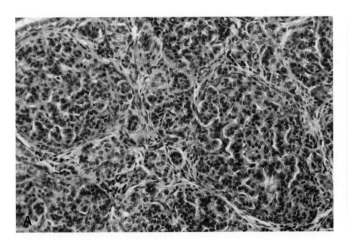
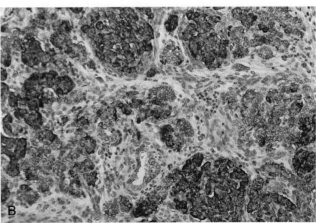

Figure 8–18. Islet hyperplasia in Beckwith-Wiedemann syndrome. *A,* H&E, ×200; *B,* Insulin immunohistochemistry stain, ×200. Crowding of the islets without fusion inside of the pancreatic lobules. (Courtesy of Dr. Ernest Lack, Washington Hospital Center, Washington, D.C.)

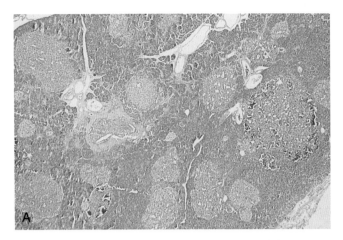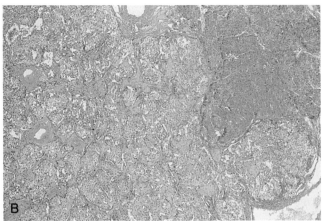

Figure 8–19. Nesidioblastosis in PNHH. *A,* Diffuse nesidioblastosis with variably sized islets that are irregularly distributed in the acinar tissue and interlobular stroma (H&E, ×50); *B,* Focal nesidioblastosis with interconnecting clusters of endocrine cells separated by strands of fibrous tissue (H&E, ×100). (Courtesy of Dr. David L. Gang, Baystate Medical Center, Springfield, MA.)

stem cells, in which small endocrine nests bud off ducts and ductules. These changes are seen in newborns with persistent neonatal hyperinsulinemic hypoglycemia (PNHH) and, extremely rarely, in adults. Nesidioblastosis may be focal or diffuse.[20, 184] Focal nesidioblastosis accounts for one-fourth to one-half of PNHH cases. The size of the focal lesion ranges 2–10 mm. The pancreas appears grossly normal if the lesion is small; larger lesions may present as an ill-defined area of increased consistency. Histologically, focal nesidioblastosis is characterized by an ill-defined accumulation of islet-like cell clusters separated from each other by rims of acinar cells or thin strands of connective tissue.[183] Ductuloinsular complexes and cells with nuclei twice as large as normal are commonly seen. Immunohistochemistry stains demonstrate insulin, glucagon, somatostatin, and PP cells that retain their normal spatial arrangement in the islet-like clusters.[20] However, the proportion of insulin-positive B cells is high and corresponds to 70%–90% of all endocrine cells (the proportion of B cells in normal newborns is about 50%). Most of the cells with enlarged nuclei are insulin-positive. Because the focal nesidioblastosis lesions are small and the remaining endocrine pancreas is histologically normal, serial sections of all available pancreatic tissue in nondiagnostic PNHH cases are required. Ultrastructurally, B cells in the lesion show increased well-organized endoplasmic reticulum and prominent Golgi's complex—signs of hyperfunction—whereas A, D, and PP cells are structurally normal.[185] Diffuse nesidioblastosis accounts for three-fourths of PNHH cases. The pancreas is grossly normal. Microscopically, the features of nesidioblastosis are seen throughout the pancreas. The hallmarks of the lesion include increased variability of islet size and shape; presence of abundant, scattered endocrine cell clusters or individual cells; prominent ductuloinsular complexes, and B-cell hypertrophy.[7, 20, 186, 187] Although some of

these changes may also be seen in the pancreas of normoglycemic newborns and infants, the presence of B cells with enlarged nuclei and prominent ductuloinsular complexes are the most useful diagnostic criteria for PNHH. In some cases, immunohistochemistry stains with pan-endocrine markers and insulin are helpful to reveal the subtle differences in the endocrine pancreas. Disseminated individual endocrine cells and cell clusters throughout the exocrine tissue in excess of those found in age-matched controls is the most frequent, but not always reliable, finding.[184, 188]

Endocrine dysplasia is defined by an endocrine cell growth less than 0.5 mm in size, which deviates from the normal architecture of the islets by having a trabecular architecture, abnormal prevalence of one of the four islet cell types, and mild cellular atypia (see Fig. 8–8D). The term "microadenoma" is applied to lesions of at least 0.5 mm in size (see Fig. 8–8B). Both dysplasia and microadenomas are nonfunctioning lesions of questionable neoplastic potential. They are frequently seen in the pancreas of patients with MEN1 (see Fig. 8–8) and are rare in non-MEN1 pancreata.[35, 107, 189]

PATHOGENESIS AND MOLECULAR ALTERATIONS

Tumors in Animals

Several animal models of pancreatic endocrine tumors have been developed. Although these models are useful in the study of some aspects of endocrine disorders, all of them suggest that animal pancreatic endocrine tumors arise from the islet cells and not from the multipotent ductular stem cells. The origin of pancreatic endocrine tumors from multipotent ductular stem cells is currently favored for humans.

In rats, islet cell tumors have been induced by irradiation,[190] and by injection of plant-derived pyrro-lizidine alkoloids,[191] and with streptozotocin-nicotinamide combination.[190, 192] Streptozotocin induced tumors resemble human pancreatic endocrine tumors. They contain insulin-, glucagon-, somatostatin-, and PP-producing cells with reduced hormone content as compared with normal islet cells. However, unlike human tumors, these experimentally induced neoplasms do not express gastrin.

Pancreatic endocrine neoplasms have been induced in mice rendered transgenic for the hybrid insulin/simian virus (SV) 40 or glucagon/SV40 oncogene.[193-195] Selective transformation and growth of islet B or A cells occurs. All subsequent steps in mouse tumorigenesis can be followed: (1) minute foci of intrainsular hyperplastic-dysplastic changes, (2) multiple B or A microadenomas, (3) macroadenomas with additional islet cell populations, and (4) metastatic tumors with islet and nonislet ("ectopic") tumor cell populations.[194, 195] This model reveals that in mice the multitypic (multicellular) endocrine tumors develop through the early monotypic growth from transformation of intrainsular mature cells.

MEN1 tumor suppressor mouse knockout model was generated through homologous recombination of the mouse homolog *MEN1*.[196] Homozygous mice die in utero at embryonic days 11.5–12.5, whereas heterozygous mice develop features remarkably similar to those of the human disorder. As early as 9 months, pancreatic islets show a range of lesions from hyperplasia to insulin-producing islet cell tumors, and parathyroid adenomas are also frequently observed. Larger, more numerous tumors involving pancreatic islets, parathyroids, thyroid, adrenal cortex, and pituitary are seen by 16 months. All the tumors tested to date show loss of the wild-type *MEN1* allele, further supporting its role as a tumor suppressor gene.

In mice, the pancreatic lesions morphologically vary from normal islets to large islets, to large islets with dysplasia, and finally to pancreatic islet cell tumors. It is hypothesized that the gradual enlargement of pancreatic islets is initially nonclonal and occurs as a consequence of a dosage effect resulting from reduced amounts of menin protein (50%). Presumably, the subsequent transition from hyperplastic islets with dysplasia to islet cell tumor is the result of loss of the wild-type *MEN1* allele.

Although many lesions in *MEN1* tumor suppressor mouse knockout model are similar to human tumors in MEN1, several differences are noted. Parathyroid tumors are frequent in humans and the mouse model; however, elevated serum calcium level is not observed in mice. Gastrinomas, the most common enteropancreatic functioning tumor in humans with MEN1, are not detected in these animals. Human MEN1 pancreata show nesidioblastosis and endocrine dysplasia, whereas mouse pancreata show enlarged and/or hyperplastic islets. Moreover, it is presently believed that in humans, pancreatic tumors arise from multipotent ductular stem cells.

Molecular Genetic Alterations in Human Pancreatic Endocrine Tumors

Unlike most nonendocrine epithelial tumors, pancreatic endocrine neoplasms do not generally carry significant alterations in known oncogenes (*ras, myc, fos, Jun, Src*) or common tumor suppressor genes (*p53, Rb*). Therefore, until recently, their molecular pathogenesis was almost completely unknown.

Hereditary syndromes such as MEN1, VHL and von Recklinghausen's disease are associated with the development of pancreatic endocrine tumors (see Table 8–3). The gene mutated in each of these diseases has been identified; however, the role of the protein in normal tissues remains unclear. All three syndromes are caused by a tumor suppressor gene. For example, MENIN, a 610–amino acid nuclear protein is altered in MEN1, is a nuclear protein, and is widely distributed in normal tissues but its function is unclear.[197] The *VHL* gene encodes a 213–amino acid protein that is important in cell growth regulation and differentiation.[198] MEN1 and VHL germline mutations are documented in patients with MEN1 and VHL disease, respectively. The initial event of pancreatic endocrine tumorigenesis in each syndrome requires a loss of the second wild-type allele of the gene.

The role of the *MEN1* gene in sporadic gastrinomas and insulinomas as well as other enteropancreatic endocrine tumors has been documented.[104] Somatic *MEN1* mutations accompanied by loss of the wild-type allele of the gene were found in 27%–39% of these tumors (with and without metastases) and suggest that the *MEN1* gene is an important initiating event in their tumorigenesis.

Somatic mutations of the *VHL* gene have not been documented in sporadic pancreatic endocrine tumors, although the loss of heterozygosity (LOH) rate on chromosome 3p is relatively high.[199]

The *p16INK4a/CDKN2A* gene (*p16INK4a*) is frequently altered by homozygous deletion, mutation, or methylation in many nonendocrine tumors, and these alterations may be predictive of recurrence, tumor growth, or aggressiveness. The *p16/MTS1* gene was found to be homozygously deleted in 41.7% of tumors in one study,[200] whereas no homozygous deletions were found by others.[201] No mutations were identified by single-strand conformation polymorphism analysis. In 52–58% of the gastrinomas, hypermethylation of a 5′-CpG island of the *p16INK4a* gene promoter was found.[200, 201] These data suggest that transcriptional silencing of *p16/MTS1* is a frequent event in these tumors. The presence or absence of methylation of the *p16INK4a* gene did not correlate with clinical characteristics of the gastrinoma, biologic behavior (gastrin release and basal or maximal acid output), the presence or absence of known prognostic factors (tumor size, gastrinoma location, lymph node metastases, liver metastases, and curability), or growth pattern of the gastrinoma postresection. Methylation of the *p16INK4a* gene is the most common gene alteration described to date in gastrinomas. Furthermore, because it is independent of the disease stage, it is probably an early event in gastrinoma pathogenesis.

The possible role of chromosome 1 on pancreatic endocrine tumor formation has been studied. Ebrahimi et al. examined 29 sporadic and MEN1 pancreatic endocrine tumors for LOH, with 12 chromosome 1 microsatellite markers.[202] LOH on chromosome 1 was identified in 10 of 29 (34%) tumors studied. Allele loss occurred more frequently in tumors with hepatic metastases (7 of 8) than tumors without metastases (3 of 21) ($p = .004$). Tumors in patients with lymph node involvement and patients with MEN1 did not demonstrate LOH for chromosome 1 markers. The authors suggest that loss of chromosome 1 is associated specifically with the development of hepatic metastases in patients with sporadic pancreatic endocrine tumors.

In summary, although some progress has been made in recent years to uncover pathogenesis of pancreatic endocrine tumors, the mechanism of tumorigenesis and steps in transformation from benign to malignant neoplasm remain largely unknown.

TREATMENT

Surgery remains the definitive treatment modality for pancreatic endocrine tumors because of its potential to correct local and hormonal effects. However, curative surgery is not always possible because of the extent of the tumor, tumor multiplicity, and inability to localize or isolate the lesion. Furthermore, surgery may be deferred if complications of hormone production are severe or life-threatening. Such complications include hypoglycemic coma, bleeding or perforated gastric ulcers, and electrolyte imbalance secondary to profound watery diarrhea.[203] Medical treatment is used when surgery cannot be performed.[56, 203–205]

Surgery

The success of the surgical procedure depends on the localization and complete removal of the tumor. The location of the tumor and degree of local invasion dictates the type of resection.[23, 206–208] Surgical options include local resection of the tumor, or distal, subtotal, or total (Whipple's) pancreatectomy.[207, 208] (Fig. 8–20). Small insulin-producing tumors in the head of the pancreas are frequently benign and can be removed by enucleation.[103, 208] Other pancreatic endocrine tumors have a higher malignant potential and are treated with more thorough resection. Because the clinical course of many pancreatic endocrine tumors is indolent, whereas the morbidity of a Whipple pancreatoduodenectomy is high, the procedure is only used for removal of the large or definitely malignant tumors.[91, 209]

Medical Treatment

Pancreatic endocrine tumors of each subtype are rare and, therefore, it is difficult to establish optimal treatment methods in clinical trials. Antisecretory medications for each functioning tumor subtype as well as general antitumor agents are available. However, they are variably or transiently effective, and patients may become resistant to their effects.

The long-lasting somatostatin analog octreotide can be used in management of symptoms caused by hormone hypersecretion by the tumor. The treatment is based on the fact that native pancreatic somatostatin inhibits release of many peptides.[210] The synthetic somatostatin analog has a half-life 30 times longer than that of native somatostatin and is administered subcutaneously.[204, 210] Although octreotide lowers plasma concentrations of peptides secreted by pancreatic endocrine tumors, it has a partial direct effect in that the degree of reduction does not

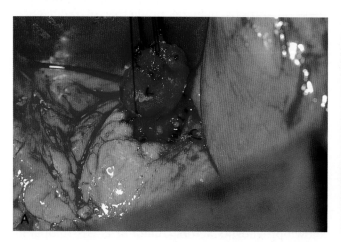 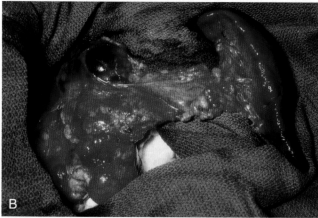

Figure 8–20. Surgical treatment of pancreatic endocrine tumors. *A,* Enucleation of insulinoma from the head of the pancreas; *B,* Endocrine tumors and a microcystic adenoma of the pancreas in VHL patient. (Intraoperative photographs courtesy of Dr. Steven K. Libutti, Surgery Branch, National Cancer Institute, Bethesda, MD.)

always parallel the degree of clinical improvement.[204, 210] The highest benefit of octreotide treatment has been seen in symptomatic relief in VIP-producing tumors and in the carcinoid syndrome.[204, 205, 211] It may be beneficial in patients with glucagon- and GHRH-producing tumors, Cushing's syndrome, and other rare hormone-hypersecretion syndromes.[204, 212] A role of octreotide treatment in the management of insulin- and gastrin-producing tumors is less clear because of the effectiveness of other therapeutic modalities,[204] e.g., diazoxide for insulinoma and histamine H$_2$-receptor blocker omeprazole for Zollinger-Ellison syndrome. Percutaneous liver needle biopsy can be used to measure somatostatin receptor status in metastatic endocrine tumors and predict therapeutic effect of octreotide in individual patients.[213] The antineoplastic effect of octreotide suggested by animal studies is not as clear in clinical practice.[210–212]

Metastases of pancreatic endocrine tumors may be treated with surgical debulking or by hepatic arterial devascularization by embolization. Single agent or combination chemotherapy with octreotide, streptozotocin, doxorubicin, 5-fluorouracil, 5-dimethyltriazeno-4-carboxamide, and α-interferon are also used.[44, 210, 213, 214]

The management of patients with a pancreatic endocrine tumor depends on whether the tumor is sporadic or part of the MEN1 or VHL disease.[43, 215–218] A negative family history does not exclude the possibility of the hereditary syndrome. The majority of MEN1 patients have had or have hyperthyroidism prior to or at the time of presentation with pancreatic endocrine tumors.[215] Pituitary adenomas are another manifestation of MEN1 that require treatment consideration. The diagnosis of MEN1 may influence the extent of surgery.[70, 217, 218] In MEN1 patients, the pancreatic and duodenal tumors are multiple and associated with multifocal nesidioblastosis and endocrine dysplasia. Therefore, subtotal pancreatectomy and duodenotomy are advocated by some authors in the attempt to achieve biochemical cure.[218] Other authors argue that in the 70% of MEN1 patients with pancreatic tumors and duodenal gastrinomas, even extensive surgery with duodenal exploration and removal of positive lymph nodes does not result in a cure because of tumor multiplicity and extensive gastrinoma metastases.[217]

Patients with VHL disease commonly present with retinal hemangiomas, hemangioblastomas of the central nervous system, and renal neoplasia before the pancreatic tumors are found. Surgical resection based on tumor size criteria has resulted in the successful management of VHL patients with nonfunctioning pancreatic endocrine tumors.[43] Pancreatic tumors larger than 2.5 cm were associated with liver metastases in some VHL patients. Screening VHL patients for solid pancreatic endocrine tumors by imaging studies and their resection before they reach 2–3 cm in size may prevent the development of hepatic metastases.[43]

References

1. Like AA, Orci L: Embryogenesis of the human pancreatic islets: A light and electron microscopic study. Diabetes 1972; 21:511.
2. Solcia E, Capella C, Klöppel G: Tumors of the Endocrine Pancreas. In Rosai J, ed.: Tumors of the Pancreas. Atlas of Tumor Pathology. Armed Forces Institute of Pathology, Washington, D.C., 1995.
3. Heitz PU, Kloppel G, Hacki WH, et al.: Nesidioblastosis: The pathologic basis of persistent hyperinsulinemic hypoglycemia in infants: Morphologic and quantitative analysis of seven cases based on specific immunostaining and electron microscopy. Diabetes 1977; 26:632.
4. Liu HM, Potter EL: Development of the human pancreas. Arch Pathol 1962; 74:439.
5. Moore KL: The Developing Human. WB Saunders, Philadelphia, 1982, p. 234.
6. Githens S: Development of duct cells. In Lebenthal E, ed.: Human Gastrointestinal Development. Raven Press, New York, 1989, p. 669.
7. Rahier J, Falt K, Muntefering H, et al.: The basic structural lesion of persistent neonatal hypoglycaemia with hyperinsulinism: Deficiency of pancreatic D cells or hyperactivity of B cells? Diabetologia 1984; 26:282.
8. Rahier J, Wallon J, Gepts W, et al.: Localization of pancreatic polypeptide cells in a limited lobe of the human neonate pancreas: Remnant of the ventral primordium? Cell Tissue Res 1979; 200:359.
9. Chen J, Baithun SI, Pollock DJ, et al.: Argyrophilic and hormone immunoreactive cells in normal and hyperplastic pancreatic ducts and exocrine pancreatic carcinoma. Virchows Arch A Pathol Anat Histopathol 1988; 413:399.
10. Goossens A, Heitz PU, Klöppel G: Pancreatic endocrine cells and their nonneoplastic proliferations. In Dayal Y, ed.: Endocrine Pathology of the Gut and Pancreas. CRC Press, Boca Raton, 1991, p. 69.
11. Capella C, Solcia E, Frigerio B, et al.: The endocrine cells of the pancreas and related tumours: Ultrastructural study and classification. Virchows Arch A Pathol Anat Histol 1977; 373:327.
12. Conklin JL: Cytogenesis of the human fetal pancreas. Am J Anat 1962; 11:181.
13. Klöppel G, In't Veld PA, Stamm B: The endocrine pancreas. In Kovacs K, Asa SL, eds.: Functional Endocrine Pathology. Blackwell Scientific Publications, Boston, 1991, p. 396.
14. Grube D, Bohn R: The microanatomy of human islets of Langerhans, with special reference to somatostatin (D-) cells. Arch Histol Jpn 1983; 46:327.
15. Sundler F, Alumets J, Hakanson R, et al.: Peptidergic (VIP) nerves in the pancreas. Histochemistry 1978; 5:173.
16. Ravazzola M, Orci L: Glucagon and glicentin immunoreactivity are topologically segregated in the alpha granule of the human pancreatic A cell. Nature 1980; 284:66.
17. Solcia E, Fiocca R, Capella C, et al.: Glucagon- and PP-related peptides of intestinal L cells and pancreatic/gastric A or PP cells: Possible interrelationships of peptides and cells during evolution, fetal development and tumor growth. Peptides 1985; 63:223.
18. Orci L, Ravazzola M, Storch MJ, et al.: Proteolytic maturation of insulin is a post-Golgi event which occurs in acidifying clathrin-coated secretory vesicles. Cell 1987; 49:865.
19. Hutton JC, Peshavaria M, Johnston CF, et al.: Immunolocalization of betagranin: A chromogranin A–related protein of the pancreatic B cell. Endocrinology 1988; 122:1014.
20. Johnson KH, O'Brien TD, Betsholtz C, et al.: Islet amyloid, islet-amyloid polypeptide, and diabetes mellitus. N Engl J Med 1989; 321:513.
21. Fiocca R, Sessa F, Tenti P, et al.: Pancreatic polypeptide (PP) cells in the PP-rich lobe of the human pancreas are identified ultrastructurally and immunocytochemically as F cells. Histochemistry 1983; 77:511.
22. Buchanan KD, Johnston CF, O'Hare MM, et al.: Neuroendocrine tumors: A European view. Am J Med 1986; 81:14.
23. Schein P: Islet cell tumors: Current concepts and management. Ann Intern Med 1973; 79:239.

24. Grimelius L, Hultquist GT, Stenkvist B: Cytological differentiation of asymptomatic pancreatic islet cell tumours in autopsy material. Virchows Arch A Pathol Anat Histol 1975; 365:275.

25. Kimura W, Kuroda A, Morioka Y: Clinical pathology of endocrine tumors of the pancreas: Analysis of autopsy cases. Dig Dis Sci 1991; 36:933.

26. Nichols AG: Simple adenoma of pancreas arising from an island of Langerhans. J Med Res 1902; 8:385.

27. Fabozzi S: Ueber die Histogenese des primaren Krebses des Pankreas. Beitrage zur Pathologie 1903; 34:90.

28. Wilder RM, Allan FN, Power MH, et al.: Carcinoma of the islands of the pancreas: Hyperinsulin and hypoglycemia. JAMA 1927; 89:348.

29. Zollinger RM, Ellison EH: Primary peotic ulcerations of the jejunum associated with islet cell tumors of the pancreas. Ann Surg 1955; 142:709.

30. Larsson LI: Endocrine pancreatic tumors. Hum Pathol 1978; 9:401.

31. Heitz PU, Kasper M, Polak JM, et al.: Pancreatic endocrine tumors. Hum Pathol 1982; 13:263.

32. Bendayan M: Presence of endocrine cells in pancreatic ducts. Pancreas 1987; 2:393.

33. Weichert RF, Roth LM, Krementz ET, et al.: Carcinoid-islet cell tumors of the duodenum: Report of twenty-one cases. Am J Surg 1971; 121:195.

34. Pearse AG, Polak JM, Heath CM: Polypeptide hormone production by "carcinoid" apudomas and their relevant cytochemistry. Virchows Arch B Cell Pathol 1974; 16:95.

35. Heitz PU: Pancreatic endocrine tumors. In Klöppel G, Heitz PU, eds.: Pancreatic Pathology. Churchill Livingstone, Edinburgh, 1984, p. 206.

36. Jensen RT, Norton JA: Endocrine tumors of the pancreas. In Yamada T, Alpers BH, Owyang C, et al., eds.: Textbook of Gastroenterology. Lippincott, Philadelphia, 1995, p. 2131.

37. Padberg B, Schröder S: Multiple endocrine neoplasia type 1 (MEN1) revisited. Virchows Arch 1995; 426:541.

38. Pipeleers-Marichal M, Donow C, Heitz PU, et al.: Pathologic aspects of gastrinomas in patients with Zollinger-Ellison syndrome with and without multiple endocrine neoplasia type I. World J Surg 1993; 17:481.

39. Thompson NW, Lloyd RV, Nishiyama RH, et al.: MEN I pancreas: A histological and immunohistochemical study. World J Surg 1984; 8:561.

40. Binkovitz LA, Johnson CD, Stephens DH: Islet cell tumors in von Hippel-Lindau disease: Increased prevalence and relationship to the multiple endocrine neoplasias. Am J Roentgenol 1990; 155:501.

41. Neumann HPH, Dinkel E, Brambs H, et al.: Pancreatic lesions in the von Hippel-Lindau syndrome. Gastoenterology 1991; 101:465.

42. Lubensky IA, Pack S, Ault A, et al.: Multiple neuroendocrine tumors of the pancreas in von Hippel-Lindau disease patients: Histopathological and molecular genetic analysis. Am J Pathol 1998; 153:223.

43. Libutti SK, Choyke PL, Bartlett DL, et al.: Pancreatic neuroendocrine tumors associated with von Hippel-Lindau disease: Diagnostic and management recommendations. Surgery 1998; 124:1153.

44. Apel RL, Asa SL: Endocrine tumors of the pancreas. Pathol Annu 1995; 30:305.

45. Solcia E, Sessa F, Rindi G, et al.: Pancreatic endocrine tumors: General concepts; non-functioning tumors and tumors with uncommon function. In Dayal Y, ed.: Endocrine Pathology of the Gut and Pancreas. CRC Press, Boca Raton, 1991, p. 105.

46. Mukai K, Grotting JC, Greider MH, et al.: Retrospective study of 77 pancreatic endocrine tumors using the immunoperoxidase method. Am J Surg Pathol 1982; 6:387.

47. Nauck M, Creutzfeldt W: Insulin producing tumors and insulinoma syndrome. In Dayal Y, ed.: Endocrine Pathology of the Gut and Pancreas. CRC Press, Boca Raton, 1991, pp. 195–225.

48. Clark ES, Carney JA: Pancreatic islet cell tumor associated with Cushing's syndrome. Am J Surg Pathol 1984; 8:917.

49. Solcia E, Klöppel G, Sobin LH, et al.: Histological Typing of Endocrine Tumours. World Health Organization, International Histological Classification of Tumours, Springer-Verlag, Berlin-Heidelberg, 2000.

50. Capella C, La Rosa S, Solcia E: Criteria for malignancy in pancreatic endocrine tumors. Endocr Pathol 1997; 8:87.

51. Yu F, Venzon DJ, Serrano J, et al.: Prospective study of the clinical course, prognostic factors, causes of death, and survival in patients with longstanding Zollinger-Ellison syndrome. J Clin Oncol 1999; 17:615.

52. Stridsberg M, Oberg K, Li Q, et al.: Measurements of chromogranin A, chromogranin B (secretogranin I), chromogranin C (secretogranin II) and pancreastatin plasma and urine from patients with carcinoid tumours and endocrine pancreatic tumours. J Endocrinol 1995; 144:49.

53. Nobels FR, Kwekkeboom DJ, Bouillon R, et al.: Chromogranin A: Its clinical value as marker of neuroendocrine tumours. Eur J Clin Invest 1998; 28:431.

54. Tomassetti P, Migliori M, Simoni P, et al.: Diagnostic value of plasma chromogranin A in neuroendocrine tumours. Eur J Gastroenterol Hepatol 2001; 13:55.

55. Goebel SU, Serrano J, Yu F, et al.: Prospective study of the value of serum chromogranin A or serum gastrin levels in the assessment of the presence, extent, or growth of gastrinomas. Cancer 1999; 85:1470.

56. Boden G: Glucagonomas and insulinomas. Gastroenterol Clin North Am 1989; 18:831.

57. Mallinson CN, Bloom SR, Warin AP, et al.: A glucagonoma syndrome. Lancet 1974; 2:1.

58. Solcia E, Capella C, Fiocca R, et al.: The gastroenteropancreatic endocrine system and related tumors. Gastroenterol Clin North Am 1989; 18:671.

59. Bordi C, Ravazzola M, Baetens D, et al.: A study of glucagonomas by light and electron microscopy and immunofluorescence. Diabetes 1979; 28:925.

60. Lokich J, Anderson N, Rossini A, et al.: Pancreatic alpha cell tumors: Case report and review of the literature. Cancer 1980; 45:2675.

61. Larsson LI, Hirsch MA, Holst JJ, et al.: Pancreatic somatostatinoma: Clinical features and physiological implications. Lancet 1977; 1:666.

62. Ganda OP, Weir GC, Soeldner J, et al.: "Somatostatinoma": A somatostatin-containing tumor of the endocrine pancreas. N Engl J Med 1977; 296:963.

63. Krejs GJ, Orci L, Conlon JM, et al.: Somatostatinoma syndrome: Biochemical, morphologic and clinical features. N Engl J Med 1979; 301:285.

64. Howard JM, Gohara AF, Cardwell RJ: Malignant islet cell tumor of the pancreas associated with high plasma calcitonin and somatostatin levels. Surgery 1989; 105:227.

65. Dayal Y, Ganda OP: Somatostatin-producing tumors. In Dayal Y, ed.: Endocrine Pathology of the Gut and Pancreas. CRC Press, Boca Raton, 1991, p. 241.

66. Gower WR, Fabri PJ: Endocrine neoplasms (non-gastrin) of the pancreas. Semin Surg Oncol 1990; 6:98.

67. Brand SJ, Fuller PJ: Differential gastrin gene expression in rat gastrointestinal tract and pancreas during neonatal development. J Biol Chem 1988; 263:5341.

68. Stamm B, Hacki WH, Klöppel G, et al.: Gastrin-producing tumors and the Zollinger-Ellison syndrome. In Dayal Y, ed.: Endocrine Pathology of the Gut and Pancreas. CRC Press, Boca Raton, 1991, p. 155.

69. Norton JA, Doppman JL, Collen MJ, et al.: Prospective study of gastrinoma localization and resection in patients with Zollinger-Ellison syndrome. Ann Surg 1986; 204:468.

70. Jensen RT: Pancreatic endocrine tumors: Recent advances. Ann Oncol 1999; 10:170.

71. Dayal Y: Hyperplastic proliferations of endocrine cells: Review. Endocrine Pathol 1994; 5:4.

72. Solcia E, Bordi C, Creutzfeldt W, et al.: Histopathological classification of nonantral gastric endocrine growths in man. Digestion 1988; 41:185.

73. Cadiot G, Lehy TH, Mignon M: Gastric endocrine cell proliferation and fundic argyrophil carcinoid tumors in patients with the Zollinger-Ellison syndrome. Acta Oncol 1993; 32:135.

74. Norton JA, Doppman JL, Jensen RT: Curative resection in Zollinger-Ellison syndrome: Results of a 10-year prospective study. Ann Surg 1992; 215:8.

75. Wolfe MM, Jensen RT: Zollinger-Ellison syndrome: Current concepts in diagnosis and management. N Engl J Med 1987; 317:1200.

76. Lundqvist G, Krause U, Larsson LI, et al.: A pancreatic-polypeptide-producing tumour associated with the WDHA syndrome. Scand J Gastroenterol 1978; 13:715.

77. Larsson LI, Schwartz T, Lundqvist G, et al.: Occurrence of human pancreatic polypeptide in pancreatic endocrine tumors: Possible implication in the watery diarrhea syndrome. Am J Pathol 1976; 85:675.

78. Ooi A, Kameya T, Tsumuraya M, et al.: Pancreatic endocrine tumours associated with WDHA syndrome: An immunohistochemical and electron microscopic study. Virchows Arch A Pathol Anat Histopathol 1985; 405:311.

79. Bloom SR, Christofides ND, Delamarter J, et al.: Diarrhoea in vipoma patients associated with cosecretion of a second active peptide (peptide histidine isoleucine) explained by single coding gene. Lancet 1983; 2:1163.

80. Hutcheon DF, Bayless TM, Cameron JL, et al.: Hormone-mediated watery diarrhea in a family with multiple endocrine neoplasms. Ann Intern Med 1979; 90:932.

81. Clark ES, Carney JA: Pancreatic islet cell tumor associated with Cushing's syndrome. Am J Surg Pathol 1984; 8:917.

82. O'Neal LW, Kipnis DM, Luse SA, et al.: Secretion of various endocrine substances by ACTH-secreting tumors: Gastrin, melanotropin, norepinephrine, serotonin, parathormone, vasopressin, glucagon. Cancer 1968; 21:1219.

83. Asa SL, Kovacs K, Vale W, et al.: Immunohistologic localization of corticotrophin-releasing hormone in human tumors. Am J Clin Pathol 1987; 87:327.

84. Guillemin R, Brazeau P, Bohlen P, et al.: Growth hormone-releasing factor from a human pancreatic tumor that caused acromegaly. Science 1982; 218:585.

85. Ezzat S, Ezrin C, Yamashita S, et al.: Recurrent acromegaly resulting from ectopic growth hormone gene expression by a metastatic pancreatic tumor. Cancer 1993; 71:66.

86. Kaplan EL: The carcinoid syndromes. In Friesen SR, ed.: Surgical Endocrinology: Clinical Syndromes. Lippincott, Philadelphia, 1978, p. 120.

87. Arps H, Dietel M, Schulz A, et al.: Pancreatic endocrine carcinoma with ectopic PTH-production and paraneoplastic hypercalcaemia. Virchows Arch A Pathol Anat Histopathol 1986; 408:497.

88. Miraliakbari BA, Asa SL, Boudreau SF: Parathyroid hormone–like peptide in pancreatic endocrine carcinoma and adenocarcinoma associated with hypercalcemia. Hum Pathol 1992; 23:884.

89. Maton PN, Gardner JD, Jensen R, et al.: Cushing's syndrome in patients with the Zollinger-Ellison syndrome. N Engl J Med 1986; 315:1.

90. Mao C, el Attar A, Domenico DR, et al.: Carcinoid tumors of the pancreas: Status report based on two cases and review of the world's literature. Int J Pancreatol 1998; 23:153.

91. Maurer CA, Glaser C, Reubi J, et al.: Carcinoid of the pancreas. Digestion 1997; 58:410.

92. Mao C, Carter P, Schaefer P, et al.: Malignant islet cell tumor associated with hypercalcemia. Surgery 1995; 117:37.

93. Drucker DJ, Asa SL, Henderson J, et al.: The parathyroid hormone–like peptide gene is expressed in the normal and neoplastic human endocrine pancreas. Mol Endocrinol 1989; 3:1589.

94. Liu TH, Zhu Y, Cui QC, et al.: Nonfunctioning pancreatic endocrine tumors: An immunohistochemical and electron microscopic analysis of 26 cases. Pathol Res Pract 1992; 188:191.

95. Venkatesh S, Ordonez NG, Ajani J, et al.: Islet cell carcinoma of the pancreas: A study of 98 patients. Cancer 1990; 65:354.

96. Thompson GB, van Heerden JA, Grant C, et al.: Islet cell carcinomas of the pancreas: A twenty-year experience. Surgery 1988; 104:1011.

97. Vinik AI, Moattari AR: Treatment of endocrine tumors of the pancreas. Endocrinol Metab Clin North Am 1989; 18:483.

98. Deveney CW, Deveney KE, Stark D, et al.: Resection of gastrinomas. Ann Surg 1983; 198:546.

99. Friesen SR, Kimmel JR, Tomita T: Pancreatic polypeptide as screening marker for pancreatic polypeptide apudomas in multiple endocrinopathies. Am J Surg 1980; 139:61.

100. Adrian TE, Uttenthal LO, Williams SJ, et al.: Secretion of pancreatic polypeptide in patients with pancreatic endocrine tumors. N Engl J Med 1986; 315:287.

101. Tomita T, Friesen SR, Kimmel JR, et al.: Pancreatic polypeptide-secreting islet-cell tumors: A study of three cases. Am J Pathol 1983; 113:134.

102. Tomita T, Friesen SR, Pollack HG: PP-producing tumors (Ppomas). In Dayal Y, ed.: Endocrine Pathology of the Gut and Pancreas. CRC Press, Boca Raton, 1991, p. 279.

103. Chandrasekharappa SC, Guru SC, Manickam P, et al.: Positional cloning of the gene for multiple endocrine neoplasia-type 1. Science 1997; 276:404.

104. Zhuang Z, Vortmeyer AO, Pack S, et al.: Somatic mutations of the MEN1 tumor suppressor gene in sporadic gastrinomas and insulinomas. Cancer Res 1997; 57:4682.

105. Weil R, Vortmeyer A, Huang S, et al.: 11q13 allelic loss in pituitary tumors in patients with multiple endocrine neoplasia syndrome, type 1. Clinical Cancer Res 1998; 7:1673.

106. Debelenko LV, Zhuang Z, Emmert-Buck MR, et al.: Allelic deletions on chromosome 11q13 in MEN 1-associated and sporadic gastrinomas and pancreatic endocrine tumors. Cancer Res 1997; 57:2238.

107. Klöppel G, Willemer S, Stamm B, et al.: Pancreatic lesions and hormonal profile of pancreatic tumors in multiple endocrine neoplasia type I: An immunocytochemical study of nine patients. Cancer 1986; 57:1824.

108. Le Bodic MF, Heymann MF, Lecomte M, et al.: Immunohistochemical study of 100 pancreatic tumors in 28 patients with multiple endocrine neoplasia, type I. Am J Surg Pathol 1996, 20:1378.

109. Shepherd JJ, Challis DR, Davies PF, et al.: Multiple endocrine neoplasm, type I: Gastrinomas, pancreatic neoplasms, microcarcinoids, the Zollinger-Ellison syndrome, lymph nodes, and hepatic metastases. Arch Surg 1993; 128:1133.

110. Debelenko LV, Emmert-Buck MR, Zhuang Z, et al.: The *MEN 1* gene locus is involved in the pathogenesis of type II gastric carcinoids. Gastroenterology 1997; 113:773.

111. Rindi G, Luinetti O, Cornaggia M, et al.: Three types of gastric argyrophil carcinoid and the gastric neuroendocrine carcinoma: A clinicopathologic study. Gastroenterology 1993; 104:994.

112. Lamiell JM, Salazar FG, Hsia YE: Von Hippel-Lindau disease affecting 43 members of a single kindred. Medicine (Baltimore) 1989; 68:1.

113. Mohr V, Vortmeyer AO, Zhuang Z, et al.: Histopathology and molecular genetics of multiple cysts and microcystic (serous) adenomas of the pancreas in von Hippel-Lindau patients. Am J Pathol 2000; 157:1615.

114. Mao C, Shah A, Hanson DJ, et al.: Von Recklinghausen's disease associated with duodenal somatostinoma: Contrast of duodenal versus pancreatic somatostinomas. J Surg Oncol 1995; 59:67.

115. Doppman JL, Shawker TH, Miller DL: Localization of islet cell tumors. Gastroenterol Clin North Am 1989; 18:793.

116. Rossi P, Allison DJ, Bezzi M, et al.: Endocrine tumors of the pancreas. Radiol Clin North Am 1989; 27:129.

117. Gunther RW, Klose KJ, Ruckert K, et al.: Islet-cell tumors: Detection of small lesions with computed tomography and ultrasound. Radiology 1983; 148:485.

118. Wise SR, Johnson J, Sparks J, et al.: Gastrinoma: The predictive value of preoperative localization. Surgery 1989; 106:1087.

119. Doherty GM, Doppman JL, Shawker TH, et al.: Results of a prospective strategy to diagnose, localize, and resect insulinomas. Surgery 1991; 110:989.

120. Vinik AI, Delbridge L, Moattari R, et al.: Transhepatic portal vein catheterization for localization of insulinomas: A ten-year experience. Surgery 1991; 109:1.

121. Fedorak IJ, Ko TC, Gordon D, et al.: Localization of islet cell tumors of the pancreas: A review of current techniques. Surgery 1993; 113:242.

122. Grant CS, van Heerden J, Charboneau JW, et al.: Insulinoma: The value of intraoperative ultrasonography. Arch Surg 1988; 123:843.

123. Norton JA, Cromack DT, Shawker TH, et al.: Intraoperative ultrasonographic localization of islet cell tumors: A prospective comparison to palpation. Ann Surg 1988; 207:160.

124. Galiber AK, Reading CC, Charboneau JW, et al.: Localization of pancreatic insulinoma: Comparison of pre- and intraoperative US with CT and angiography. Radiology 1988; 166:405.

125. Kvols LK, Brown ML, O'Connor MK, et al.: Evaluation of a radiolabeled somatostatin analog (l-123 octreotide) in the detection and localization of carcinoid and islet cell tumors. Radiology 1993; 187:129.

126. Krenning EP, Kwekkeboom DJ, Bakker WH, et al.: Somatostatin receptor scintigraphy with [¹¹¹In-DTPA-D-Phe1]- and [¹²³I-Tyr3]-octreotide: The Rotterdam experience with more than 1000 patients. Eur J Nucl Med 1993; 20:716.

127. Reubi JC, Kvols LK, Waser B, et al.: Detection of somatostatin receptors in surgical and percutaneous needle biopsy samples of carcinoids and islet cell carcinomas. Cancer Res 1990; 50:5969.

128. van Eijck CH, Lamberts SW, Lemaire L, et al.: The use of somatostatin receptor scintigraphy in the differential diagnosis of pancreatic duct cancers and islet cell tumors. Ann Surg 1996; 224:119.

129. Gibril F, Reynolds JC, Chen CC, et al.: Specificity of somatostatin receptor scintigraphy: A prospective study and effects of false-positive localizations on management in patients with gastrinomas. J Nucl Med 1999; 40:539.

130. Shaw JA, Vance RP, Geisinger KR, et al.: Islet cell neoplasms: A fine-needle aspiration cytology study with immunocytochemical correlations. Am J Clin Pathol 1990; 94:142.

131. Bell DA: Cytologic features of islet-cell tumors. Acta Cytol 1987; 31:485.

132. Zeng XJ, Zhong SX, Zhu Y, et al.: Insulinoma: 31 years of tumor localization and excision. J Surg Oncol 1988; 39:274.

133. Howard TJ, Stabile BE, Zinner MJ, et al.: Anatomic distribution of pancreatic endocrine tumors. Am J Surg 1990; 159:258.

134. Stabile BE, Morrow DJ, Passaro E Jr.: The gastrinoma triangle: Operative implications. Am J Surg 1984; 147:25.

135. Huettner PC, Bird DJ, Chang YC, et al.: Carcinoid tumor of the kidney with morphologic and immunohistochemical profile of a hindgut endocrine tumor: Report of a case. Ultrastruct Pathol 1991; 15:655.

136. Asa SL, Scheithauer BW, Bilbao JM, et al.: A case for hypothalamic acromegaly: A clinicopathological study of six patients with hypothalamic gangliocytomas producing growth hormone-releasing factor. J Clin Endocrinol Metab 1984; 58:796.

137. Cooper GJ, Willis AC, Clark A, et al.: Purification and characterization of a peptide from amyloid-rich pancreases of type 2 diabetic patients. Proc Natl Acad Sci U S A 1987; 84:8628.

138. Lukinius A, Wilander E, Westermark GT, et al.: Co-localization of islet amyloid polypeptide and insulin in the B cell secretory granules of the human pancreatic islets. Diabetologia 1989; 32:240.

139. Westermark P, Grimelius L, Polak J, et al.: Amyloid in polypeptide hormone–producing tumors. Lab Invest 1977; 37:212.

140. Ordonez NG, Manning JT Jr, Hanssen G: Alpha-1-antitrypsin in islet cell tumors of the pancreas. Am J Clin Pathol 1983; 80:277.

141. Tomita T, Bhatia P, Gourley W: Mucin-producing islet cell adenoma. Hum Pathol 1981; 12:850.

142. Guarda LA, Silva EG, Ordonez NG, et al.: Clear cell islet cell tumor. Am J Clin Pathol 1983; 79:512.

143. Sadoul JL, Saint-Paul MC, Hoffman P, et al.: Malignant pancreatic oncocytoma: An unusual cause of organic hypoglycemia. J Endocrinol Invest 1992; 15:211.

144. Wilander E: Diagnostic pathology of gastrointestinal and pancreatic neuroendocrine tumours. Acta Oncol 1989; 28:363.

145. Lloyd RV, Mervak T, Schmidt K, et al.: Immunohistochemical detection of chromogranin and neuron-specific enolase in pancreatic endocrine neoplasms. Am J Surg Pathol 1984; 8:607.

146. Bordi C, Pilato FP, D'Adda T: Comparative study of seven neuroendocrine markers in pancreatic endocrine tumours. Virchows Arch A Pathol Anat Histopathol 1988; 413:387.

147. Gould VE, Wiedenmann B, Lee I, et al.: Synaptophysin expression in neuroendocrine neoplasms as determined by immunocytochemistry. Am J Pathol 1987; 126:243.

148. Chejfec G, Falkmer S, Grimelius L, et al.: Synaptophysin: A new marker for pancreatic neuroendocrine tumors. Am J Surg Pathol 1987; 11:241.

149. Hagn C, Schmid KW, Fischer-Colbrie R, et al.: Chromogranin A, B, and C in human adrenal medulla and endocrine tissues. Lab Invest 1986; 55:405.

150. Tischler AS, Mobtaker H, Mann K, et al.: Anti-lymphocyte antibody Leu-7 (HNK-1) recognizes a constituent of neuroendocrine granule matrix. J Histochem Cytochem 1986; 34:1213.

151. Rode J, Dhillon AP, Doran JF, et al.: PGP 9.5, a new marker for human neuroendocrine tumours. Histopathology 1985; 9:147.

152. Bordi C, Krisch K, Horvat G, et al.: Immunocytochemical patterns of islet cell tumors as defined by the monoclonal antibody HISL-19. Am J Pathol 1988; 132:249.

153. Ahlman H, Ahlund L, Dahlstrom A, et al.: Somatostatin analogue and tissue cultures in the study of a human malignant glucagonoma. J Surg Oncol 1990; 44:191.

154. Drucker DJ, Asa SL, Silverberg J, et al.: Molecular and cellular analysis of a neoplastic pancreatic A cell tumor. Cancer 1990; 65:1762.

155. Perkins PL, McLeod MK, Jin L, et al.: Analysis of gastrinomas by immunohistochemistry and in situ hybridization histochemistry. Diagn Mol Pathol 1992; 1:155.

156. Suzuki H, Matsuyama M: Ultrastructure of functioning beta cell tumors of the pancreatic islets. Cancer 1971; 28:1302.

157. Kenny BD, Sloan JM, Hamilton PW, et al.: The role of morphometry in predicting prognosis in pancreatic islet cell tumors. Cancer 1989; 64:460.

158. Oberg K, Wide L: hCG and hCG subunits as tumour markers in patients with endocrine pancreatic tumours and carcinoids. Acta Endocrinol (Copenh) 1981; 98:256.

159. Heitz PU, Kasper M, Kloppel G, et al.: Glycoprotein-hormone alpha-chain production by pancreatic endocrine tumors: A specific marker for malignancy: Immunocytochemical analysis of tumors of 155 patients. Cancer 1983; 51:277.

160. Kloppel G, Girard J, Polak JM, et al.: Alpha-human chorionic gonadotropin and neuron-specific enolase as markers for malignancy and neuroendocrine nature of pancreatic endocrine tumors. Cancer Detect Prev 1983; 6:161.

161. Kahn CR, Rosen SW, Weintraub BD, et al.: Ectopic production of chorionic gonadotropin and its subunits by islet-cell tumors: A specific marker for malignancy. N Engl J Med 1977; 297:565.

162. Graeme-Cook F, Nardi G, Compton CC: Immunocytochemical staining for human chorionic gonadotropin subunits does not predict malignancy in insulinomas. Am J Clin Pathol 1990; 93:273.

163. Graeme-Cook F, Bell DA, Flotte TJ, et al.: Aneuploidy in pancreatic insulinomas does not predict malignancy. Cancer 1990; 66:2365.

164. Eriksson B, Oberg K, Wilander E, et al.: Nuclear DNA distribution in neuroendocrine gastroenteropancreatic tumors before and during treatment. Acta Oncol 1989; 28:193.

165. Pelosi G, Zamboni G, Doglioni C, et al.: Immunodetection of proliferating cell nuclear antigen assesses the growth fraction and predicts malignancy in endocrine tumors of the pancreas. Am J Surg Pathol 1992; 16:1215.

166. Ruschoff J, Willemer S, Brunzel M, et al.: Nucleolar organizer regions and glycoprotein-hormone alpha-chain reaction as markers of malignancy in endocrine tumours of the pancreas. Histopathology 1993; 22:51.

167. Morohoshi T, Held G, Kloppel G: Exocrine pancreatic tumours and their histological classification: A study based on 167 autopsy and 97 surgical cases. Histopathology 1983; 7:645.

168. Reyes CV, Wang T: Undifferentiated small cell carcinoma of the pancreas: A report of five cases. Cancer 1981; 47:2500.

169. Sessa F, Bonato M, Frigerio B, et al.: Ductal cancers of the pancreas frequently express markers of gastrointestinal epithelial cells. Gastroenterology 1990; 98:1655.

170. Ibrahim NB, Briggs JC, Corbishley CM: Extrapulmonary oat cell carcinoma. Cancer 1984; 54:1645.

171. Dollinger MR, Ratner LH, Shamoian CA, et al.: Carcinoid syndrome associated with pancreatic tumors. Arch Intern Med 1967; 120:575.

172. Gordon DL, Lo MC, Schwartz MA: Carcinoid of the pancreas. Am J Med 1971; 51:412.

173. Morant R, Bruckner HW: Complete remission of refractory small cell carcinoma of the pancreas with cisplatin and etoposide. Cancer 1989; 64:2007.

174. O'Connor TP, Wade TP, Sunwoo Y, et al.: Small cell undifferentiated carcinoma of the pancreas: Report of a patient with tumor marker studies. Cancer 1992; 70:1514.

175. Nonomura A, Mizukami Y, Matsubara F, et al.: Duct-islet cell tumor of the pancreas: A case report with immunohistochemical and electron microscopic findings. Acta Pathol Jpn 1989; 39:328.

176. Arihiro K, Inai K: Malignant islet cell tumor of the pancreas with multiple hormone production and expression of CEA and CA19-9: Report of an autopsy case. Acta Pathol Jpn 1991; 41:150.

177. Reid JD, Yuh SL, Petrelli M, et al.: Ductuloinsular tumors of the pancreas: A light, electron microscopic and immunohistochemical study. Cancer 1982; 49:908.

178. Ichihara T, Nagura H, Nakao A, et al.: Immunohistochemical localization of CA 19-9 and CEA in pancreatic carcinoma and associated diseases. Cancer 1988; 61:324.

179. Weidenheim KM, Hinchey WW, Campbell WG: Hyperinsulinemic hypoglycemia in adults with islet-cell hyperplasia and degranulation of exocrine cells of the pancreas. Am J Clin Pathol 1983; 79:14.

180. Ray MB, Zumwalt R: Islet-cell hyperplasia in genetic deficiency of alpha-1-proteinase inhibitor. Am J Clin Pathol 1986; 85:681.

181. Hardwick DF, Dimmick JE: Metabolic cirrhoses of infancy and early childhood. Perspect Pediatr Pathol 1976; 3:103.

182. Stefan Y, Bordi C, Grasso S, et al.: Beckwith-Wiedemann syndrome: A quantitative, immunohistochemical study of pancreatic islet cell populations. Diabetologia 1985; 28:914.

183. Solcia E, Capella C, Klöppel G: Tumor-like lesions of the exocrine pancreas. In Rosai J, ed: Tumors of the Pancreas. Atlas of Tumor Pathology. Armed Forces Institute of Pathology, Washington, D.C., 1995, p 237.

184. Goossens A, Gepts W, Saudubray JM, et al.: Diffuse and focal nesidioblastosis: A clinicopathological study of 24 patients with persistent neonatal hyperinsulinemic hypoglycemia. Am J Surg Pathol 1989; 13:766.

185. Klöppel G, Altenahr E, Menke B: The ultrastructure of focal islet cell adenomatosis in the newborn with hypoglycemia and hyperinsulinism. Virchows Arch A Pathol Anat Histol 1975; 366:223.

186. Gould VE, Memoli VA, Dardi LE, et al.: Nesidiodysplasia and nesidioblastosis of infancy: Structural and functional correlations with the syndrome of hyperinsulinemic hypoglycemia. Pediatr Pathol 1:7.

187. Jaffe R, Hashida Y, Yunis EJ: Pancreatic pathology in hyperinsulinemic hypoglycemia of infancy. Lab Invest 1980; 42:356.

188. Witte DP, Greider MH, DeSchryver-Kecskemeti K, et al.: The juvenile human endocrine pancreas: Normal versus idiopathic hyperinsulinemic hypoglycemia. Semin Diagn Pathol 1984; 1:30.

189. Pilato FP, D'Adda T, Banchini E, et al.: Nonrandom expression of polypeptide hormones in pancreatic endocrine tumors: An immunohistochemical study in a case of multiple islet cell neoplasia. Cancer 1988; 61:1815.

190. Boschetti AE, Moloney WC: Observations on pancreatic islet cell and other radiation-induced tumors in the rat. Lab Invest 1966; 15:565.

191. Schoental R, Fowler ME, Coady A: Islet cell tumors of the pancreas found in rats given pyrrolizidine alkaloids from *Amsinckia intermedia* Fisch and Mey and from *Heliotropium supinum L.* Cancer Res 1970; 30:2127.

192. Volk BW, Wellmann KF, Brancato P: Fine structure of rat islet cell tumors induced by streptozotocin and nicotinamide. Diabetologia 1974; 10:37.

193. Hanahan D: Heritable formation of pancreatic beta-cell tumours in transgenic mice expressing recombinant insulin/simian virus 40 oncogenes. Nature 1985; 315:115.

194. Rindi G, Bishop AE, Murphy D, et al.: A morphological analysis of endocrine tumour genesis in pancreas and anterior pituitary of AVP/SV40 transgenic mice. Virchows Arch A Pathol Anat Histopathol 1998; 412:255.

195. Rindi G, Efrat S, Ghatei MA, et al.: Glucagonomas of transgenic mice express a wide range of general neuroendocrine markers and bioactive peptides. Virchows Arch A Pathol Anat Histopathol 1991; 419:115.

196. Crabtree JS, Scacheri PC, Ward JM, et al.: A mouse model of multiple endocrine neoplasia, type 1, develops multiple endocrine tumors. Proc Natl Acad Sci U S A 2001; 98:1118.

197. Guru SC, Goldsmith PK, Burns A, et al.: Menin, the product of the *MEN1* gene, is a nuclear protein. Proc Natl Acad Sci U S A 1998; 95:1630.

198. Kaelin WG Jr, Maher ER: The VHL tumour-suppressor gene paradigm. Trends Genet 1998; 14:423.

199. Chung DC, Smith AP, Louis DN, et al.: A novel pancreatic endocrine tumor suppressor gene locus on chromosome 3p with clinical prognostic implications. J Clin Invest 1997; 100:404.

200. Muscarella P, Melvin WS, Fisher WE, et al.: Genetic alterations in gastrinomas and nonfunctioning pancreatic neuroendocrine tumors: An analysis of *p16/MTS1* tumor suppressor gene inactivation. Cancer Res 1998; 58:237.

201. Serrano J, Goebel SU, Peghini PL, et al.: Alterations in the *p16INK4a/CDKN2A* tumor suppressor gene in gastrinomas. J Clin Endocrinol Metab 2000; 85:4146.

202. Ebrahimi SA, Wang EH, Wu A, et al.: Deletion of chromosome 1 predicts prognosis in pancreatic endocrine tumors. Cancer Res 1999; 59:311.

203. Ajani JA, Levin B, Wallace S: Systemic and regional therapy of advanced islet cell tumors. Gastroenterol Clin North Am 1989; 18:923.

204. Maton PN: The use of the long-acting somatostatin analogue, octreotide acetate, in patients with islet cell tumors. Gastroenterol Clin North Am 1989; 18:897.

205. O'Dorisio TM, Mekhjian HS, Gaginella TS: Medical therapy of VIPomas. Endocrinol Metab Clin North Am 1989; 18:545.

206. Norton JA, Fraker DL, Alexander HR, et al.: Surgery to cure the Zollinger-Ellison syndrome. N Engl J Med 1999; 341:635.

207. Grama D, Eriksson B, Martensson H, et al.: Clinical characteristics, treatment and survival in patients with pancreatic tumors causing hormonal syndromes. World J Surg 1992; 16:632.

208. Park BJ, Alexander HR, Libutti SK, et al.: Operative management of islet-cell tumors arising in the head of the pancreas. Surgery 1998; 124:1056.

209. Broughan TA, Leslie JD, Soto J, et al.: Pancreatic islet cell tumors. Surgery 1986; 99:671.

210. Wynick D, Bloom SR: Clinical review 23: The use of the long-acting somatostatin analog octreotide in the treatment of gut neuroendocrine tumors. J Clin Endocrinol Metab 1991; 73:1.

211. Kvols LK, Moertel CG, O'Connell M, et al.: Treatment of the malignant carcinoid syndrome: Evaluation of a long-acting somatostatin analogue. N Engl J Med 1986; 315:663.

212. Souquet JC, Sassolas G, Forichon J, et al.: Clinical and hormonal effects of a long-acting somatostatin analogue in pancreatic endocrine tumors and in carcinoid syndrome. Cancer 1987; 59:1654.

213. Eriksson B, Oberg K: An update of the medical treatment of malignant endocrine pancreatic tumors. Acta Oncol 1993; 32:203.

214. Bajetta E, Zilembo N, Di Bartolomeo M, et al.: Treatment of metastatic carcinoids and other neuroendocrine tumors with recombinant interferon-alpha-2a: A study by the Italian Trials in Medical Oncology Group. Cancer 1993; 72:3099.

215. Demeure MJ, Klonoff DC, Karam JH, et al.: Insulinomas associated with multiple endocrine neoplasia type I: The need for a different surgical approach. Surgery 1991; 110:998.

216. Jensen RT: Management of the Zollinger-Ellison syndrome in patients with multiple endocrine neoplasia type 1. J Intern Med 1998; 243:477.

217. MacFarlane MP, Fraker DL, Alexander HR, et al.: Prospective study of surgical resection of duodenal and pancreatic gastrinomas in multiple endocrine neoplasia type 1. Surgery 1995; 118:973.

218. Thompson NW: Current concepts in the surgical management of multiple endocrine neoplasia type 1 pancreatic-duodenal disease: Results in the treatment of 40 patients with Zollinger-Ellison syndrome, hypoglycaemia or both. J Intern Med 1998; 243:495.

CHAPTER 9

Gastrointestinal Tract

Emma E. Furth, M.D.

EMBRYOLOGY OF THE GUT AND ENTEROENDOCRINE CELLS

General Considerations

The discovery of gut neuroendocrine cells or enterochromaffin cells actually followed the initial descriptions of carcinoid tumor. After the initial description of these tumors in 1888 and the subsequent adaptation of the term "carcinoid" in 1907, the identification of the enterochromaffin cell and the hypothesis that these cells were the cell of origin of carcinoids rested upon the use of argentaffin staining performed in midgut tumors. The embryologic origin of the cells initially was thought to be from the neural crest, with migration into the gut. This hypothesis aimed at developing a unifying theory of derivation for all APUD (amine precursor uptake and decarboxylation) cells. However, upon emergence of molecular biology techniques, it is clear that all gut neuroendocrine cells are derived from gut stem cells, with no role of migration from the neuroectoderm.

Using chimera animal models, it has been shown that the gut ganglion cells indeed are derived from the neural crest, whereas the enterochromaffin cells are derived from gut endoderm. Although chimeric mouse models have shown a common embryologic origin of gastric endocrine and epithelial cells, it is not clear whether within a given crypt there is a common stem cell for usual gut epithelial cells and the enterochromaffin cells. However, X-linked enzyme analysis has shown that each crypt is monoclonal.[1] Despite this clonality, clear-cut lineage-specific differentiation lines clearly exist within each crypt, as lineage ablation studies for Paneth cells have been possible.[2] Thus, the study of gut epithelial development and differentiation is important in elucidating critical factors involved in the control of enteroendocrine cells. Understanding normal control mechanisms naturally leads to understanding consequences of perturbation of these systems, which we term disease.

The development of the fetal intestine is complete by gestation week 13, with full motility by week 36. This process involves numerous steps, including epithelial and mesenchymal development and organization, which proceed cranially to caudally. It is interesting to note that this development is independent of luminal and hormonal factors, since human fetal small and large bowel segments xenografted to *scid* mice develop normally.[3] Gut endocrine cells appear as early as 8 weeks' gestation, as does the formation of villi. Within the initially stratified layer of undifferentiated epithelial cells, the endocrine cells may be found representing beginning differentiation from a common epithelial stem cell. With epithelial differentiation, cytokeratin 20 is expressed in the absorptive and goblet cells but not in Paneth and endocrine cells.[4]

The development of the gut involves differentiation at numerous levels. From the cranial to caudal aspect, the gut must differentiate into the esophagus, stomach, small bowel, and colon. Even among these regions, there is further differentiation. For example, the duodenum and ileum are both small bowel but have clear morphologic and embryologic differences. The coordination of this process requires numerous factors. The *hox* genes are a crucial set of genes involved in this axial differentiation. The initial identification of these homeotic genes came from work with *Drosophila,* in which their protein product transcription factors were found to control segmentation and pattern formation through a conserved homeobox sequence.

Thus, the small bowel and colon are composed of a series of clonal "turnover units." The crypts house the stem cells, which proliferate and give rise to daughter cells, which have additional replicative ability. It is not entirely known when cell lineage specificity is defined. Although each crypt is monoclonal, each villus is derived from several crypts. It is interesting that the cells derived from one crypt do not mix with those from another crypt, leading to bands or ribbons of cells along a villus that can be detected only with chimeric or transgenic mouse

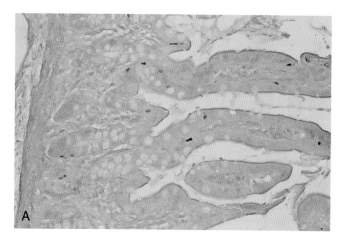
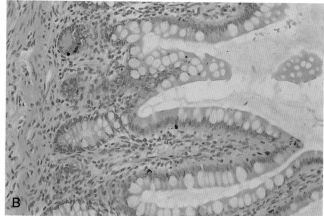

Figure 9–1. Enteroendocrine cells in the small bowel. The enteroendocrine cells are terminally differentiated and distributed throughout the villous structure. They are derived from the same stem cell as the rest of the epithelium. The Grimelius *(A)* and Fontana *(B)* stains highlight these cells (×50.) The Grimelius stain uses exogenous reducing agents in the reaction, which results in silver precipitation; cells that stain are termed "argyrophil" cells. The Fontana stain does not have exogenous reducing agents, and thus for a cell to stain it must contain the proper reducing compounds; cells that stain are termed "argentaffin" cells. The Grimelius stain will stain all argentaffin cells, assuming proper fixation, whereas the Fontana stain may stain only a subset of Grimelius-positive cells.

systems. In contrast to these ribbons, cells within a crypt can indeed mix. Thus, while there is an orderly progression of differentiation along the crypt to the villous axis, this process does not occur in a "conveyer belt" fashion. The endocrine cells represent at most 1% of the total epithelial cell population and are turned over in about 5 days, as are the enterocytes and goblet cells, whereas the Paneth cells survive for several weeks.

Serotonin cells are the most frequent type of gut neuroendocrine cell. Lineage specificity is defined, but the endocrine products of a given endocrine cell can change with migration along the crypt to the villous axis. Specifically, cells expressing substance P may switch to expressing serotonin in the villus. Not all endocrine cells migrate to the surface as do the enterocytes and goblet cells, which further adds to the evidence arguing against the conveyer belt concept of gut epithelial migration. For example, many of the endocrine cells are found at the base or mid-crypt (Figs. 9–1 and 9–2).

Transcription Factors

Numerous transcription factors are involved in the development of the gut. Transcription factors are proteins that promote the transcription (i.e., mRNA synthesis) of genes. Each gene contains a promoter, which is not transcribed or synthesized into proteins but rather serves as the starting point for RNA synthesis. This promoter region, and in many instances upstream sequences, contains genomic sequences that specifically bind only certain transcription factors. Thus, transcriptional regulation and consequently protein expression are controlled by the specificity of the transcription factors. Hepatic nuclear

factor 3beta (HNF-3beta), a member of the related forkhead/winged helix *Drosophila* genes, is important to the formation of the foregut and midgut, as shown in mouse knock-out experiments.[5] The expression of HNF-3alpha and beta is dependent upon cellular differentiation both in vivo and in vitro, with increased expression paralleling increased cellular differentiation. In contrast, HNF-11 is reciprocally expressed with high levels in the base of the intestinal crypts where the proliferative, less differentiated cells reside.[6–8]

A plethora of intestine-specific transcription factors have been identified, yet those responsible for enteroendocrine cellular differentiation have not been very well defined. However, recent work has identified the basic helix-loop-helix protein BETA2 transcription as a controlling factor for the transcription of the secretin gene.[9] Secretin cells are terminally differentiated endocrine cells found in the villous epithelium of the small bowel. The basic-helix-loop-helix (bHLH) proteins form a family of transcription factors that are involved in controlling cellular differentiation in myogenic and B cells. BETA2, also known as neuroD because of its expression in neurons during differentiation, is also important in pancreatic islet development and function. Specifically, BETA2 is an activator of insulin gene transcription. BETA2's role in secretin cell differentiation was shown by BETA2 knock-out mice that failed to develop secretin and cholycystokinin cells while maintaining the other sets of endocrine cells.

BETA2 exerts transcriptional regulation by binding to the E box sequence in the secretin gene in a heterodimeric state with the ubiquitously expressed bHLH proteins E12/E47, with interaction from the cAMP response, element-binding, protein-related transcription coactivator p300. The transcription of secretin is coordinated with cell cycle

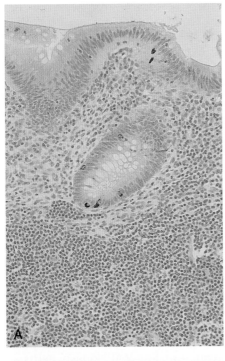

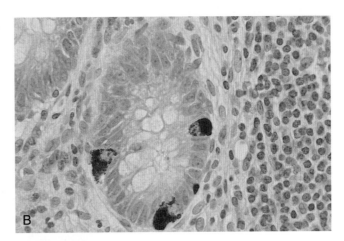

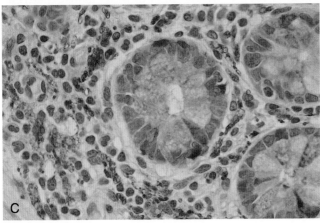

Figure 9-2. Enteroendocrine cells in the appendix. *A, B,* As with the small bowel, the endocrine cells are distributed throughout the crypt compartments and stain with chromogranin. *C,* S-100 is also expressed by endocrine cells and also by dendritic cells in the lamina propria. (×100, 400.)

arrest, perhaps through activation of the cyclin-dependent kinase inhibitor p21. BETA2 activated the p21 gene in transfection assays with concomitant cessation of proliferation and induction of apoptosis.

Further evidence to support the coordinate control of cell cycle and secretin transcription is the observation that the adenovirus protein E1A or the large T cell antigen of SV40 induced re-entry into the cell cycle with a concomitant block in secretin transcription. It is interesting that p300 is known to associate with E1A. Protein-mapping studies using binding assays and mammalian two-hybrid systems have shown that the carboxy terminus of p300 is needed for interaction with BETA2. In addition, the BETA2 binding domain of p300 overlaps with the E1A binding region of p300.

Additional elegant studies with BETA2–beta-galactosidase fusion protein transgenic mice have elucidated the cell populations normally expressing BETA2. In this model system, the regulatory elements of BETA2 are placed in front of the beta-galactosidase gene. Beta-galactosidase expression can then be visualized with a colometric reaction. In BETA-2 heterozygous mice, secretin cells were normal, and most cells expressing beta-galactosidase also expressed p21, with no expression of the proliferation marker PCNA. In contrast, in BETA2 homozygous mice, the galactosidase-positive cells did not express p21; they expressed PCNA and had no secretin cells.

The pancreatic-duodenal homeobox 1 gene (*pdx1*) is expressed in the cells of the distal stomach and duodenum in gastrin-, somatostatin-, and serotonin-secreting cells. *Pdx1* is essential for gastrin cell differentiation, as *pdx1* knock-out mice were essentially deficient in gastrin cells but maintained normal numbers of somatostatin cells and increased numbers of serotonin cells.[10]

Transgenic mice have allowed further dissection of gut epithelial lineage differentiation. These studies have shown that the small bowel and colon have differences in the mechanisms of enteroendocrine cell differentiation. By fusing a reporter gene with that of the 5' flanking control sequence of a specific gene, the expression may be followed. Because the liver fatty acid–binding protein is expressed not only in hepatocytes but also in a subset of gut epithelial cells, including endocrine cells, its 5' flanking sequence was fused with the human growth hormone, which served as the reporter gene. By means of dual immunohistochemistry for human growth hormone and various gut hormones, the cell lineages showing dual expression were identified. In the small bowel, co-expression was found in cholecystokinin, gastric inhibitory polypeptide, secretin, and glucagon cells. Although the small bowel showed dual expression in 30% of peptide YY and serotonin cells, the colon showed no co-expression in these cells but did show similar co-expression patterns in the other hormones.[11]

Stomach

The stomach is composed of three mucosal types: cardiac, fundic or oxyntic, and antral. The enteroendocrine cells of the stomach are composed of seven types, with differing distributions in the varying mucosa types. Gastrin is a peptide hormone secreted by G cells located in the antrum, which regulates acid production but also has a role in gastric epithelial development and maintenance. Gastrin receptors are G-coupled proteins expressed on enterochromaffin-like (ECL) cells of the gastric body, parietal cells, and chief cells, but not gut foveolar cells. There are at least seven types of endocrine cells in the stomach; ECL cells represent half of these, with the majority located in the fundus. Specifically, these cells constitute 35% of endocrine cells in the oxyntic mucosa. Enterochromaffin cells, which secrete 5-hydroxytryptophan, are found in the antrum and fundus, representing 25% of endocrine cells in the fundus. Uniformly distributed in the antrum and fundus are the D cells that secrete somatostatin; in the fundus these cells are 25% of the endocrine cell population. X cells are found only in the oxyntic mucosa and produce amylin, but the true function of these cells is not known. P and D1 cells are found in both the antrum and fundus.[12]

The control of gastric acid secretion is complex, with input from differing endocrine cells. The ECL cells play a key role in the regulation of gastric acid secretion. The cholecystokinin-B/gastrin receptor on the ECL cells is a member of a family of receptors linked to phospholipase C. After receptor stimulation, phospholipase C generates phosphatidylinositol, which increases free cytosolic calcium levels with subsequent activation of protein kinase C. When stimulated by amidated gastrin, a series of events is set off, including the release of histamine and the activation and induction of the enzyme histidine decarboxylase,[13] which catalyzes the decarboxylation of L-histidine and is the rate-limiting step in the production of histamine. Histamine secreted by ECL cells is the major acid secretagogue in the stomach, leading to HCl secretion by the parietal cells through histamine receptors. In contrast, somatostatin secreted by the D cells inhibits acid secretion. Gastrin stimulates acid secretion from parietal cells not only directly but also indirectly by enhancing histamine release from ECL cells through gastrin receptors (Fig. 9–3).[14, 15] Although gastrin receptors are present in both ECL and parietal cells, they activate the Ras-MAP kinase pathway only in ECL cells.[16]

The ECL cells thus play a key role in the regulation of gastric acid secretion. Therefore the molecular mechanisms of gastrin's regulation of ECL function are critical to understand. When the histamine content of ECL cells was depleted by means of pharmacologic agents, histidine decarboxylase and chromogranin A mRNA increased in these cells by a gastrin-independent mechanism, implying a role for histamine auto-feedback inhibition.[17] Other work points toward a central role of gastrin in regulating the transcription of this enzyme. The induction of immediate early genes is a response to many hormones. The genes activated include *c-fos* and *c-jun* through a protein kinase C pathway. C-fos and c-jun proteins function as transcription factors, forming a heterodimeric complex termed AP-1, which binds to specific DNA enhancer elements.

Gastrin regulates the transcription of the histidine decarboxylase gene through AP-1.[18] However, activation of the histidine decarboxylase promoter by AP-1 appears to be indirect. Raf-1 kinase and extracellular signal-regulated kinase-related signaling pathways (ERKs) are regulated by gastrin and are

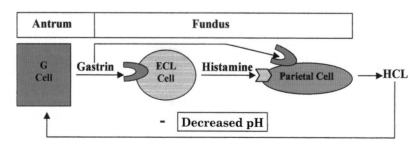

Figure 9–3. The control of gastric acid secretion.

important in activation of the histidine decarboxylase promoter in a cell culture model system.[19] In addition to regulation of histamine decarboxylase in ECL cells by gastrin, it also regulates the expression of the acidic protein chromogranin A, whose expression in the stomach is primarily in the ECL cells. Using transfection reporter assays with the chromogranin A promoter, gastrin was shown to increase the level of the transcription factor Sp1 and CRE (cyclic AMP-responsive element)-binding (CREB) proteins, which act through consensus sequences in the chromogranin promoter.[20] The transcription factors Sp1 and phosphorylated CREB act cooperatively to upregulate chromogranin A.

In a gastrin receptor knock-out mouse, the stomach had decreased parietal and ECL cells, showing that gastrin has an important role in gastric development.[21] With targeted knock-out of the gastrin gene in mice, the mice had atrophic gastric mucosa in the oxynic mucosa with decreased numbers of ECL, parietal, and chief cells, as confirmed by immunohistochemistry for chromogranin A, a parietal cell–specific H^+,K^+-ATPase, and intrinsic factor, respectively.[22] It is interesting that the mucous neck cells were increased, as confirmed by immunohistochemistry for a trifoil peptide. The remaining parietal cells appeared morphologically normal, and the decreased cell numbers in the stomach were not explained by changes in proliferative rates. However, these animals did show decreased proliferation of colonic epithelium despite the fact that these cells do not express gastrin receptors. These results show that gastrin has an important role in cell lineage differentiation in the stomach.

The GATA transcription factors have been found to be important in ECL cells. These transcription factors contain two zinc finger-binding domains and form a family of factors that are *trans*-activating, which bind specifically to *cis*-regulatory elements of (A/T)GATA(A/G) sequence.[23] Of the six known factors in this family, factors 4, 5, and 6 are involved in the control of gene expression in gut epithelial development.[24] The GATA-4 and GATA-6 factors are expressed in the parietal and ECL cells, respectively.[25] The promoter regions of the genes for the alpha and beta subunits of the gastric proton pump and histidine decarboxylase, expressed in parietal and ECL cells, respectively, contain GATA sequences.[26] In the rat, GATA-6 is increased with feeding.

Thus, we now understand that enteroendocrine cells are derived from the same stem cell population as the other gut epithelial cells (Fig. 9–4). The control mechanisms determining cell lineage specificity involve specific transcription factors, DNA-binding sites, and enhancer sequences. Cell lineage specificity involves the generation of pluripotential daughter cells, with further specificity of progressive generations. Therefore, given these events, it is easy to understand how in epithelial malignancies of the gastrointestinal tract, pure cell lineage fidelity may not always hold. Adenocarcinomas may have endocrine and/or Paneth cells scattered in the tumor.

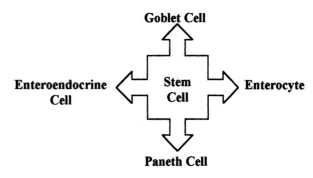

Figure 9–4. The endocrine cells of the gut are derived from the same stem cells as the other gut epithelial cells.

Carcinoid tumors may have mucin production and gland formation. Hybrid tumors such as the goblet cell carcinoid exist. What may have once appeared to be a paradox is now beginning to be understood.

CARCINOID AND NEUROENDOCRINE TUMORS

General Considerations

The carcinoid tumors of the gastrointestinal tract are a diverse group of tumors with both heterogeneous biologic potentials and essentially unknown etiologies. Thus, although the term "carcinoid" is used, one should in no way assume uniformity of these diverse tumors. Carcinoid tumors accounted for 2% of all malignant tumors in a large series of reported registered tumors, among which 74% were found in the gastrointestinal tract[27] (Fig. 9–5). However, these incidence figures represent reported tumors and hence do not take into account truly asymptomatic tumors. In another study, which included autopsy material, the incidence of carcinoid tumors was fourfold higher than that of the earlier study,[28] implying that most tumors are asymptomatic. Despite their derivation from gut epithelial cells, these tumors have striking morphologic, biologic, and genetic differences compared with adenocarcinomas. For example, most carcinoids are indolent tumors although fully capable of metastatic behavior. Additionally, mutations in the *APC* gene, although critical for colon and small bowel adenocarcinoma progression, are not involved in neoplastic transformation of the enteroendocrine cell. For example, patients with familial adenomatous polyposis

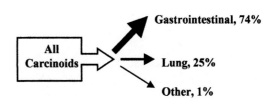

Figure 9–5. Most carcinoid tumors are in the gastrointestinal tract.

are born with a germline mutation in the *APC* gene. These patients develop numerous colonic and small bowel adenomas and eventually carcinomas but have no increased risk of neuroendocrine tumors compared with nonaffected patients. Conversely, patients with multiple endocrine neoplasia (MEN-I) are born with a germline mutation in the *MEN-I* gene and are prone to develop neuroendocrine tumors, including gastrinomas; however, these patients are not at increased risk for adenocarcinomas.

Because these tumors are derived from endocrine cells, they may continue to secrete hormones in an unregulated fashion, which may lead to functional consequences. These consequences are at times more devastating than the tumor mass itself. For example, the gastrin secreted by gastrinomas may cause parietal cell hypertrophy, increased gastric output, and duodenal ulcerations. Secretion of histamine and serotonin may lead to flushing and cardiac problems as part of the "carcinoid syndrome."

Based upon embryologic development, carcinoids are divided into those from the foregut (lung, stomach, first part of the duodenum), midgut (Figs. 9–6 and 9–7) (duodenum, jejunum, ileum, appendix, right colon), hindgut (Fig. 9–8) (transverse colon, left colon, rectum). These designations do correlate somewhat with morphology and staining characteristics. In general, foregut carcinoids may produce 5-hydroxytryptophan, tachykinins, gastrin, ACTH, and human chorionic gonadotropin. The liberation of histamine by foregut tumors may result in the atypical carcinoid syndrome characterized by generalized flushing, diarrhea, cutaneous edema, bronchoconstriction, and tearing. Midgut tumors may produce serotonin. Hindgut carcinoids may produce tachykinins, somatostatin, pancreatic polypeptide, 5-hydroxytryptophan, dopamine, and neurotensin.[29]

A study in 1997 of 8305 carcinoid tumors has yielded important epidemiologic and biologic behavior information.[27] Table 9–1 shows the frequency distribution of carcinoids in the luminal gastrointestinal tract. The small bowel is the most frequent site of carcinoid development, followed closely by the colon. Small bowel carcinoid tumors are the second most common tumor in that site, preceded by small bowel adenocarcinomas. Carcinoids in the stomach are relatively rare (4.3% of gut carcinoids), and esophageal carcinoid tumors are exceedingly rare. The terminal ileum and appendix were the most frequent specific gut sites of

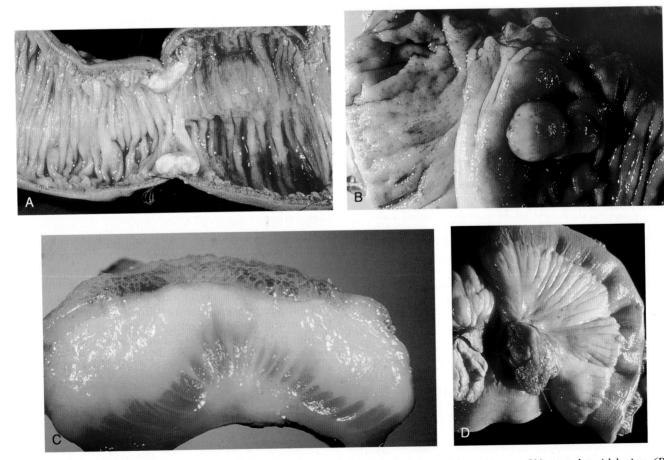

Figure 9–6. Midgut carcinoid tumor. Carcinoid tumors may present as a mural-based mass *(A)* or polypoid lesion *(B)* with extensive infiltration into the small bowel wall *(C). D,* Mesenteric involvement by tumor may result in fibrosis and tethering of the mesentery.

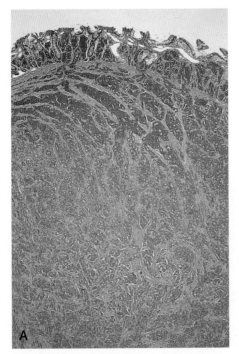

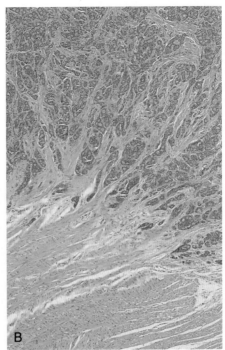

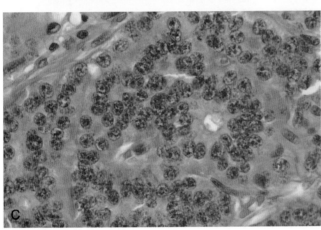

Figure 9–7. Terminal ileal carcinoid. Although the carcinoid tumor may involve the mucosa, the bulk of the tumor is in the submucosa *(A)* and gut wall *(B). C,* Carcinoid tumors have a variety of morphologies and may display glandular architecture.

carcinoid development (21% and 25.6%, respectively). There appears to be an inverse relationship to the frequency of adenocarcinomas and carcinoids along the small bowel, with adenocarcinomas occurring mostly in the proximal small bowel. However, the rectum comprised 17% of carcinoid tumors, representing over 50% of total colonic carcinoid tumors. The average age of patients with appendiceal carcinoids was 42 years, whereas that of the patients with carcinoid tumors in the remainder of the gut was 60 years. In contrast, the average age of noncarcinoid tumors in these sites was 62 and 67 years, respectively. Thus, carcinoid tumors were found in a younger age group than noncarcinoid tumors. African–Americans had a higher probability of rectal carcinoids than whites, with an African-American–to–white ratio of 0.34, compared with an overall ratio of 0.13. Carcinoid tumors were found associated with other tumors in 16.6% of

small bowel, 13.1% colonic (excluding appendix), 14.6% appendix, 7.8% gastric, and 9.2% rectal cases.

Despite the apparent indolent nature of typical carcinoid tumors, they do have the ability to metastasize and kill patients. The metastatic propensity is related to a number of factors, including the site of their derivation. In the large study of carcinoid tumors,[27] 63% of carcinoids of the appendix were localized lesions, with 28.5% having regional metastasis and 8.5% having distant spread. Rectal carcinoids were localized in 72.2% of cases, had regional spread in 7.1%, and distant metastasis in 7.1% of cases (the remainder of cases were unstaged). In contrast, carcinoids of the small bowel and colon were localized in only 25% and 22.8% of cases, respectively (Fig. 9–9). These sites had regional spread in 39.3% and 36.3% and distant metastasis in 31.4% and 37.8%, respectively. Figure 9–10 shows that the 5-year survival was dependent upon the stage of the tumor.

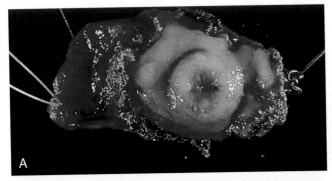

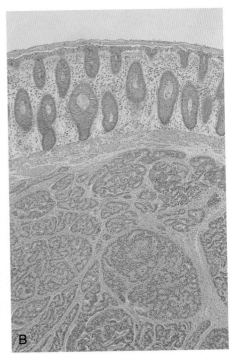

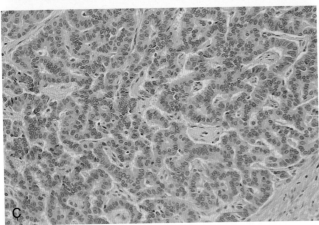

Figure 9–8. Hindgut carcinoid tumors. *A,* These tumors may present as polypoid masses. They may present in many locations, but the rectum is a common colonic site. *B,* Histologically, as with all gut carcinoid tumors, the bulk of the tumor is submucosal. *C,* The trabecular ribboning pattern is another architectural variant of these tumors.

Immunohistochemistry

With the exception of appendiceal carcinoid tumors, most gastrointestinal carcinoid tumors stain with antibodies to chromogranin, neuron-specific enolase (NSE), cytokeratin, and glycoproteins. Carcinoid tumors may demonstrate mucin production.

Table 9–1. Frequency of Distribution of Gastrointestinal Carcinoid Tumors

Carcinoid Site	% Cases
Esophagus	0.05
Stomach	4.3
Small bowel	39
(Ileum)	(21)
Appendix	25.6
Colon	31
(Rectum)	(17)

In general, gastrointestinal adenocarcinomas express carcinoembryonic antigen (CEA), which is a high-molecular-weight glycoprotein, and polymorphic epithelial mucins (PEMs), which are high in serine/threonine carbohydrate chains. The monoclonal antibody B72.3 was originally developed against human breast cancer and reacts with a specific PEM (Neu-Acalpha2 → 6GalNAcalpha1 → O-Ser/Thr(sialo-Tn). It is now known not to be specific for breast cancer as it reacts with adenocarcinomas from many sites. B72.3 was found to react with 31% of carcinoid tumors, including those from the appendix, jejunoileum, rectum, and cecum.[30] In this same study, the authors generated a novel antibody, ACT19, against short carbohydrate chains, including the same sequence recognized by B72.3; however, this antibody recognized a distinct epitope from that of B72.3. ACT19 was found to react with 74% of carcinoid tumors from the earlier listed sites. A monoclonal antibody to CEA reacted weakly with 26% of cases.

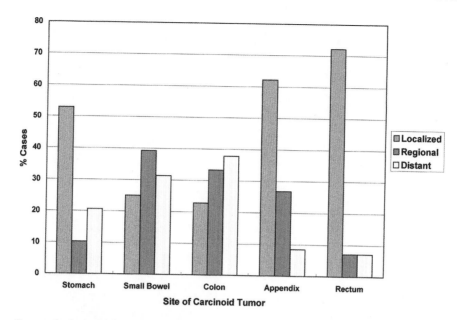

Figure 9–9. Stage of carcinoid tumors from differing gastrointestinal locations. (From Modin IM, Sandor A: An analysis of 8305 cases of carcinoid tumors. Cancer 1997; 79:813.)

Carcinoid tumors stain with cytokeratin, with the exception of most appendiceal tumors. However, the molecular weights of keratin expressed in these lesions differ from those expressed by adenocarcinomas and the non-neoplastic epithelium. For example, cytokeratin 20 stains intestinal epithelial cells exclusive of the enteroendocrine cells. In keeping with their non-neoplastic counterparts, carcinoid tumors also do not stain with cytokeratin 20 (personal observations) (Fig. 9–11). However, adenocarcinomas do express cytokeratin 20. Cytokeratin 18 is expressed in the intestinal epithelium and also heavily expressed in intestinal carcinoids but not in appendiceal carcinoids.[31] Because pheochromocytomas also lack cytokeratin 18 expression, Wilander and Schelbenpflug[31] claim that appendiceal carcinoids are more akin to pheochromocytomas than are other intestinal carcinoids. Additionally, most

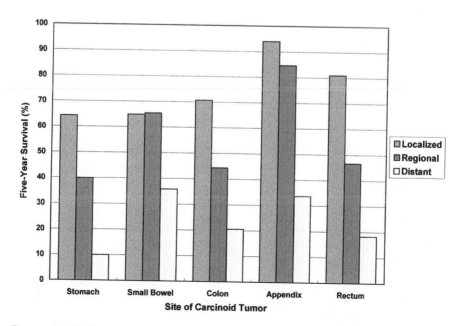

Figure 9–10. Five-year survival of patients with carcinoid tumors dependent upon stage and site. The most important parameter of survival appears to be the stage of the tumor. (From Modin IM, Sandor A: An analysis of 8305 cases of carcinoid tumors. Cancer 1997; 79:813.)

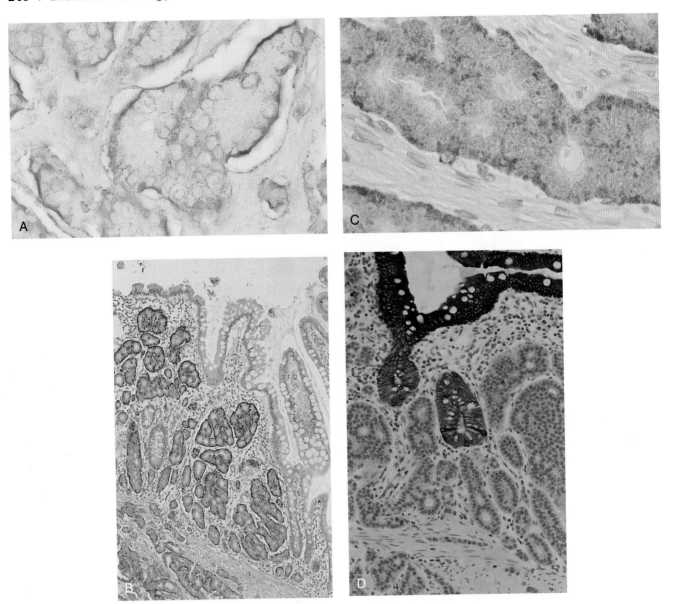

Figure 9–11. Staining of carcinoid tumors. Carcinoid tumors may stain with Grimelius *(A)* and Fontana *(B)* stains. *C,* Synaptophysin is expressed by virtually all gut carcinoid tumors. *D,* Enteroendocrine cells and carcinoid tumors do not express cytokeratin 18, which is strongly expressed by the rest of the gut epithelium. (×400, 50, 400).

appendiceal carcinoids are thought to arise from subepithelial endocrine cells rather than from epithelial endocrine cells.

S-100 is an acidic calcium-binding protein expressed in neural crest tissues, such as astrocytes, oligodendrocytes, Schwann cells, adrenal medulla, and sustentacular cells.[32] S-100 was expressed in the great majority of appendiceal carcinoid tumors but in only a minority of carcinoid tumors of the rest of the gastrointestinal tract.[33–35] The cells expressing S-100 in carcinoid tumors were slender and were located at the periphery of the tumor cluster aggregates with occasional interdigitation in the tumor nests. However, occasional tumors showed clear staining in the actual tumor cells. Additionally, the great majority of appendiceal carcinoids expressed serotonin.

Chromogranin A (CgA) is a 49-kDa acidic protein, is a member of the granin/secretogranin family, and is expressed in endocrine and neuroendocrine cells. It serves a regulatory role in the secretion of peptide hormones and neurotransmitters. Specifically, CgA can be secreted and processed into the bioactive hormone pancreastatin, which inhibits insulin secretion from islet cells and acid secretion from parietal cells.[36] Additionally, CgA plays an important intracellular role because it binds calcium and catecholamines. A consensus cAMP element and a TATA-box motif in the area of the transcription site are important for neuroendocrine cell-specific expression and basal and cAMP-induced expression of CgA.[37] Chromogranin was found to be expressed in 88% of foregut, 100% of midgut, and 60% of hindgut carcinoids.

Synaptophysin is a membrane protein located in 30- to 50-nm vesicles in neurons and neuroendocrine cells. In neurons, this protein is located in synaptic vesicles. Although it constitutes 7% of total vesicle protein, its function is not clearly understood, because mutation studies have shown that its disruption did not interfere with synaptic transmission or the phenotype in mutant mice.[38, 39] Additionally, the lack of this protein did not disrupt the assembly of the small vesicles as they were visible with electron microscopy. Synaptophysin, unlike chromogranin, was universally expressed in all carcinoid tumors of the gastrointestinal tract.[35]

The neural cell adhesion molecule (N-CAM) is a member of the immunoglobulin (Ig) superfamily and serves as a homophilic and heterophilic cell adhesion molecule. While its role in neuronal migration and dendritic sprouting is clear, N-CAM is also essential for normal segregation and structure of pancreatic islet cells.[40] N-CAM was expressed in 76.5%, 58%, and 20% of foregut, midgut, and hindgut carcinoids, respectively.[35] N-CAM was expressed in sustentacular cells or tumor cells. Of the midgut tumors staining for N-CAM, only 50% showed tumor staining.

Carcinoembryogenic antigen (CEA) is a 180-kDa cell surface glycoprotein anchored by a glycophatidyl inositol linkage, which has a role in cell adhesion and is a member of the Ig supergene family. The N-domain has been shown to mediate homotypic cell adhesion.[41] This antigen is upregulated during colonic neoplastic transformation,[42] with virtually all gastrointestinal adenocarcinomas expressing CEA. In keeping with the derivation from an identical stem cell, carcinoid tumors as well may be CEA positive, although the percentage of positive cases is well below 100%. Specifically, 26% of gastrointestinal carcinoid tumors expressed CEA.[30] It is interesting that CEA expression is not limited to gastrointestinal carcinoid tumors; it is expressed in the normal C cells of the thyroid and in their neoplastic counterparts. Thyroid follicles and thyroid carcinomas, however, do not express CEA.[43, 44] The homophilic binding property of CEA may give cancer cells metastatic ability; increased CEA expression enhanced colon carcinoma cell aggregates and liver metastasis in an in vitro and in vivo model system, respectively.[45] Similarly, carcinoid tumors with CEA expression seem to have a higher rate of metastasis than do CEA-negative tumors.[46, 47]

Presentation

Patients with carcinoid tumors may present as a result of symptoms caused by hormone production, metastatic disease, or gut obstruction (see Fig. 9–3), or as an incidental finding. With the advent of endoscopy, carcinoid tumors may present as polypoid/submucosal masses that may invoke a limited differential diagnosis (Table 9–2). Patients may present primarily with a metastatic lesion. For example,

Table 9–2. Differential Diagnosis of a Submucosal Mass

Carcinoid
Lipoma
Metastatic tumor
Lymphoma
Brunner gland

a solitary cervical metastasis was found in the soft tissue of one patient, with the ileal primary found only 4 years later after further presentation with carcinoid syndrome.[48] Similarly, gut carcinoids have been reported to present as a primary breast tumor.[49] It is important to note that patients with carcinoid tumors of unknown primary have a survival rate similar to that of patients with midgut tumors with distant spread. Additionally, patients with carcinoid tumors of unknown primary had hormone levels of urinary 5-hydroxyindoleacetic acid and serotonin similar to those of patients with midgut tumors.[50]

Specific Types and Sites

Gastric

Gastric carcinoid tumors are divided into three types to reflect underlying hypergastrinemia, etiology, and biologic behavior. Types I and II are both associated with hypergastrinemia, with the underlying conditions of chronic atrophic gastritis and Zollinger-Ellison syndrome (multiple endocrine neoplasia-I), respectively. Type III carcinoids, in contrast, are sporadic and not associated with hypergastrinemia. Hypergastrinemia drives the ECL cell population, leading to proliferation and carcinoid formation; thus, types I and II carcinoids are composed of ECL cells and surrounding ECL hyperplasia (Fig. 9–12).[51] Carcinoid tumors of types I and II are usually less than 1 cm in size and are multiple. They have a relatively benign behavior, although local and liver metastasis may occur in 9% to 23% and 3% to 5% of patients with types I and II, respectively.[52–55] The size of type I carcinoids correlates with invasiveness. Specifically, tumors less than 1 cm may be managed endoscopically, whereas tumors greater than 2 cm may warrant surgical excision.[56] In contrast, type III carcinoid tumors are usually larger than 1 cm, are composed of multiple endocrine cell types, and therefore are not restricted to ECL cells, are not associated with ECL hyperplasia, and are biologically aggressive.[57]

Hypergastrinemia is thought to drive the proliferation of the ECL cells, leading eventually to carcinoid formation, but other factors must also be operative. Specifically, patients with Zollinger-Ellison (ZE) syndrome of the sporadic type, a hypertrophic gastropathy of the parietal cell type due to hypergastrinemia, rarely develop gastric carcinoid tumors (0% to 0.6%), whereas patients with this same

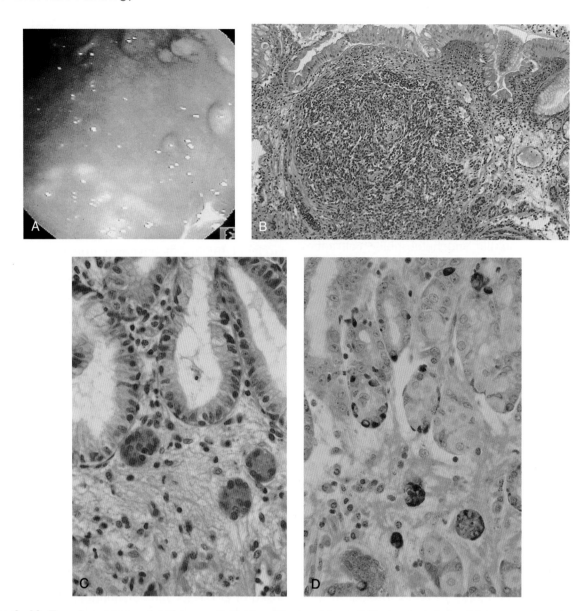

Figure 9–12. Type I gastric carcinoid tumor. Patients with atrophic gastritis have prolonged hypergastrinemia, which is trophic to the enterochromaffin-like (ECL) cells. *A,* Macrocarcinoid tumors, typically multiple, may develop and present as small nodules as seen with endoscopy. *B,* Histologically, these lesions are composed of a mass of ECL cells. Surrounding the macrocarcinoids are microcarcinoids and ECL hyperplasia. *C,* The microcarcinoid tumors are seen as small clusters of slightly eosinophilic cells, preferentially located at the base of the glands. *D,* The ECL hyperplasia is seen only with a chromogranin stain, which highlights the microcarcinoids but now shows abundant positive cells in the gastric glands.

syndrome with MEN-I frequently develop gastric carcinoid tumors (13% to 30%).[58, 59] In ZE-MEN-I, the gastrinomas were located in the duodenum in 80% of patients, with the remainder located in the pancreas. In patients with ZE without MEN-I, the primary gastrinomas were found in the duodenum (36%), pancreas (30%), and other sites. Liver metastasis developed in 11% and 5% of patients with and without MEN-I, respectively; however, there was no significant difference between the two groups. The overall 15-year survival was 93% in patients with ZE-MEN-I and 68% in sporadic cases. Patients with ZE in MEN-I had the onset of their disease at 33.7 years of age and were diagnosed by 37.8 years, whereas the age of onset and diagnosis for patients with sporadic ZE was 43.1 and 48.9 years, respectively.[59, 60] Both sets of patients had similar serum gastrin levels, gastric acid output, and rates of peptic ulceration. Additionally, men and women were equally frequent in both sets of patient groups. The most striking difference between ZE-MEN-I and sporadic ZE was the prevalence of gastric carcinoid tumors, which was 37% and 2%, respectively.

Because of the excellent long-term survival of patients with ZE-MEN-I, the surgical treatment of their gastrinomas is debated. Even with lymph node metastasis, which occurred in 78% of patients, survival was excellent. Lymph node metastasis also did not decrease survival in sporadic ZE patients.[60, 61] Additionally, the gastrinomas in ZE-MEN-I tend to be multiple, making surgical cure difficult. In contrast, surgical excision of sporadic gastrinomas is warranted as the operation may be curative, with the rate of liver metastasis decreased and survival prolonged. Pancreatic gastrinomas greater than 3 cm had a high association with liver metastasis and decreased survival in ZE-MEN-I patients.[62] Also, surgical excision of the pancreatic tumor did not seem to improve survival or risk for liver metastasis. The fraction of cells in S-phase, as determined by flow cytometry of sporadic gastrinomas, correlated with disease extent.[63]

Somatostatin receptor scintigraphy is excellent for the evaluation of metastatic disease and primary duodenal gastrinomas. However, small duodenal tumors may be missed.[64]

Patients with pernicious anemia develop hypergastrinemia as a response to decreased gastric acid secondary to the primary destruction of their parietal cells. Over time, 2% to 9% of these patients will develop gastric carcinoid tumors.[65]

Certain pharmacologic drugs result in hypergastrinemia and have raised concern about their ability to induce gastric carcinoid formation. Omeprazole is a proton pump inhibitor used to lower gastric acid secretion for the treatment of peptic ulcer disease. Because of its ability to interfere with gastric acid secretion, serum gastrin is increased. Gastrin levels stabilize at two to four times baseline levels at an initial peak 2 to 4 months after initiation of therapy. Gastrin levels of greater than 500 ng/L are seen in only 11% of patients. Omeprazole has no effect on plasma gastrin in achlorhydric patients, which is consistent with its hypergastrinemic effect being entirely secondary to acid inhibition.[66] Thus, there is a theoretic risk in this hypergastrinemic state of causing ECL hyperplasia and carcinoid formation. Rats given omeprazole developed hypergastrinemia, ECL hyperplasia, and gastric carcinoids.[67] However, long-term treatment (5 years) in humans has not resulted in gastric carcinoid formation.[68-70] Although carcinoid formation has not been observed, ECL hyperplasia has been seen, with microcarcinoid prevalence increasing from 2.5% to 20% after daily treatment for 36 to 64 months.[70] However, overall, the risk of neoplastic development in this drug-induced hypergastrinemic state is not increased. The reason for the risk not being increased in comparison to the increased risk seen in ZE and pernicious anemia may relate to the higher gastrin levels present in those conditions.

Helicobacter pylori has been reported to cause hypergastrinemia, but there is no association with carcinoid formation. Specifically, two patients were found to have fasting hypergastrinemia, gastric acid hypersecretion, and *H. pylori* gastritis without evidence for ZE syndrome. Eradication of the *H. pylori* infection resulted in resolution of the hypergastrinemia.[71]

Somatostatinomas

Somatostatinomas are endocrine tumors that secrete somatostatin. These tumors are exceedingly rare, representing at most 1% of all endocrine tumors of the gut and pancreas.[72] Most of these tumors (75%) are found in the pancreas, with the great majority of the remainder localized to the duodenum. It is interesting that the somatostatin syndrome, defined by weight loss, diarrhea, diabetes mellitus, and gallstone disease, is seen only with pancreatic tumors, whereas the duodenal tumors may present with pain and/or jaundice, particularly if localized to the ampullary region.[73] Often these duodenal tumors are found incidentally.[74] The pancreatic tumors also seem to differ from the duodenal tumors in that they are usually larger in size, are more common in women, and have a worse prognosis.[75]

Histologically, duodenal somatostatinomas invariably contain the characteristic psammoma bodies (Fig. 9–13) composed of calcium apatite crystals,[74] which are not found in pancreatic somatostatinomas or other duodenal neuroendocrine tumors.[73] Rarely, amyloid deposition is seen in pancreatic somatostatinomas, which may represent a novel amyloid as it does not react with antibodies to the amyloid P component, islet amyloid peptide, somatostatin, or other hormones.[76] However, this amyloid has not been reported in duodenal somatostatinomas. These tumors stain with neuron-specific enolase, chromogranin, and somatostatin.

These tumors are rare, but the duodenal tumors have been associated with von Recklinghausen's disease and the pancreatic tumors weakly associated with MEN-I.[72, 77]

Because of the small size and clinical presentation of the duodenal tumors, their detection is made mostly by endoscopy. Octreotide, a synthetic somatostatin analogue, labeled with indium 111

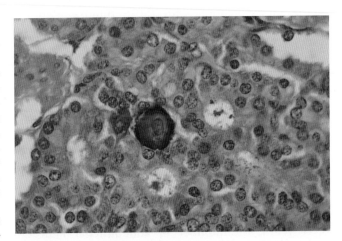

Figure 9–13. Somatostatinoma, duodenum. These rare tumors have characteristic psammoma bodies. Although the psammoma bodies are specific to this neuroendocrine tumor in the duodenum, they are not specific in pancreatic endocrine tumors. (×400).

(OctreoScan), has been used to localize somatostatin receptor–bearing tumors. Although the efficacy of this detection system for somatostatinomas is limited, this scan has been effective in the detection of pancreatic tumors but has failed to detect duodenal tumors.[78] The duodenal tumors may remain localized but do have the ability to metastasize to lymph nodes and the liver. However, the pancreatic tumors seem to have a higher liver metastatic rate than do duodenal tumors. Local resection is the current treatment.

Appendix

In contrast to the rest of the luminal gastrointestinal tract, carcinoid tumors are the most frequent tumors of the appendix, representing 77.3% of tumors at this site. There was a twofold female predominance in appendiceal carcinoid tumors in the study of 8305 cases of carcinoid tumors.[27] One may initially attribute this striking female predominance to a selection bias based upon incidental appendectomies during gyneocologic procedures, but this hypothesis does not hold when one considers that the frequency of noncarcinoid appendiceal tumors was essentially equal in men and women (male/female = 1:15).

Most of these tumors are discovered incidentally. In a study of histologic abnormalities in incidental appendectomies in urologic patients, two carcinoid tumors were found in 38 specimens. Additionally, fibrous obliteration was seen in 35 of the 38 cases.[79] Some appendices are removed incidentally, others are removed for appendicitis. The etiologic role of carcinoid tumors in the clinical presentation of appendicitis is not known but most likely is minimal at best, especially when one considers that 75% of carcinoid tumors are present at the tip. It seems more plausible to consider that the 10% of tumors present at the base of the appendix may account for appendicitis in association with these tumors. Patients presenting with disseminated appendiceal carcinoid tumor are the exception.

The endocrine cells of the appendix can be classified according to their location relative to the mucosal glands. Endocrine cells within the epithelium are called epithelial neuroendocrine cells and those separate from the epithelium, usually located in the deep lamina propria, are termed subepithelial neuroendocrine cells. The claim that the cell of origin of appendiceal carcinoids is the subepithelial neurosecretory cell is based upon circumstantial evidence. The subepithelial neuroendocrine cells stain with antibodies to serotonin and are argentaphilic.[80] Whereas the appendix reaches adult size by the age of 4 years, the number of subepithelial neuroendocrine cells continues to increase with age. Specifically, appendices from patients aged 9 years showed only occasional subepithelial neurosecretory cells. The number of these cells increased with age, reaching a plateau by age 30 years.[81, 82] A subset of appendices showed no increase in subepithelial endocrine cells with age. In contrast, the number of epithelial endocrine cells does not vary with age. The density of subepithelial neuroendocrine cells was maximal at the appendiceal tip, paralleling the site of appendiceal carcinoid tumors. In contrast, the epithelial endocrine cells (both Grimelius argyrophilic and Masson-Fontana argentaphilic showed no site variation along the appendix. Immunohistochemistry for S-100 showed positivity in the classic organoid carcinoid tumor consistent with a subepithelial neuroendocrine origin while tubular and goblet cell carcinoids were negative for S-100, arguing for an epithelial endocrine cell origin.[83]

Grossly, most carcinoid tumors present as a yellow nodule. The measurement of this nodule is important, as the size is directly proportional to the probability of metastatic disease. However, diffuse apendiceal involvement with carcinoid tumor is occasionally seen. Histologically, the carcinoids may have a trabeculated or nesting pattern. As with other carcinoid tumors, the cells have a low mitotic rate and the typical stippled chromatin pattern. These features are in contrast to those seen in the more aggressive adenocarcinoid tumors. Despite the indolent nature of the great majority of appendiceal carcinoid tumors, most have lymphatic permeation. Sixty-five percent of the tumors invade into and through the muscle wall, with peritoneal surface involvement, and 18% invade the mesoappendix.[84] The biologic behavior of most appendiceal carcinoids is benign. When these tumors have developed distant metastasis, the size of the original tumor was greater than 2 cm after formalin fixation.[85] However, rare cases of disseminated tumor have been reported in tumors of less than 2 cm.[86] Fortunately, 70% to 90% of tumors are less than 1 cm in diameter, 4% to 25% are 1 to 2 cm, and only a few are greater than 2 cm.[87] Simple appendectomy is usually sufficient to treat carcinoid tumors of the appendix even when there is involvement of the peritoneum and/or mesoappendix.[88–90] Right hemicolectomy may be warranted for tumors greater than 2 cm in diameter.

Goblet Cell Carcinoid/Adenocarcinoid/Crypt Cell Carcinoma

This tumor is a distinctive, albeit rare, type of neoplasia that displays both glandular and neuroendocrine morphologies. Because of its dual morphology, this enigmatic lesion goes under a variety of names in the literature, including goblet cell carcinoid, adenocarcinoid, and crypt cell carcinoma. Unlike "typical" carcinoid tumors whose biologic behavior is fairly indolent, these tumors may act more aggressively. In keeping with this more aggressive behavior, these tumors may show increased atypia and mitotic activity. These tumors are rare; they occur most commonly in the appendix but represent only 5% of primary appendiceal tumors.[91] Although

Table 9-3. Histologic Features of Adenocarcinoid Tumors

Lack of overlying surface epithelial dysplasia
Tumor located below the crypts
Apparent mucin production
Goblet cell and/or tubular morphology
Neuroendocrine differentiation (e.g., argyrophilic granules)

the appendix is the most common site of presentation, goblet cell carcinoid tumors have been found in the periampullary area of the duodenum.[92]

The histologic diagnosis of this tumor is based upon several criteria (Table 9–3). An adenomatous or dysplastic epithelial precursor is lacking. The tumors are located below the crypts and, unlike typical carcinoid tumors, do not usually form a discrete mass but involve the wall rather diffusely. The most striking feature is the glandular morphology, which has led to the plethora of names given to this lesion.

The glandular morphology may be either a goblet cell feature or tubular and glandular structures with mucin production (Fig. 9–14). However, this morphologic distinction is somewhat artificial as most tumors contain a spectrum of both morphologies.

Several pitfalls in the histologic diagnosis should be avoided. First, the finding of mucin alone in no way negates the diagnosis of a typical carcinoid, nor does its presence equate with a diagnosis of adenocarcinoid or adenocarcinoma. Specifically, carcinoid tumors themselves may have mucin.[93] Second, the goblet cell morphology should not mislead one to diagnose the tumor as a signet ring carcinoma, either primary or metastatic. On the other hand, one should consider this lesion when faced with an ovary with an apparent metastatic "signet ring" carcinoma, as these tumors have a propensity for ovarian spread.[94]

The goblet cell morphology may be striking (see Fig. 9–14), with groups of cells having distended, mucin-filled cells. These cells may group and cluster,

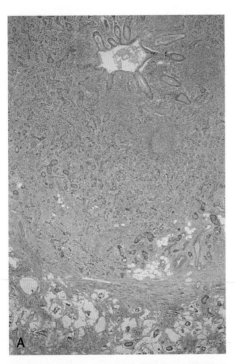
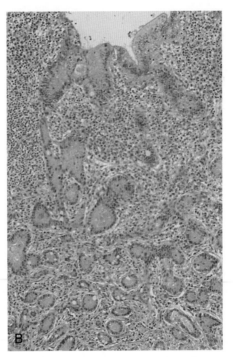
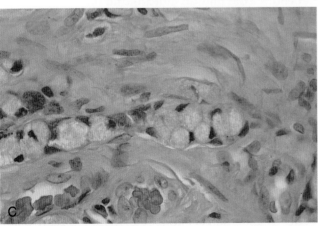

Figure 9-14. Goblet cell carcinoid, appendix. Goblet cell carcinoid tumors display more glandular phenotype and may be more aggressive than typical carcinoid tumors. *A, B,* These tumors may infiltrate the wall of the appendix rather than forming a discrete mass. *C, D,* The name "goblet cell carcinoid" is derived from areas of signet ring morphology with mucin production. The signet ring morphology may be confused with a signet ring carcinoma. *E,* Other areas of the tumor show carcinoid architecture but may show readily identifiable mitotic figures that are not seen in typical carcinoid tumors. *F,* The spectrum of cytologic atypia may be wide within the same tumor, with areas verging on small cell carcinoma identified. *G,* Occasional staining with chromogranin is seen. (*A,* ×25, *B,* ×50, *C,* ×630. *D,* mucicarmine.)

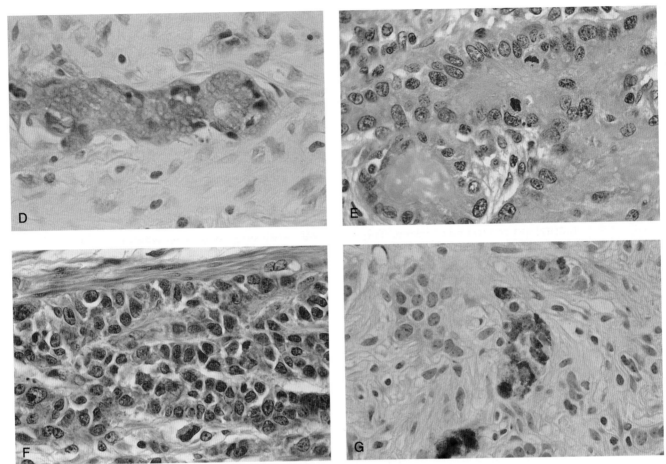

Figure 9–14. Continued.

form glands, and/or stream. This streaming pattern may also be somewhat confusing and may, again, raise in one's mind the possibility of signet ring carcinoma. The goblet cell morphology is more common than the tubular type present in 30 of 39 cases in one series.[95] Neuroendocrine differentiation is evident by their cytology but also by markers (argentaffin/argyrophil), which are positive in 56% and 88% of cases, respectively.[96] Paneth cells may also be seen in this lesion, with one study detecting them in 9 of 39 cases. It is interesting that Paneth cells may also be seen in metastatic lesions.[96] The goblet cell morphology and endocrine differentiation do not appear to be mutually exclusive as both types of cells are found in metastasis. Additionally, co-expression by the same cell of neuroendocrine and goblet features has been demonstrated by electron microscopy, showing mucin droplets and dense core granules in the same cell.[97]

The presentation of patients with appendiceal adenocarcinoids differs from that for the usual appendiceal carcinoid tumors, which are usually incidental lesions. In the aforementioned study,[97] 23 of 39 patients presented with acute appendicitis: 9 incidentally, 2 as a mass, 1 with obstruction, 2 as an autopsy finding, and 2 for which there was no information. An additional study examining 10 cases found a similar spectrum of presentations: 5 patients presented with acute appendicitis, and 5 with an abdominal mass.[97]

Adenocarcinoid tumors may be aggressive tumors. In the report of Edmunds and associates,[97] 11 patients (13%) of 86 cases died of disease, and 3 had persistent disease. Such a percentage is in marked contrast to appendiceal carcinoid tumors, which have essentially no ability to kill the patient, with the very rare exception of those tumors greater than 2 cm. When these tumors do disseminate, it is mostly by the intra-abdominal route, with liver metastasis being rare. The risk for metastasis may depend on the mitotic index of the tumor, as at least one mitosis per high-power field was found in all tumors with metastasis.[95] Additionally, the stage of the tumor undoubtedly is an important factor. Nuclear atypia was found to correlate with aggressive behavior as well.

Thus, given the potentially more aggressive behavior of these tumors compared with the usual appendiceal carcinoid tumors, the therapy for these tumors is debated.[98] Some of the patients who were free of disease had simple appendectomies. On the other hand, right hemicolectomy has been advocated for the treatment of these tumors. It must be stressed, however, that a complete stage by stage comparison of differing treatments has not been done. In general, recommendations for a right hemicolectomy may be given if the tumor shows greater than one mitosis per 10 high-power fields, nuclear atypia, or spread beyond the appendix.[99] In further contrast to carcinoid tumors, goblet cell carcinoid tumors were found to stain with anti-p53 antibodies whereas carcinoid tumors did not show this reactivity,[100] implying that mutations in p53 are involved in the neoplastic progression in goblet cell carcinoid but not in that of carcinoids.

Neuroendocrine Carcinoma

Poorly differentiated carcinoma with neuroendocrine features is a rare but aggressive tumor with variable association with adenomatous epithelium (Fig. 9–15). This tumor displays neuroendocrine differentiation with variable staining, with staining for S-100, synaptophysin, and chromogranin. The variable association with adenomatous epithelium leads to a dilemma regarding the origin of this tumor. Molecular studies have now shown that this poorly differentiated carcinoma has the same loss of heterozygosity in the *APC* gene as the adenomatous epithelium. It is important to note that carcinoid tumors showed no loss of heterozygosity at the *APC* locus.[101] Thus, these tumors are best viewed as a poorly differentiated component along the adenocarcinoma sequence rather than along the carcinoid pathway.

Genetics

Colon Cancer Genes and Relationship to Neuroendocrine Tumor Formation

The development of molecular biology has led to an explosion in our understanding of both normal cellular homeostasis and neoplastic development.

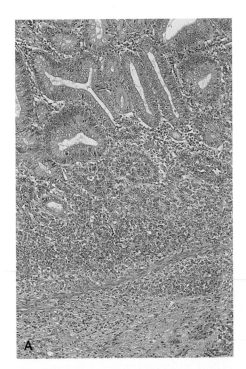

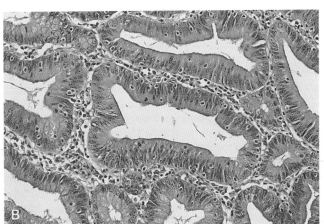

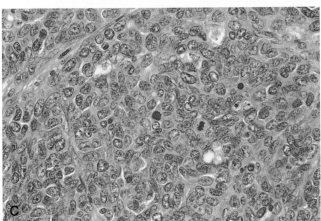

Figure 9–15. Neuroendocrine carcinoma arising in association with a villous adenoma. These biologically aggressive tumors are actually poorly differentiated adenocarcinomas with neuroendocrine features. *A,* These tumors originally were thought to be a composite tumor, as the overlying adenomatous component appeared distinctive from the underlying, poorly differentiated carcinoma. The overlying adenoma *(B)* shows nuclear features, which are different from the high-grade nuclei present in the carcinoma *(C).* Molecular studies have shown that the adenoma and the carcinoma are clonal with loss of the adenomatous polyposis coli gene. In addition, a merging of these components may at times be seen *(A).*

The identification of familial syndromes and their underlying germline mutations has allowed the identification of numerous key genes in these processes. Despite our advances, we still are fairly ignorant about the important genes involved in gut carcinoid development, with the exception of the *MEN* genes. One might think that because the enteroendocrine cells are epithelial cells derived from the same stem cell as the other cell lineages, the same mechanisms of neoplastic progression leading to adenocarcinoma would apply to the neoplastic progression in gut endocrine tumors. Unfortunately, we may not apply this logic to these tumors.

The adenomatous polyposis coli (*APC*) gene is a key component of the control of intestinal epithelial cell homeostasis. This gene was first identified through family linkage studies from patients with familial adenomatous polyposis (FAP). In this autosomal dominant disorder, patients develop hundreds to thousands of adenomatous colon polyps, with eventual progression to colon cancer. Additionally, these patients develop small bowel adenomas and cancers, albeit fewer in number than in the colon. The cloning of this gene and the protein identification that followed are leading to an explosion in the understanding of the mechanisms involved in normal intestinal epithelial cell biology and colon carcinogenesis. Patients are born with a germline mutation in one of the *APC* genes and are initially phenotypically normal, with normal gut differentiation and cellular components, including enteroendocrine cells. When the one functional *APC* gene is mutated, leading to the complete loss of APC function, an adenoma develops. Specifically, APC is now known to be an intricate member of factors involved in the control of the transcription factor Tcf-4. APC becomes phosphorylated by glycogen synthase kinase 3beta after appropriate Wnt signaling and then complexes with axin/conductin and beta-catenins. This complex targets beta-catenins for proteolysis, with subsequent diminution in the free monomeric cytoplasmic pool of beta-catenins. If there is increased monomeric beta-catenins, they may complex with Tcf-4 and serve as transcription factors with increased expression of c-myc, a protein important in control of cellular proliferation. In the intestine, APC is normally expressed highly in the surface cells, which are not proliferating, and less so in the base of the crypts.

Despite APC's ubiquitous expression and crucial role in cellular homeostasis and neoplastic progression in colon and small bowel adenocarcinomas, it does not seem to have an impact of neoplastic progression in enteroendocrine cells. Patients with FAP do not have an increased risk of developing neuroendocrine tumors.

The "deleted in colon cancer" (DCC) protein was once thought to be a key component in the neoplastic progression of colon cancer but is now known not to be involved directly in this process. Currently it is thought to function in axonal chemotaxis by serving as part of a receptor complex, which mediates the effects of netrin-1.[102] Specifically, inactivating the mouse homologue of DCC did not result in increased tumors. Additionally, DCC inactivation in the Min mouse (the mouse FAP equivalent) did not change the size of adenomas. In terms of gut development, the loss of DCC did not result in abnormalities of substance P and serotonin enteroendocrine cells, either in quantity or spatial distribution. The loss of DCC was shown not to change the rate of crypt cell production, loss, or spatial distribution in chimeric mice. As expected, however, abnormalities in brain development were seen.

The Lynch syndrome, or hereditary nonpolyposis coli, is an autosomal dominant disorder due to a germline mutation in one of the genes involved in DNA mismatch repair, with the most common genes affected being *MSH2* and *MLH.* These patients develop right-sided colon cancers in their fourth decade of life. However, they do not have an increased risk of developing gut neuroendocrine tumors.

Activating mutations in the ras family of proto-oncogenes are seen in a wide array of malignancies. Mutations in K-ras, particularly in codon 12, are present in about 20% to 40% of colon cancers.[103] Although these same point mutations were also seen in 14% of duodenal adenocarcinomas, they were not detected in small bowel carcinoids or adenocarcinomas of the ileum or jejunum.[104] In addition, mutations in the other ras family members—H-ras, N-ras—were not seen.

P53 is located on chromosome 17 and is one of the most important genes involved in neoplastic progression in most malignancies except carcinoid tumors. Functional p53 is an important component of cell cycle control, causing cell cycle arrest and in some circumstances inducing cellular apoptosis. Point mutations may result in inactivation and an accumulation of the abnormal protein. Therefore, immunohistochemical detection usually, but not always, equates with mutation in this gene. Immunohistochemical detection of *p53* was found in the great majority of adenocarcinomas of the colon and anal/rectal region and anal squamous carcinomas but in none of carcinoid tumors of the ileum, appendix, or colon, despite some of these tumors showing metastatic ability.[105] In contrast, the rare goblet cell carcinoid tumor has been shown to stain with *p53.*[100] An alternative method to detect genetic changes in genes is single-strand conformational analysis. Using this technique, only 1 of 33 gastrointestinal carcinoid tumors was found to have a *k-ras* mutation (codon 283, CGC to CCC) in a clinically benign rectal carcinoid tumor.[106] Thus, despite *p53*'s clear importance in cell cycle control and its prevalent role in neoplastic progression in numerous organ systems, it seems to play no role in neuroendocrine tumor development.

Multiple Endocrine Neoplasia Type I (MEN-I)

Multiple endocrine neoplasia type I is an autosomal dominant disorder affecting 1 in 10,000 to

100,000 people. These patients develop endocrine tumors of the parathyroid, pancreatic islets, anterior pituitary, or foregut. The *MEN-I* gene is located on chromosome 11q13 and is composed of 10 exons with a 2.8-kilobase transcript and a 610-amino acid protein termed "menin".[107] The *MEN-I* gene is most likely a tumor suppressor, based upon family and loss of heterozygosity studies. The function of the protein product menin is not known. However, using N-terminal tagged menin, menin was found to be located in the nuclei of nondividing cells, with cytoplasmic localization in proliferating cells.[108] Using a yeast two-hybrid system, menin directly interacted with the transcription JunD but not with other members of the Jun or Fos family members.[109] Menin repressed JunD's activation of an AP1-responsive reporter. Mutations in menin disrupted its ability to repress JunD. These missense mutations are known to occur naturally. The murine homologue of MEN-I is 97% homologous to the human protein and was detected in thymus, skeletal muscle, brain, and testis.[110] In the mouse, menin was found in nerve cell nuclei and spermatogonia in a perinuclear distribution. This wide distribution of menin implies a broad and diverse function for this protein.

The role of the *MEN-I* gene in the development of endocrine tumors in patients with germline mutations in MEN-I is clear, and a significant role of these mutations in sporadic carcinoid tumors is also becoming evident. Although patients with MEN-I do not have an increased risk of midgut and hindgut carcinoid tumors compared with nonaffected patients, mutations and allelic deletions have been found in 16.6% of sporadic hindgut/midgut tumors and in 15.2% of sporadic foregut tumors.[111]

REG

The *Reg*alpha gene (*Reg*) encodes a secretory protein proposed to be a growth factor regulating islet cell and gastric mucous cell growth.[112, 113] Specifically, Reg is a mitogen for gastric mucous cells. In the stomach, *Reg* is expressed in gastric enterochromaffin-like (ECL) cells and chief cells. The related protein, PAP-1, conferred resistance to apoptosis in a pancreatic cell line (AR4-2J cells).[114] The ECL hyperplasia seen with hypergastrinemia is also associated with an upregulation of Reg expression. Further evidence for the role of this growth factor in gastric carcinoid formation is the fact that mutations in *Reg* are associated with ECL cell carcinoid tumors. Reg is thought to balance gastrin-stimulated growth of ECL cells and possibly parietal and chief cells, with growth of mucous neck and surface gastric epithelial cells.[115]

Transgenic Models of Carcinoid Formation

Transgenic animals have been important not only in elucidating the mechanisms of normal cellular dif-ferentiation but also in dissecting the mechanisms involved in neoplastic transformation. Whereas several transgenic and knock-out mice models exist for the development of gut adenocarcinomas, few such models exist for the study of intestinal endocrine tumors. Glucagon is a hormone expressed in the pancreas and L cells of the intestine. The glucagon-like peptide (GLP-1) is involved in glucose-dependent insulin secretion. This peptide is only one of several proglucagon-derived peptides that are synthesized by the L cells in the large and small bowel.

Tissue-specific post-translational modification results in a number of differing peptides. One of these peptides, glucagon-like peptide 2, induces small bowel epithelial proliferation.[116] Transgenic mice expressing the SV40 large T antigen under the control of 2000 base pairs of the 5' flanking sequence of the glucagon gene developed endocrine tumors in the colon and pancreas.[117] It is interesting that a 1300 base pair sequence resulted in expression in the brain and pancreas but not the gut, implying the existence of a critical upstream *cis*-acting regulatory element. Some of these tumors (12 of 38 animals) developed metastatic ability with lymph node involvement.

The appearance of the tumors in these transgenic mice was preceded by hyperplasia of cells expressing GLP-1 and SV40 antigen; in the colon, this hyperplasia was most prominent in the cecum.[118] Additionally, an excised tumor from the transgenic mouse was grown in a nude mouse, with the subsequent isolation of a cell line capable of in vitro growth. In vitro, these cells maintained endocrine differentiation and expressed the proglucagon and cholecystokinin genes.[119] Proglucagon gene expression was regulated by a protein kinase-C–dependent pathway.

Transgenic mice with adenovirus E1A and E1B genes under the control of human renin developed gut carcinoid tumors although these tumors did not have metastatic ability. N-myc and c-jun mRNA were markedly increased in these tumors compared with non-neoplastic gut.[120]

Systemic Predisposing Conditions

Inflammatory Bowel Diseases

Ulcerative colitis and Crohn's disease are idiopathic inflammatory bowel diseases that have an increased risk for the development of adenocarcinoma, compared with nonaffected patients. Especially in the case of ulcerative colitis, the risk of colon cancer is directly linked to the disease duration. The mechanisms involved in the neoplastic progression involve mutations in the *TGF-beta II* receptor and *APC* genes. The etiology for these genetic changes may involve free radical production from inflammation or increased epithelial turnover due to epithelial loss. Case reports of carcinoids arising in association with inflammatory bowel diseases exist,[121, 122] with some claims that the inflammatory condition was a predisposing factor for the endocrine tumor development. However, despite this global epithelial insult to which the enteroendocrine cells are not immune, more extensive studies have shown that these patients do not have an increased risk for the development of gut neuroendocrine tumors.[123, 124]

On the other hand, patients with ileal carcinoid tumors may be mistakenly diagnosed with Crohn's disease.[125] One can understand such an error when one considers that Crohn's disease commonly involves the terminal ileum, which is also the most common site for small bowel carcinoids. Additionally, when carcinoid tumors invade the muscularis propria, they incite a tethering reaction that may cause stricture formation; this stricturing may cause symptoms mimicking those of Crohn's disease. An ileal stricture secondary to numerous etiologies (e.g., endometriosis) may be confused with strictures caused by Crohn's disease. This misdiagnosis was seen in 2.3% of ileal carcinoids in one series.[125] In this study, the mean time from symptoms to the correct diagnosis was 2 years.

Although carcinoid tumors are not associated with inflammatory bowel disease but may mimic Crohn's disease, the enteroendocrine cells may play a role in the pathogenesis of ulcerative colitis and Crohn's disease.[126]

Graft vs Host Disease

Graft vs host disease may occur following transplantation, particularly with bone marrow transplantation. The gastrointestinal tract may be affected, and the patient may present with diarrhea. Histologically, the gastrointestinal epithelium is infiltrated with a mild amount of lymphocytes, with epithelial apoptosis present in the bases of the crypts. However, the enterochromaffin cells are not killed in this process and seem to be selectively spared.[127] Because of this sparing, collections of these cells may be seen resembling microcarcinoids. However, true carcinoid tumor formation does not follow.

Detection

The detection of carcinoid tumors is important for diagnosis, treatment, and staging. Although increased urinary 5-hydroxytryptamine (5-HIAA) may be found in patients with carcinoid tumors, particularly of midgut origin, this test does not localize the tumor and does not equate with metastatic disease. Somatostatin receptor scintigraphy (SRS) is an imaging modality that has taken advantage of the fact that many carcinoid tumors express the somatostatin receptor. The peptide somatostatin exists in a 14-amino acid and a 28-amino acid molecular form and is abundantly present in endocrine cells and neurons in the gastrointestinal tract, with highest concentrations in the stomach, upper small intestine, and pancreas.

Both these molecular forms bind with high affinity to the five different somatostatin receptor subtypes (sst_1, sst_2, sst_3, sst_4, and sst_5). These receptors belong to the G protein–coupled receptor superfamily. Octreotide is a short-chain somatostatin analogue that binds sst_2 receptors with high affinity, sst_3 and sst_5 receptors with intermediate affinity, and sst_1 and sst_4 receptors with little or nonexistent affinity. Most gastroenteropancreatic neuroendocrine tumors, with the exception of insulinomas, contain an abundance of sst_2 messenger RNA and express a high density of sst_2 receptors; consequently, they avidly bind radiolabeled octreotide.[128]

SRS is an excellent modality for the detection of metastatic disease, finding 95% of liver metastases. However, its ability to detect primary carcinoid tumors in the duodenogastric area is not as good, with a detection rate of 50%. When combined with endoscopic ultrasound, 90% of primary tumors were found. CT imaging has not proved effective, detecting only 5% of primary tumors.[129] Thus, SRS is superior to CT and ultrasonography for determining the extent of the disease in patients with gastrinomas or gut carcinoids; it is not helpful, however, in patients with pancreatic insulinomas and nonfunctional pancreatic endocrine tumors.[130] High-resolution MRI was able to detect a 1-cm primary duodenal carcinoid tumor in a case report. Thus, there is a possibility that breath-hold contrast-enhanced MRI is capable of evaluating disease of the small bowel.[131]

Carcinoid Syndrome

The carcinoid syndrome is manifested by diarrhea (83%), flushing (49%), dyspnea (20%), wheezing (6%), and heart valve dysfunction. These symptoms are the result of histamine, other 5-HIAA metabolites, serotonin, kinins, and prostaglandins released from the tumor. Although most patients with carcinoid syndrome have metastatic disease, it is the minority of patients with metastatic disease who actually develop this syndrome. Carcinoid syndrome develops in less than 10% of patients with carcinoid tumors.[132] The endocardium, particularly in the area of the tricuspid valve, may become fibrotic, leading to valve dysfunction and right-sided heart failure. The somatostatin analogue octreotide is effective in relieving symptoms by blocking the release of the hormones.[133] More than 50% of patients receiving octreotide developed cholelithiasis; however, only a minority of patients developed symptoms. Thus, while the risk of gallstone formation is great, prophylactic cholecystectomy is not indicated.[134]

Hepatic artery embolization may also decrease symptoms in 80% of patients.[135] However, overall survival is probably not prolonged, and the procedure itself carries a high degree of morbidity and possible mortality.

Not all patients presenting with symptoms attributable to the carcinoid syndrome have underlying carcinoid tumors. A group of male patients with flushing and increased urinary 5-HIAA levels were found to have hypogonadism after screening for carcinoid tumor. Resolution of flushing and normalization of 5-HIAA was achieved with testosterone treatment. The term "pseudocarcinoid syndrome" has been applied to this clinical situation.[136] Additionally, one patient presenting with flushing and diarrhea was found to have a duodenal adenoma with serotonin-positive endocrine cells populating the tumor. The patient's symptoms resolved after the adenoma was removed.[137] Although the carcinoid syndrome is a rare event secondary to an adenoma, the presence of endocrine cells in adenomas and carcinomas of the small bowel is not unusual. Additionally, the endocrine cells found in the tumors reflect the types and frequency of those found in the neighboring non-neoplastic epithelium.[138]

Treatment

Because gut neuroendocrine tumors are a diverse group of neoplastic lesions with divergent biologic behaviors, clinical treatment modalities must be specifically tailored. Additionally, treatment options must also take into account the stage of the disease and the presence of symptoms related to tumor hormone production. The goals of therapy may range from curative to relieving symptoms. For example, the great majority of appendiceal carcinoids are of little clinical consequence, as their metastatic ability is essentially zero for tumors less than 2 cm in size. Thus, simple appendectomy is sufficient. On the other hand, a small bowel carcinoid tumor should be removed and properly staged, for the probability of metastatic disease is definitely above zero. Patients with carcinoid syndrome are treated with agents aimed at decreasing the effects of products released from the tumor.

Hepatic artery chemoembolization improves symptoms of carcinoid syndrome, has a high tumor response rate, and improves short-term quality of life in this group of patients with advanced hepatic carcinoid disease.[139] Untreated carcinoid liver metastases double after 1 year of follow-up.[140] The cardiac manifestations of the carcinoid syndrome may have morbid consequences as right-sided valvular lesions occur frequently and may lead to right-sided heart failure. Forty-five percent of patients with carcinoid syndrome were found to have cardiac involvement, most of which involved the tricuspid valves with thickening and shortening. Additionally, the pulmonary valve was affected half as frequently as the tricuspid with thickening and shortening. Balloon valvotomy was only palliative, with surgery being the most effective treatment apart from the treatment of the underlying condition.[141]

Endoscopic treatment of rectal carcinoid tumors was found to be appropriate when the tumor measured 1 cm or less in diameter, did not infiltrate beyond the submucosal layer, and had no histologic atypia.[142] Atypical histopathologic features and a tumor size greater than 1 cm were associated with aggressive behavior; however, extensive surgery had no survival advantage over local excision.[143] DNA ploidy does not appear to be a useful prognostic factor for rectal carcinoid tumors.[144]

Liver transplantation for metastatic neuroendocrine tumors was effective in relieving symptoms from the carcinoid syndrome; however, by 11 months post-transplantation, more than 50% of patients had tumor recurrence. By 1 year post-transplantation, 82% of patients were alive, and by 5 years, 57% were alive. It is interesting that the tumor recurrence did not always result in return of the carcinoid syndrome.[145]

References

1. Griffiths DF, Davies SJ, Williams D, et al.: Demonstration of somatic mutation and colonic crypt clonality by x-linked enzyme histochemistry. Nature 1988; 333:461.
2. Garabedian EM, Roberts LJ, McNevin MS, et al.: Examining the role of Paneth cells in the small intestine by lineage ablation in transgenic mice. J Biol Chem 1997; 272:23729.
3. Savidge TC, Morey AL, Ferguson DJ, et al.: Human intestinal development in a severe combined immunodeficient xenograft model. Differentiation 1995; 58:361.
4. Moll R, Zimbelmann R, Goldschmidt MD, et al.: The human gene encoding cytokeratin 20 and its expression during fetal development and in gastrointestinal carcinomas. Differentiation 1993; 53:75.
5. Si S, Rossant J: HNF-3beta is essential for node and notocord formation in mouse development. Cell 1994; 78:561.
6. Ye H, Kelly TF, Samadani U, et al.: Hepatocyte nuclear factor 3/fork head homolog 11 is expressed in proliferating epithelial and mesenchymal cells of embryonic and adult tissues. Mol Cell Biol 1997; 17:1626.
7. Rausa F, Samadani U, Ye H, et al.: The gut-homeodomain transcriptional activator HNF-6 is coexpressed with its target gene HNF-3beta in the developing murine liver and pancrease. Dev Biol 1997; 192:228.
8. Samadani U, Costa RH: The transcriptional activator hepatocyte nuclear factor 6 regulates liver gene expression. Mol Cell Biol 1996; 16:6273.
9. Mutoh H, Naya FJ, Tsai MJ, et al.: The basic helix-loop-helix protein BETA2 interacts with p300 to coordinate differentiation of secretin-expressing enteroendocrine cells. Genes Dev 1998; 12:820.
10. Larsson LI, Madsen OD, Serup P, et al.: Pancreatic-duodenal homeobox 1—role in gastric endocrine patterning. Mech Dev 1996; 60:175.
11. Mutoh H, Fung BP, Naya FJ, et al.: The basic helix-loop-helix transcription factor BETA2-NeuroD is expressed in mammalian enteroendocrine cells and activates secretin gene expression. Proc Natl Acad Sci U S A 1997; 94:3560.
12. Gilligan CJ, Lawton G, Tang L, et al.: Gastric carcinoid tumors: The biology and therapy of an enigmatic and controversial lesion. Am J Gastroenterol 1995; 90:338.
13. Lee YM, Beinborn M, McBride EW, et al.: The human brain cholecystokinin-B/gastrin recptor: Cloning and characterization. J Biol Chem 1993; 268:8164.
14. Waldum HL, Sandvik AK, Brenna E, et al.: Gastrin-histamine sequence in the regulation of gastric acid secretion. Gut 1991; 32:698.
15. Chiba T, Fisher SK, Park J, et al.: Carbamoylcholine and gastrin induce inositol lipid turnover in canine gastric parietal cells. Am J Physiol 1988; 255:G99.

16. Yoshikazu O, Hirohisa N, Kiyohiko K, et al.: A comparison of the signal transduction pathways activated by gastrin in enterochromaffin-like and parietal cells. Gastroenterology 1998; 115:93.

17. Andersson K, Lindstrom E, Chen D, et al.: Depletion of enterochromaffin-like cell histamine increases histidinedecarboxylase and chromogranin A mRNA levels in rat stomach by a gastrin-independent mechanism. Scand J Gastroenterol 1996; 31:959.

18. Hocker M, Zhang Z, Merchant JL, et al.: Gastrin regulates the human histidine decarboxylase promoter through an AP-1-dependent mechanism. Am J Physiol 1997; 272:G822.

19. Hocker M, Henihan RJ, Rosewicz S, et al.: Gastrin and phorbol 12-myristate 13-acetate regulate the human histidine decarboxylase promoter through Raf-dependent activation of extracellular signal-regulated kinase-related signaling pathways in gastric cancer cells. J Biol Chem 1997; 272:27015.

20. Hocker M, Raychowdhury R, Plath T, et al.: Sp1 and CREB mediate gastrin-dependent regulation of chromogranin A promoter activity in gastric carcinoma cells. J Biol Chem 1998; 273:34000.

21. Langhans N, Rindi G, Chiu M, et al.: Abnormal gastric histology and decreased acid production in cholecystokinin-B/gastrin receptor-deficient mice. Gastroenterology 1997; 112:280.

22. Koh TJ, Goldenring JR, Ito S, et al.: Gastrin deficiency results in altered gastric differentiation and decreased colonic proliferation in mice. Gastroenterology 1997; 113:1015.

23. Orkin SH: GATA-binding transcription factors in hematopoietic cells. Blood 1992; 80:575.

24. Laverriere AC, MacNeill C, Muellers C, et al.: GATA-4/5/6, a subfamily of three transcription factors transcribed in developing heart and gut. J Biol Chem 1994; 269:23177.

25. Dimaline R, Campbell BJ, Watson F, et al.: Regulated expression of GATA-6 transcription factor in gastric endocrine cells. Gastroenterology 1997; 112:1559.

26. Tamura S, Wang XH, Maeda M, et al.: Gastric DNA-binding proteins recognize upstream sequence motifs of parietal cell-specific genes. Proc Natl Acad Sci U S A 1993; 90:10876.

27. Modlin IM, Sandor A: An analysis of 8305 cases of carcinoid tumors. Cancer 1997; 79:813.

28. Berge T, Linell F: Carcinoid tumors; Frequency in a defined population during a 12-year period. Acta Pathol Microbiol Scand 1976; 84:322.

29. Creutzfeldt W, Falkner S: Carcinoids and carcinoid syndrome. Am J Med 1987; 82:4.

30. Moyana TN, Xiang J: Expression of the tumor-associated polymorphic epithelial mucin and carcinoembryonic antigen in gastrointestinal carcinoid tumors. Cancer 1995; 75:2836.

31. Wilander E, Schelbenpflug L: Cytokeratin expression in small intestinal and appendiceal carcinoids: A basis for classification. Acta Oncol 1993; 32:131.

32. Kahn HJ, Marks A, Thom H, et al.: Role of antibody to S-100 protein in diagnostic pathology. Am J Clin Pathol 1983; 79:341.

33. Wilander E, Lindqvist M, Zmovin T: S-100 protein in carcinoid tumors of appendix. Acta Neuropathol 1985; 66:306.

34. Moyana TN, Satunam N: A comparative immunohistochemical study of jejunoileal and appendiceal carcinoids for histogenesis and pathogenesis. Cancer 1992; 70:1081.

35. Al-Khafaji B, Noffisinger A, Miller MA, et al.: Immunohistologic analysis of gastrointestinal and pulmonary carcinoid tumors. Hum Pathol 1998; 29:992.

36. Iacangelo A, Fischer-Colbrie R, Koller KJ, et al.: The sequence of porcine chromogranin A can serve as the precursor for the biologically active hormone, pancreastatin. Endocrinology 1988; 122:2339.

37. Canaff L, Bevan S, Wheeler DG, et al.: Analysis of molecular mechanisms controlling neuroendocrine cell-specific transcription of the chromogranin A gene. Endocrinology 1998; 139:1184.

38. McMahon HT, Bolshakov VY, Janz R, et al.: Synaptophysin, a major synaptic vesicle protein, is not essential for neurotransmitter release. Proc Natl Acad Sci U S A 1996; 93:4760.

39. Eshkind LG, Leube RE: Mice lacking synaptophysin reproduce and form typical synaptic vesicles. Cell Tissue Res 1995; 282:423.

40. Esni F, Taljedal IB, Perl AK, et al.: Neural cell adhesion molecule (N-CAM) is required for cell type segregation and normal ultrastructure in pancreatic islets. Cell Biol 1999; 144:325.

41. You YH, Hefta LJ, Yazaki PJ, et al.: Expression, purification, and characterization of a two-domain carcinoembryonic antigen minigene (N-A3) in pichia pastoris. The essential role of the N-domain. Anticancer Res 1998; 18:3193.

42. Ilantzis C, Jothy S, Alpert LC, et al.: Cell-surface levels of human carcinoembryonic antigen are inversely correlated with colonocyte differentiation in colon carcinogenesis. Lab Invest 1997; 76:703.

43. Osamura RY, Yasuda O, Kawakami T, et al.: Immunoelectron microscopic demonstration of regulated pathway for calcitonin and constitutive pathway for carcinoembryonic antigen in the same cells of human medullary carcinomas of thyroid glands. Mod Pathol 1997; 10:7.

44. Dasovic-Knezevic M, Bormer O, Holm R, et al.: Carcinoembryonic antigen in medullary thyroid carcinoma: An immunohistochemical study applying six novel monoclonal antibodies. Mod Pathol 1989; 2:610.

45. Kim JC, Roh SA, Park KC: Adhesive function of carcinoembryonic antigen in the liver metastasis of KM-12c colon carcinoma cell line. Dis Colon Rectum 1997; 40:946.

46. Yonemura Y, Hashimoto T, Shima Y, et al.: A study of malignancy in gastrointestinal carcinoids, with special reference to the association of the prognosis and peptide hormone or oncofetal protein producing pattern. Nippon Geka Gakkai Zasshi (J Japan Surg Soc) 1986; 87:1324.

47. Federspiel BH, Burke AP, Shekitka KM, et al.: Carcinoembryonic antigen and carcinoids of the gastrointestinal tract. Mod Pathol 1990; 3:586.

48. Naschitz JE, Yeshurun D, Nash E, et al.: Cervical soft tissue metastasis of typical carcinoid tumor preceding diagnosis of ileal primary by 4 years. Am J Gastroenterol 1992; 87:1665.

49. Rubio IT, Korourian S, Brown H, et al.: Carcinoid tumor metastatic to the breast. Arch Surg 1998; 133:1117.

50. Kirshbom PM, Kherani AR, Onaitis MW, et al.: Carcinoids of unknown origin: Comparative analysis with foregut, midgut, hindgut carcinoids. Surgery 1998; 124:1063.

51. Rindi G, Luinetti O, Cornaggia M, et al.: Three subtypes of gastric argyrophil carcinoids and the gastric neuroendocrine carcinoma: A clinicopathologic study. Gastroenterology 1993; 104:994.

52. Solcia E, Capella C, Sessa F, et al.: Gastric carcinoids and related endocrine growths. Digestion 1986; 35(suppl 1):3.

53. Solcia E, Capella C, Fiocca R, et al.: The gastroenteropancreatic endocrine system and related tumors. Gastroenterol Clin North Am 1989; 18:671.

54. Solcia E, Bordi C, Creutzfeldt W, et al.: Histopathological classification of nonantral gastric endocrine growths in man. Digestion 1988; 41:185.

55. Granberg D, Wilander E, Stridsberg M, et al.: Clinical symptoms, hormone profiles, treatment, and prognosis in patients with gastric carcinoids. Gut 1998; 43:223.

56. Rindi G, Bordi C, Rappel S, et al.: Gastric carcinoids and neuroendocrine carcinomas: Pathogenesis, pathology, and behavior. World J Surg 1996; 20:168.

57. Bordi C, Baggi MT, Davoli C, et al.: Gastric carcinoids and their precursor lesions. A histologic and immunohistochemical study of 23 cases. Cancer 1991; 67:663.

58. Solcia E, Capella C, Fiocca R, et al.: Gastric argyrophil carcinoids in patients with Zollinger-Ellison syndrome due to type 1 multiple endocrine neoplasia. A newly recognized association. Am J Surg Pathol 1990; 14:503.

59. Cadiot G, Vissuzaine C, Potet F, et al.: Fundic argyrophil carcinoid tumor in a patient with sporadic Zollinger-Ellison syndrome. Gut 1994; 35:275.

60. Jensen RT: Management of the Zollinger-Ellison syndrome in patients with multiple endocrine neoplasia type 1. J Intern Med 1998; 243:477.

61. Weber HC, Venzon DJ, Lin JT, et al.: Determinants of metastatic rate and survival in patients with Zollinger-Ellison syndrome: A prospective long-term study. Gastroenterology 1995; 108:1637.

62. Cadiot G, Vuagnat A, Doukhan I, et al.: Prognostic factors in patients with Zollinger-Ellison syndrome and multiple endocrine neoplasia type 1. Gastroenterology 1999; 116:286.

63. Metz DC, Kuchnio M, Fraker DL, et al.: Flow cytometry and Zollinger-Ellison syndrome: Relationship to clinical course. Gastroenterology 1993; 105:799.

64. Cadiot G, Lebahi R, Sardra L, et al.: Prospective detection of duodenal gastrinomas and pancreatic lymph nodes by somatostatin receptor scintigraphy. Gastroenterology 1996; 111:845.

65. Borch K, Renvall H, Liedberg G: Gastric endocrine cell hyperplasia and carcinoid tumors in pernicious anemia. Gastroenterology 1985; 88:638.

66. Banerjee S, Ardill JE, Beattie AD, et al.: Effect of omeprazole and feeding on plasma gastrin inpatients with achlorhydria. Aliment Pharmacol Ther 1995; 9:507.

67. Axelson J, Ekelund M, Sundler F, et al.: Enhanced hyperplasia of gastric enterochromaffin-like cells in response to omeprazole-evoked hypergastrinemia in rats with portacaval shunts. An immunocytochemical and chemical study. Gastroenterology 1990; 99:635.

68. Freston JW: Omeprazole, hypergastrinemia, and gastric carcinoid tumors. Ann Intern Med 1994; 121:232.

69. Berlin RG: Omeprazole. Gastrin and gastric endocrine cell data from clinical studies. Dig Dis Sci 1991; 36:129.

70. Klinkenberg-Knol EC, Festen HP, Jansen JB, et al.: Efficacy and safety of long-term treatment with omeprazole for refractory reflux esophagitis. Ann Intern Med 1994; 121:161.

71. Metz DC, Weber HC, Orbuch M, et al.: *Helicobacter pylori* infection: A reversible cause of hypergastrinemia and hyperchlorhydria which may mimic Zollinger-Ellison syndrome. Dig Dis Sci 1995; 40:153.

72. Blaser A, Vajda P, Rosset P: Duodenal somatostatinomas associated with von Recklinghausen disease. Schweiz Med Wochensch 1998; 128:1984.

73. O'Brien TD, Chejfec G, Prinz RA: Clinical features of duodenal somatostatinomas. Surgery 1993; 114:1144.

74. Albrecht S, Gardiner GW, Kovacs K, et al.: Duodenal somatostatinoma with psammoma bodies. Arch Pathol Lab Med 1989; 113:517.

75. Fulfaro F, Quagliuolo V, De Conno F, et al.: Carcinoid somatostatinoma of the duodenum. Eur J Surg Oncol 1998; 24:601.

76. Ohsawa H, Kanatsuka A, Tokuyama Y, et al.: Amyloid protein in somatostatinoma differs from human islet amyloid polypeptide. Acta Endocrinol 1991; 124:45.

77. Tan CC, Hall RI, Semeraro D, et al.: Ampullary somatostatinoma associated with von Recklinghausen's neurofibromatosis presenting as obstructive jaundice. Eur J Surg Oncol 1996; 22:298.

78. Tjon A, Tham RT, Jansen JB, et al.: Imaging features of somatostatinoma: MR, CT, US, and angiography. J Comput Assist Tomogr 1994; 18:427.

79. Leibovitch I, Avigad I, Nativ O, et al.: The frequency of histological abnormalities in incidental appendectomies in urologic patients. J Urol 1992; 148:41.

80. Rode J, Dhillon AP, Papadaki L: Serotonin-immunoreactive cells in the lamina propria plexus of the appendix. Hum Pathol 1983; 14:464.

81. Dhillon AP, Williams RA, Rode J: Age, site and distribution of subepithelial neurosecretory cells in the appendix. Pathology 1992; 24:56.

82. Shaw P: The topographical and age distribution of the neuroendocrine cells in the normal human appendix. J Pathol 1991; 164:235.

83. Goddard MJ, Lonsdale RN: The histogenesis of appendiceal carcinoid tumours. Histopathology, 1992; 20:345.

84. Moertel C, Dockerty M, Judd E: Carcinoid tumors of the vermiform appendix. Cancer 1992; 21:270.

85. Anderson J, Wilson B: Carcinoid tumors of the appendix. Br J Surg 1985; 72:545.

86. Thirlby R, Kasper C, Jones R: Metastatic carcinoid tumor of the appendix: Report of a case and review of the literature. Dis Colon Rectum 1984; 27:42.

87. Stinner B, Kisker O, Zielke A, et al.: Surgical management for carcinoid tumors of the small bowel, appendix, colon, and rectum. World J Surg 1996; 20:183.

88. Moertel C, Dockerty M, Judd E: Carcinoid tumors of the vermiform appendix. Cancer 1968; 21:270.

89. Lyss A: Appendiceal malignancies. Semin Oncol 1988; 15:129.

90. Svedendsen L, Bulow S: Carcinoid tumors of the appendix in young children. Acta Chir Scand 1980; 146:137.

91. Jones RA, MacFarlane A: Carcinomas and carcinoid tumors of the appendix in a district general hospital. J Pathol 1976; 29:687.

92. Burke A, Lee YL: Adenocarcinoid (goblet cell carcinoid) of the duodenum presenting as gastric outlet obstruction. Hum Pathol 1990; 21:238.

93. Dockerty MB, Ashburn FS: Carcinoid tumors (so-called) of the ileum: Report of thirteen cases in which there was metastasis. Arch Surg 1943; 47:221.

94. Ikeda E, Tsutsumi Y, Yoshida H, et al.: Goblet cell carcinoid of the vermiform appendix with ovarian metastasis mimicking mucinous cystadenocarcinoma. Acta Pathol Japonica 1991; 41:455.

95. Warkel RL, Cooper PH, Helwig EB: Adenocarcinoma, a mucin-producing carcinoid tumor of the appendix: A study of 39 cases. Cancer 1978; 42:2781.

96. Watson PH, Alguacil-Garcia A: Mixed crypt cell carcinoma. Virchows Arch A 1987; 412:175.

97. Edmunds P, Merino M, LiVolsi VA, et al.: Adenocarcinoid (mucinous carcinoid) of the appendix. Gastroenterology 1984; 86:302.

98. Butler JA, Houshiar A, Lin F, et al.: Goblet cell carcinoid of the appendix. Am J Surg 1994; 168:685.

99. Bak M, Asschenfeldt J: Adenocarcinoid of the vermiform appendix: A clinicopathologic study of 20 cases. Dis Colon Rectum 1988; 31:605.

100. Horiuchi S, Endo T, Shimoji H, et al.: Goblet cell carcinoid of the appendix endoscopically diagnosed and examined with *p53* immunostaining. J Gastroenterol 1998; 33:582.

101. Vortmeyer AO, Lubensky IA, Merino MJ, et al.: Concordance of genetic alterations in poorly differentiated colorectal neuroendocrine carcinomas and associated adenocarcinomas. J Nat Cancer Inst 1997; 89:1448.

102. Fazeli A, Dickinson SL, Hermiston ML, et al.: Phenotype of mice lacking functional deleted in colorectal cancer (*DCC*) gene. Nature 1997; 386:796.

103. Bos JL: The *ras* gene family and human carcinogenesis. Mutat Res 1988; 195:255.

104. Younes N, Fulton N, Tanaka R, et al.: The presence of K-12 *ras* mutations in duodenal adenocarcinomas and the absence of *ras* mutations in other small bowel adenocarcinomas and carcinoid tumors. Cancer 1997; 79:1804.

105. O'Dowd G, Gosney JR: Absence of overexpression of *p53* protein by intestinal carcinoid tumours. J Pathol 1995; 175:403.

106. Lohmann DR, Funk A, Niedermeyer HP, et al.: Identification of *p53* gene mutations in gastrointestinal and pancreatic carcinoids by nonradioisotopic SSCA. Virchows Arch B 1993; 64:293.

107. Chandrasekharappa C, Guru SC, Manickam P, et al.: Positional cloning of the gene for multiple endocrine neoplasia–type 1. Science 1997; 276:404.

108. Huang SC, Zhuang Z, Weil RJ, et al.: Nuclear/cytoplasmic localization of the multiple endocrine neoplasia type 1 gene product, menin. Lab Invest 1999; 79:301.

109. Agarwal SK, Guru SC, Heppner C, et al.: Menin interacts with the AP1 transcription factor JunD and represses JunD-activated transcription. Cell 1999; 96:143.

110. Stewart C, Parente F, Piehl F, et al.: Characterization of the mouse MENI gene and its expression during development. Oncogene 1998; 17:2485.

111. Gortz B, Roth J, Krahenmann A: Mutations and allelic deletions of the *MENI* gene are associated with a subset of sporadic endocrine pancreatic and neuroendocrine tumors and not restricted to foregut neoplasms. Am J Pathol 1999; 154:429.

112. Watanabe T, Yonemura Y, Yonekura H, et al.: Pancreatic beta-cell replication and amelioration of surgical diabetes by *reg* protein. Proc Natl Acad Sci U S A 1994; 91:3589.

113. Fukui H, Kinoshita Y, Maekawa T, et al.: Regenerating gene protein may mediate gastric mucosal proliferation induced by hypergastrinemia in rats. Gastroenterology 1998; 115:1483.

114. Ortiz EM, Dusetti NJ, Vasseur S, et al.: The pancreatitis-associated protein is induced by free radicals in AR4-2J cells and confers cell resistance to apoptosis. Gastroenterology 1998; 114:808.

115. Higham A, Bishop L, Dimaline R, et al.: Mutations of *RegI* are associated with enterochromaffin-like cell tumor development in patients with hypergastrinemia. Gastroenterology 1999; 116:1310.

116. Drucker DJ, Ehrlich P, Asa SL, et al.: Induction of intestinal epithelial proliferation by glucagon-like peptide 2. Proc Natl Acad Sci U S A 1996; 93:7911.

117. Lee YC, Asa SL, Drucker DL: Glucagon gene 5′-flanking sequences direct expression of simian virus 40 large T antigen to the intestine, producing carcinoma of the large bowel in transgenic mice. J Biol Chem 1992; 267:10705.

118. Asa SL, Lee YC, Drucker DJ: Development of colonic and pancreatic endocrine tumors in mice expressing a glucagon-Sv40 T antigen transgene. Virchows Arch 1996; 427:595.

119. Drucker DJ, Jin TJ, Asa SL, et al.: Activation of proglucagon gene transcription by protein kinase-A in a novel mouse enteroendocrine cell line. Mol Endocrinol 1994; 8:1646.

120. Sagara M, Sugiyama F, Horiguchi H, et al.: Activation of the nuclear oncogenes *N-myc* and *c-jun* in carcinoid tumors of transgenic mice carrying the human adenovirus type 12 E1 region gene. DNA Cell Biol 1995; 14:95.

121. McNeely B, Owen DA, Pezim M: Multiple microcarcinoids arising in chronic ulcerative colitis. Am J Clin Pathol 1992; 98:112.

122. Kortbeek J, Kelly JK, Preshaw RM: Carcinoid tumors and inflammatory bowel disease. J Surg Oncol 1992; 49:122.

123. Greenstein AJ, Balasubramanian S, Harpaz N, et al.: Carcinoid tumor and inflammatory bowel disease: A study of eleven cases and review of the literature. Am J Gastroenterol 1997; 92:682.

124. McNeely B, Owen DA, Pezim M: Multiple carcinoids arising in chronic ulcerative colitis. Am J Clin Pathol 1992; 98:112.

125. Hsu EY, Feldman JM, Lichtenstein GR: Ileal carcinoid tumors simulating Crohn's disease: Incidence among 176 consecutive cases of ileal carcinoid. Am J Gastroenterol 1997; 92:2062.

126. Kuhn M, Kulaksiz H, Cetin Y, et al.: Circulating and tissue guanylin immunoreactivity in intestinal secretory diarrhoea. Eur J Clin Invest 1995; 25:899.

127. Lampert IA, Thorpe P, van Noorden S, et al.: Selective sparing of enterochromaffin cells in graft versus host disease affecting the colonic mucosa. Histopathology 1985; 9:875.

128. Reubi JC, Schaer JC, Waser B, et al.: Expression and localization of somatostatin receptor SSTR₁, SSTR₂, and SSTR₃ messenger RNAs in primary human tumors using in situ hybridization. Cancer Res 1994; 54:3455.

129. Lebtahi R, Cadiot G, Sarda L, et al.: Clinical impact of somatostatin receptor scintigraphy in the management of patients with neuroendocrine gastroenteropancreatic tumors. J Nucl Med 1997; 38:853.

130. Kisker O, Bartsch D, Weinel RJ, et al.: The value of somatostatin-receptor scintigraphy in newly diagnosed endocrine gastroenteropancreatic tumors. J Am Coll Surg 1997; 184:487.

131. Whitfill CH, Siegelman ES, Rosato EF, et al.: Primary carcinoid of the duodenum: Detection and characterization by magnetic resonance imaging. J Magn Reson Imag 1998; 8:1175.

132. Napolitano G, Bucci I, Lio S, et al.: An overview on the management of carcinoid tumors. J Nucl Biol Med 1991; 35:337.

133. Arnold R, Frank M, Kajdan U: Management of gastroenteropancreatic endocrine tmours: The place of somatostatin analogues. Digestion 1995; 55:107.

134. Trendle MC, Moertel CG, Kvols LK: Incidence and morbidity of cholelithiasis in patients receiving chronic octreotide for metastatic carcinoid and malignant islet cell tumors. Cancer 1997; 79:830.

135. Moertel CG, Johnson CM, McKusick MA, et al.: The management of patients with advanced carcinoid tumors and islet cell carcinomas. Ann Intern Med 1994; 120:302.

136. Shakir KM, Jasser MZ, Yoshihashi AK, et al.: Pseudocarcinoid syndrome associated with hypogonadism and response to testosterone therapy. Mayo Clin Proc 1996; 71:1145.

137. Betchen SA, Cirigliano M, Furth EE, et al.: Tubulovillous adenoma of the duodenum: A new etiology for flushing and urinary 5-HIAA elevation. Dig Dis Sci 1998; 43:1474.

138. Iwafuchi M, Watanabe H, Ishihara N, et al.: Neoplastic endocrine cells in carcinomas of the small intestine: Histochemical and immunohistochemical studies of 24 tumors. Hum Pathol 1987; 18:185.

139. Drougas JG, Anthony LB, Blair TK, et al.: Hepatic artery chemoembolization for management of patients with advanced metastatic carcinoid tumors Am J Surg 1998; 175:408.

140. Skinazi F, Zins M, Menu Y, et al.: Liver metastases of digestive endocrine tumours: Natural history and response to medical treatment. Eur J Gastroenterol Hepatol 1996; 8:673.

141. Moyssakis IE, Rallidis LS, Guida GF, et al.: Incidence and evolution of carcinoid syndrome in the heart. J Heart Valve Dis 1997; 6:625.

142. Higaki S, Nishiaki M, Mitani N, et al.: Effectiveness of local endoscopic resection of rectal carcinoid tumors. Endoscopy 1997; 29:171.

143. Koura AN, Giacco GG, Curley SA, et al.: Carcinoid tumors of the rectum: Effect of size, histopathology, and surgical treatment on metastasis-free survival. Cancer 1997; 79:1294.

144. Fitzgerald SD, Meagher AP, Moniz-Pereira P, et al.: Carcinoid tumor of the rectum; DNA ploidy is not a prognostic factor. Dis Colon Rectum 1996; 39:643.

145. Routley D, Ramage JK, McPeake J, et al.: Orthotopic liver transplantation in the treatment of metastatic neuroendocrine tumors of the liver. Liver Transplant Surg 1995; 1:118.

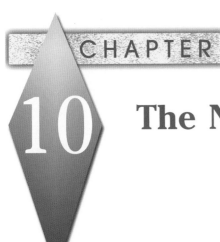

The Neuroendocrine Lung

Constantine A. Axiotis

The dispersed neuroendocrine (NE) system is represented in the epithelium of the bronchopulmonary tract by two components: (1) uninnervated solitary and clustered pulmonary neuroendocrine cells (PNECs), and (2) organized clusters of innervated PNECs called neuroepithelial bodies (NEBs). PNECs have the capability to synthesize, package, and transport biologically active neuroamines, neuropeptides, and related substances. The expression of pan-NE markers and the presence of dense-core granules (DCGs) characterize both PNECs and NEBs. Solitary PNECs are thought to have a paracrine regulatory function, whereas, NEBs are thought to act as intrapulmonary chemoreceptors sensitive to hypoxia. Starting in the early 1990s, clinical and experimental studies have steadily consolidated evidence that the neural component of the pulmonary NE system is sensory, that PNECs stimulate airway development and epithelial cell differentiation, that a specific membrane oxygen receptor is present in NEBs, and that PNECs play a significant role in the pathogenesis of a variety of adult and pediatric chronic pulmonary diseases.[1]

For the pathologist, the endocrine aspects of the lung are most familiar in the context of the pulmonary neoplasms that show NE differentiation. Knowledge about lung tumors that have NE differentiation has increased explosively in recent years. This chapter surveys the development, anatomy, physiology, pathophysiology, and pathology of the pulmonary NE system. Aspects of phylogeny, ontogeny, development, reaction to hypoxic and non-hypoxic injury, and proliferation are reviewed. Particular emphasis is given to the concept of NE differentiation in pulmonary tumors and its biologic and clinical implications. Finally, this chapter presents a detailed exposition of the spectrum of specific bronchopulmonary neoplasms that display overt NE differentiation and puts forward a practical algorithm for their diagnosis and classification.

DEVELOPMENT

Human fetal PNECs are the first lung epithelial cell type to differentiate. They have been identified either singly or in pairs in a basal location in the epithelium of large proximal airways at 7 to 8 weeks' gestation.[2, 3] These early or pre-PNECs exhibit definitive proof of endocrine differentiation by the presence of single or few randomly distributed DCGs of 90-nm mean diameter. In addition, they exhibit weak argyrophilia and immunoreactivity to neuron-specific enolase (NSE).[4] Between 10 and 16 weeks of gestation, the overall number of PNECs increases. They form prominent dendrite-like processes along the basement membrane and differentiate into three distinct PNEC types characterized by vesicular and spherical DCGs of varying density ranging from 110- to 180-nm mean diameter (Fig. 10–1).[5] These PNECs become strongly positive for NSE and develop immunoreactivity for bombesin-like peptides (BLPs) and serotonin (5-HT), as well as focal cytoplasmic staining for low-molecular-weight keratin.[6]

All three PNEC types have been identified in bronchiolar epithelium in the fetus at 14 to 24 weeks. Clusters of three to five PNECs appear at airway branching points, sometimes in contact with rare nerve endings.[7] Rare PNECs also have been observed in developing submucosal glands.[8] After 25 weeks, and particularly at the time of birth, there is an increase and peak in the number of PNECs due mainly to their development in peripheral airways up to the level of the respiratory bronchiole. Various studies show that the secretory products of PNECs in the fetal lung have an orderly appearance, indicating a relationship to the stages of pulmonary development. 5-HT and BLPs appear first, at approximately 8 to 9 weeks. BLPs eventually predominate (Fig. 10–2). Recent studies support the view that gastrin-releasing peptide (GRP) is chiefly present in human PNECs and is cross-reactive to a variety of antibodies to BLPs.[9] Calcitonin (CT) and calcitonin gene-related peptide (CGRP) do not appear until much later, around 20 weeks of gestation.[10]

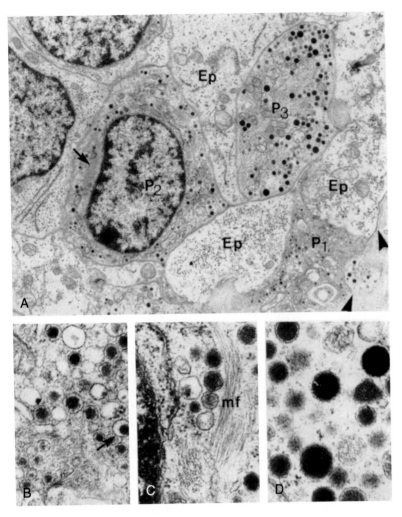

Figure 10-1. A, Different types of NE cells between processes of epithelial cells (Ep). P_1 cell near basement membrane *(arrowheads),* P_2 cell with nucleus and perinuclear filaments *(arrow),* and process of P_3 cell. Human fetal lung at 14 weeks' gestation. (Transmission electron microscope [TEM] ×8500.) *B,* Close-up of dense-core granules (DCGs) in P_1 cell, average size 110 nm, with occasional eccentric cores *(arrow).* (TEM ×59,500.) *C,* DCGs of P_2 cell are larger, average size 130 nm, and moderately electron-dense. Bundle of microfilaments (mf) closely associated. (TEM ×59,500.) *D,* DCGs in P_3 cell are the largest, average size 180 nm, and most electron-dense. (TEM ×59,500.) (From McDowell EM: Lung Carcinomas, Churchill Livingstone, 1987, p. 16.)

Fetal lungs show a greater diversity and density of PNECs than at any subsequent time in life. The number and activity of PNECs diminish after birth, possibly reflecting a wider dispersion and redistribution in the growing lung rather than an absolute decrease.[11] An absolute diminution in PNEC density and wider distribution occur in the adult in comparison with the lungs of fetuses and neonates. Few studies have examined the changing patterns of PNEC distribution with aging in healthy, mature lungs. It appears that PNECs cells are more often arranged in the form of clusters in younger adults than in elderly people, in whom clusters are extremely rare.[12]

Studies on the ontogeny of PNECs favor derivation from an endodermal stem cell rather than migration from the neural crest, although it has been suggested that CT-containing pulmonary PNECs potentially could share their origin with neural crest–derived thyroid C-cells.[13, 14] Arguments

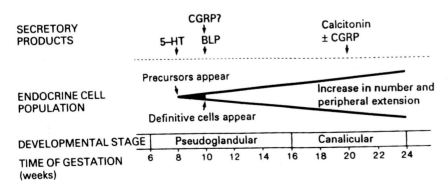

Figure 10-2. Development of PNECs in the human fetal lung. Precursor cells appear at about 8 weeks of gestation and definitive cells at 10 weeks. 5-HT is the first secretory product demonstrable, closely followed by BLP and later (20 weeks) by CGRP. (From Gosney JR: Pulmonary Endocrine Pathology, Butterworth Heinemann, 1992, p. 28.)

favoring an endodermal or epithelial origin are supported by tissue culture studies of fetal airway epithelium without mesenchyme, indicating that they derive from airway epithelium.[15] Arguments for a neuroectodermal origin have been supported by recent studies on the human homologue to the *Drosophila* achaete-scute (*hASH1*) family of helix-loop-helix transcription factors, which play a critical role in neural development in vertebrates (Fig. 10–3). They are essential for PNEC differentiation and are selectively expressed in normal fetal PNECs. When the *hASH1* gene is disrupted, no PNECs can be detected.[16] In addition, expression of neural cell adhesion molecules (NCAM), which are expressed mostly in cells of neuroectodermal origin, has been demonstrated in human infant PNECs.[17]

The precocious differentiation of PNECs preceding other airway epithelial cells is unique to the fetal period and is not recapitulated in the adult lung, where PNEC differentiation is a late event after respiratory epithelial injury. However, there are parallels between the differentiation of fetal PNECs and NE neoplasms. The paucity of DCGs and absent or infrequent immunoreactivity to GRP, chromogranin (ChrA), and other neuropeptides found in early PNECs are also encountered in poorly differentiated NE neoplasms of the lung, such as small cell lung carcinoma (SCLC). In contrast, more

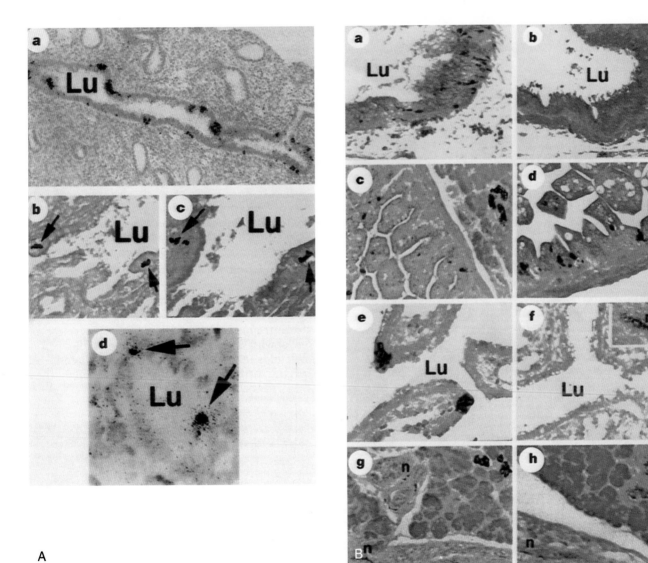

Figure 10–3. A, Data suggesting that *ASH1* is instrumental for the development of the pulmonary NE phenotype. *a,* Mouse *ASH1* RNA/RNA in situ hybridization from mouse embryo in multiple NEBs and solitary NE cells adjacent to airway lumen (Lu). *b–c,* Serial sections show mouse *ASH1* and CGRP co-localized to same NEBs. *d,* *hASH1* in situ hybridization of 18-week-old human fetal lung shows similar NE pattern. B, Data illustrating the specific role of *ASH1* in PNEC differentiation. *a, e,* Normal and heterozygous mice show NEBs and solitary NE cells staining for chromogranin and CGRP. *b, f, ASH1*Δ transgenic knock-out mice showed no detectable NEBs or isolated PNECs. *f, (inset, n)* Persistent synaptophysin and CGRP-reactive autonomic neurons in lungs of mutant mice, and persistent chromogranin (*c, d*) and CGRP (*e, h*) immunoreactive enteric neurons and NE cells in the gut and pancreas. (From Borges et al 1997, Nature 386:852–855.)

Occurrence of Argyrophil Cells in Bronchi, Bronchioles, and Bronchial Glands			
	No. Cases With Argyrophil Cells		
Sites	Women; %	Men; %	Total; %
1, lobar bronchus	5; 25.0	1; 4.0	6; 13.3
2	8; 40.0	1; 4.0	9; 20.0
3, segmental bronchus	11; 55.0	8; 32.0	19; 42.2
4, subsegmental bronchus	13; 65.0	11; 44.0	24; 53.3
5	14; 70.0	14; 56.0	28; 62.2
6	16; 80.0	17; 68.0	33; 73.3
7, bronchioles	18; 90.0	23; 92.2	41; 91.1
Terminal bronchioles	0; 0.0	1; 4.0	1; 2.2
Glandular ducts	1; 5.0	0; 0.0	1; 2.2
Glandular acini	0; 0.0	0; 0.0	0; 0.0

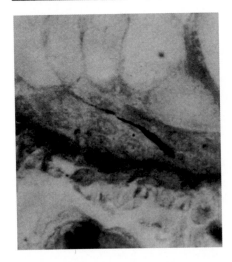
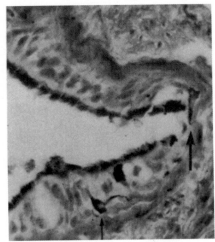

Figure 10–4. The distribution of PNECs in a given site of bronchus in human adult lungs. The number of PNECs increases as the caliber of the bronchus decreases, but they are rarely found in the terminal bronchioles. PNECs lie along the basement membrane (*thick arrow*) and have long dendritic processes interdigitating among other epithelial cells. Some are bipolar (*arrow*). Subsegmental bronchus (Bodian's stain). (From Tateishi et al 1973 Arch Pathol Lab Med 96:198–202.)

numerous DCGs and increased expression of neuropeptides present in late fetal or neonatal PNECs are likewise found in better-differentiated NE tumors, such as bronchial carcinoids.[2, 18] The expression of low-molecular-weight keratins in both fetal PNECs and NE neoplasms draws a further parallel between the differentiation of PNECs in the fetal lung and neoplasia.[19]

MICROSCOPIC ANATOMY

Solitary PNECs are rare; they are columnar, triangular, or bottle-shaped basal cells that occur in both surface epithelium and submucosal glands. They have an overall concentration of 1 PNEC cell for every 2500 epithelial cells.[20] In the adult human lung, PNECs occur mostly singly, although clusters of up to 12 cells occasionally may be encountered. The number of PNECs increases inversely to the caliber of the bronchus (Fig. 10–4). They are rarely found at or distal to terminal bronchioli and alveoli.[21] PNEC–mucous cell transitional forms have also been found in the bronchi.[22] On hematoxylin and eosin sections, PNECs have a clear to slightly eosinophilic cytoplasm. The appearance of aggregates of PNECs is variable and irregular (Fig. 10–5). When these clusters are organized and innervated,

they are termed NEBs. They are more frequent and well developed in the lungs of fetuses and neonates. NEBs are intramucosal, spherical-to-ovoid groups of basal cells with clear cytoplasm whose apical portion protrudes above the level of the ciliated cell lining of the bronchial or bronchiolar lumen; they

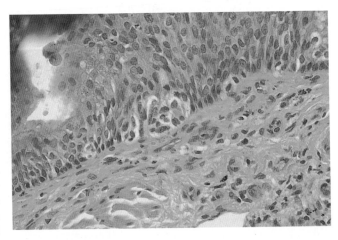

Figure 10–5. Cluster and single PNECs adjacent to basement membrane of segmental bronchiectatic bronchus. Note hyperplasia of epithelial cells. (hematoxylin and eosin.)

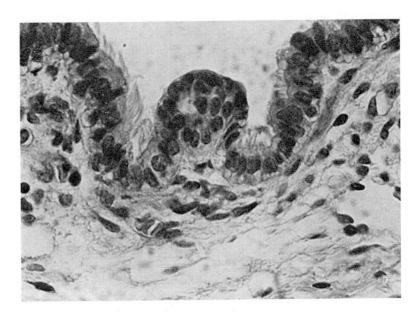

Figure 10–6. NEB protruding slightly above surrounding ciliated cells. It consists of large oval cells with clear cytoplasm. The apical part is lined by flattened, nonciliated cells. Human infant lung. (Hematoxylin and eosin.) (From Lauweryns et al Anat Rec 1972; 172:471–482.)

consist of nonciliated cuboidal cells (Fig. 10–6).[23-26] NEBs have a complex innervation of afferent and efferent unmyelinated nerve fibers corresponding to the adrenergic, cholinergic, and noncholinergic divisions of the pulmonary nervous system. They penetrate the basal lamina beneath the NEBs and make morphologic synaptic specializations.[9]

The ultrastructure of pulmonary PNECs and NEBs is essentially the same and is characterized by three salient features: (1) the presence of numerous spherical, cytoplasmic DCGs of neurosecretory type, (2) the presence of small, clear vesicles similar to the synaptic vesicles of neurons, and (3) the presence of cytoplasmic, pseudopod-like DCG containing extensions that interdigitate between neighboring cells for variable distances and often reach the lumen (Fig. 10–7). The DCGs are uniform in appearance and size, averaging 110 to 140 nm in diameter, and have a prominent electron-dense core always surrounded by a less electron-dense halo beneath the enclosing unit membrane (Fig. 10–8). Occasionally the DCGs may exhibit a lamellar or crystalloid pattern.[27-29] In the adult lung, one type of DCG is present corresponding morphologically to the fetal P_2 cell.[30] Synapsis-like vesicles are clear, membrane-bound vesicles averaging 40 to 80 nm in diameter.

PNECs and NEBs are also characterized by the demonstration of a variety of specific pan-NE markers (Table 10–1). These markers include cytoplasmic enolases, proteases, and carboxylases, as well as membrane glycoproteins and secretory granule matrix proteins (Fig. 10–9). The demonstration of a specific pan-NE marker such as ChrA or synaptophysin (SY38) by immunohistochemistry is considered sufficient for the identification of the NE phenotype. Pan-NE cell markers, because of their independence from specific hormone production, are particularly important in tumor diagnosis when neoplastic NE cells may not be producing or secreting distinct products. SY38, an integral membrane

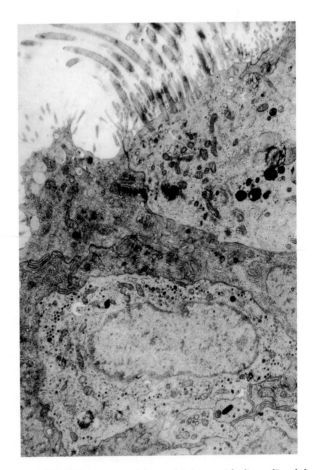

Figure 10–7. Segment of bronchiolar epithelium lined by ciliated cell (upper right) and cell with surface pseudopods (upper left). Subjacent and not reaching the bronchiolar lumen is a PNEC with large numbers of DCGs. (TEM ×9300.) (Courtesy of Dr. Klaus Bensch; from Gmelich et al 1967 Lab Invest 17:88–98.)

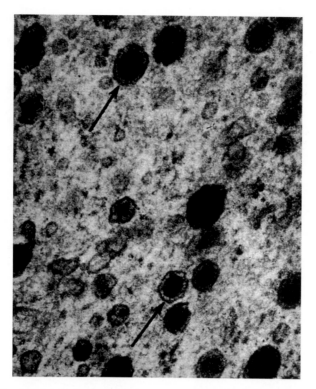

Figure 10–8. DCGs of bronchial PNECs exhibiting characteristic prominent electron-dense core always surrounded by a less electron-dense halo beneath the enclosing unit membrane. (TEM ×66,000.) (From Bensch et al 1965 J Ultrastruct Res 12:665–686.)

glycoprotein that occurs in the small clear vesicles of NE cells,[31] is considered the most specific of the pan-NE markers because it is expressed independent of secretory granule products,[32] notably the ChrA, whose immunostaining correlates directly with the number of DCGs. ChrA may not be expressed immunohistochemically in PNECs that have undergone exocytosis of DCGs secondary to hypoxia or in poorly differentiated NE neoplasms with degranulation or a paucity of DCGs. Chromogranin mRNA, however, may be detected by Northern blot or in situ hybridization (Fig. 10–10).[33]

PNECs and NEBs also produce a variety of regulatory neuropeptides and biogenic amines.[34] There is correlation between DCG morphology and content. Co-storage of peptide and amine in the same cell or even the same granule is characteristic of neoplastic NE cells; however, it is uncertain whether co-storage of peptides derived from different genes occurs in normal PNECs. Co-localization was rarely found in normal fetuses; it was most frequently found in newborn infants with acute lung disease, usually hyaline membrane disease (HMD), or with the development of chronic lung disease in the first weeks or months after birth (Fig. 10–11).[35] Co-localization to the same DCG has been shown in humans for GRP and CT, CT and CGRP, and GRP and CGRP. However, it is possible that these lungs were not absolutely normal.[36, 37] Vasoconstrictors such as endothelin have also been co-localized with GRP in human PNECs.[38] Finally, the epithelial nature of PNECs and NEBs is highlighted by the consistent expression of desmoplakins and low-molecular-weight keratins, such as keratins 8, 18, and 19 in solitary PNECs and in at least some NEBs.[39, 40]

PHYSIOLOGY

PNECs may be considered as modified neurons or *paraneurons*[41] that have a dual receptor-effector function. On the one hand, they exhibit obvious connections via NEBs with nerves and may be viewed as receptors and participants in neurotransmission; on the other hand, because of their well-known capacity to produce, store, and secrete various hormones, they may be viewed as paracrine effector cells.

The concept that the lung contained receptors for monitoring the composition of inspired air had been put forth by Frölich in the late 1940s.[23] However, it was not until 1973, when Lauweryns and Cokelaere demonstrated the degranulation of innervated NEBs in neonatal rabbits under hypoxic conditions, that experimental evidence documented that NEBs served a chemoreceptor function.[42, 43] Since the

Table 10–1. Immunocytochemical Markers of Pulmonary Neuroendocrine Cells and Neuroepithelial Bodies

Localization	Marker
	Pan-NE Markers
Cytosolic markers	NSE-γ; PGP 9.5; 7B2
DCG-associated markers	Chromogranins A, B, C; CD57 (HNK1)
Small vesicle–associated markers	Synaptophysin
Cell surface markers	Neural cell adhesion molecules (NCAM)
	Biogenic Amines and Neuropeptides
NE cell secretory products	GRP (BLPs); CT; CGRP; 5-HT; dopamine; leu-enkephalin*; somatostatin; cholecystokinin; substance P

* Present only in solitary NE cells.
BLP, bombesin-like peptides; CGRP, calcitonin gene-related peptide; CT, calcitonin; DCG, dense-core granule; GRP, gastrin-releasing peptide; 5-HT, serotonin; NE, neuroendocrine; NSE, neuron-specific enolase; PGP, protein gene product.

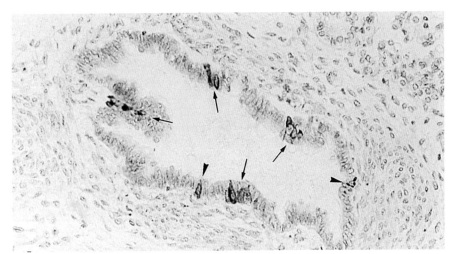

Figure 10-9. NEBs (*arrows*) and single PNECs (*arrowheads*) demonstrating CD57 immunoreactivity. Fetal bronchiole. (Immunoperoxidase, hematoxylin ×100.) (From Lauweryns et al 1987 J Histochem Cytochem 35:687–691.)

early 1990s, experiments have firmly established that NEBs carry a specific membrane oxygen receptor.[1, 44, 45] It appears that hypercapnia has no significant effect on exocytosis from NEBs,[46] although recent studies have demonstrated that elevated concentrations of carbon dioxide may result in PNEC proliferation and an increase in the transcription of the growth-promoting gene *c-fos*.[47]

NEBs are innervated by morphologic afferent- and efferent-like synaptic specializations and may be involved in both chemoreception and secretion. Activation of certain neural pathways may control the release of biogenic substances to influence physiologic airway functions. Although the precise functional implications of NEB innervation remain unclear,[9] experiments have confirmed that vagal stimulation

increases the amount of 5-HT in rabbit NEBs while decreasing their rate of degranulation. This is prevented by both supranodosal and infranodosal vagotomy, suggesting that vagal efferents are responsible.[48, 49] The ultimate effects of centripetal transmission of impulses in the afferent nerves of NEBs are unknown.[50]

Studies that have looked at the effects on NEBs of long-term existence at natural high altitude have confirmed that hypoxic chemoreception is their primary role. Studies of Bolivian highlanders showed an increase in the number of clusters of NEBs compared with controls living at sea level. It is noteworthy that in every case the increase in PNECs was largely due to larger number of clusters rather than solitary cells. Although no study confirms

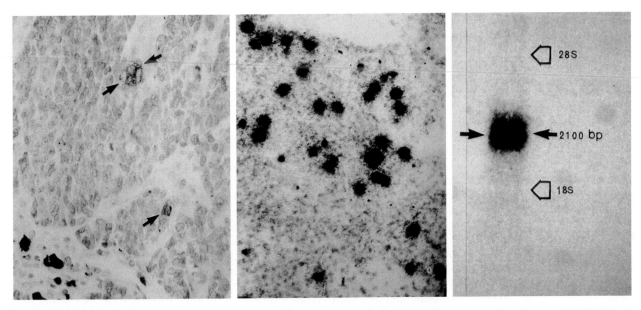

Figure 10-10. Expression of ChrA in a poorly differentiated neuroendocrine carcinoma, small cell type (PDNEC-SC). Left panel, PDNEC-SC with few cells immunostaining (*arrows*) for ChrA. Middle panel, exhibiting intense labeling on in situ hybridization with cRNA probe. Right panel, Northern blot analysis showing intense single band (2.1 kb) corresponding to ChrA. Arrows labeled 18S and 28S show position of ribosomal RNA markers. (From Hamid et al 1991 J Pathol 163:293–297.)

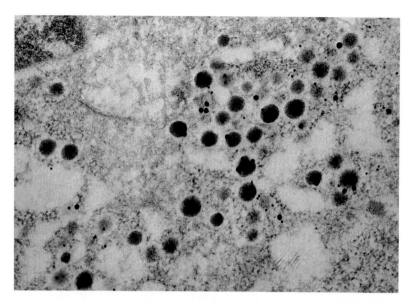

Figure 10–11. Co-storage of peptides derived from different genes occurs in normal PNECs. Double gold immunolabeling using anti-GRP and anti-CGRP as primary antibodies and secondary antibodies labeled with different-size gold spheres (*large spheres,* GRP; *small spheres,* CGRP) show co-localization in the same PNEC. Newborn infant. (From Stahlman et al 1993 Anat Rec 236:206–212.)

these clusters as NEBs by demonstrating their innervation, illustrations of them, where provided, generally show the orderly structure typical of NEBs.[18]

A major role of PNECs is to maintain pulmonary homeostasis by regulating the growth of pulmonary tissues during development and following injury. These trophic effects are gradually emerging as the most important PNEC paracrine function. CT, 5-HT, CGRP, and GRP are the established secretory products of PNECs. Cholecystokinin, somatostatin (ST), substance P, leu-enkephalin, and others have been less consistently demonstrated.[34] In adult human lungs, about 65% of PNECs contain GRP, and the majority of the rest contains CT.[20]

CT is thought to be primarily involved with the pulmonary inflammatory response via its association with arachidonic acid metabolism. 5-HT appears to promote vascularization and recently has been implicated in clearing fluid from the lungs at the time of birth.[51] It is co-localized with GRP and CGRP and also may be involved with their release. CGRP is well-established as a vasodilator, a neuro transmitter, and a promoter for proliferation of airway epithelium.[52, 53]

To date, however, most definitive studies of PNEC secretory products have been on the BLP (GRP-like) family of neuropeptides. Increases in PNECs can stimulate lung development and maturation in early and late gestation by the paracrine secretion of mitogens such as GRP, which affect the growth of adjacent airway epithelial cells.[54] Signal transduction pathways activated by BLPs and by cell adhesion involving the integrins have a common point of convergence in the phosphorylation of focal adhesion kinase (p125^{FAK}), a protein tyrosine kinase that co-localizes with cellular focal adhesions.[55] In this fashion, BLPs may interact with intracellular signaling caused by cellular adhesion to the extracellular matrix, a process of known importance in morphogenesis.

PATHOPHYSIOLOGY AND PATHOLOGY

PNECs in Non-neoplastic Lung Disease

Inflammatory injury to the pulmonary epithelium causes both an increase in PNECs and an alteration in their secretory products. The increase of PNECs appears to depend on the severity and chronicity of the injury and generally proceeds according to a stereotypic morphologic progression from orderly to disordered as follows:

1. formation of interrupted rows (linear hyperplasia) of PNECs in apposition to the basement membrane,
2. formation of intraepithelial, nodular PNEC aggregates, and
3. formation of small (2 to 3 mm) submucosal aggregates of PNECs (tumorlets) discontinuous from the basement membrane, growing into the immediately subadjacent tissues, and often associated with a conspicuous fibrous stroma (Fig. 10–12).

These changes secondary to inflammatory injury, followed by regeneration and repair, need to be distinguished from those that occur in uncomplicated persistent hypoxia, in which the increase is in the number of NEBs rather than solitary PNECs.

This morphologic progression is accompanied by alterations in the amount and nature of PNEC secretory products. CT becomes the predominant peptide within interrupted rows of PNECs, explaining, perhaps, the consistently demonstrable hypercalcitoninemia and hypercalcitoninemia in patients with tuberculosis, chronic obstructive pulmonary disease, and sarcoidosis.[56, 57] Disorderly nodular PNEC aggregates often express GRP. GRP may function as a chemoattractant for monocytes in chronic bronchitis, respiratory bronchiolitis, bronchiectasis, and other specific inflammatory pulmonary disorders

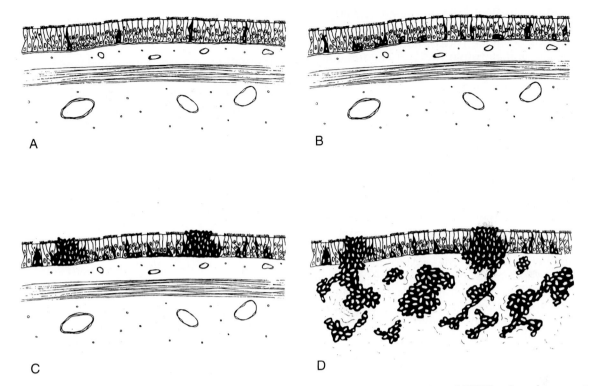

Figure 10–12. Schematic presentation of PNEC proliferation. *A,* Normal, even spacing of PNECs along basement membrane of pulmonary epithelium. *B,* Earliest change, formation of *interrupted rows* of cells along basement membrane. *C,* PNECs forming intraepithelial *nodular aggregates.* *D,* PNECs breach basement membrane and grow in subjacent tissue (formation of tumorlet). (From Gosney et al 1997 Microscopy Res Tech 37:107–113.)

associated with PNEC hyperplasia.[58, 59] Neuropeptides may exert autocrine control over PNECs in conditions characterized by vigorous regeneration, such as bronchopulmonary dysplasia in which excessive concentrations contribute to the pathogenesis of the disease.[60]

The local action of neuropeptides in the homeostasis of PNECs may be modulated by neutral endopeptidase (NEP), a cell-surface enzyme that hydrolyzes GRP and other neuropeptides. Lung diseases characterized by increased PNECs, including idiopathic diffuse hyperplasia of PNECs, respiratory bronchiolitis, and eosinophilic granuloma, have increased levels of NEP, reflecting a compensatory increase that may mitigate high levels of neuropeptides.[61] Alternatively, low NEP expression could increase neuropeptide-induced autocrine effects by increasing local levels of neuropeptides. Experimental evidence indicates that NEP inhibition leads to increases in PNECs and decreased apoptosis.[62] Low or undetectable NEP is also present in many primary NE and non-NE lung cancers and cell lines. These differences may represent disrupted or intact feedback mechanisms in malignant and benign disorders, respectively.[63]

Although the mechanism of this reactive increase in PNECs has often been referred to as "hyperplasia" or proliferation, such terms may not really be appropriate, since they imply that cell division is responsible. Recent evidence points to transdifferentiation of non-NE cells as the most important mechanism underlying the increase of PNECs in diseased lungs. Mitoses are rarely, if ever, found in the PNECs of adult lungs.[64] PNECs appear late in the process of re-epithelialization after injury.[65] In experimental animals, tritiated thymidine is first taken up by Clara-like cells immediately adjacent to PNECs and then after about 8 hours by the PNECs themselves. These results suggest that the adjacent first-labeled non-NE cells divided and subsequently developed a NE phenotype.[66]

A recent report highlighted the close relationship between Clara cells and PNECs by demonstrating dual CC 10/CGRP cells in the mouse airway after injury.[67] Further studies have shown that both Clara cell–specific protein and CGRP-containing cells within NEBs undergo proliferation after injury.[68] Whether transdifferentiation of non-PNEC cells is the predominant mechanism involved, resulting in increased numbers of PNECs, is unknown. Most likely the processes of differentiation, proliferation, and apoptosis combine to determine PNEC numbers. Morphometric studies in animal models have demonstrated that the PNEC hyperplasia caused by airway epithelial injury is accompanied by a combination of increased proliferation and decreased apoptosis.[62] Nodular aggregates of PNECs and tumorlets are also associated with the expression of various aberrant products, such as adrenocorticotropic hormone (ACTH), ST, vasoactive intestinal polypeptide (VIP), β-endorphin, human growth hormone (hGH), and subunits of human chorionic gonadotropin (hCG).[69] The function of these ectopic peptides is unclear and may best be interpreted as markers of increasingly disordered PNEC proliferation akin to that seen in bronchial neoplasms.

Inflammatory and Fibrotic Pulmonary Disease

Linear increases and more disorganized focal aggregates of PNECs have been well documented in chronic bronchitis, bronchiectasis, and interstitial fibrosis (Fig. 10–13). In patients with chronic bronchitis and emphysema, the PNEC number and arrangement, as well as the proportion containing GRP and CT, differ considerably from those in controls. The overall population of PNECs is uniformly increased approximately fivefold, compared with control lungs. In acute inflammatory lung disease, the increase in PNECs is not uniform but rather was more pronounced in the areas of pneumonia.[70] Apart from the secretion of CT and GRP, secretion of ectopic neuropeptides like ACTH, ST, and VIP has been described in bronchiectatic lungs in association with a decrease in the size of the Golgi apparatus and the number of the DCGs. Ectopic neuropeptides tend to appear when the increase of PNECs is particularly florid and disorganized.[18]

On the other hand, patients who develop bronchiolitis obliterans subsequent to lung transplantation have decreased numbers of PNECs and NEBs. This decrease in NE cells is considered to be a primary contributing factor to the development of bronchiolitis obliterans. It is thought that the absence of PNECs inhibits epithelial regeneration after injury, which in turn leads to chronic fibrosis.[71]

Idiopathic Diffuse Hyperplasia of PNECs

Idiopathic diffuse hyperplasia of PNECs (IDH-PNC), in the absence of preexisting lung disease or hypoxia, is a clinicopathologic entity characterized by a diffuse hyperplasia of NE cells involving distal bronchi and bronchioles. The pathogenesis of this syndrome remains unknown. The hyperplastic PNECs contain multiple neuropeptides that stimulate proliferation of fibroblasts in a paracrine fashion and PNEC proliferation in an autocrine manner.[61, 72–74] The pathologic hallmark is a diffuse intraepithelial proliferation of PNECs. The hyperplastic PNECs may be associated with mild to moderate degrees of interstitial and peribronchial fibrosis and the presence of tumorlets. A unique case has been described with aggregates of PNECs filling the alveolar spaces without interstitial invasion and only moderate interstitial fibrosis (Fig. 10–14).[75] Increased NEP expression has been reported in lung tissue from patients with IDHPNC and may reflect a compensatory increase that partly counteracts the abundant neuropeptides present in this disorder.[61]

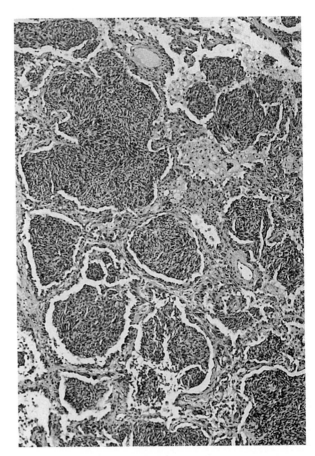

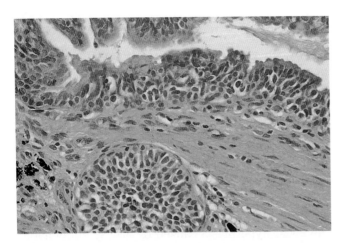

Figure 10–13. Linear increases and disorganized focal aggregates of PNECs in subsegmental bronchus of bronchiectatic lung. Note submucosal PNEC aggregate. (Hematoxylin and eosin.)

Figure 10–14. Diffuse idiopathic hyperplasia of PNECs. PNECs filling the alveolar spaces without interstitial invasion and only moderate interstitial fibrosis. (From Armas et al 1995 Am J Surg Pathol 19;963–970.)

Neonatal Pulmonary Disease

Hyaline membrane disease (HMD) and the sometimes subsequent exaggerated process of regeneration and repair, bronchopulmonary dysplasia (BPD), are two neonatal conditions in which there are marked alterations of PNECs. In HMD there is a marked decrease in the numbers of GRP, CT, and 5-HT–immunoreactive PNECs accompanying the destructive changes to the alveolar and bronchiolar epithelium, whereas infants who develop BPD demonstrate a disordered increase in PNECs accompanying the florid proliferation of epithelial and mesenchymal elements.[76] The presence of large numbers of CGRP immunoreactive cells has also been noted in infants with BPD.[77, 78] Similar changes have also been seen with Wilson-Mikity syndrome, sometimes considered a variant of BPD.[79] These findings document an association between hyperoxia, airway remodeling, and PNEC hyperplasia and imply that PNEC products may contribute to the pathogenesis of oxygen-related pulmonary diseases such as BPD.[80]

Pulmonary hypoplasia, often accompanied by other congenital abnormalities such as diaphragmatic hernia, has also been associated with reduction in percentage of GRP-immunoreactive PNECs.[81] The increased GRP and CGRP immunostaining observed in some cases of congenital diaphragmatic hernia might reflect a compensatory mechanism related to impaired lung development or failure of neuropeptide secretion during neonatal adaptation or both.[82] Because CGRP exhibits growth factor–like properties for endothelium and epithelial cells, the lack of this factor during a crucial developmental stage may be causally related to lung hypoplasia.[53]

Pulmonary Hypertension

Hypertensive pulmonary vascular disease with plexiform lesions caused by a variety of conditions has been associated with increased numbers of PNECs, which, in many cases, show irregular aggregation. The number of PNECs appears related to the degree of activity of myofibroblasts. The PNECs are most prominent in the preplexiform stage, when smooth muscle cells migrate through gaps in the inner elastic lamina to reach the intima. Here they are transformed into myofibroblasts and proliferate. The migration of muscle cells may be related in some way to long-acting trophic factors released from the pulmonary endocrine cells into the surrounding tissues from which they reach the blood and hence the pulmonary arteries. The hyperplastic PNECs label most prominently for GRP, CT, and 5-HT. In contrast, patients with pulmonary hypertension without plexiform lesions do not show PNEC hyperplasia.[83, 84]

Tumorlets

"Tumorlets" is the term most widely used to describe the small (0.2 to 0.4 cm), often multiple submucosal aggregates of PNECs discontinuous from the basement membrane. The exact incidence of tumorlets is not known, but in one autopsy series they were found in 2 of 1900 patients with no lung disease and in 20 of 2400 lung specimens surgically removed for various causes.[85] They form focal proliferations considerably larger than intramucosal aggregates of PNECs and grow into the immediately subadjacent tissues (Fig. 10–15). The cellular aggregates are confined to the thickened bronchial and bronchiolar wall but occasionally can be found in the connective tissues surrounding dilated airways. They are recognizable only on histologic examination of lung tissue. Tumorlets are often associated with a conspicuous fibrous stroma. They frequently occur in bronchiectatic lungs,[85] lobar sequestration,[86] and other chronic pulmonary diseases associated with fibrosis.[87–90] They are also known to occur in association with bronchial neoplasms of all types.[18]

On light microscopic examination, tumorlets appear as small nests of uniform, plump cells of moderate size, with clear cytoplasm and regular, slightly hyperchromatic nuclei. Nucleoli are inconspicuous. Tumorlets share histopathologic features with carcinoid tumors (Fig. 10–16A,B); in practice, however, the difference in the size (tumorlets, less than 0.4 cm in greatest diameter) of the growths and their association with distal airways readily permit separation of the two entities. Occasionally, peripheral carcinoids may be multiple, in which case they should be differentiated from tumorlets.[91] Sometimes tumorlets have a striking resemblance to the histologic pattern of SCLC. However, nuclear irregularities, mitoses, and necrosis are absent (Fig. 10–16C,D). Ultrastructurally, tumorlet cells contain large numbers of DCGs identical to those present in PNECs (Fig. 10–17).[92]

Tumorlets express neuropeptides and biogenic amines such as 5-HT, CT, and GRP, as well as ectopic neuropeptides such as ACTH and hCG.[93] It has been suggested that local release of the products of tumorlets may provoke formation of dense, fibrous stroma.[94] A unique case of pulmonary tumorlets causing severe Cushing's syndrome owing to ectopic secretion of ACTH has been reported.[95]

Because of their close morphologic resemblance to pulmonary carcinoid tumors, the neoplastic nature of tumorlets has been debated. Some observers believe that tumorlets are microcarcinoids capable of metastasis.[96] Rare cases of tumorlets have been reported with alleged metastatic involvement of the local lymph nodes.[97, 98] Recent cytogenetic evidence using tissue microdissection techniques has shown that the 11q13 region (Int-2) allelic imbalance significantly associated with carcinoids is not present in tumorlets. Furthermore, in patients having both carcinoids and tumorlets, the latter showed allelic balance and were thus discordant in genotype with coexisting carcinoid, excluding pathogenesis of tumorlets from intramucosal spread of carcinoids.[99]

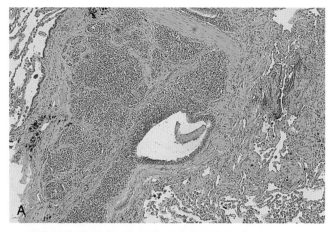

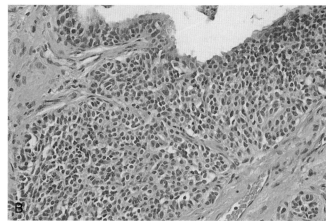

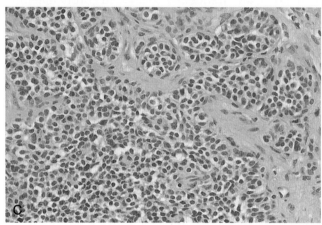

Figure 10–15. Pulmonary tumorlet. *A,* Solid tumorlet aggregates confined to the thickened bronchiolar wall in area of pulmonary fibrosis. *B,* Area of continuity with intraepithelial PNEC proliferation. *C,* Solid, infiltrative area with sclerosis. (Hematoxylin and eosin.)

CARCINOGENESIS AND MOLECULAR BIOLOGY OF NEUROENDOCRINE NEOPLASIA

NE carcinogenesis appears to be the result of multiple genetic alterations subsequent to critical exposure of the pulmonary epithelium to two environmental initiating agents, most commonly cigarette smoke and less commonly radon.[100] Although it is well known that over 95% of patients with SCLC are either current or ex-smokers, the initial molecular changes associated with NE carcinogenesis have been difficult to study experimentally because of the paucity of identifiable early lesions and the existence of few appropriate animal models. Much of the information on the genetic and molecular changes in pulmonary NE neoplasia is derived from studies of advanced human lesions and NE cancer cell lines, largely of SCLC. Considerably less is known about the molecular pathology of other NE tumors.

Although NE tumors of the lung share common phenotypic features, suggesting a genotypic relationship, they differ remarkably in their cytogenetic characteristics, highlighting an early fundamental molecular divergence during their development. The frequent loss of 11q material represents a characteristic genetic alteration in both typical carcinoid (TC) and atypical carcinoid (AC) that is rarely found in SCLC and large cell neuroendocrine carcinoma

(LCNEC). Losses of 10q and 13q sequences permit further cytogenetic differentiation between TC and AC. In contrast, SCLC and LCNEC are characterized by losses and gains primarily in 3p, 5q, 5p, and 13q.[101, 102] Although some AC may resemble LCNEC morphologically, it is still unclear whether there are similarities at the genetic level.[103, 104]

The development of NE pulmonary tumors is associated with both the overexpression of oncogenes and the inactivation of antioncogenes (tumor suppressor oncogenes). The *myc* family of dominant oncogenes, which play a pivotal role in controlling cell growth and differentiation and are likely to be involved in the apoptosis pathway, has been shown to be important in the progression of SCLC. It is the oncogene most consistently found to correlate with the end-stage behavior of SCLC, and in particular with survival after chemotherapeutic treatment. It appears that *c-myc* oncogene modulation also affects differentiation of SCLC. *c-myc* amplification occurs in cultures of the variant SCLC, mixed small cell/large cell (SC/LC) subtype, and may be responsible for the development of variant lines in culture and, by implication, of SC/LC tumors in vivo. SC/LC has been associated with rapid growth in vitro and in vivo, with radioresistance, and with poor survival.[105, 106] The activation of the dominant proto-oncogenes *c-myb, c-kit, c-jun,* and *c-src* has also been described in SCLC.

Altered expression of two tumor suppressor genes, *p53* and the retinoblastoma (Rb) gene product, has been demonstrated in NE neoplasms. *p53* is progressively overexpressed in AC, SCLC, and LC-NEC.[107-109] NE carcinomas have also been reported to show a loss of heterozygosity at the Rb locus and in the inactivation of this gene, and the reduced or absent expression of the encoded protein occurs in most SCLC and LCNEC.[110] TC and AC show heterogeneous expression of Rb-encoded protein. These findings suggest that all SCLCs and LCNECs have abnormalities in the p16:Rb pathway, as do at least certain ACs, whereas the p16:Rb pathway is normal in TCs.[111, 112] Karyotypic and molecular genetic studies have demonstrated that another tumor suppressor gene, *3p14.2* FHIT, is not expressed in the majority of SCLCs whereas TCs, similar to normal lung epithelia, are strongly positive for the cytoplasmic Fhit protein. ACs appeared to express an intermediate level of Fhit protein between TC and SCLC on the basis of extent of loss of 3p alleles and reduced expression of Fhit protein.[102]

Recent evidence suggests that the genetic regulation of apoptosis is also of critical importance during NE tumorigenesis. Oncogene and tumor suppressor genes can regulate the rate or susceptibility of PNECs to undergo apoptosis. A recent study investigated the expression of *Bcl-2* protein in SCLC, AC, and TC, and compared it with *p53* expression. *Bcl-2* immunoreactivity was present in the majority of SCLCs, ACs, and TCs. Western and Northern blot analysis also revealed that TC expressed the *26 kD* protein and *bcl-2* transcripts. Although a large number of SCLCs studied displayed *p53* protein immunoreactivity, *p53* expression was not found in any of the carcinoid tumors. Differences in *Bcl-2* and *p53* expression between SCLCs and carcinoid tumors suggest that disregulation of the genetic mechanisms controlling apoptosis is a critical step in the multistep tumorigenesis of SCLC.[113]

DNA synthesis/repair genes have also been implicated in pulmonary NE tumorigenesis. A recent study demonstrated that upregulation of the RNA component (hTR) of telomerase occurs in the majority of human SCLCs, whereas TCs had a significantly lower frequency of hTR expression. When hTR expression was compared with the well-characterized biologic targets *p53* and *Bcl-2*, hTR was expressed

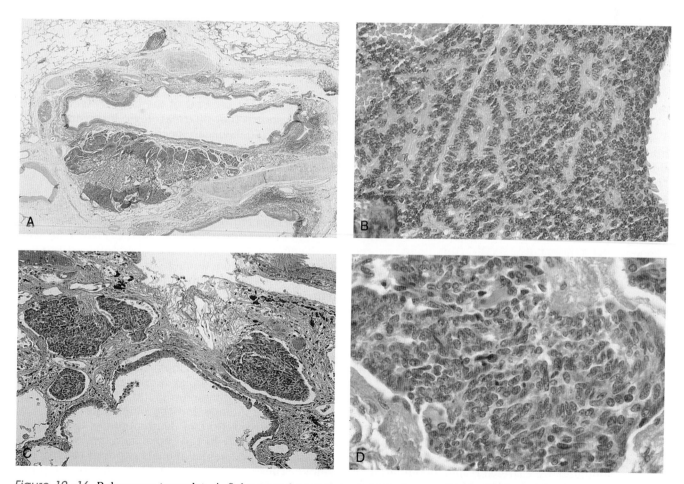

Figure 10–16. Pulmonary tumorlet. *A,* Submucosal tumorlet aggregate is associated with bronchiectatic airway. *B,* Uniform, plump cells with clear cytoplasm arranged in trabecular and organoid pattern histologically indistinguishable from typical carcinoid. *C,* Tumorlets may have a striking resemblance to the histologic pattern of PDNEC-SC. *D,* Lack of nuclear irregularities, mitoses, or necrosis distinguishes tumorlets from PDNEC-SC. (Hematoxylin and eosin.)

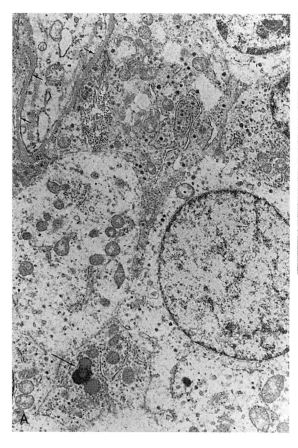

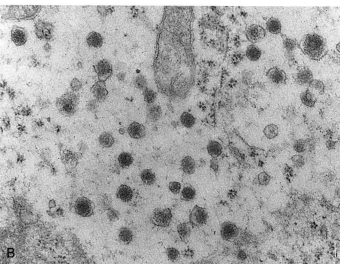

Figure 10–17. Pulmonary tumorlet. *A,* Several tumorlet cells with numerous DCGs. Residual bodies (*arrow*). Junction between tumorlet and connective tissue demarcated by well-defined basement membrane (*arrowheads*). (TEM × 16,000.) *B,* DCGs in tumorlet averaging 110 to 140 nm in diameter, surrounded by well-defined limiting membrane and clear halo. (From Bonikos et al 1976 Human Pathol 7:461–470.)

more frequently, indicating that therapies directed at hTR may be useful in SCLC.[114]

Autocrine growth factors are important in promoting the growth of pulmonary NE tumors. Bombesin/gastrin releasing peptide (BN/GRP), insulin-like growth factor I (IGF-I), and transferrin have been identified as autocrine growth factors in SCLC. High levels of GRP mRNA and immunoreactivity are present in SCLC cells. The secretion rate of GRP from SCLC cells is increased by VIP, which elevates the intracellular cAMP. GRP binds to cell surface receptors, elevates cytosolic calcium, and stimulates the growth of SCLC cells. IGF-I binds with high affinity to SCLC cells and stimulates tyrosine kinase activity and growth. Transferrin binds with high affinity to SCLC cells and stimulates iron transport and growth. Synthetic peptide antagonists and monoclonal antibodies have been identified that disrupt autocrine growth pathways and inhibit SCLC growth.[115]

It has been shown that SCLC cells express low levels of the metalloendopeptidase CD10/neutral endopeptidase 24.11 (CD10/NEP, common acute lymphoblastic leukemia antigen), and that this enzyme hydrolyzes GRP. The growth of GRP-dependent SCLC is inhibited by CD10/NEP and potentiated by CD10/NEP inhibition. Because SCLC occurs almost exclusively in cigarette smokers and cigarette smoke inactivates CD10/NEP, decreased cell surface CD10/NEP enzymatic activity may be causally related to

the development of SCLC of the lung.[116] Recent studies have shown that pharmacologic intervention targeting the biochemical mechanisms necessary for synthesis and activation of peptide growth factors, or immunotherapy directly targeting GRP, has promising results in SCLCs that are dependent on autocrine growth loops.[117, 118]

Tobacco appears to play a dual role in the genesis and development of SCLC. It stimulates the secretion of autocrine growth factors by the PNECs as well as facilitates the occurrence of mitotic mutations. This autocrine functioning also gives a selective advantage to cells going through transformation or immortalization. The procarcinogenic or carcinogenic agents contained in tobacco smoke contribute to the accumulation of mutations affecting both suppressor genes and oncogenes.[119]

PNECs and neuropeptides, which serve both as coordinators of lung development and mediators of pulmonary injury, also play a critical role in the earliest stages of NE tumor promotion. Abnormalities in both the morphology and the number of the PNECs and in the secretion of neuropeptides have been found consistently in the proximal airways of smokers and in experimental animals exposed to cigarette smoke. These abnormalities have been attributed primarily to the effect of nicotine and nitrosamines. Chronic stimulation of nicotinic receptors by nicotine and nitrosamines in cigarette smokers has been proposed as one of the molecular events responsible for PNEC proliferation and, ultimately, the development of lung tumors with NE differentiation. Model systems have shown that exposure to the tobacco-specific nitrosamine 4-(methylnitrosamino)-1-(3-pyridyl)-1-butanone can cause NE lung tumors in hyperoxic hamsters. These tumors manifest cytologic, histologic, immunologic, and ultrastructural features of NE differentiation.

Abnormal pulmonary oxygen levels may be an essential factor for the induction of NE tumors. Exposure of experimental animals to nitrosamines under eupoxic conditions may cause proliferation of PNECs and/or the induction of non-NE neoplasms but not NE tumors akin to those naturally occuring in the human lung. Data support the hypothesis that chronic stimulation of nicotinic acetylcholine receptors in an environment of impaired pulmonary oxygenation contributes to the carcinogenic burden associated with exposure to cigarette smoke and provides selective growth advantage for lung tumors with a NE phenotype.[120–124] Other studies, however, have not reproduced these observations, finding instead only a marked but transient proliferation of PNECs.[125]

PULMONARY NEOPLASMS WITH NEUROENDOCRINE DIFFERENTIATION

Neuroendocrine Characteristics in Lung Tumors

Lung carcinomas are traditionally classified into discrete histologic subtypes; however, there is ample evidence for plasticity of cell phenotype at the cellular and molecular level. Lung tumors in general, and NE tumors in particular, represent a continuum of cell types, where transition among the cell types is possible, both spontaneously and after therapeutic intervention. Spontaneous phenotypic conversion of NE tumors into non-NE squamous, large cell, and adenocarcinomas is observed (1) in human NE neoplasms, in which tumor histology at the time of clinical presentation is different from that found at autopsy following tumor progression, (2) in the hamster model of NE carcinoma, in which tumors have been consistently induced by the administration of nitrosamines in the presence of hypoxia or hyperoxia, and (3) in the transgenic mice model, in which the *ras* gene is expressed specifically in PNECs.[126–128] Post-treatment histologic heterogeneity has also been observed in SCLC.[129] Despite the phenotypic heterogeneity present in human lung cancer, important segregating features such as growth factors, differentiation markers, proto-oncogenes, and tumor suppressor genes distinguish NE neoplasms from nonsmall cell lung carcinomas (NSCLCs).[130]

Pulmonary neoplasms that share a common phenotype characterized by the capability to synthesize, package, and transport biologically active neuroamines, neuropeptides, and related substances are considered to exhibit NE differentiation. The mechanisms that regulate the NE phenotype in these tumors and their cellular precursors are not well understood. A common functional link distinguishing PNECs and lung tumors with NE differentiation from cells and neoplasms without NE phenotype is the human achaete-scute homologue-1 (*hASH1*), a basic helix-loop-helix transcription factor that is homologous to *Drosophila* neural determination proteins. Lung tumors with NE features constitutively express *hASH1*, whereas NSCLC tumors do not.[16, 131, 132] Depletion of this transcription factor from lung cancer cells by antisense oligonucleotides results in a significant decrease in the expression of neuroendocrine markers.[16] Modulation of *hASH1* may contribute to the plasticity of lung cancer phenotypes and the observed transition of SCLC to NSCLC.

The overtly NE tumors manifest easily recognizable common morphologic features by light and electron microscopy. The histologic appearance of organoid growth with sheets, ribbons, trabeculae, nests, pseudoglandular formations, rosette-like areas, mosaicism, and peripheral palisading, coupled with the particular cytology of scant cytoplasm, uniform nuclei, finely granular chromatin, inconspicuous nucleoli, and nuclear molding, creates a distinctive continuum of differentiation from the well-differentiated carcinoid tumor at one end to the poorly differentiated NE carcinoma at the other. Ultrastructural studies have consistently shown that tumors with the aforementioned histologic and cytologic features have variable numbers of DCGs, more numerous in the better-differentiated tumors and scantier in less-differentiated ones.

Neoplasms with the aforementioned classic NE histology do not need ancillary techniques to discern NE differentiation. These adjunctive methods include histochemical procedures, electron microscopy, immunohistochemistry, and molecular and genetic analyses. Histochemical techniques based on silver reduction are obsolescent and have for the most part been supplanted by immunohistochemistry. The Grimelius and Cherukian-Schenk modifications of the argyrophylic reaction are usually positive only in cases in which the histology is strongly suggestive of NE differentiation. The presence of DCGs is considered the gold standard characteristic of NE differentiation, and their presence in morphologically non-NE neoplasms is considered indicative of NE differentiation. Furthermore, DCGs may be seen even in suboptimally formalin-fixed tissues or in samples removed from paraffin-embedded blocks. In appropriately sampled material, the finding of DCGs by electron microscopy may be the most sensitive as well as the most specific indicator for NE differentiation.[133]

NE differentiation in pulmonary tumors is best characterized by the demonstration of a panel of specific pan-NE markers by immunohistochemistry. Pan-NE cell markers, because of their independence from specific hormone production, are particularly important in tumor diagnosis when neoplastic NE cells may not be producing or secreting distinct products. The different methods and antibodies used in various clinical studies make it difficult to know with certainty which markers and how many of them are needed to identify a tumor as having NE differentiation. A useful panel in the delineation of the NE phenotype should include NSE, Leu-7 (CD57), ChrA, SY38, and NCAM.[134, 135] The immunohistochemical demonstration of two or more is considered sufficient for the identification of the NE phenotype. In situ hybridization and Northern blot techniques have not been of practical value in delineating NE differentiation in pulmonary tumors.

CLASSIFICATION

Few human neoplasms have been studied, have been written about, or have managed to elicit so much controversy with respect to their terminology, origin, and nature as much as the NE neoplasms of the lung. The multiple and often complex classifications of pulmonary NE neoplasms are potentially confusing. Traditionally, light microscopic evaluation has been the cornerstone for classification of NE tumors because it has been shown to be important in determining the clinical outcomes of patients. A useful classification of NE tumors must be able to identify easily recognizable, reproducible, and clinically relevant morphologic categories while at the same time maintain simplicity and minimize the number of unclassifiable lesions.

The practical application of morphologic classifications of NE neoplasms is particularly difficult for the nonsmall cell types without access to electron microscopy and immunohistochemistry. In addition, tumor heterogeneity at both the light and electron microscopic level can lead to problems in interpreting NE features. The significance of large or small areas of NE differentiation in tumor classification remains unclear, and definitive classification may require large quantities of tissue not available with bronchial and aspiration biopsies. Finally, a standardized panel of NE markers needs to be devised and uniformly applied if immunohistochemistry is to become a tool in NE tumor classification.[136]

In general, pulmonary NE neoplasms can be divided into two groups: (1) those that show overt NE differentiation by light microscopy, and (2) those that manifest NE differentiation or "features" only by electron microscopy and/or immunohistochemistry. The former group, traditionally classified as NE neoplasms, constitutes a pathobiologic continuum of tumors that manifests a wide variety of morphologic appearances both within and between particular taxonomic categories, often distinguished from each other only by subtle cytologic and histologic differences. The latter group, recently separated from the group of large cell, squamous, and adenocarcinomas, represents a category of tumors whose biologic and clinical implications are not fully understood. Since the mid-1970s, the application of new techniques, including electron microscopy, cell culture, immunohistochemistry, and more recently molecular biology, has greatly added to our understanding of the origin, pathogenesis, and behavior of these neoplasms. These investigations have validated what constitute the light microscopic characteristics of the NE phenotype and have also revealed the NE nature of neoplasms otherwise unsuspected by morphology alone.

The following discussion presents, compares, and highlights the problems of the major histologic classifications of NE tumors in light of the current understanding of the biology and clinical implications of NE differentiation and proposes a practical morphologicofunctional algorithm for their classification and diagnosis, with reproducible categories best reflective of pathobiology, clinical behavior, and prognosis (Table 10–2).

Table 10–2. Comparison of Major Classifications of NE Neoplasms with Approximate Interrelationships

WHO 1981	WHO/IASLC	WHO 1999[144]	Gould et al.[18, 145]	Present
Carcinoid*	Carcinoid*	Carcinoid Atypical carcinoid	Carcinoid WDNEC, Grade I, II WDNEC, Grade III	Carcinoid WDNEC MDNEC
SCLC, oat cell SCLC, intermediate	SCLC	SCLC	NEC, small cell type	PDNEC-SC
	SC/LC	LCNEC†	NEC, intermediate	PDNEC, SC/LC PDNEC-LC
SCLC, combined	SCLC, combined	SCLC, combined	SCLC, combined	PDNEC-SC, combined
		NSCLC-NE		NSCLC-NE

* WHO 1981 does not classify atypical carcinoid separately.
† LCNEC includes cases combined with adenocarcinoma.
IASLC, International Association for the Study of Lung Cancer; LCNEC, large cell neuroendocrine carcinoma; MDNEC, moderately differentiated neuroendocrine carcinoma; NEC, neuroendocrine carcinoma; NSCLC-NE, nonsmall cell lung carcinoma with endocrine differentiation; PDNEC-LC, poorly differentiated neuroendocrine carcinoma, large cell type; PDNEC-SC, poorly differentiated neuroendocrine carcinoma, small cell type; SC/LC, small cell/large cell; SCLC, small cell lung carcinoma; WDNEC, well-differentiated neuroendocrine carcinoma; WHO, World Health Organization.

Neoplasms with NE Differentiation by Light Microscopy

To date, the most widely used current classification of NE tumors of the lung is that of the World Health Organization (WHO), a 1981 classification with revisions suggested by the International Association for the Study of Lung Cancer (WHO-IASLC).[137, 138] It is based exclusively on morphologic criteria by light microscopy and attempts to relate morphologic categories to natural history, biology, and response to therapy, particularly in regard to SCLC. The WHO-IASLC classification divided NE tumors into carcinoid tumors (TC and AC are not separated), SCLC, SC/LC, and combined SCLC (SCLC-C).

The major contributions of this classification have been the recognition that oat cell and intermediate (polygonal, fusiform) subtypes of SCLC[139, 140] can be combined under the designation SCLC because of identical clinical behavior and prognosis,[141] and the recognition that SC/LC is a subtype of SCLC, containing in addition to its SCLC component a variable population of cells resembling those of large cell lung carcinoma.[142, 143] Two major inadequacies of the WHO-IASLC classification have been the placement of TC and AC in a single category and the failure to address explicitly the spectrum of tumors with a significant or predominantly large cell NE component. The WHO 1999 *Classification of Pulmonary and Pleural Tumors*[144] partially addresses these issues. WHO 1999 separated AC from TC, retained the term "SCLC," discarded the category of SC/LC, and introduced the category of large cell neuroendocrine carcinoma (LCNEC) for tumors with vague organoid features composed of predominantly large undifferentiated cells.

The second major classification of NE lung tumors is that of Gould and colleagues.[18, 145] They proposed a new taxonomy of pulmonary NE neoplasms based on extensive histologic, ultrastructural, and immunochemical studies that explicitly emphasized their biologic spectrum and recognized that the morphology of pulmonary NE tumors was both a reflection of their degree of differentiation and their behavior and prognosis. In this fashion, they delineated two wide spectra of NE differentiation, exemplified at one end by the highly differentiated TC with a continuum toward SCLC, and at the other pole by the poorly differentiated SCLC with a continuum toward LCNEC. This explicit recognition within a systematic classificatory scheme of a morphologic NE spectrum between TC, SCLC, and LCNEC, simultaneously predictive of clinical behavior and based on biologic principles, represented a significant advance in the understanding of pulmonary NE neoplasms.

The first major problem in the classification of pulmonary NE tumors is the identification and taxonomy of AC. Although morphologically atypical and biologically aggressive carcinoid tumors had been long recognized sporadically,[146] it was Arrigoni and associates[147] who first separated AC from TC, utilizing defined morphologic features, and recognized their intermediate biologic behavior between TC and SCLC. Shortly after the distinction of AC from TC by Arrigoni and colleagues, it became clearly evident that these tumors were more pleomorphic than initially recognized. Retaining a distinctly organoid architecture evocative of carcinoid, AC manifested a broad range of nuclear largeness and atypia, mitotic activity, fibrosis, infarct-like necrosis, and even in some series microscopic foci resembling SCLC,[148–150] while still maintaining a significantly better prognosis than that of SCLC.[150–153]

Gould and colleagues[154] critically examined the issue of AC. They defined TC very precisely as a highly differentiated neoplasm with overt NE features, rare, if any, mitoses, and a minimal propensity for low-grade malignant behavior. They placed AC, which constituted a morphologic continuum between TC and SCLC, in a heterogeneous category designated as well-differentiated NE carcinoma (WDNEC).[145, 155–157] Warren and associates[157] subsequently subclassified WDNEC into three subsets based upon the degree of pleomorphism, local and vascular invasion, stromal fibrosis, mitoses, and extent of tumor necrosis. Although WDNEC, with the most aggressive histologic features (subset III), had a distinctly worse clinical course than that of tumors displaying blander features (subsets I and II), it had a significantly longer survival than similarly treated stages I and II SCLC.[157]

The WHO 1999 classification[144] retained the name AC for those tumors that differed minimally from TC. The definitional criteria of 2 to 10 mitoses/10 hpf and minimal necrosis, employed by WHO 1999 for inclusion of neoplasms in the AC category, appears too restrictive and excludes a significant number of tumors that manifest ultrastructural, immunohistochemical, histologic, and clinical features intermediate between those of TC and SCLC. In practice, only a minority of AC differ minimally from TC. The majority of AC has readily discernible morphologic differences from both TC and SCLC.

I believe that tumors with the morphologic spectrum of AC are classified best as well- or moderately differentiated NE carcinomas (WDNEC or MDNEC). They share the NE differentiation of TC, particularly the pronounced organoid architecture, but are distinguished from TC by variable degrees of tumor necrosis, nuclear enlargement, mitotic activity, and a distinctly worse prognosis. Neoplasms with the low-power light microscopic appearance of a TC having 2 to 10 mitoses/10 hpf, mild to moderate nuclear pleomorphism, and focal necrosis are classified best as WDNEC, whereas neoplasms with the low-power light microscopic appearance of a TC with 11 or more mitoses/10 hpf, marked nuclear pleomorphism (with or without foci reminiscent of SCLC), and conspicuous areas of central necrosis are classified best as MDNEC (Table 10–3). It is evident that the perpetuation of the term AC retains only historical interest and is not reflective of biology, histology, and clinical behavior.

Table 10-3. Practical Algorithm for the Histologic Diagnosis of Neuroendocrine Lung Tumors

Low-Power Appearance of Carcinoid?
YES
Carcinoid, WDNEC, or MDNEC
No mitoses or necrosis
Carcinoid
5–10 mitoses/10 HPF, mild to moderate nuclear pleomorphism, focal necrosis
WDNEC
≥11 mitoses per 10 HPF, marked nuclear pleomorphism, and conspicuous areas of central necrosis
MDNEC
NO
PDNEC-SC, PDNEC-SC/LC, PDNEC-LC, or NSCLC
Vague NE Pattern, Many Mitoses, Hyperchromatic Nuclei, Geographic Necrosis?
YES
PDNEC-SC, PDNEC-SC/LC, PDNEC-LC
Scant cytoplasm, 1.5×–4× lymphocyte, finely granular chromatin, and absent or inconspicuous nucleoli
PDNEC-SC*
Intermixed large cells 2× SC with vesicular nuclei, prominent nucleoli, and moderate host response
PDNEC-SC/LC
Large cell component constitutes the entire tumor, with marked host response
PDNEC-LC†
NO
NSCLC
NE Differentiation by Immunohistochemistry or Electron Microscopy?
YES
NSCLC-NE
NO
NSCLC

* If distinct squamous or adenocarcinomatous foci are present, the neoplasm is considered PDNEC-SC, combined.
† May require corroboration of NE differentiation by immunohistochemistry or electron microscopy.
HPF, high-power field; MDNEC, moderately differentiated neuroendocrine carcinoma; NE, neuroendocrine; NSCLC, nonsmall cell lung carcinoma; NSCLC-NE, nonsmall cell lung carcinoma with endocrine differentiation; PDNEC-LC, poorly differentiated neuroendocrine carcinoma, large cell type; PDNEC-SC, poorly differentiated neuroendocrine carcinoma, small cell; SC/LC, small cell, large cell; WDNEC, well-differentiated neuroendocrine carcinoma.

The second major problem in pulmonary NE tumor classification is the taxonomic position of NE tumors with a significant or predominant complement of large cells. Awareness of this second spectrum of NE differentiation emerged from studies of SCLC that noted that some contained a distinct population of much larger cells with more cytoplasm, vesicular nuclei, and often eosinophilic nucleoli.[137] In some cases, these larger cells were interspersed within the obvious SCLC complement; in others they formed distinct island aggregates; and in yet others the large cell complement predominated. The presence of large undifferentiated tumor cells in SCLC is concordant with tissue culture studies demonstrating that NE tumors develop along two main lines: (1) a classic SCLC cell line with expression of DCGs and secretion of neuropeptides, and (2) a variant cell line composed of larger cells with a weaker expression of NE markers.[106, 158]

The classification and interpretation of this morphologic continuum of differentiation within SCLC has been a major source of debate and confusion for a variety of reasons. First, the WHO-IASCL category of SCLC does not explicitly address tumors with a significant or predominant large cell component. The criteria for defining large cells are open to wide interpretation and are applied differently even among experts. For example, when small cells predominate, the large cells of SCLC may be interpreted as intermediate SCLC cells,[139] thereby classifying a tumor as SCLC, or conversely, when the large cells predominate, they may be interpreted as undifferentiated, non-NE large cells, thereby classifying a tumor as large cell carcinoma (LCC). Furthermore, examination of the heterogeneous group of so-called pure undifferentiated or LCC has yielded divergent conclusions concerning their NE differentiation, and their interpretation requires considerable caution.

Second, large cell neoplasms characterized in the literature as either LCNEC[144, 159–161] or NE carcinoma of intermediate type (NEC-I),[18] when examined critically also contain overlapping features faintly reminiscent of SCLC or WDNEC. WHO 1999[144] has defined LCNEC as a high-grade, biologically aggressive tumor with definite neuroendocrine morphology consisting of organoid nesting, peripheral palisading, rosettes, and trabeculae, as well as 11 or more mitoses/10 hpf and significant areas of necrosis that have a prognosis similar to that of SCLC. These inclusion criteria, however, significantly overlap with those of the WDNEC, subtype III, of Gould and associates[157] and AC as described by Mills and colleagues.[150] In addition, the WHO 1999 classification broadens the criteria of LCNEC in the opposite direction to include tumors that have large cells with fine nuclear chromatin and lack nucleoli, reminiscent of intermediate SCLC cells or the large cells described in SC/LC.

Other studies further expand the definition of LCNEC[162] and describe high-grade, large cell neoplasms with less prominent NE (organoid) morphology reminiscent of large cell carcinomas with NE differentiation (LCC-NE) or non-SCLC (squamous and adenocarcinomas) with NE differentiation (NSCLC-NE). It is also noteworthy that LCNEC, as originally described by Travis and associates,[159] WDNEC, subtype III,[152] and AC[150] all had a distinctly *better* prognosis than SCLC. Finally, the decision of WHO 1999 to classify LCNEC as a subtype of LCC on the basis of putative increased resistance to chemotherapy is contrary to the morphologic, cytogenetic, and molecular evidence.[102, 104, 163]

The NEC-I of Gould and coworkers[157] is also problematic. It is likewise too inclusive, encompassing large cell tumors that have no evidence of NE differentiation by light microscopy, tumors with a vaguely organoid pattern morphologically similar to LCNEC, and tumors that have a mixture of medium and small cells similar to those of SC/LC. Furthermore the term "intermediate" causes semantic confusion with the intermediate (polygonal, fusiform) subtypes of SCLC.

I believe that poorly differentiated NE neoplasms of the lung are classified best as poorly differentiated neuroendocrine carcinomas of small cell, small cell/large cell, and large cell type (PDNEC-SC, PDNEC-SC/LC, and PDNEC-LC). They share the common features of a vague NE pattern, many mitoses, hyperchromatic nuclei, and areas of geographic necrosis but are distinguished from each other by nuclear chromatin pattern and the number and character of the large cell component. Neoplasms containing cells with scant cytoplasm, finely granular chromatin, absent or inconspicuous nucleoli, and nuclei 1.5 to 4 times the size of lymphocytes are classified best as PDNEC-SC. Neoplasms containing a complement of single, small aggregates, or clusters of intermixed large cells with vesicular nuclei and prominent nucleoli, twice the size of SCLC cells and having a moderate host response, are classified best as PDNEC-SC/LC. Neoplasms in which the large cell component constitutes the entire tumor and is surrounded by a marked host response are classified best as PDNEC-LC (see Table 10–3).

There is general agreement that combined SCLC (C-SCLC) is a variant of SCLC in which there is a significant, well-defined separate component of either squamous, large cell, or adenocarcinoma. Although distinctly rare at initial diagnosis, this variant of SCLC is seen more often with the passage of time at autopsy, especially after chemotherapy. No known clinical significance is associated with C-SCLC.[130] Although the WHO 1999 classification has proposed that C-SCLC may include areas of LCNEC, I believe that combinations of SCLC and LCNEC are best classified in the PDNEC category.

Neoplasms with NE Differentiation by Electron Microscopy or Immunohistochemistry or Both

Pulmonary neoplasms that display NE differentiation only by electron microscopy or immunohistochemistry can be divided into two groups: (1) large cell carcinomas, and (2) squamous or adenocarcinomas.[164–168] Collectively, they comprise approximately 10% to 15% of all NSCLC.[130, 169] The former group has been termed "large cell carcinomas with NE differentiation" (LCC-NE), and the latter has been termed "non-SCLC with NE differentiation" (NSCLC-NE). NE differentiation is more common in large cell carcinomas and adenocarcinomas than in squamous cell carcinomas. The practical implication of NE differentiation in NSCLC pulmonary neoplasms is whether or not they will behave aggressively like classic SCLC and respond to chemotherapy. NE differentiation may merely reflect the well-known heterogeneity of lung tumors and the general plasticity and pluripotential nature of transformed cells without necessarily being indicative of clinical behavior. Some studies have suggested that LCC-NE and NSCLC-NE may be responsive to SCLC chemotherapy regimens,[170, 171] but other studies have indicated no correlation between the presence of NE differentiation and either response to chemotherapy or time to disease progression.[172]

PATHOLOGY OF NEUROENDOCRINE NEOPLASMS

Carcinoid Tumors

The TC is a well-differentiated NE neoplasm, more than 0.5 cm in greatest diameter, characterized by an organoid, trabecular, rosette-like, palisading, or spindle growth of uniform cells with moderate granular eosinophilic cytoplasm, finely granular chromatin, inconspicuous nucleoli, and less than 2 mitoses per 10 hpf. Often mixed histologic patterns are present. Foci of exocrine differentiation, mucin production, stromal fibrosis, and hyalinization are common. No necrosis should be present. TCs are designated as *central* when they arise in association with large airways and *peripheral* when they arise as in the periphery of the lung, often subpleural, or associated with subsegmental bronchi and distal bronchioles. TCs are rare tumors that represent less than 2% of all pulmonary neoplasms.

Central Carcinoids

Central TCs are most prevalent in middle-age, with peak incidence in the fifth decade. There is a slight female predominance.[173, 174] They most commonly arise in proximal airways (80% to 90%) and present as well-demarcated, solitary endobronchial polyps. The overlying epithelium is intact or sometimes

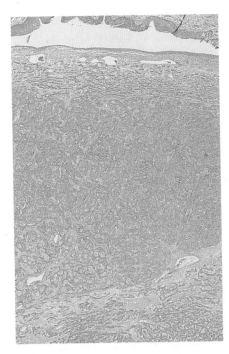

Figure 10-18. Central carcinoid. Tumor mass compressing large airway. Organoid, trabecular, and insular histology. Note squamous metaplasia of bronchial mucosa. (Hematoxylin and eosin.)

may demonstrate squamous metaplasia. Infiltrative growth around cartilaginous plates and into surrounding lung parenchyma is frequent (Figs. 10-18, 10-19). TCs range generally from 2 to 4 cm in greatest diameter at presentation. They display a yellow or red-brown color and a homogeneous appearance on cut section without hemorrhage or necrosis. The clinical presentation is that of a localized obstruction whose symptoms and signs develop insidiously due to the slow growth. Hemoptysis and persistent cough are the most common presenting symptoms.

Development of carcinoid syndrome is rare unless there is metastatic liver disease.[175] Occasionally, Cushing's syndrome due to ectopic ACTH hormone production is caused by TCs.[176, 177] Other paraneoplastic syndromes are rare.[178]

In addition to the aforementioned histologic patterns, TCs may display a papillary, clear cell, and oncocytic morphology. Rare cases with melanocytic differentiation have also been described.[179-182] Ultrastructurally, the most conspicuous characteristic of TCs is the large number DCGs between 150 and 250 nm in diameter, similar to the granules seen in normal PNECs.[183] Heterogeneous DCGs have been described in TCs; however, single cells appear to contain only one type of granule.[184, 185] Basal lamina, cytoplasmic processes, well-formed desmosomes, and paranuclear aggregates of intermediate filaments are also consistently present.[186] The heterogeneous granule populations seen by electron microscopy reflect the multiple expression of secretory products. Most TCs contain more than one secretory product. 5-HT, GRP, CT, and CGRP are most commonly expressed.[186-188] TCs have the highest percentage, distribution, and intensity of immunohistochemical staining for both pan-NE and hormonal markers of all NE neoplasms. Almost all TCs are reactive for the pan-NE markers ChrA, SY-38, NCAM, and CD57. Low-molecular-weight cytokeratins, particularly keratin 19, are expressed in most cases.[40]

Peripheral Carcinoids

Peripheral TCs tend to occur in older patients than do their central counterparts. Because of their peripheral location, they do not produce symptoms and signs of bronchial obstruction but rather present as asymptomatic pulmonary nodules, often with calcification (Figs. 10-20, 10-21). Occasionally they may be multiple and have also been found in

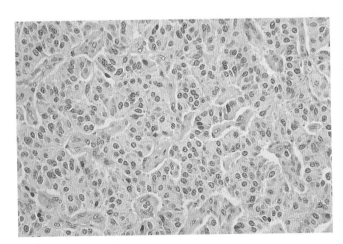

Figure 10-19. Central carcinoid. Characteristic histology pattern and cytologic features. Organoid growth of uniform cells with moderate, granular eosinophilic cytoplasm, finely granular chromatin, and inconspicuous nucleoli. (Hematoxylin and eosin.)

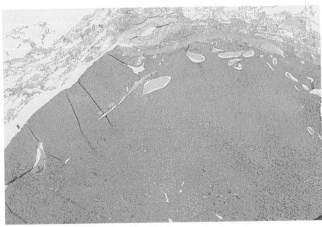

Figure 10-20. Peripheral carcinoid. Circumscribed, nonencapsulated peripheral pulmonary nodule not anatomically related to airway. The tumor is very cellular and exhibits no necrosis. (Hematoxylin and eosin.)

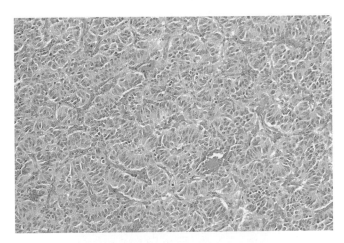

Figure 10-21. Peripheral carcinoid. Tumor cells similar to central carcinoid. Tumor cells have a propensity toward spindling. Note prominent vascular channels. (Hematoxylin and eosin.)

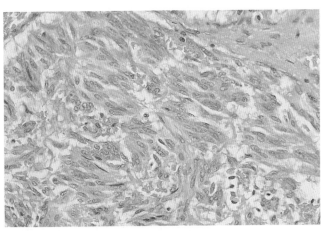

Figure 10-23. Peripheral carcinoid. Overt spindle cell pattern reminiscent of mesenchymal neoplasm. Note absence of necrosis and mitoses. (Hematoxylin and eosin.)

conjunction with pulmonary tumorlets.[28, 189] Histologically, ultrastructurally, and immunohistochemically, peripheral TCs are similar to those of centrally located tumors, although they tend to have a spindle cell or papillary morphology and a more pronounced vascular sclerosis (Figs. 10–22 through 10–25).[91, 181, 190]

Behavior

TCs strictly defined according to the preceding criteria may be considered extremely indolent tumors that rarely give rise to distant metastases. Recurrence after complete excision is unlikely, even in cases of large tumors with local lymph node metastases. The more aggressive prognosis associated with these tumors in some studies is undoubtedly due to the inclusion of histologically less-differentiated lesions.[191] Most often peripheral NE neoplasms

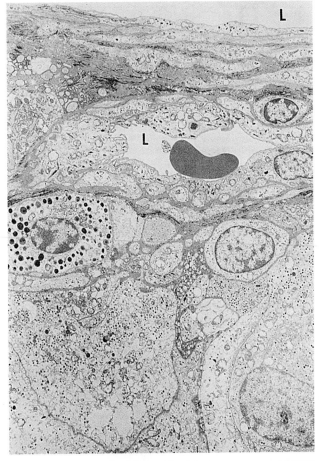

Figure 10-24. Peripheral carcinoid. Tumor cells embedded in a rich vascular stroma in close proximity with one or two vessels. Note numerous DCGs distributed evenly throughout tumor cell cytoplasm. L, vascular lumina. (TEM ×6960.) (From Bonikos et al 1976 Cancer 37:1977–1998.)

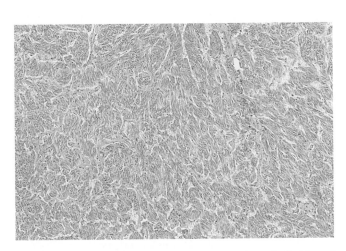

Figure 10-22. Peripheral carcinoid. Mixed epithelioid and spindle cell pattern. (Hematoxylin and eosin.)

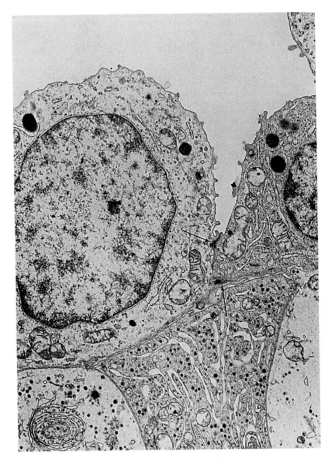

Figure 10-25. Peripheral carcinoid. Tumor cells with numerous DCGs subjacent to a continuous layer of alveolar lining cells held together by well-formed desmosomes (*arrows*). No specialized attachments between alveolar lining cells and tumor cells. (TEM ×16,200.) (From Bonikos et al 1976 Cancer 37:1977–1998.)

with spindle cell morphology, mitotic activity, and/or small foci of necrosis have been inappropriately classified as TCs rather than WDNECs. On the other hand, the peripheral location, spindle cell pattern, and finding of metastases in an otherwise TC are not adequate criteria in themselves to classify the lesion as WDNEC.

No histopathologic indicators predict which TCs are likely to metastasize. Flow cytometric DNA analysis does not provide clinically useful information additional to the results of routine histologic examination.[192, 193]

Neuroendocrine Carcinoma

WDNEC and MDNEC constitute approximately 0.5% of all lung tumors. They present most commonly in men during the sixth decade as solitary, large, peripheral lung nodules, which range generally from 2 to 5 cm in greatest diameter and display extensive hemorrhage or necrosis on cut section (Fig. 10–26). Approximately half the cases have regional lymph node metastases at presentation.

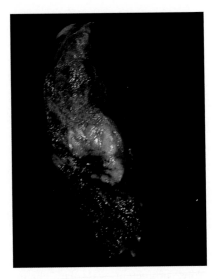

Figure 10-26. WDNEC. Subpleural nodule with anthracotic scar and focal necrosis. Note infiltrative border.

Well Differentiated

WDNEC is a well-differentiated neoplasm with a distinctly organoid or "carcinoid-like" growth pattern. It has an apparent loss of architectural organization, between 2 and 10 mitoses per hpf, and small foci of necrosis. WDNEC most closely resembles the "atypical carcinoid" as originally described by Arrigoni and associates.[147] and recently modified by WHO 1999[144] and the WDNEC, subsets I and II, of Gould and colleagues (Fig. 10–27).[157] The number of mitoses and the presence of necrosis are the most important criteria separating WDNEC from TC. Invariably, necrosis is present and can be readily demonstrated in adequately sampled tumors. The characteristic pattern is that of punctate central necrosis of cell groups (Fig. 10–28). Other more subjective features of WDNEC are increased cellularity, mild to moderate cellular and nuclear pleomorphism, nucleoli, and a spindle cell form (Fig. 10–29).

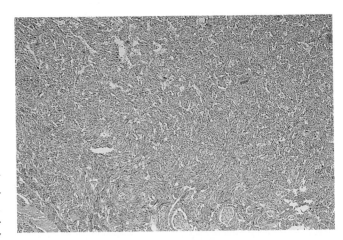

Figure 10-27. WDNEC. Distinctly organoid architecture evocative of TC on low power. Note scattered foci of punctate nerosis. (Hematoxylin and eosin.)

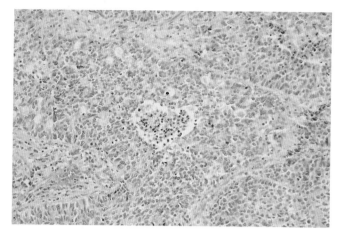

Figure 10–28. WDNEC. Mitoses, mild to moderate nuclear pleomorphism, and focal necrosis distinguish WDNEC from TC. (Hematoxylin and eosin.)

Moderately Differentiated

MDNEC is a moderately differentiated neoplasm with a distinctly organoid or "carcinoid-like" growth pattern. It has a prominent loss of architectural organization and cellular discohesion, 11 or more mitoses/10 hpf, and conspicuous areas of central necrosis. MDNEC most closely resembles the "atypical carcinoid" described by Mills and coworkers,[150]

the WDNEC, type III, of Gould and colleagues,[157] and a number of cases designated as LCNEC by WHO 1999 (Fig. 10–30A,B).[144] The distinct, organoid architecture of MDNEC is the cardinal feature that separates it from PDNEC-SC and LCNEC.

The neoplastic cells are pleomorphic with abundant cytoplasm and nuclei with granular to coarsely clumped chromatin and often conspicuous nucleoli. Sometimes the mitotic count may be as high as in PDNEC-SC. The neoplastic cells are arranged in discrete clusters or anastomosing trabeculae, with prominent peripheral palisading, and are separated by varying degrees of fibroblastic stroma containing chronic inflammatory cells. Rosette-like structures and true lumina are not uncommon. Occasionally small foci of PDNEC-SC-like areas may be present adjacent to areas of necrosis.

Ultrastructurally, WDNEC and MDNEC exhibit smaller (140 to 180 nm) and less numerous DCGs than does TC (Fig. 10–30C). The percentage, distribution, and intensity of immunohistochemical staining for both pan-NE and hormonal markers are less than in TC.

Behavior

WDNEC and MDNEC strictly defined according to the preceding criteria exhibit an intermediate behavior between those of TC and PDNEC-SC.

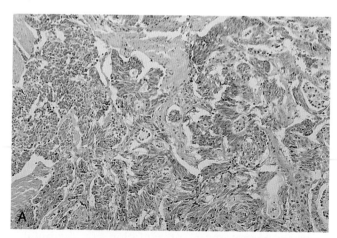

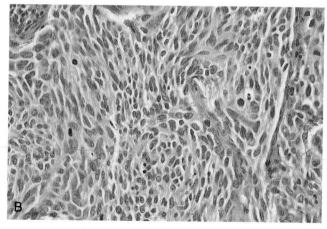

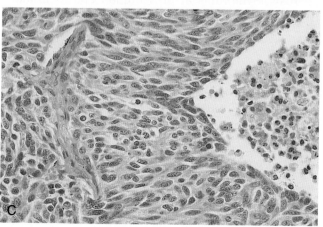

Figure 10–29. WDNEC. *A,* Peripheral nodule with mixed spindle cell and organoid pattern, having the low-power appearance of spindle cell peripheral carcinoid. *B,* Hyperchromatic spindle cells with inconspicuous nucleoli, a moderate amount of cytoplasm, and numerous mitoses. *C,* Discrete area of necrosis. The lack of finely granular ("salt and pepper") nuclear chromatin and the absence of extensive areas of necrosis distinguish this tumor from PDNEC-SC. (Hematoxylin and eosin.)

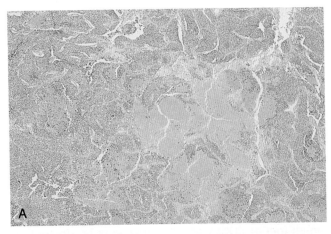

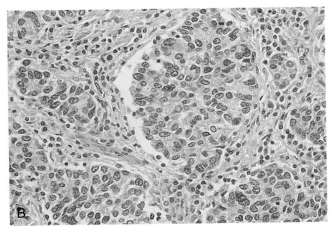

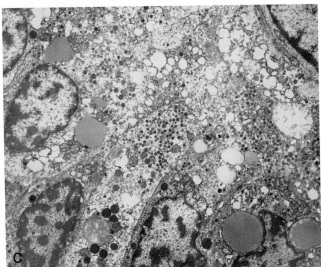

Figure 10–30. MDNEC. *A,* Distinctly organoid or "carcinoid-like" growth pattern, with areas of geographic necrosis. *B,* Nests of pleomorphic tumor cells with abundant cytoplasm and nuclei, with granular to coarsely clumped chromatin and often conspicuous nucleoli. Sometimes the mitotic town may be as high as in PDNEC-SC. The neoplastic cells are separated by varying degrees of fibroblastic stroma containing chronic inflammatory cells. The lack of vesicular nuclei, prominent nucleoli, and a marked-to-moderate host response around tumor nests distinguish MDNEC from PDNEC-LC. (Hematoxylin and eosin.) *C,* Nuclei with granular to coarsely clumped, irregular chromatin and often conspicuous nucleoli. Number of DCGS are less than TC but more than PDNEC-SC. (TEM ×200.) (Courtesy of William Thelmo, M.D.)

Approximately 70% metastasize, and the 5-year survival rate ranges from 25% to 68% (Table 10–4). Although MDNEC has a distinctly worse clinical course than that of WDNEC, it has a significantly longer survival than similarly treated stage I and stage II SCLC.[157] Recently, large tumor size, large cell or mixed SC/LC morphology, peripheral localization, and advanced stage have been shown to be adverse prognostic indicators, whereas mitotic activity and the presence of necrosis did not appear to influence stage or behavior.[148]

Poorly Differentiated

Small Cell Type

PDNEC, small cell type (PDNEC-SC), occurs predominantly among men in the seventh and eighth decades of life and accounts for approximately 25% of all lung cancers. Most cases arise in major bronchi and present as a perihilar mass (Fig. 10–31). The tumor is gray-white, with extensive necrosis. Symptoms at presentation are attributable to the primary growth, to metastatic disease, or

Table 10-4. Prognosis of Well-differentiated Neuroendocrine Carcinoma (WDNEC)

References	No. Cases	WDNEC*,†	SCLC	2-yr Survival (%)	> 5-yr Survival (%)
Arrigoni et al.[147]	23	23		70	
Mills et al.[150]	17	17		53	
Carter et al.[153]	15	15		57	
Warren et al.[152]	23	12	11	75/9	25/0
Lequaglie et al.*[151]	16	16		80	68

* Includes cases of moderately differentiated neuroendocrine carcinoma.
† Stage I (T1N0, T2N0)
SCLC, small cell lung carcinoma.

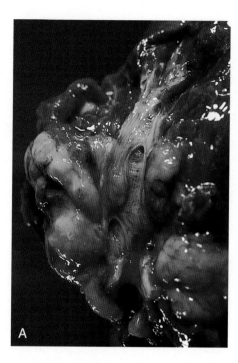

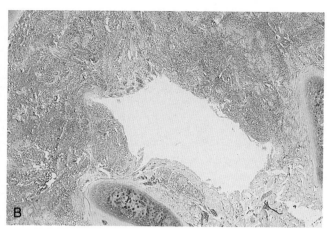

Figure 10–31. PDNEC-SC. Perihilar mass. *A,* Large, gray-white mass compressing the central airway. *B,* Sheets of hyperchromatic tumor cells infiltrate bronchial mucosa and extend into bronchial cartilage.

less commonly to paraneoplastic syndrome. Endobronchial lesions are unusual, and less than 5% present as peripheral nodules.

PDNEC-SC is a poorly differentiated tumor consisting of hyperchromatic cells with scant cytoplasm, finely granular ("salt and pepper") nuclear chromatin, and absent or inconspicuous nucleoli (Fig. 10–32). The cells may be ovoid, polygonal, or fusiform, often show prominent nuclear molding, and range in size from 1.5 to 4 times the diameter of a lymphocyte. The tumor cells correspond to the oat cell and intermediate cell types of the WHO 1981[139] classification (Fig. 10–33). Mitoses are abundant. The tumor cells grow in sheets without a particular pattern. Sometimes rudimentary trabeculae,

tubular formations, and rosettes are present. Tumor cells may palisade around blood vessels, forming "pseudo-rosettes" (Fig. 10–34). A desmoplastic or inflammatory reaction is minimal or absent. Extensive necrosis is common. Two properties—crush artifact, a coalescing and basophilic smearing of groups of tumor cells, and the impregnation of vessel walls by the released tumor DNA of necrotic tumor cells (Azzopardi's effect)—are characteristic and practically pathognomonic features of this tumor (Fig. 10–35).[194–196]

DCGs can generally be found in PDNEC-SC, provided the material is sufficient for evaluation.[197] They are small, uniform, and approximately 120 nm in diameter. In most cases they are sparse and found clustered in dendritic processes (Fig. 10–36). The SC/LC variant contains fewer DCGs and more desmosomes.[198] The LC variant shows prominent nucleoli, more DCGs than in SC, and prominent cytoplasmic lumina and desmosomal attachments (Fig. 10–37). Immunohistochemistry for pan-NE markers and hormonal markers is readily demonstrable, in PDNEC-SC, -SC/LC, and -LC, although often focally and less intensively than in TC.

Mixed Small Cell/Large Cell

PDNEC, mixed small cell/large cell (PDNEC-SC/LC), is characterized by an admixture of larger cells approximately twice the size of PDNEC-SC, with abundant eosinophilic cytoplasm and vesicular nuclei with prominent nucleoli. They show marked pleomorphism, polygonal or fusiform shape, and very numerous mitoses. These larger cells may intermingle with the small cell component, may form distinct areas, or may constitute a significant proportion of the tumor (Fig. 10–38). Architecturally, solid clus-

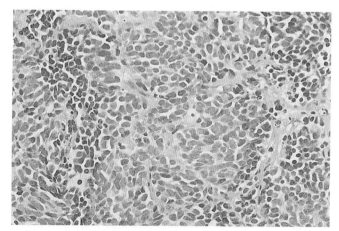

Figure 10–32. PDNEC-SC. Hyperchromatic cells with scant cytoplasm, finely granular ("salt and pepper") nuclear chromatin, and absent or inconspicuous nucleoli. (Hematoxylin and eosin.)

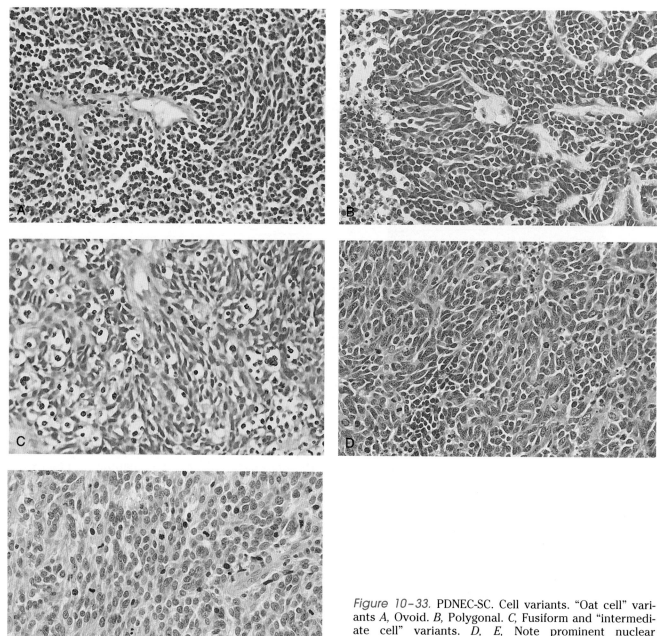

Figure 10–33. PDNEC-SC. Cell variants. "Oat cell" variants *A*, Ovoid. *B*, Polygonal. *C*, Fusiform and "intermediate cell" variants. *D*, *E*, Note prominent nuclear molding in the polygonal cell variant. The intermediate cell variant shows larger cells with more vesicular nuclear chromatin, conspicuous nucleoli, and cytoplasm. (Hematoxylin and eosin.)

ters of large cells often display central necrosis and peripheral palisading.

Large Cell Type

PDNEC, large cell type (PDNEC-LC), is a subtype of PDNEC in which the large cell component constitutes the entire tumor. PDNEC-LC may be either central or peripheral, or they may extensively replace large areas of the lung. Usually they present as large, circumscribed masses, with extensive areas of hemorrhage and necrosis characterized by solid clusters of loosely arranged tumor cells and

peripheral palisading. These clusters are often separated by stromal fibrosis with a marked chronic inflammatory infiltrate (Fig. 10–39). Extensive infarct-like central necrosis is present (Fig. 10–40). Often, in adequately sampled lesions, a SC component is discernible (Fig. 10–41). Foci of adenomatous or squamous differentiation may be present (Fig. 10–42). This tumor most closely resembles certain LCNEC described by Travis and associates[159] and a proportion of the "NE carcinomas of intermediate type" described by Gould and colleagues.[18] The main morphologic feature that distinguishes these tumors from WDNEC and MDNEC is the noncohesive

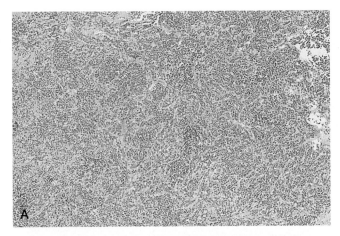

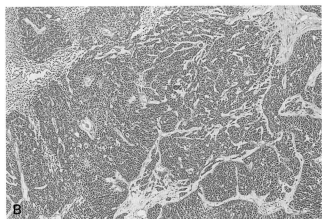

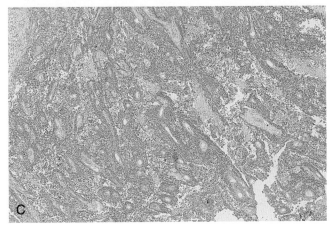

Figure 10–34. PDNEC-SC. Histologic patterns. *A,* Monotonous sheets of small, uniform hyperchromatic cells in sheets without a particular pattern. *B,* Sometimes rudimentary trabeculae, tubular formations, and rosettes are present. *C,* Well-preserved tumor cells may palisade around blood vessels, forming "pseudorosettes." Note pyknotic tumor cells undergoing necrosis away from vessels. (Hematoxylin and eosin.)

sheets of high-grade neoplastic cells that lack a distinct organoid architecture. The main morphologic feature that distinguishes PDNEC-LC from non-NE large cell carcinoma is the vaguely NE appearance manifest by the nuclear features and the peripheral palisading of the tumor cells. Sometimes the ambiguities of morphologic NE features require immunohistochemistry and electron microscopy to clarify the presence of NE differentiation.

Figure 10–35. PDNEC-SC. Impregnation of vessel walls by the released tumor DNA of necrotic tumor cells (Azzopardi's effect). (Hematoxylin and eosin.)

Combined

PDNEC, combined (PDNEC-C), contains in addition to the SC component a significant, separate area of squamous carcinoma or adenocarcinoma (Fig. 10–43). This phenomenon has been seen in PDNEC-SC, either with disease progression or in response to chemotherapy.[129] PDNEC-C is the least frequent variant of PDNEC-SC, and it has been reported to constitute about 5% of all PDNEC-SC at the time of diagnosis. The exact frequency is difficult to ascertain because of the small tumor sample size at the time of initial surgical biopsy. It is seen much more frequently in autopsy series.

Behavior

PDNEC-SC is an extremely aggressive neoplasm, with a median survival of patients of less than 2 years. There is some evidence to suggest that PDNEC-SC/LC are more aggressive and more chemoresistant than PDNEC-SC, but other studies do not show any significant difference in their behavior. Whether PDNEC-C has a worse or better prognosis than purely small cell lesions is unclear.[199] Although the response to chemotherapy and median survival is similar, prolonged survival has been observed in patients with PDNEC-C who underwent resection.[200] PDNEC-LC identified by histologic examination have a remarkably

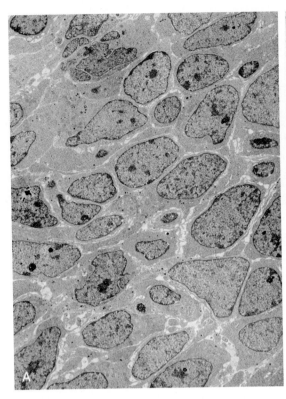

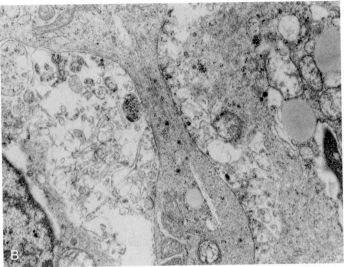

Figure 10-36. PDNEC-SC. *A,* Cells with high nuclear-to-cytoplasmic ratio, characteristic nuclear chromatin, and paucity of organelles. (TEM ×3500.) *B,* Few DCGs are present in the cytoplasmic process. (TEM ×23,000.) (From Mackay B, Lukeman JM, Ordóñez NG: Tumors of the Lung. WB Saunders, Philadelphia, 1991, pp. 226, 228.)

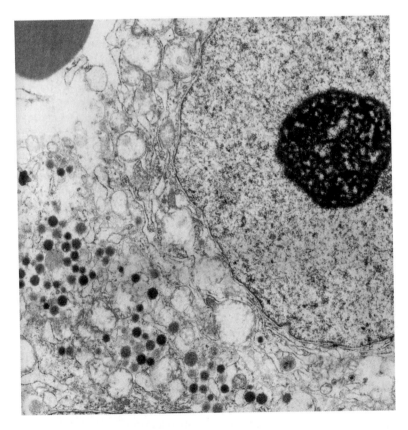

Figure 10-37. PDNEC-LC. Tumor cell with huge nucleolus and numerous DCGs in cytoplasm. (TEM ×43,000.) (From Dail DH, Hammar SP: Pulmonary Pathology. Springer-Verlag, 1994, p. 1235.)

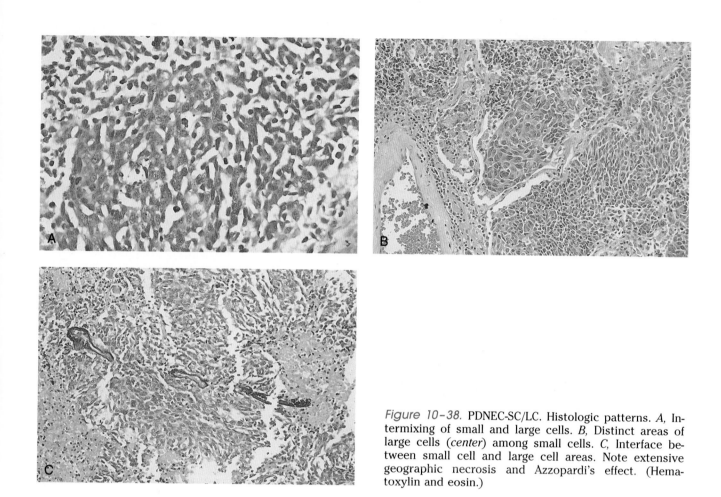

Figure 10–38. PDNEC-SC/LC. Histologic patterns. *A,* Intermixing of small and large cells. *B,* Distinct areas of large cells (*center*) among small cells. *C,* Interface between small cell and large cell areas. Note extensive geographic necrosis and Azzopardi's effect. (Hematoxylin and eosin.)

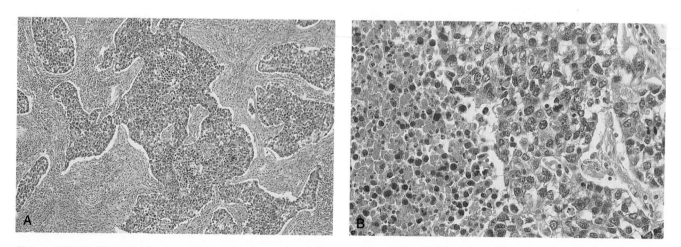

Figure 10–39. PDNEC-LC. *A,* Solid clusters of loosely arranged tumor cells with vague peripheral palisading and separated by stromal fibrosis with a marked chronic inflammatory infiltrate. *B,* Tumor clusters composed of large cells with prominent nucleoli and vesicular chromatin twice the size of SCLC cells. (Hematoxylin and eosin.)

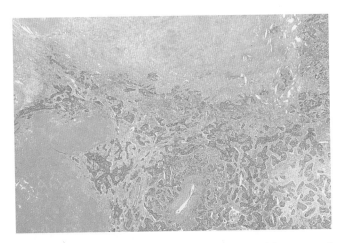

Figure 10–40. PDNEC-LC. Extensive, infarct-like, central necrosis. (Hematoxylin and eosin.)

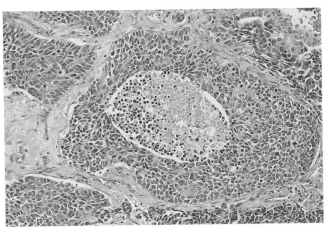

Figure 10–41. PDNEC-LC. Area of PDNEC-SC. Note the minimal desmoplasia and "intermediate" SC cytology. (Hematoxylin and eosin.)

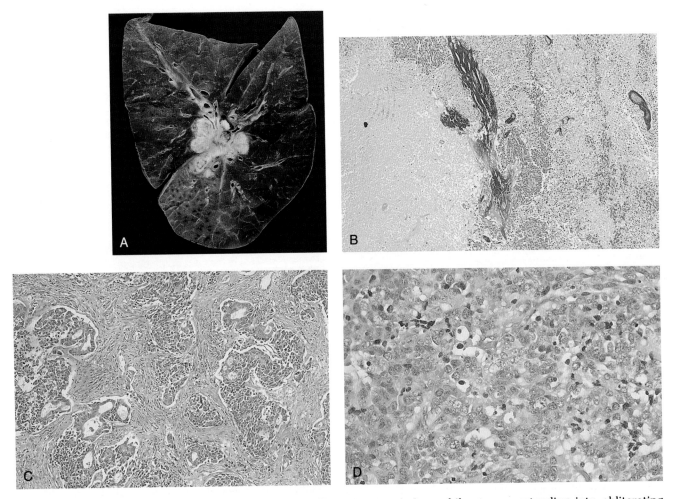

Figure 10–42. PDNEC. Plasticity of differentiation in NE carcinoma. *A,* Large hilar tumor extending into obliterating main stem bronchus and extending into lung parenchyma and hilar lymph nodes. *B,* Area of PDNEC-SC with extensive necrosis and Azzopardi's effect. *C,* Area of SC and adenocarcinoma. *D,* Area of large cell carcinoma. (Hematoxylin and eosin.)

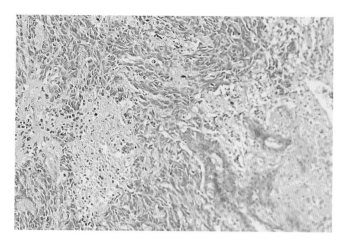

Figure 10–43. PDNEC-C. Mixed PDNEC-SC and adenocarcinoma. (Mucicarmine.)

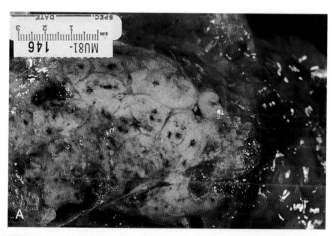

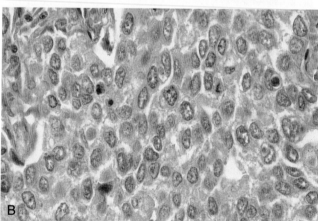

Figure 10–44. NSCLC-NE. *A,* Large, lobulated peripheral lung mass with necrosis and hemorrhage. *B,* Large, undifferentiated tumor cells with prominent nucleoli and abundant cytoplasm. No evidence of NE differentiation on light microscopy. Tumor cells were positive for SY38 and ChrA by immunohistochemistry. (Hematoxylin and eosin.)

poor prognosis, similar to that of PDNEC-SC even in very early-stage disease.[201] Adjuvant therapy did not improve survival.[202, 203]

Non-SCLC with NE Differentiation

NSCLC-NE is defined as a lung carcinoma that does not show NE differentiation by light microscopy but rather demonstrates evidence of NE differentiation by immunohistochemistry or electron microscopy (Fig. 10–44). NSCLC-NE includes tumors with overt squamous carcinoma and adenocarcinoma differentiation, as well as those with undifferentiated LC morphology. A number of neoplasms previously described as "atypical endocrine tumors" would be included in this category.[168, 204] Approximately 10% to 15% of NSCLCs will show NE differentiation if examined by immunohistochemistry or electron microscopy.[100, 166] NSCLC-NE expresses *hASH1* and should be regarded as a neoplasm that shares a characteristic NE phenotype with TCs, WD-NECs, MDNECs, and PDNECs.[16]

The significance of NE differentiation in NSCLC is unclear. Some studies suggest that expression of NE markers may be an unfavorable prognostic factor,[171, 205] whereas others do not.[206, 207] Similarly, some evidence, especially from in vitro studies of cell lines, has suggested that NSCLC-NE may be responsive to chemotherapy;[130] however, recent clinical studies have shown this not to be the case.[208]

Acknowledgment

To my mentor and friend, Professor Dionysios S. Bonikos, MD, who first introduced me to the marvels of the neuroendocrine lung.

References

1. Van Lommel A, Bolle T, Fannes W, et al.: The pulmonary neuroendocrine system: The past decade. Arch Histol Cytol 1999; 62:1.
2. Cutz E: Neuroendocrine cells of the lung. An overview of morphologic characteristics and development. Exp Lung Res 1982; 3:185.
3. Watanabe H: Pathological studies of neuroendocrine cells in human embryonic and fetal lung. Light microscopical, immunohistochemical, and electron microscopical approaches. Acta Pathol Jpn 1988; 38:59.
4. Sheppard MN, Marangos PJ, Bloom SR, et al.: Neuron specific enolase: A marker for the early development of nerves and endocrine cells. Life Sci 1984; 34:265.
5. Hage E: Electron microscopic identification of several types of endocrine cells in the bronchial epithelium of human foetuses. Z Zellforsch 1973; 141:401.
6. Cutz E: Cytomorphology and differentiation of airway epithelium in developing human lung. In McDowell EM, ed.: Lung Carcinomas. Churchill Livingstone, Edinburgh, 1987, p. 11.
7. Stahlman MT, Gray ME: Ontogeny of neuroendocrine cells in human fetal lung. I. An electron microscopic study. Lab Invest 1984; 51:449.
8. Jeffrey PK, Reid LM: Ultrastructure of airway epithelium and submucosal glands during development. In Hodson WA, ed.:

Development of the Lung. Marcel Dekker, New York, 1977, p. 67.

9. Scheuermann DW: Comparative histology of pulmonary neuroendocrine cell system in mammalian lungs. Microsc Res Tech 1997; 37:31.

10. Gosney JR: Development and distribution of the pulmonary endocrine system. In Pulmonary Endocrine Pathology. Butterworth-Heinemann, Oxford, 1992, p. 25.

11. Cutz E, Gillan JE, Track NS, eds.: Pulmonary Endocrine Cells in the Developing Human Lung and During Neonatal Adaptation. WB Saunders, Philadelphia, 1984.

12. Gosney JR: Neuroendocrine cell populations in postnatal human lungs: Minimal variation from childhood to old age. Anat Rec 1993; 236:177.

13. Weston JA: The embryonic neural crest. Migration and differentiation and possible contributions to the development of the lung. In Becker KI, Gazdar AF, eds.: Endocrine Lung in Health and Disease. WB Saunders, Philadelphia, 1984, p. 79.

14. Sorokin SP, Hoyt RF Jr, Shaffer MJ: Ontogeny of neuroepithelial bodies: Correlations with mitogenesis and innervation. Microsc Res Tech 1997; 37:43.

15. Ito T, Nogawa H, Udaka N, et al.: Development of pulmonary neuroendocrine cells of fetal hamster in explant culture. Lab Invest 1997; 77:449.

16. Borges M, Linnoila RI, van de Velde HJ, et al.: An achaete-scute homologue essential for neuroendocrine differentiation in the lung. Nature 1997; 386:852.

17. Yeger H, Speirs V, Youngson C, et al.: Pulmonary neuroendocrine cells in cultures of human infant airway mucosa from postmortem tissues. Am J Respir Cell Mol Biol 1996; 15:232.

18. Gould VE, Linnoila I, Memoli VA, et al.: Biology of disease: Neuroendocrine components of the bronchopulmonary tract: Hyperplasias, dysplasias, and neoplasms. Lab Invest 1983; 49:519.

19. Blobel GA, Gould VE, Moll R, et al.: Coexpression of neuroendocrine markers and epithelial cytoskeletal proteins in bronchopulmonary neuroendocrine neoplasms. Lab Invest 1985; 52:39.

20. Gosney JR, Sissons MCJ, Allibone R: Neuroendocrine cell populations in normal human lungs. A quantitative study. Thorax 1988; 43:878.

21. Tateishi R: Distribution of argyrophil cells in adult human lungs. Arch Pathol 1973; 96:198.

22. Terzakis JA, Sommers SC, Andersson B: Neurosecretory appearing cells of human segmental bronchi. Lab Invest 1972; 26:127.

23. Frölich F: "Helle zelle" der Bronchialschleimhaut und ihre Beziehungen zum Problem der Chemoreceptoren. Frankfurt Ztschr Z Pathol 1949; 60:517.

24. Feyrter F: Zur Pathologie der argyrophilen Helle-Zelle-Organes im Bronchialbaum des Menschen. Virchous Arch [Anat Pathol] 1954; 325:723.

25. Glorieux R: Les cellules argentaffines du poumon et leurs connexions avec le système nerveux. Arch Biol 1963; 74:377.

26. Lauweryns JM, Peuskens JC: Neuro-epithelial bodies (neuroreceptor or secretory organs?) in human infant bronchial and bronchiolar epithelium. Anat Rec 1972; 172:471.

27. Bensch KG, Gordon GB, Miller LR: Studies on the bronchial counterpart of the Kultschitzky (argentaffin) cell and innervation of bronchial glands. J Ultrastruct Res 1965; 12:668.

28. Gmelich JT, Bensch KG, Liebow AA: Cells of Kultchitsky type in bronchioles and their relation to the origin of peripheral carcinoid tumor. Lab Invest 1967; 17:88.

29. Bonikos DS, Bensch KG: Endocrine cells of bronchial and bronchiolar epithelium. Am J Med 1977; 63:765.

30. Scheuermann DW: Morphology and cytochemistry of the endocrine epithelial system of the lung. Int Rev Cytol 1987; 106:35.

31. Wiedenmann B, Franke WW, Kuhn C, et al.: Synaptophysin: A marker protein for neuroendocrine cells and neoplasms. Proc Natl Acad Sci U S A 1986; 83:3500.

32. Schmitt-Graff A, Muller H, Rancso C, et al.: [Molecules of regulated secretion are differentiation markers of neuroendocrine tumors.] Verh Dtsch Ges Pathol 1997; 81:157.

33. Hamid Q, Corrin B, Sheppard MN, et al.: Expression of chromogranin A mRNA in small cell carcinoma of the lung. J Pathol 1991; 163:293.

34. Polak JM, Becker KL, Cutz E, et al.: Lung endocrine cell markers, peptides, and amines. Anat Rec 1993; 236:169.

35. Stahlman MT, Gray ME: Colocalization of peptide hormones in neuroendocrine cells of human fetal and newborn lungs: An electron microscopic study. Anat Rec 1993; 236:206.

36. Stahlman MT, Gray ME: Immunogold EM localization of neurochemicals in human pulmonary neuroendocrine cells. Microsc Res Tech 1997; 37:77.

37. Van den Steen P, Verbeken EK, Van Lommel A, et al.: Immunoreactivity for the alpha-subunit of the pituitary glycoprotein hormones in pulmonary neuroendocrine cells of developing human lung and various perinatal diseases. Regul Pept 1997; 70:37.

38. Giaid A, Polak JM, Gaitonde V, et al.: Distribution of endothelin-like immunoreactivity and mRNA in the developing and adult human lung. Am J Respir Cell Mol Biol 1991; 4:50.

39. Lee I, Gould VE, Moll R, et al.: Synaptophysin expressed in the bronchopulmonary tract: Neuroendocrine cells, neuroepithelial bodies, and neuroendocrine neoplasms. Differentiation 1987; 34:115.

40. Yuminamochi T, Ishii Y, Nakazawa K, et al.: [Immunohistochemical study on keratin no. 8, 18 and 19 expression of carcinoid tumors.] Rinsho Byori 1998; 46:163.

41. Fujita T: Concept of paraneurons. Arch Histol Jpn 1977; 10(suppl):1.

42. Lauweryns JM, Cokelaere M: Intrapulmonary neuro-epithelial bodies: Hypoxia-sensitive neuro(chemo-)receptors. Experientia 1973; 29:1384.

43. Lauweryns JM, Cokelaere M: Hypoxia-sensitive neuro-epithelial bodies. Intrapulmonary secretory neuroreceptors, modulated by the CNS. Z Zellforsch Mikrosk Anat 1973; 145:521.

44. Wang D, Youngson C, Wong V, et al.: NADPH-oxidase and a hydrogen peroxide–sensitive K+ channel may function as an oxygen sensor complex in airway chemoreceptors and small cell lung carcinoma cell lines. Proc Natl Acad Sci U S A 1996; 93:13182.

45. Youngson C, Nurse C, Yeger H, et al.: Oxygen sensing in airway chemoreceptors. Nature 1993; 365:153.

46. Lauweryns JM, Tierens A, Decramer M: Influence of hypercapnia on rabbit intrapulmonary neuroepithelial bodies: Microfluorimetric and morphometric study. Eur Respir J 1990; 3:182.

47. Miller MS, Fan M, Schuller HS: Induction of *c-fos* expression following stimulation of pulmonary neuroendocrine cell proliferation by alterations in $CO_2/C.O.$ concentration. Int J Oncol 1996; 8:423.

48. Lauweryns J, Van Lommel A: Effect of various vagotomy procedures on the reaction to hypoxia of rabbit neuroepithelial bodies: Modulation by intrapulmonary axon reflexes? Exp Lung Res 1986; 11:319.

49. Lauweryns JM, De Brock V, Decramer M: Effects of unilateral vagal stimulation on intrapulmonary neuroepithelial bodies. J Appl Physiol 1987; 63:1781.

50. Gosney JR: Physiology of pulmonary endocrine system. In Pulmonary Endocrine Pathology. Butterworth-Heineman, Oxford, 1992, p. 42.

51. Chua BA, Perks AM: The pulmonary neuroendocrine system and drainage of the fetal lung: Effects of serotonin. Gen Comp Endocrinol 1999; 113:374.

52. Sakamoto N, Doi M, Ohashi N, et al.: [Immunohistochemical study on pulmonary neuroendocrine cells containing calcitonin gene-related peptide in sudden infant death syndrome.] Nippon Hoigaku Zasshi 1998; 52:27.

53. Ijsselstijn H, Hung N, de Jongste JC, et al.: Calcitonin gene-related peptide expression is altered in pulmonary neuroendocrine cells in developing lungs of rats with congenital diaphragmatic hernia. Am J Respir Cell Mol Biol 1998; 19:278.

54. Aguayo SM, Schuyler WE, Murtagh JJ Jr, et al.: Regulation of lung branching morphogenesis by bombesin-like peptides and neutral endopeptidase. Am J Respir Cell Mol Biol 1994; 10:635.

55. Zachary I, Rosengurt E: Focal adhesion kinase (p125^{FAK}): A point of convergence in the action of neuropeptides, integrins, and bombesin-like peptides. Cell 1992; 71:891.

56. Becker KL, Nash D, Silva OL, et al.: Increased serum and urinary calcitonin levels in patients with pulmonary disease. Chest 1981; 79:211.

57. Yiakoumakis E, Proukakis C, Raptis G, et al.: Calcitonin concentrations in lung cancer and non-malignant pulmonary diseases. Oncology 1987; 44:145.

58. Meloni F, Bertolett R, Corsico A, et al.: Bombesin/gastrin releasing peptide levels of peripheral mononuclear cells, monocytes, and alveolar macrophages in chronic bronchitis. Int J Tissue React 1992; 14:195.

59. Aguayo SM.: Neuroendocrine cells and airway wall remodelling in chronic airflow obstruction: A perspective. Monaldi Arch Chest Dis 1994; 49:243.

60. Sunday ME, Yoder BA, Cuttitta F, et al.: Bombesin-like peptide mediates lung injury in a baboon model of bronchopulmonary dysplasia. J Clin Invest 1998; 102:584.

61. Cohen AJ, King TE Jr, Gilman LB, et al.: High expression of neutral endopeptidase in idiopathic diffuse hyperplasia of pulmonary neuroendocrine cells. Am J Respir Crit Care Med 1998; 158:1593.

62. Willett CG, Shahsafei A, Graham SA, et al.: CD10/neutral endopeptidase inhibition augments pulmonary neuroendocrine cell hyperplasia in hamsters treated with diethylnitrosamine and hyperoxia. Am J Respir Cell Mol Biol 1999; 21:13.

63. Cohen AJ, Miller YE: Neuroendocrine differentiation, neuropeptides, and neprilysin. Am J Respir Cell Mol Biol 1999; 21:1.

64. Cutz E, Gillan JE, Bryan AC: Neuroendocrine cells in the developing human lung: Morphologic and functional considerations. Pediatr Pulmonol 1985; 1(suppl.):S21.

65. Di Augustine RP, Jahnke GD, Talley F: Endocrine cells of the guinea pig upper airways. Morphology, distribution and disposition after xenotransplantation in the nude mouse. In Becker KL, Gazdar AF, eds.: The Endocrine Lung in Health and Disease. WB Saunders, Philadelphia, 1984, p. 232.

66. Linnoila RI: Effects of diethylnitrosamine on lung neuroendocrine cells. Exp Lung Res 1982; 3:225.

67. Reynolds SD, Giangreco A, Power JHT, et al.: Two spatially related stem cell populations participate in the generation of the airway following Clara cell ablation [abstract]. Am J Respir Crit Care Med 1999; 159:A439.

68. Reynolds SD, Giangreco A, Power JH, et al.: Neuroepithelial bodies of pulmonary airways serve as a reservoir of progenitor cells capable of epithelial regeneration. Am J Pathol 2000; 156:269.

69. Sheard JDH, Gosney JR: Endocrine cells in tumor-bearing lungs. Thorax 1996; 51:721.

70. Gosney JR: The pulmonary endocrine system in diseased lungs. In Pulmonary Endocrine Pathology. Butterworth-Heinemann, Oxford, 1992, p. 52.

71. Yousem SA, Isaacs A: Pulmonary neuroendocrine cells in the airways of lung allografts. Transplantation 1995; 59:1070.

72. Alshehri M, Cutz E, Banzhoff A, et al.: Hyperplasia of pulmonary neuroendocrine cells in a case of childhood pulmonary emphysema. Chest 1997; 112:553.

73. Johnson JE: Idiopathic hyperplasia of pulmonary neuroendocrine cells [letter; comment]. N Engl J Med 1993; 328:581.

74. Aguayo SM, Miller YE, Waldron JA Jr, et al.: Brief report: Idiopathic diffuse hyperplasia of pulmonary neuroendocrine cells and airways disease [see comments]. N Engl J Med 1992; 327:1285.

75. Armas OA, White DA, Erlandson RA, et al.: Diffuse idiopathic pulmonary neuroendocrine cell proliferation presenting as interstitial lung disease. Am J Surg Pathol 1995; 19:963.

76. Johnson DE, Kulik TJ, Lock JE, et al.: Bombesin-, calcitonin-, and serotonin-immunoreactive pulmonary neuroendocrine cells in acute and chronic neonatal lung disease. Pediatr Pulmonol 1985; 1(3 Suppl):S13.

77. Johnson MD, Gray ME, Stahlman MT: Calcitonin gene-related peptide in human fetal lung and in neonatal lung disease. J Histochem Cytochem 1988; 36:199.

78. Johnson DE, Wobken JD: Calcitonin gene-related peptide immunoreactivity in airway epithelial cells of the human fetus and infant. Cell Tissue Res 1987; 250:579.

79. Gillan JE, Cutz E: Abnormal pulmonary bombesin immunoreactive cells in Wilson-Mikity syndrome (pulmonary dysmaturity) and bronchopulmonary dysplasia. Pediatr Pathol 1993; 13:165.

80. Shenberger JS, Shew RL, Johnson DE: Hyperoxia-induced airway remodeling and pulmonary neuroendocrine cell hyperplasia in the weanling rat. Pediatr Res 1997; 42:539.

81. Durbin J, Thomas P, Langston C, et al.: Gastrin-releasing peptide in hypoplastic lungs. Pediatr Pathol Lab Med 1996; 16:927.

82. Ijsselstijn H, Gaillard JL, de Jongste JC, et al.: Abnormal expression of pulmonary bombesin-like peptide immunostaining cells in infants with congenital diaphragmatic hernia. Pediatr Res 1997; 42:715.

83. Heath D, Yacoub M, Gosney JR, et al.: Pulmonary endocrine cells in hypertensive pulmonary vascular disease. Histopathology 1990; 16:21.

84. Heath D, Madden B, Yacoub M: Pulmonary endocrine cells in plexogenic pulmonary arteriopathy. Physiol Bohemoslov 1990; 39:309.

85. Whitwell F: Tumorlets of the lung. J Pathol Bacteriol 1955; 70:529.

86. Pelosi G, Zancanaro C, Sbabo L, et al.: Development of innumerable neuroendocrine tumorlets in pulmonary lobe scarred by intralobar sequestration. Immunohistochemical and ultrastructural study of an unusual case. Arch Pathol Lab Med 1992; 116:1167.

87. Nagai S, Katakura H, Okazaki T, et al.: [A pulmonary tumorlet with caseous granuloma associated with atypical mycobacterium.] Nihon Kokyuki Gakkai Zasshi 1998; 36:464.

88. Ramon-Capilla M, Arnau Obrer A, Navarro Ibanez R, et al.: [Pulmonary tumorlet. Report of 5 cases.] Arch Bronconeumol 1996; 32:489.

89. Resl M, Kral B, Simek J: [Carcinoid tumorlets and pulmonary hypoxia.] Cesk Patol 1995; 31:84.

90. Klinke F, Bosse U, Hofler H: [The tumorlet carcinoid in bronchiectasis-changed lungs. An example of a multifocal, endocrine tumor.] Pneumologie 1990; 44:607.

91. Bonikos DS, Bensch KG, Jamplis RW: Peripheral pulmonary carcinoid tumors. Cancer 1976; 37:1977.

92. Bonikos DS, Archibald R, Bensch KG: On the origin of the so-called tumorlets of the lung. Hum Pathol 1976; 7:461.

93. Gosney J, Green AR, Taylor W: Appropriate and inappropriate neuroendocrine products in pulmonary tumourlets. Thorax 1990; 45:679.

94. Ranchod M: The histogenesis and development of pulmonary tumorlets. Cancer 1977; 39:1135.

95. Arioglu E, Doppman J, Gomes M, et al.: Cushing's syndrome caused by corticotropin secretion by pulmonary tumorlets. N Engl J Med 1998; 339:883.

96. Churg A, Warnock ML: Pulmonary tumorlet: A form of peripheral carcinoid. Cancer 1976; 37:1469.

97. D'Agati VD, Perzin KH: Carcinoid tumorlets of the lung with metastasis to a peribronchial lymph node: Report of a case and review of the literature. Cancer 1985; 55:2472.

98. Hausman DH, Weimann RB: Pulmonary tumorlets with hilar lymph node metastases. Cancer 1967; 20:1515.

99. Finkelstein SD, Hasegawa T, Colby T, et al.: 11q13 allelic imbalance discriminates pulmonary carcinoids from tumorlets. A microdissection-based genotyping approach useful in clinical practice. Am J Pathol 1999; 155:633.

100. Yesner R: Lung cancer: Pathogenesis and pathology. Clin Chest Med 1993; 14:17.

101. Walch AK, Zitzelsberger HF, Aubele MM, et al.: Typical and atypical carcinoid tumors of the lung are characterized by 11q deletions as detected by comparative genomic hybridization. Am J Pathol 1998; 153:1089.

102. Kovatich A, Friedland DM, Druck T, et al.: Molecular alterations to human chromosome 3p loci in neuroendocrine lung tumors. Cancer 1998; 83:1109.

103. Ullman R, Petzman S, Sharma A, et al.: CGH analysis of large cell neuroendocrine carcinomas reveals patterns of

chromosomal aberrations comparable to SCLC and some atypical carcinoids. Lab Invest 2000; 80:217A.

104. Ullmann R, Schwendel A, Klemen H, et al.: Unbalanced chromosomal aberrations in neuroendocrine lung tumors as detected by comparative genomic hybridization. Hum Pathol 1998; 29:1145.

105. van Waardenburg RC, Meijer C, Pinto-Sietsma SJ, et al.: Effects of c-myc oncogene modulation on differentiation of human small cell lung carcinoma cell lines. Anticancer Res 1998; 18:91.

106. Cook RM, Miller YE, Bunn PA Jr: Small cell lung cancer: Etiology, biology, clinical features, staging, and treatment. Curr Probl Cancer 1993; 17:69.

107. Roncalli M, Doglioni C, Springall DR, et al.: Abnormal p53 expression in lung neuroendocrine tumors. Diagnostic and prognostic implications. Diagn Mol Pathol 1992; 1:129.

108. Barbareschi M, Girlando S, Mauri FA, et al.: Tumour suppressor gene products, proliferation, and differentiation markers in lung neuroendocrine neoplasms. J Pathol 1992; 166:343.

109. Brambilla E, Negoescu A, Gazzeri S, et al.: Apoptosis-related factors p53, Bcl2, and Bax in neuroendocrine lung tumors. Am J Pathol 1996; 149:1941.

110. Harbour JW, Lai SL, Whang-Peng J, et al.: Abnormalities in structure and expression of the human retinoblastoma gene in SCLC. Science 1988; 241:353.

111. Cagle PT, el-Naggar AK, Xu HJ, et al.: Differential retinoblastoma protein expression in neuroendocrine tumors of the lung. Potential diagnostic implications. Am J Pathol 1997; 150:393.

112. Dosaka-Akita H, Cagle PT, Hiroumi H, et al.: Differential retinoblastoma and p16(INK4A) protein expression in neuroendocrine tumors of the lung. Cancer 2000; 88:550.

113. Wang DG, Johnston CF, Sloan JM, et al.: Expression of Bcl-2 in lung neuroendocrine tumours: Comparison with p53. J Pathol 1998; 184:247.

114. Sarvesvaran J, Going JJ, Milroy R, et al.: Is small cell lung cancer the perfect target for anti-telomerase treatment? Carcinogenesis 1999; 20:1649.

115. Moody TW, Cuttitta F: Growth factor and peptide receptors in small cell lung cancer. Life Sci 1993; 52:1161.

116. Shipp MA, Tarr GE, Chen CY, et al.: CD10/neutral endopeptidase 24.11 hydrolyzes bombesin-like peptides and regulates the growth of small cell carcinomas of the lung. Proc Natl Acad Sci USA 1991; 88:10662.

117. Iwai N, Martinez A, Miller MJ, et al.: Autocrine growth loops dependent on peptidyl alpha-amidating enzyme as targets for novel tumor cell growth inhibitors [in process citation]. Lung Cancer 1999; 23:209.

118. Johnson BE, Kelley MJ: Autocrine growth factors and neuroendocrine markers in the development of small-cell lung cancer. Oncology 1998; 12:11.

119. Levy R, Andrieu JM, Even P: [Biology of small-cell bronchogenic carcinoma: Recent advances.] Bull Cancer 1992; 79:25.

120. Schuller HM, McGavin MD, Orloff M, et al.: Simultaneous exposure to nicotine and hyperoxia causes tumors in hamsters. Lab Invest 1995; 73:448.

121. Schuller HM: Nitrosamine-induced lung carcinogenesis and Ca2+/calmodulin antagonists. Cancer Res 1992; 52:2723S.

122. Schuller HM, Witschi HP, Nylen E, et al.: Pathobiology of lung tumors induced in hamsters by 4-(methylnitrosamino)-1-(3-pyridyl)-1-butanone and the modulating effect of hyperoxia. Cancer Res 1990; 50:1960.

123. Nylen ES, Becker KL, Joshi PA, et al.: Pulmonary bombesin and calcitonin in hamsters during exposure to hyperoxia and diethylnitrosamine. Am J Respir Cell Mol Biol 1990; 2:25.

124. Schuller HM, Becker KL, Witschi HP: An animal model for neuroendocrine lung cancer. Carcinogenesis 1988; 9:293.

125. Sunday ME, Willet CG: Induction and spontaneous regression of intense pulmonary neuroendocrine cell differentiation in a model of preneoplastic lung injury. Cancer Res 1992; 52:2677S.

126. Sunday ME, Haley KJ, Sikorski K, et al.: Calcitonin-driven v-Ha-ras induces multilineage pulmonary epithelial hyperplasias and neoplasms. Oncogene 1999; 18:4336.

127. Reznik-Schuller H: Sequential morphologic alterations in the bronchial epithelium of Syrian golden hamsters during N-nitrosomorpholine-induced pulmonary tumorigenesis. Am J Pathol 1977; 89:59.

128. Reznik-Schuller H: Ultrastructural alterations of APUD cells during nitrosamine-induced lung carcinogenesis. J Pathol 1976; 121:79.

129. Brereton HD, Mathews MM, Costa J, et al.: Mixed anaplastic small-cell and squamous-cell carcinoma of the lung. Ann Intern Med 1978; 88:805.

130. Vuitch F, Sekido Y, Fong K, et al.: Neuroendocrine tumors of the lung. Pathology and molecular biology. Chest Surg Clin North Am 1997; 7:21.

131. Chen H, Biel MA, Borges MW, et al.: Tissue-specific expression of human achaete-scute homologue-1 in neuroendocrine tumors: Transcriptional regulation by dual inhibitory regions. Cell Growth Differ 1997; 8:677.

132. Chen H, Thiagalingam A, Chopra H, et al.: Conservation of the Drosophila lateral inhibition pathway in human lung cancer: A hairy-related protein (HES-1) directly represses achaete-scute homolog-1 expression. Proc Natl Acad Sci USA 1997; 94:5355.

133. Nagle RB, Payne CM, Clark VA: Comparison of the usefulness of histochemistry and ultrastructural cytochemistry in the identification of neuroendocrine neoplasms. Am J Clin Pathol 1986; 85:289.

134. Senderovitz T, Skov BG, Hirsch FR: Neuroendocrine characteristics in malignant lung tumors: Implications for diagnosis, treatment, and prognosis [review]. Cancer Treat Res 1995; 72:143.

135. Carbone DP, Koros AM, Linnoila RI, et al.: Neural cell adhesion molecule expression and messenger RNA splicing patterns in lung cancer cell lines are correlated with neuroendocrine phenotype and growth morphology. Cancer Res 1991; 51:6142.

136. Sheppard MN: Neuroendocrine differentiation in lung tumours. Thorax 1991; 46:843.

137. Hirsch FR, Matthews MJ, Aisner S, et al.: Histopathologic classification of small cell lung cancer. Cancer 1988; 62:973.

138. Yesner R: Classification of lung cancer histology. N Engl J Med 1985; 312:652.

139. World Health Organization: Histological typing of lung tumors. In Sobin LH, ed.: International Histological Classification of Tumors, 2nd ed. World Health Organization, Geneva, 1981, p. 23.

140. Kreyberg L, Liebow AA, Vehlinger EA: Histological typing of lung tumors. In Torloni H, ed.: International Classification of Tumors. World Health Organization, Geneva, 1967, p. 21.

141. Carney DN, Matthews MJ, Ihde DC, et al.: Influence of histologic subtype of small cell carcinoma of the lung on clinical presentation, response to therapy, and survival. J Natl Cancer Inst 1980; 65:1225.

142. Fushimi H, Kikui M, Morino H, et al.: Detection of large cell component in small cell lung carcinoma by combined cytologic and histologic examinations and its clinical implication. Cancer 1992; 70:599.

143. Radice PA, Matthews MJ, Ihde DC, et al.: The clinical behavior are of "mixed" small cell/large cell carcinoma compared to "pure" small cell subtypes. Cancer 1982; 50:2894.

144. World Health Organization: Histological typing of lung and pleural tumors. In Sobin LH, ed.: International Histological Classification of Tumors. World Health Organization, Geneva, 1999, p. 1.

145. Warren WH, Gould VE: Differential diagnosis of small cell neuroendocrine carcinoma of the lung. Chest Surg Clin North Am 1997; 7:49.

146. Engelbreth-Holm J: Benign bronchial adenomas. Acta Chir Scand 1945; 90:383.

147. Arrigoni MG, Woolner LB, Burnatz PE: Atypical carcinoid tumors of the lung. J Thorac Cardiovasc Surg 1972; 64:413.

148. Valli M, Fabris GA, Dewar A, et al.: Atypical carcinoid tumour of the lung: A study of 33 cases with prognostic features. Histopathology 1994; 24:363.

149. Choplin RH, Kawamoto EH, Dyer RB, et al.: Atypical carcinoid of the lung: Radiographic features. AJR Am J Roentgenol 1986; 146:665.

150. Mills SE, Walker AN, Cooper PH, et al.: Atypical carcinoid tumor of the lung. Am J Surg Pathol 1982; 6:643.
151. Lequaglie C, Patriarca C, Cataldo I, et al.: Prognosis of resected well-differentiated neuroendocrine carcinoma of the lung [see comments]. Chest 1991; 100:1053.
152. Warren WH, Memoli VA, Jordan AG, et al.: Reevaluation of pulmonary neoplasms resected as small cell carcinomas. Significance of distinguishing between well-differentiated and small cell neuroendocrine carcinomas. Cancer 1990; 65:1003.
153. Carter D, Yesner R: Carcinomas of the lung with neuroendocrine differentiation. Semin Diagn Pathol 1985; 2:235.
154. Warren WH, Gould VE, Faber LP, et al.: Neuroendocrine neoplasms of the bronchopulmonary tract. A classification of the spectrum of carcinoid to small cell carcinoma and intervening variants. J Thorac Cardiovasc Surg 1985; 89:819.
155. Warren WH, Gould VE: Neuroendocrine neoplasms of the lung. A 10-year perspective of their classification. Zentralbl Pathol 1993; 139:107.
156. Warren WH, Faber LP, Gould VE: Neuroendocrine neoplasms of the lung. A clinicopathologic update [see comments]. J Thorac Cardiovasc Surg 1989; 98:321.
157. Warren WH, Memoli VA, Gould VE: Well-differentiated and small cell neuroendocrine carcinomas of the lung. Two related but distinct clinicopathologic entities. Virchows Arch B 1988; 55:299.
158. Gazdar AF, Carney DN, Nau MM, et al.: Characterization of variant subclasses of cell local lines derived from small cell lung cancer having distinct biochemical, morphological, and growth properties. Cancer Res 1985; 45:2924.
159. Travis WD, Linnoila RI, Tsokos MG, et al.: Neuroendocrine tumors of the lung with proposed criteria for large-cell neuroendocrine carcinoma. An ultrastructural, immunohistochemical, and flow cytometric study of 35 cases. Am J Surg Pathol 1991; 15:529.
160. Mooi WJ, Dewar A, Springall D, et al.: Non-small cell lung carcinomas with neuroendocrine features. A light microscopic, immunohistochemical and ultrastructural study of 11 cases. Histopathology 1988; 13:329.
161. Hammond ME, Sause WT: Large cell neuroendocrine tumors of the lung. Clinical significance and histopathologic definition. Cancer 1985; 56:1624.
162. Jiang SX, Kameya T, Shoji M, et al.: Large cell neuroendocrine carcinoma of the lung: A histologic and immunohistochemical study of 22 cases. Am J Surg Pathol 1998; 22:526.
163. Onuki N, Wistuba II, Travis WD, et al.: Genetic changes in the spectrum of neuroendocrine lung tumors. Cancer 1999; 85:600.
164. Visscher DW, Zarbo RJ, Trojanowski JQ, et al.: Neuroendocrine differentiation in poorly differentiated lung carcinomas: A light microscopic and immunohistologic study. Mod Pathol 1990; 3:508.
165. Linnoila RI, Mulshine JL, Steinberg SM, et al.: Neuroendocrine differentiation in endocrine and nonendocrine lung carcinomas. Am J Clin Pathol 1988; 90:641.
166. Gazdar AF, Helman LJ, Israel MA, et al.: Expression of neuroendocrine cell markers L-dopa decarboxylase, chromogranin A, and dense core granules in human tumors of endocrine and nonendocrine origin. Cancer Res 1988; 48:4078.
167. Kosinski R, Cohen P, Orenstein JM: Atypical endocrine tumors of the lung: A histologic, ultrastructural, and clinical study of 19 cases. Hum Pathol 1986; 17:1264.
168. McDowell EM, Wilson TS, Trump BF: Atypical endocrine tumors. Arch Pathol Lab Med 1981; 105:20.
169. Gazdar AF: Advances in the biology of lung cancer: Clinical significance of neuroendocrine differentiation. Chest 1989; 96:39.
170. Gazdar AF, Kadoyama C, Venzon D, et al.: Association between histological type and neuroendocrine differentiation on drug sensitivity of lung cancer cell lines. J Natl Cancer Inst Monogr 1992; 13:191.
171. Wick MR, Berg LC, Hertz MI: Large cell carcinoma of the lung with neuroendocrine differentiation: A comparison with large cell "undifferentiated" pulmonary tumors. Am J Clin Pathol 1992; 97:796.
172. Schleusener JT, Tazelaar HD, Jung SH, et al.: Neuroendocrine differentiation is an independent prognostic factor in chemotherapy-treated nonsmall cell lung carcinoma. Cancer 1996; 77:1284.
173. Yellin A, Benfield JR: The pulmonary Kulchitsky cell (neuroendocrine) cancers: From carcinoid to small cell carcinomas. Curr Probl Cancer 1985; 9:1.
174. Lawson RM, Ramanathan L, Hurley G, et al.: Bronchial adenoma: Review of an 18-year experience at the Brompton Hospital. Thorax 1976; 31:245.
175. Davila DG, Dunn WF, Tazelaar HD, et al.: Bronchial carcinoid tumors. Mayo Clin Proc 1993; 68:795.
176. Chabot V, de Keyzer Y, Gebhard S, et al.: Ectopic ACTH with Cushing's syndrome: V3 vasopressin receptor but not CRH receptor gene expression in a pulmonary carcinoid tumor. Horm Res 1998; 50:226.
177. Liu TH, Liu HR, Lu ZL, et al.: Thoracic ectopic ACTH-producing tumors with Cushing's syndrome. Zentralbl Pathol 1993; 139:131.
178. Hussein AM, Feun LG, Savaraj N, et al.: Carcinoid tumor presenting as central nervous system symptoms. Case report and review of the literature. Am J Clin Oncol 1990; 13:251.
179. Gal AA, Koss MN, Hochholzer L, et al.: Pigmented pulmonary carcinoid tumor. An immunohistochemical and ultrastructural study. Arch Pathol Lab Med 1993; 117:832.
180. Ghadially FN, Block HJ: Oncocytic carcinoid of the lung. J Submicrosc Cytol 1985; 17:435.
181. Sklar JL, Churg A, Bensch KG: Oncocytic carcinoid tumor of the lung. Am J Surg Pathol 1980; 4:287.
182. Mark EJ, Quay SC, Dickersin GR: Papillary carcinoid tumor of the lung. Cancer 1981; 48:316.
183. Bensch KG, Gordon GB, Miller LR: Electron microscopic and biochemical studies on the bronchial carcinoid tumor. Cancer 1965; 18:592.
184. Capella C, Gabrielli M, Polak JM, et al.: Ultrastructural and histological study of 11 bronchial carcinoids. Evidence for different types. Virchows Arch A 1979; 381:313.
185. Hage E: Histochemistry and fine structure of bronchial carcinoid tumours. Virchows Arch A 1973; 361:121.
186. Warren WH, Memoli VA, Gould VE: Immunohistochemical and ultrastructural analysis of bronchopulmonary neuroendocrine neoplasms. I. Carcinoids. Ultrastruct Pathol 1984; 6:15.
187. Tsutsumi Y: Immunohistochemical analysis of calcitonin and calcitonin gene-related peptide in human lung. Hum Pathol 1989; 20:896.
188. Bostwick DG, Roth KA, Evans CJ, et al.: Gastrin-releasing peptide, a mammalian analog of bombesin, is present in human neuroendocrine lung tumors. Am J Pathol 1984; 117:195.
189. Felton WLI, Liebow AA, Lindskog GE: Peripheral and multiple bronchial adenomas. Cancer 1953; 6:555.
190. Ranchod M, Levine GD: Spindle-cell carcinoid tumors of the lung. Am J Surg Pathol 1980; 4:315.
191. Warren WH, Gould VE: Long-term follow-up of classical bronchial carcinoid tumors. Scand J Thorac Cardiovasc Surg 1990; 24:125.
192. Caulet S, Capron F, Ghorra C, et al.: Flow cytometric DNA analysis of 20 bronchopulmonary neuroendocrine tumours. Eur Respir J 1993; 6:83.
193. Jones DJ, Hasleton PS, Moore M: DNA ploidy in bronchopulmonary carcinoid tumours. Thorax 1988; 43:195.
194. Sidhu GS: The ultrastructure of malignant epithelial neoplasms of the lung. In Sommers SC, Rosen PP, eds.: Pathology Annual. Appleton-Century-Crofts, Norwalk, CT, 1982.
195. Carstens PHB: Electron microscopy of small cell carcinoma with special reference to the crush phenomenon. Ultrastruct Pathol 1973; 4:253.
196. Azzopardi JG: Oat-cell carcinoma of the bronchus. J Pathol Bacteriol 1959; 78:513.
197. Mooi WJ, Dingemans KP, Van Zandwijk N: Prevalence of neuroendocrine granules in small cell lung carcinoma. Usefulness of electron microscopy in lung cancer classification. J Pathol 1986; 149:41.
198. Yokose T, Asami H, Ito Y: Immunohistochemical and ultrastructural study of mixed small cell/large cell carcinoma of the lung. Expression of sialyl LeX-i antigens and scarcity of neuroendocrine characteristics. Acta Pathol Jpn 1991; 41:540.

199. Sehested M, Hirsch FR, Osterlind K, et al.: Morphologic variations of small cell lung cancer: A histopathologic study of 104 pre-treatment and post-treatment specimens. Cancer 1986; 57:804.

200. Magnum MD, Hainsworth JD, Hande KR, et al.: Combined small-cell and non-small-cell lung cancer. J Clin Oncol 1989; 7:607.

201. Travis WD, Rush W, Flieder DB, et al.: Survival analysis of 200 pulmonary neuroendocrine tumors with clarification of criteria for atypical carcinoid and its separation from typical carcinoid. Am J Surg Pathol 1998; 22:934.

202. Rusch VW, Klimstra DS, Venkatraman ES: Molecular markers help characterize neuroendocrine lung tumors. Ann Thorac Surg 1996; 62:798.

203. Dresler CM, Ritter JH, Patterson GA, et al.: Clinical-pathologic analysis of 40 patients with large cell neuroendocrine carcinoma of the lung. Ann Thorac Surg 1997; 63:180.

204. Neal MH, Kosinski R, Cohen P, et al.: Atypical endocrine tumors of the lung: A histologic, ultrastructural, and clinical study of 19 cases. Hum Pathol 1986; 17:1264.

205. Berendsen HH, de Leij L, Poppema S, et al.: Clinical characterization of non-small-cell lung cancer tumors showing neuroendocrine differentiation features. J Clin Oncol 1989; 7:1614.

206. Wertzel H, Grahmann PR, Bansbach S, et al.: Results after surgery in undifferentiated large cell carcinoma of the lung: The role of neuroendocrine expression. Eur J Cardiothorac Surg 1997; 12:698.

207. Linnoila RI, Piantadosi S, Ruckdeschel JC: Impact of neuroendocrine differentiation in non-small cell lung cancer. The LCSG experience. Chest 1994; 106:367S.

208. Graziano SL, Kern JA, Herndon JE, et al.: Analysis of neuroendocrine markers, HER2 and CEA before and after chemotherapy in patients with stage IIIA non-small cell lung cancer: A Cancer and Leukemia Group B study. Lung Cancer 1998; 21:203.

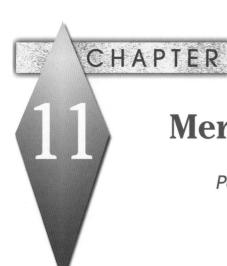

CHAPTER 11

Merkel Cell Carcinoma

Hong Wu, Rosalie Elenitsas,
Paul Zhang, and David E. Elder

Merkel cell carcinoma (MCC) was first described as a distinct clinicopathologic entity in 1972 by Toker[1] under the name "trabecular carcinoma of the skin." Before then, the tumor was often mistaken for a skin metastasis of a carcinoma from another site, or even for a malignant lymphoma. Toker originally proposed that the tumor might have derived from primitive sweat gland cells. Subsequently, in 1978, Tang and Toker[2] described three new cases studied with the electron microscope. The tumor cells were found to have cytoplasmic electron-dense granules that were identical to neurosecretory granules in neuroendocrine cells. Thus, the cutaneous Merkel cell was postulated as a possible progenitor cell for MCC.[2] For the same reason, other commonly used names for MCC include "primary neuroendocrine carcinoma of the skin" or "cutaneous neuroendocrine carcinoma."[3-9] Even though the histogenesis of MCC is not entirely proved, the current most commonly used name is "Merkel cell carcinoma," which accurately describes the immunohistochemical and ultrastructural similarities between the tumor cells of MCC and normal Merkel's cells. In a broad sense, the tumor could either derive from or differentiate toward Merkel's cells.[10]

Merkel's cells were identified in 1875 by Friedrich Merkel as specific terminal touch-sensitive cells in the skin. Electrophysiologic and ultrastructural studies have since proved that Merkel's cells are a type of mechanoreceptor associated with nerve fibers.[11] They are specialized epithelial cells that are most commonly found in skin with high hair density, in glabrous epithelium of the digits and lips, and in regions of the oral cavity. Specifically, Merkel's cells are localized at the basal cell layer of the epidermis or mucosa and in the outer root sheath of the hair follicle in the bulge area.[12] Without special staining, Merkel's cells cannot be distinguished from the surrounding cells by light microscopy. The cells appear paler than surrounding basal cells after fixation with glutaraldehyde-osmium followed by toluidine blue stain. However, even with this special technique, Merkel's cells can still be confused with basal cells and Langerhans' cells.

The most definitive identification of Merkel's cells is by electron microscopy.[11] In silver-impregnated sections, a Merkel cell can be seen as a Merkel disc, which is a minute neural terminal that covers the basal portion of each Merkel cell. Immunohistochemically, Merkel's cells are positive for simple epithelial cytokeratin (CK8, 18, and 19) but negative for cytokeratins of the stratified squamous epithelium. The cells also express neuroendocrine markers, including neuron-specific enolase (NSE), chromogranin, and synaptophysin; however, in contrast to MCC, they do not contain neurofilament (NF).[13] Ultrastructurally, Merkel's cells contain electron-dense, membrane-bound neurosecretory granules that are 80 to 200 nm in diameter, with perinuclear strands of intermediate filaments that resemble tonofilaments and also contain small desmosomes.[10, 11, 13] Putative neurotransmitters have also been localized to the dense core granules, including vasoactive intestinal polypeptide (VIP) and met-enkephalin.[14] Embryologically, Merkel's cells arise in fetal epidermis between 8 and 12 weeks of gestational age. However, the origin of Merkel's cells has been a subject of debate. They may derive in situ from the epidermis, or they may have migrated from the neural crest.

CLINICAL FEATURES

MCC is an uncommon malignant primary skin tumor. There is no report of a population-based annual incidence of the tumor. In the literature, cumulatively over 600 cases have been reported worldwide.[15] However, the numbers of cases described in most series, which were based on data from one medical center or a single region, are limited to 10 to 30 cases, usually over 5 to 10 years.[5, 16-20] In general, MCC is a much less common tumor than basal cell carcinoma (BCC) or even malignant melanoma. A 1985 report from a British pathology department described seeing five cases of MCC over 5 years, which corresponded to 2% and 0.3% of the total numbers of malignant melanomas and BCC seen in the same period, respectively.[21] MCC occurs predominantly in the elderly population, with reported average/mean ages of 66 to 79 years.[3, 5-8, 20, 22-24] However, rare cases have been reported in teenagers as well.[25, 26] Whites are more commonly affected than other races.[6] It has been reported in Asians and blacks.[27] Men and women are equally affected,[3, 5-8, 20, 22-24] although in some series there is a female predominance (Table 11-1).[23, 24] The tumor has a predilection for sun-exposed skin. The most common site of occurrence is the head and neck region (34% to 67%), followed by the upper or lower extremities (10% to 30%) and the trunk (5% to 20%) (see Table 11-1).[3, 5-8, 20, 22, 23, 28] In the head and neck region, the periorbital area has been described as a commonly involved site.[29, 30] One of 43 patients in the study of Sibley and associates[8] was described as having two primary sites of the tumor, one on the forearm and the other on the buttock, the latter lesion occurring 10 years after the first lesion.

Clinically, the tumor often presents as a small dermal nodule or indurated plaque averaging 2 to 3 cm in diameter (see Table 11-1). The overlying skin often shows pink, red, or violaceous discoloration, sometimes with associated telangiectasia.[8] Occasionally MCC presents as a papule or a skin ulcer.[24, 31] It is interesting that, among 132 cases studied at the Armed Forces Institute of Pathology (AFIP), a considerable number (37 cases, 28%) were described as having skin ulceration.[3] Most often the lesion is asymptomatic.[13, 24] MCC tends to develop fairly rapidly. The average length of time between a patient's first noticing the lesion and histologic diagnosis is often less than 6 months.[5, 6, 28] Unfortunately, there are no reliable clinical features to distinguish MCC from other dermal lesions. As a result, MCC is rarely suspected prior to histologic examination.[3]

MCC has also been reported to occur in unusual locations, including the vulva, scrotum, submandibular gland, and labial mucosa.[13, 32] A certain percentage (12% to 29%) of patients have regional lymph node metastases at the time of diagnosis, i.e., present with stage II disease.[5, 6, 10, 13, 28] Rare cases present initially with distant metastases.[2, 28] There is no known consistently associated precursor lesion for MCC. Several reports have documented that MCC occurred within or near lesions of squamous cell carcinoma (SCC), BCC, Bowen's disease, actinic keratoses, sweat gland tumors, and psoriasis (reviewed in references 15 and 28). Two of 43 cases (5%) in the study of Sibley and associates[8] showed typical Bowen's disease in the epidermis overlying MCC. Bowenoid change and solar elastosis were also found in 9% and 30% of 132 cases studied at the AFIP, respectively.[3]

Because a high percentage of the tumor occurs in sun-exposed areas and whites have the highest incidence of the disease, ultraviolet radiation is considered a significant etiologic factor for MCC.[13, 33] In addition, MCC has also been reported in patients who are immunosuppressed for organ transplantation or treatment of collagen vascular disease.[34-37] Some investigators have also noted occurrences in patients with chronic lymphocytic leukemia, chronic renal failure, polycythemia vera, and other lymphoproliferative disorders.[28] However, it is difficult to compare the incidence in immunosuppressed patients with that in the general population.

Table 11-1. Clinical Data for Merkel Cell Carcinoma

Reference	Year	Mean or Average Age/Yrs (Range)	Gender (F/M)	Head/Neck No. (%)	Upper Limb No. (%)	Lower Limb No. (%)	Trunk No. (%)	Others No. (%)
Parrado et al.[5]	1998	72 (20–91)	12/13	10 (40)	7 (28)	3 (12)	1 (4)	buttock, 4 (16)
Schmidt et al.[22]	1998	72 (41–90)	40/36	26 (34)	17 (22)	10 (13)	12 (16)	
Skelton et al.[3]	1997	71 (15–92)	64/68	57 (43)	33 (25)	13 (10)	10 (7.6)	buttock & thigh, 19 (14.4)
Al-Ghazal et al.[24]	1996	79.3 (68–86)	10/3	5 (39)	2 (15)	6 (46)	0	
Smith et al.[6]	1995	66 (32–82)	9/26	20 (57)	7 (20)	5 (14)	3 (9)	
Brinkschmidt et al.[23]	1995	70.5 (50–87)	13/5	12 (67)	5 (27)	0	1 (6)	
Yiengpruksawan et al.[64]	1992	66 (38–88)	31/39	19 (27)	9 (13)	26 (37)	3 (4)	buttock, 13 (19)
Pitale et al.[28] (review of 309 cases 1972–89)	1992	68 (18–92)	53/47	(53)	upper & lower limb (35)		0	others (9); multiple primaries (3)
Visscher et al.[7]	1989	76.4 (54–90)	9/12	12 (57)	1 (2)	7 (33)	0	buttock, 1 (2)
Sibley et al.[8]	1985	69.7 (39–89)	22/21	17 (40)	11 (26)	13 (30)	2 (4.5)	
Reviewed in Sibley et al. (146 cases)[8]	1985	67 (23–93)	62/38	(48)	(14)	(27)	(11)	
Kroll and Toker[20]	1982	68 (37–92)	15/15	13 (43)	8 (27)	5 (17)	3 (10)	multiple sites, 1 (3)

HISTOPATHOLOGY

Morphology

Grossly, MCC usually appears as a gray-white mass confined to the dermis and subcutis. Most reported cases range in size from 0.3 to 6 cm (average, 2 to 3 cm) in diameter.[6, 8, 20, 28] It is important for pathologists to document the size of the lesion, since several reports have described its size as a potential prognostic factor.[3, 8]

On a low-power view, MCC usually appears as a bluish, densely cellular lesion in the dermis (Fig. 11–1), sometimes with extension to the subcutaneous fat.[23] Rarely, the lesion is entirely located in the subcutis, with sparing of the dermis.[10] Typically, the epidermis is not involved, with a zone of dermal tissue separating the tumor from the epidermis. However, there have been multiple reports of MCC with an intraepidermal component that presents as either pagetoid changes or Pautrier-like microabscesses.[38-40] In a large series conducted at the AFIP, 12 of 132 cases (9%) showed epidermal involvement.[3] Six cases described by LeBoit and colleagues[38] showed a dermal component that would be seen typically in MCC, whereas the epidermis shows various histologic changes, including junctional nest formation at the dermoepidermal junction and pagetoid spread of single cells at all levels. Immunohistochemical (IHC) findings were characteristic of neuroendocrine carcinoma. Furthermore, in two cases intraepidermal tumor volume exceeded that in the dermis. The researchers pointed out that, among the various pagetoid skin lesions. MCC with epidermal involvement is most likely to be confused with malignant melanoma and cutaneous T-cell lymphoma (CTCL) with pagetoid features, since the cells in these three types of tumors may contain little cytoplasm.[38] Cases of MCC with epidermal involvement had been misdiagnosed by referring pathologists.[38] In fact, one of us (RE) managed a

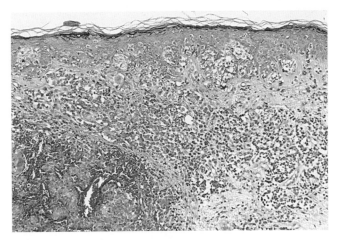

Figure 11–2. MCC with epidermal pagetoid growth pattern may superficially simulate a malignant melanoma (100×).

case of MCC with prominent junctional nests and pagetoid growth pattern in the periphery of a superficial dermal tumor, closely resembling the silhouette of a superficial spreading type of malignant melanoma (Fig. 11–2).

MCC may exhibit a variety of histologic patterns. The classic trabecular pattern, for which the tumor was originally designated, is characterized by interconnecting trabeculae separated by strands of connective tissue (Fig. 11–3A and B).[1, 20] However, this histologic pattern is least common in most reported series. Only 10% to 25% of the cases have the trabecular pattern as the predominant histologic feature.[8, 30] On the other hand, it is not uncommon to see the trabecular pattern as a part of the lesion, especially at the periphery of a central solidly cellular tumor.[8] More commonly, the tumor cells are arranged in solid sheets (see Fig. 11–3C) or large, compact nests (see Fig. 11–3D). In some cases, the cells are discohesive and hence have a striking resemblance to lymphoma or leukemia. This discohesive "leukemia-like" pattern is often observed at the periphery of a more solid tumor (see Fig. 11–3E). Uncommonly, rosette formation or organoid structures with pseudoglandular patterns are also seen[8, 24, 30, 31] (see Fig. 11–3F). In a large lesion, there are often areas of different histologic patterns. MCC characteristically has a very high mitotic rate and also contains numerous apoptotic nuclear fragments.[8-11] Among 132 cases in the study of Skelton and group,[3] 67% and 22% contained 6 to 10 mitoses per high-power field (hpf) and greater than 10 mitoses per hpf, respectively.[3] Variable areas of necrosis may also be present (see Fig. 11–3G).[8, 41]

Cytologically, within a given lesion the cells are usually fairly uniform in size and shape. The cell size ranges from small to medium, with the small cells in general twice or three times the size of mature lymphocytes.[3, 24] The cells have a very high nuclear-cytoplasmic ratio, with a narrow rim of amphophilic cytoplasm. The nuclei are usually round to ovoid,

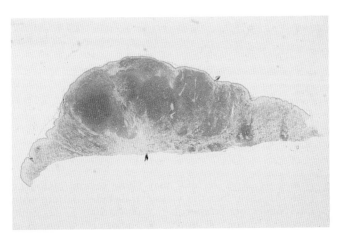

Figure 11–1. A low-power view shows a densely cellular tumor in the dermis, with a zone of dermal tissue separating the tumor from the epidermis (1×).

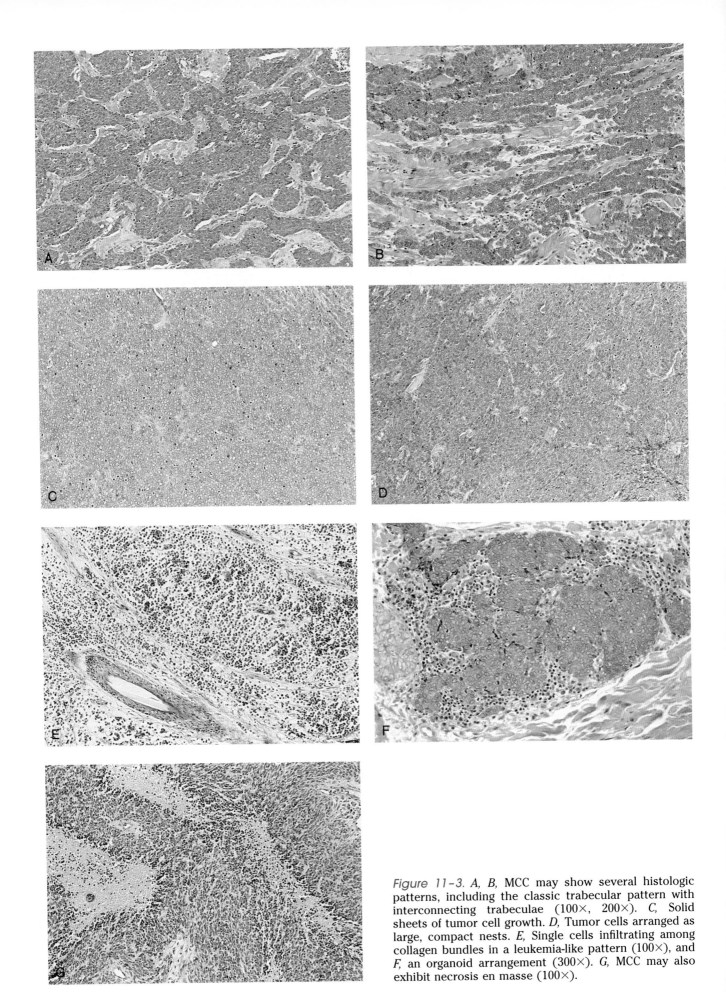

Figure 11–3. A, B, MCC may show several histologic patterns, including the classic trabecular pattern with interconnecting trabeculae (100×, 200×). *C,* Solid sheets of tumor cell growth. *D,* Tumor cells arranged as large, compact nests. *E,* Single cells infiltrating among collagen bundles in a leukemia-like pattern (100×), and *F,* an organoid arrangement (300×). *G,* MCC may also exhibit necrosis en masse (100×).

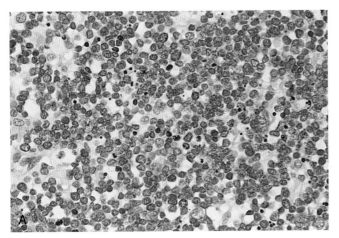
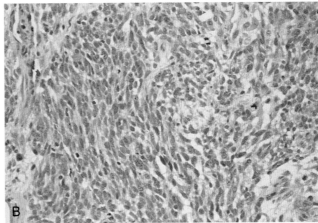

Figure 11–4. A, The tumor cells in MCC typically have a high nuclear-cytoplasmic ratio, scant cytoplasm, and finely dispersed stippled chromatin, with frequent pyknotic and mitotic figures. *B,* Some cases may show spindled cells with hyperchromatic nuclei (400×).

with finely dispersed, stippled ("dusty," "powdery") nuclear chromatin and either inconspicuous or multiple small nucleoli (Fig. 11–4A).[24, 29, 42] In some cases, the cells are spindle shaped and have hyperchromatic nuclei (see Fig. 11–4B).[8, 24, 41] Nuclear molding has been observed in some cases.[24, 41] This change was seen in 22% of 132 cases in the study of Skelton and associates.[3]

Angiolymphatic invasion is very commonly seen in MCC, often at the periphery of the tumor or immediately beneath the epidermis.[7, 8, 10, 41] Sibley and colleagues[8] described angiolymphatic invasion in 84% of their 43 cases. The presence of angiolymphatic invasion should be documented, since it is believed to have important prognostic implications.[13] A lymphoplasmacytic infiltrate is commonly seen within the tumor; sometimes it may be difficult to differentiate infiltrating lymphocytes from small, hyperchromatic tumor cells. This could potentially cause diagnostic difficulty, especially when frozen sections are used for evaluation of resection margins.[30] Satellite lesions can also be present. Furthermore, positive margins can be seen in a significant number of cases.[6]

Some cases of MCC may show foci of squamous (Fig. 11–5A) or eccrine (see Fig. 11–5B) differentiation.[1, 20, 43, 44] Of the 42 MCC cases studied by Gould and coworkers,[43] two cases showed numerous tubular formations within otherwise typical sheets and nests of MCC cells. The ducts are morphologically similar to eccrine ducts and also are positive for carcinoembryonic antigen (CEA).[43] Five percent (6 of 132 cases) in the study of Skelton and associates[3] showed squamous differentiation. We have observed a few cases in which numerous atypical squamous islands are present within MCC. Particularly if the change is limited to the superficial dermis, it may be difficult to differentiate tumor-induced pseudoepitheliomatous hyperplasia from tumor-derived squamous differentiation (see Fig. 11–5C).

Immunohistochemistry

The finding of a small blue cell tumor in the skin elicits a broad range of differential diagnoses, including metastatic neuroendocrine tumor (carcinomas or carcinoid) primary to other sites, lymphoma, leukemia, poorly differentiated skin adnexal tumors, amelanotic melanoma, atypical BCC, and even metastatic neuroblastoma and Ewing's sarcoma.[8, 13, 16] The histologic distinction between MCC and malignant lymphoma is not difficult when the tumor cells of MCC exhibit cohesiveness and focal organoid arrangement. In well-preserved sections, the cytologic features of MCC differ from those of lymphoma or leukemia. In general, either small or large lymphoma cells would not have a finely stippled chromatin pattern as is characteristic of neuroendocrine carcinomas.[41] However, discohesiveness and poor preservation may cause diagnostic difficulty. In one study, a significant number of cases were initially misdiagnosed as lymphoma by pathologists.[45]

The most difficult differential diagnosis is, perhaps, from metastatic neuroendocrine tumors that are primary to other sites. Although it has been stated in some studies that the nuclei of MCC cells appear somewhat larger and less hyperchromatic than is usually seen in metastatic small cell carcinoma of the lung,[24] a distinction based purely on histology can be very unreliable. Aside from a detailed clinical investigation to uncover other primary tumors, immunohistochemical (IHC) studies offer very important information. MCC cells, in the great majority of cases and with rare exceptions, are positive for low-molecular-weight (LMW) cytokeratin (CK) (exemplified by CAM 5.2, which is against CK8, 18, and 19). In contrast, the tumor cells are negative for high-molecular-weight (HMW) cytokeratin.[3, 5, 9, 16, 22, 23, 45] In addition, in a very high percentage (up to 90%) of cases, the CK immunostain shows a distinct paranuclear dotlike

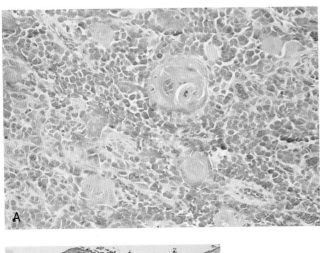
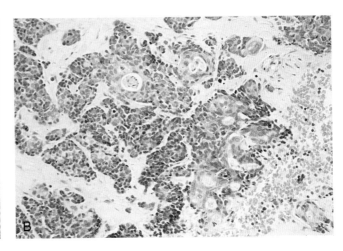
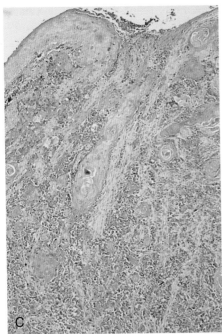

Figure 11–5. A, Squamous and *B,* eccrine differentiation can be seen in some cases of MCC (200×). *C,* Squamous differentiation in the superficial dermis may be difficult to differentiate from tumor-induced pseudoepitheliomatous hyperplasia (50×).

pattern, resembling a cytoplasmic inclusion body (Fig. 11–6A) (Table 11–2). In some cases, there may be a combined paranuclear dotlike reactivity as well as diffuse cytoplasmic immunostaining for cytokeratin.[22] This dotlike CK-staining pattern was previously thought a distinct feature of MCC that could be used as a distinguishing feature from metastatic small cell carcinoma of the lung.[22, 45] However, a 1997 report found that up to 35% of small cell carcinoma of the lung exhibited a similar paranuclear CK-staining pattern (see Table 11–2).[4] The same study also found this CK-staining pattern in small cell carcinoma arising in various sites; specifically, in 60% (three of five cases) of salivary gland, 44% (4/9) of gastrointestinal, 60% (3/5) of sinonasal and pharyngeal, 22% (2/9) of laryngeal, 33% (1/3) of thymic, and 9% (1/11) of cervical small cell carcinoma.[4] Thus, a paranuclear dotlike immunostaining with LMW CK alone is not sufficient evidence of MCC.

In a study published in 1995, Miettinen[46] reported cytokeratin 20 (CK20) reactivity in all five cases of MCC studied. CK20 is a 46-KDa type I LMW cytokeratin that is mainly distributed in glandular epithelium, chiefly of gastrointestinal epithelium, urothelium, and their tumors. In addition to the consistent reactivity in MCC cases, more importantly the tumor cells in six cases of small cell carcinoma and eight cases of carcinoid of the lung show no reactivity with CK20.[46] As early as 1985, Moll and Franke[47] had previously reported the differential expression of the same 46-KDa cytoskeletal protein in cutaneous and pulmonary neuroendocrine neoplasms. In both studies by Moll and colleagues,[47, 48] frozen tissue was used for the IHC stain for CK20. In combination, 100% (24/24) of MCC cases were positive for CK20, in contrast to only 13% (3/23) of small cell carcinoma of the lung, using the same testing conditions.

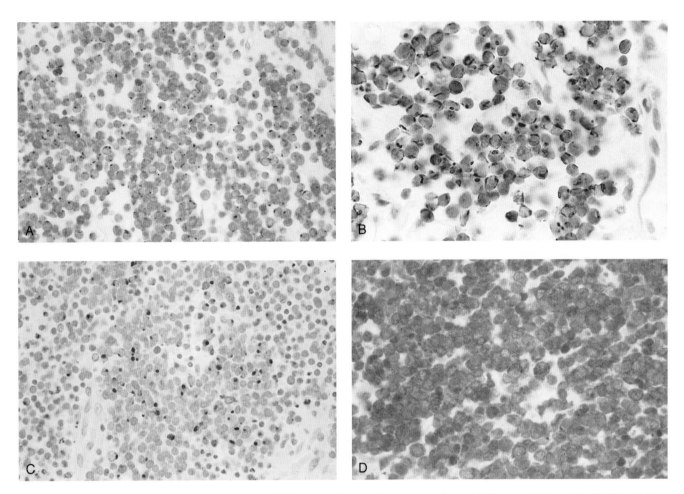

Figure 11-6. Immunohistochemical stains in MCC typically reveal a paranuclear dotlike reactivity with LMW cytokeratin (CAM 5.2) (*A,* 300×) and CK20 (*B,* 400×). *C,* Some cases may show a similar dotlike staining pattern with neurofilament (300×). *D,* Nearly all cases show diffuse cytoplasmic positivity for NSE (400×).

Chan and associates[4] published a larger series in 1997 and showed that all but one of 33 MCC cases were CK20-positive. Moreover, almost 100% of the tumor cells were reactive, and 30 of the 33 showed a paranuclear dotlike pattern. In contrast, only rare cases of pulmonary and cervical small cell carcinomas showed CK20 positivity (see Table 11–2). It is interesting that three of five salivary gland small cell carcinomas had uniform CK20 positivity.[4] The workers concluded that CK20 positivity is a strong predictor for MCC in a small cell carcinoma of uncertain origin. According to Chan and associates,[4] a negative CK20 reaction can practically rule out MCC, provided an effective antigen retrieval technique is used and appropriate staining is obtained with other cytokeratin antibodies.

Several other studies also observed a very high percentage (90% or higher) of CK20-positive MCC (see Table 11–2).[23, 49, 50] Nevertheless, note that the percentage of CK20-positive MCC varies among different reports. Several reports failed to show a near-90% positivity (see Table 11–3).[5, 22] Even so, the overall positive rate in the various

studies is in the range of 80% or higher (see Table 11–3).

Another important feature of CK20 staining in MCC is the extent and intensity of the positive reaction in the tumor cells.[4] In a recent study, Scott and Helm[49] also emphasized that 78% (7/9) of CK20-positive MCC cases were strongly positive, with 25% to 90% of the cells reactive. In addition, most of the CK20-positive cases showed a paranuclear dotlike staining pattern (see Fig. 11–6B).[4, 49] Both Chan and associates[4] and Scott and Helm[49] noticed that occasional MCC cases (two cases in each study) showed less CK20 reactivity, with 5% to 30% of positive tumor cells. Also, it is worth noticing that rare cases of small cell carcinoma of the lung may show limited CK20 reactivity (1 case with 40% positive cells, among 37 cases studied).[4] The reactivity of CK20 in carcinoids has been controversial (see Table 11–2). CK20 reactivity has also been tested against other cutaneous tumors. Cumulatively from three studies, the reactivity was not observed in SCC (19 cases), BCC (14 cases), melanoma (10 cases), spiradenoma (4 cases),

Table 11-2. Immunohistochemical Characteristics of Merkel Cell Carcinoma in Comparison with Other Tumors

Reference (Year)	Cytokeratin 20 Reactivity				Paranuclear Dotlike CK Staining				Neurofilament Reactivity				
	MCC	SCCL	Carcinoid	SCC of Salivary Gland	MCC	SCCL	Carcinoid	Undiff. Ca.	MCC	SCCL	Carcinoid	Undiff. Ca.	NE Ca. of Lung
Scott & Helm[49] (1999)	9/10 (90%)	0/6	0/5	ND	7/9 (78%)	ND	ND	ND	ND	ND	ND	ND	ND
Schmidt et al.[22] (1998)	43/50 (77%)	0/20	ND	ND	63/71 (89%)	1/21	ND	ND	25/40	0/22	ND	ND	ND
Miettinen[46] (1995)	5/5 (100%)	0/6	5/6 (scattered pos. cells)	ND	3/5 (60%)	ND	ND	ND	ND	ND	ND	ND	ND
Chan et al.[4] (1997)	33/34 (97%)	1/37 (3%)	ND	3/5 (60%)	30/33 (91%)	13/37 (35%)	ND	ND	ND	0/28	0/85	ND	0/37
Shah et al.[16] (1993)	ND	ND	ND	ND	ND	ND	ND	ND	9/9 (100%)	0/10	0/20	0/10	ND
Battifora & Silva[45] (1986)	ND	ND	ND	ND	18/25 (72%)	ND	2/20 (10%)	0/10	5/26 (19%)	ND	ND	ND	ND
*Moll et al.[48] (1992)	9/9 (100%)	0/8	ND	ND	ND	ND	ND	ND	ND	ND	ND	ND	ND
*Moll & Franke[47] (1985)	15/15 (100%)	3/15 (20%)	2/2 (100%)	ND	ND	ND	ND	ND	ND	ND	ND	ND	ND

* Frozen tissue was used for immunohistochemistry.
MCC, Merkel cell carcinoma; ND, not determined; NE, neuroendocrine; SCC, small cell carcinoma; SCCL, small cell carcinoma of lung; Undiff Ca., undifferentiated carcinoma.

Table 11-3. Immunohistochemical Features of Merkel Cell Carcinoma

Reference	Year	Keratin LMW (pos/ tested case)	CK20 (pos/ tested case)	NSE (pos/ tested case)	Syn. (pos/ tested case)	Chr. (pos/ tested case)	NF (pos/ tested case)	S100 (pos/ tested case)	LCA (pos/ tested case)	Vimentin (pos/ tested case)	EMA (pos/ tested case)	Others (pos/ tested case)	Comment
Parrado et al.[5]	1998	19/25 (76%) (CK8, 18, 19)	18/23 (88%)	21/24 88%	24/24 100%	21/24 (88%)	ND	ND	ND	ND	11/25 (44%)	NCAM, 9/24 (38%)	Only 1 case neg. for both keratin and CK20
Schmidt et al.[22]	1998	71/76 (93%)	43/56 (77%)	ND	ND	ND	25/40 (63%)	ND	ND	ND	ND	BER-EP4, 48/50 (96%)	91/132 with paranuclear dotlike CK staining
Skelton et al.[3]	1997	132/132 (100%)	ND	132/132 (100%)	ND	30/75 (41%)	ND	0/131	ND	ND	17/17 (100%)	Leu7, 2/75 (3%) Ber-EP4, 48/50 (96%)	
Al-Ghazal et al.[24]	1996	13/13 (10%)	ND	13/13 (100%)	ND	10/13 (77%)	See comment	0/13	0/13	See comment	ND		NF and vimentin were neg. in few cases tested
Brinkschmidt et al.[23]	1995	18/18 (100%)	17/18 (94%)	18/18 (100%)	7/18 (39%)	12/18 (67%)	ND	ND	ND	ND	14/18 (78%)		
Shah et al.[16]	1993	9/9 (100%)	ND	9/9 (100%)	ND	3/8 (38%)	9/9 (100%)	2/9 (22%)	0/8	1/9 (11%)	7/8 (87%)	CD15, 0/9 CEA, 1/9 (11%)	
Visscher et al.[7]	1989	21/21 (100%)	ND	9/21 (43%)	6/21 (29%)	11/21 (52%)	9/21 (43%)	ND	ND	ND	ND		100% paranuclear CK staining
Battifora & Silva[45]	1986	25/26 (96%)	ND	12/22 (55%)	ND	7/21 (33%)	5/26 (19%)	0/26	0/26	ND	ND		
Leong et al.[41]	1986	10/10 (100%)	ND	13/13 (100%)	ND	ND	7/10 (70%)	ND	0/13	ND	ND	VIP, 5/10 (50%) calcitonin, 4/10 (40%) HMW CK neg. in all cases	
Sibley & Dahl[19]	1985	16/21 (76%)	ND	11/21 (52%)	ND	ND	10/21 (48%)	ND	ND	ND	ND	VIP, 7/21 (33%)	

CEA, carcinoembryonic antigen; Chr., chromogranin; CK20, cytokeratin 20; EMA, epithelial membrane antigen; HMW, high molecular weight; LCA, leukocyte common antigen; Leu7, leucine; LMW, low molecular weight; NCAM, natural cell adhesion molecule; ND, no data; NF, neurofilament; NSE, neuron-specific enalase; Syn, synaptophysin; VIP, vasoactive intestinal polypeptide.

sebaceous carcinoma (3 cases), eccrine carcinoma (3 cases), or hidradenoma (4 cases).[46, 48, 49]

Another stain of special differential diagnostic value is neurofilament (NF). MCC, in contrast to normal Merkel cells, also expresses NF. NF has been found in significant numbers of MCC, often exhibiting a dotlike pattern similar to the CK or CK20 staining pattern (see Fig. 11–6C). The numbers of NF-positive cases vary among different studies, ranging from 19% to 100%, though more commonly in the range of 40% to 70% (see Table 11–2). NF has not been found in neuroendocrine tumors from other sites (see Table 11–3).[16, 22, 45] Shah and associates made an interesting observation that, with regard to intermediate filament expression, MCC differs from the neuroendocrine tumors that express only NF (such as pheochromocytoma and paraganglioma), and from those that express only CK (neuroendocrine carcinomas and carcinoids of various sites). Thus, the finding of coexpression of CK and NF in a neuroendocrine tumor is another strong predictor of MCC.

Nearly all MCC shows positivity for NSE (see Table 11–3) (see Fig. 11–6D). A significant proportion, though far less than 100%, is also positive for synaptophysin (20% to 100%) and chromogranin (33% to 88%) (see Table 11–3). In addition, epithelial membrane antigen (EMA) is also found in a high percentage of the cases (see Table 11–3). S100 and leukocyte common antigen (LCA) are consistently negative in all cases studied (see Table 11–3).

Schmidt and associates[22] recommended an algorithm for using IHC in differentiating MCC from small cell carcinoma of the lung. First of all, CK20 positivity strongly suggests MCC. If CK20 is negative, coexpression of CK and NF would strongly favor MCC. When these two tests fail, a paranuclear dotlike CK staining pattern that is present in most of the cells would argue in favor of MCC.[4, 22, 49] On the other hand, diffuse CK reactivity and negative reaction for CK20 or NF suggest a small cell carcinoma of the lung.[22] However, rare cases of MCC may be negative for all CK, in which case there could be a diagnostic dilemma.[5, 22, 45]

In Battifora and Silva's[45] study, two cases with overfixation in formalin were originally negative for all CK stainings, prior to prolonged enzyme treatment. Thus, lack of CK reactivity cannot be the sole reason for which a diagnosis of MCC is excluded. Even though CK-negative MCC cases are very uncommon with good techniques, such cases do exist. One case in the study of Parrado and colleagues[5] was negative for CK8, 18, 19, and 20 and positive for NSE, chromogranin, and synaptophysin. The diagnosis of MCC was also supported in this case by a negative chest CT scan.

Another case in the study of Battifora and Silva[45] was negative for all CKs tested and also showed no reactivity to any other antibodies tested; however, there were electron microscopic findings compatible with MCC. Similarly, four of five CK-negative cases in the study of Sibley and associates[9] also did not show reactivity for any other markers tested. In general practice, because small cell carcinomas of the lung have little tendency to cutaneous metastasis (2% at the time of diagnosis and 11% in advanced cases), a solitary neuroendocrine tumor in the skin is more likely to be a primary MCC than a metastatic small cell carcinoma of the lung.[16, 22]

In summary, with the combination of histology, CK20 and NF positivity, paranuclear dotlike CK staining pattern and, most importantly, an adequate clinical history, a differential diagnosis of MCC from metastatic neuroendocrine carcinoma of other sites can be confidently reached in most cases.

Ultrastructural Studies

Electron microscopic examination of MCC cells has invariably demonstrated membrane-bound, electron-dense granules that are indistinguishable from neurosecretory granules. The granules are 80 to 300 nm in diameter (reviewed in ref. 8). In many cases, a clear zone surrounds the dense core.[8] Another important feature is the presence of paranuclear or juxtanuclear whorls of intermediate filaments in many or most of the reported cases.[8, 41] This typical appearance of perinuclear intermediate filaments is the most important ultrastructural feature for differentiating MCC from a metastatic neuroendocrine tumor. In the report by Sibley and associates,[8] 91% of 77 cases reviewed, as well as 39 of 40 cases studied, showed this ultrastructural feature. In contrast, fewer than 10% of neuroendocrine tumors from other sites studied by Sibley and associates showed collections of filaments, which are usually difficult to find except in paraganglioma or medullary carcinoma of the thyroid.[8]

In one report, tumor cells are connected by complex intercellular junctions that are not identical to desmosomes.[8] Another study showed that in some cases the cells may also be connected by desmosomes.[2] Some cases also contain cytoplasmic spinous or microvillous projections.[8, 41] Moreover, an immunoelectron microscopic case study correlated light microscopic findings of paranuclear CK staining with positive keratin-labeled filaments arranged in paranuclear aggregates, as well as synaptophysin- and chromogranin-positive granules.[51] The close similarity at the ultrastructural level is the main reason that led to the hypothesis that MCC may be derived from Merkel's cells.[2]

MCC as Metastases

Surgical pathologists may encounter MCC as regional or distant metastases. Regional lymph node metastasis is the most common form. The affected lymph nodes may contain only limited foci of tumor cells in the subcapsular sinuses (Fig. 11–7A). More frequently the lymph node contains large aggregates of tumor (see Fig. 11–7B) or even becomes entirely

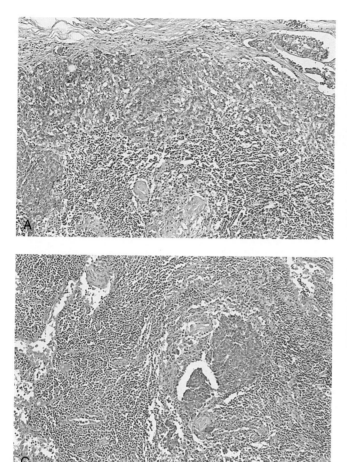

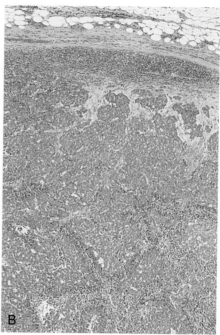

Figure 11–7. A, Metastatic MCC in a lymph node may appear as limited foci of tumor cells in the subcapsular sinuses (200×). *B,* They may also appear as easily identifiable large aggregates of tumor cells (50×). *C,* They may intermingle with surrounding lymphocytes, simulating a germinal center (200×).

replaced by the tumor. Occasionally, the tumor cells may appear to intermingle with surrounding lymphocytes imperceptibly and can be difficult to appreciate under a low-power view (see Fig. 11–7C). In cases without a known history of MCC, appropriate IHC studies may prove to be very important in reaching a correct diagnosis. Chan and colleagues[4] described two metastatic MCC in lymph nodes that were originally labeled as "metastatic small cell carcinoma of unknown primary." Owing to the strong CK20 positivity uncovered in the study, a more thorough review of the history and previous biopsies revealed that both patients had primary cutaneous MCC.

Several reports have documented rare cases of MCC within lymph nodes in the absence of an associated primary skin tumor. Eusebi and coworkers[52] in 1992 reported eight cases of neuroendocrine carcinoma found within inguinal, axillary, and submandibular lymph nodes. After extensive clinical investigation, no primary tumor was identified. All cases showed effacement of the lymph nodes by a tumor that morphologically closely resembled MCC. IHC studies showed that the cells were positive for LMW CK with a paranuclear dotlike pattern while negative for HMW CK. By electron microscopy, cytoplasmic paranuclear globular aggregates of intermediate filaments were seen in all cases. CK20 was

not tested in these cases. It is interesting that 5 of the 8 patients were alive and well through the follow-up period of 6 to 26 months. The investigators postulated that lymph nodes could be a de novo site for MCC-like carcinoma.[52] On the other hand, these cases could also represent a metastatic MCC in which the primary tumor has undergone spontaneous regression, very much like some cases of malignant melanoma.[5, 52] Similar cases have been reported sporadically (summarized in ref. 30). Stringent histologic and immunohistochemical criteria and rigorous clinical examinations should be applied to the diagnosis of primary lymph node MCC. Patients presenting with multiple lesions should be considered as having metastases from an unknown primary.[30, 52] It seems that the survival rates of the reported cases are more similar to those of MCC than to metastatic neuroendocrine tumor of other sites. Disease limited to a single lymph node appeared to have a better prognosis than cases involving more than one node (summarized in ref. 30).

Distant metastases have been observed in a significant number of patients with MCC. In rare cases, patients have presented with metastases without a prior recognized cutaneous primary. The common sites for distant metastases include liver (Fig. 11–8) bone, lungs, pancreas, parotid gland, brain, and meninges.[8, 20] Other reported sites are

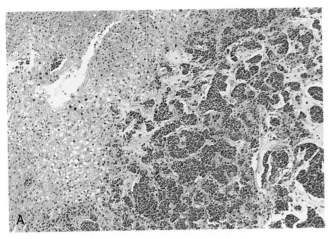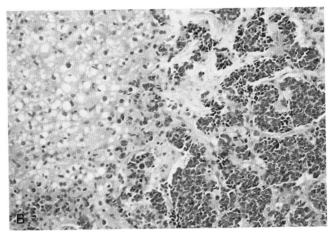

Figure 11-8. A and B, Metastatic MCC in the liver appears as a densely cellular tumor mass that is in sharp contrast with the adjacent liver parenchyma (A, 100×, B, 200×).

adrenal gland, kidney, urinary bladder, parathyroid, retroperitoneum, mediastinum, chest wall, stomach, eye, peritoneum, tonsil, ovary, and testicles.[8, 13, 20, 53, 54] Involvement of the parotid gland can be due to either direct extension of a skin lesion or to salivary gland invasion secondary to a positive intraparotid lymph node.[8] Histologically, it is difficult to distinguish a metastasis from MCC versus that from neuroendocrine tumors of other sites, or from other poorly differentiated tumors. With a known clinical history, metastatic MCC can usually be diagnosed by recognizing a metastatic, poorly differentiated tumor with neuroendocrine features, in combination with appropriate IHC profiles. On the other hand, characterization of such a metastasis without a pertinent clinical history can be very challenging.

Among the panel of IHC markers that are usually applied to a poorly differentiated tumor with unknown primary, LMW cytokeratin may yield a characteristically paranuclear dotlike staining pattern (see Table 11-2).[4, 22, 45] In combination with other features, including negative stains for HMW keratin, S100, and LCA, a differential diagnosis should include MCC. Further investigations, including IHC stains for CK20, NF, EMA, and NSE, will greatly facilitate a diagnosis of MCC. Needless to say, an appropriate clinical history would be most valuable.

MCC has been diagnosed by fine-needle aspiration, based on cytologic features, in combination with appropriate IHC stains.[42]

Histologic Features in Relation to Prognosis

Several reports have attempted to associate certain histologic features with prognosis. Skelton and coworkers[3] reviewed 132 cases seen at the Armed Forces Institute of Pathology and categorized the tumors based on cell sizes. In the small cell variant,

the cells are 14 μm or less in diameter, which is approximately twice the size of mature lymphocytes. They have scant cytoplasm and tend to form sheets and trabeculae with little organoid growth. The intermediate cell size group has cells larger than 14 μm, with more discernible cytoplasm, and shows a more organoid growth pattern. The definition of large cell variant, however, is not clearly delineated. Seventy-eight percent of the cases are classified as small cell variant. Univariate analysis showed that small cell size, high mitotic rate (over 10/hpf), and large tumor size were associated with a low survival rate. The intermediate cell variant showed more differentiation and was associated with a better prognosis.

Multivariate analysis within each cell-type group showed that when the tumor is the small cell variant, the other factors do not significantly affect the prognosis, whereas for the intermediate cell variant, the mitotic rate is a significant risk factor (other factors, including gender, age, and tumor location, were not significant in the study).[3]

Sibley and associates[8] emphasized the importance of tumor size. In relation to regional lymph node metastasis, tumor size in patients who developed regional lymph node metastases was 2.4 cm (0.3 to 6 cm), compared with 1.5 cm (0.8 to 3.0 cm) in those without metastases. Furthermore, the patients who died of the tumor had larger primary tumors (average, 2.5 cm) than those living at the time of follow-up (with tumors averaging 1.9 cm). In the same study, 50% (3/6) of cases with spindle- or oat-shaped cells, in comparison with 32% (12/37) of cases with round cells, died of tumor at an average follow-up of 19.3 months, although the difference is not statistically significant.[8] Parrado and associates[5] described several histologic patterns as "aberrant MCC," including "anaplastic type" with exaggerated cellular and nuclear pleomorphism, "atypical carcinoid-like," "pseudorosette-forming," and "neuroblastoma-like" variants. It seems that more patients

(4/7) with "aberrant MCC" had a fatal outcome than those with the classic histologic pattern (1/18 died of disease).[5]

In general, the histologic features that may predict unfavorable outcomes include large tumor size (greater than 2 cm), advanced stage, vascular or lymphatic invasion, high mitotic rate (more than 10 per hpf), and small cell size (summarized in ref. 30). In several reviews, IHC markers were not seen to be consistently useful in predicting clinical outcome.[17, 18, 55]

Cytogenetics of MCC

Cytogenetically, variable structural and numerical chromosome anomalies involving multiple chromosomes have been described in MCC. Structural anomalies are most frequently identified involving chromosome 1, which contains genes relevant to the differentiation of neural crest–derived tissue.[56–58] Karyotypes that are similar to small cell carcinomas of the lung and peripheral neuroectodermal tumors are also found in some MCC.[59, 60] Certain karyotypes such as t(1;17) and trisomy 6 might play a role in tumor progression.[61–63]

TREATMENT AND PROGNOSIS

Because of the rarity of the disease, it is difficult to obtain prospective studies to compare different modalities of treatment. Most therapeutic recommendations are based on retrospective studies or researchers' experience. Most investigators recommend a wide local excision of the primary site, specifically 3 cm or greater for lateral margins.[64] For clinically palpable lymph nodes, regional lymph node dissection is followed by radiotherapy to both postsurgical bed and lymph node basin.[15] However, the role of elective lymph node dissection in the absence of clinically evident lymph nodes still remains controversial. Several studies emphasized the importance of an early prophylactic lymph node dissection.[6, 33, 64] Yiengpruksawan and associates[64] noticed that most distant metastases were preceded by metastases to local regional lymph nodes and proposed that MCC metastasizes primarily via the lymphatics in a predictable "cascade" pattern. This observation has been used to justify an elective lymph node dissection; however, it is also possible that lymph node metastases are markers of tumors that have the capacity for distant metastases. In most of the cases, distant metastases are invariably associated with fatal outcomes. At an advanced stage, neither radiation nor chemotherapy is effective in obtaining long-term survival.[8, 19] Since most of the recurrences and metastases occur within a relatively short period of time (less than 2 years), close follow-up within the first 2 years of initial treatment is considered to be important.[8, 64] Monthly follow-up evaluation has been recommended in the first 6 months after completion of therapy, followed by follow-up every 3 months for the next 2 years.[13]

MCC is an aggressive disease, with 26% to 44% of patients developing local recurrences, 50% to 65% with synchronous or metachronous regional lymph node metastases, and, most significantly, 25% to 34% of patients developing distant metastases (Table 11–4). The mean time to local recurrences and regional lymph node metastases occurs within 2 years of the diagnosis.[64] Some patients may experience multiple local recurrences.[8] Fifteen percent of 309 cases reviewed by Pitale and coworkers[28] developed

Table 11–4. Clinical Follow-up and Outcome of Merkel Cell Carcinoma

Reference	Year	Average F/U	Total No.	Local Rec. (%)	RLNM (%)	Dmet (%)	Death (%)	Comment
Parrado et al.[5]	1998	38 mo	25	8 (32)	11 (44)	5 (20)	5 (20)	
Skelton et al.[3]	1997	1–10 yr	122	37 (30)	RLNM & Dmet 43 (35)		28 (23)	Most met. were to RLN
Smith et al.[6]	1995		34	8 (24)	8 (24)		8 (24)	Projected 5-yr survival 62%
Yiengpruksawan et al.[64]	1992	28 mo	70	18 (26)	46 (66)	20 (29)	19 (27)	Overall 5-yr survival rate, 64%; median F/U of 51 mo for ones free of disease
Reviewed in Pitale et al.[28] (1972–89)	1992		309	(44)	(55)	(34)	(28)	
Visscher et al.[7]	1989	26 mo	19	6 (32)	6 (32)	3 (16)	4 (22)	
Sibley et al.[8]	1985	34.2 mo	43	14 (33)	28 (65)	17 (40)	15 (35)	
Reviewed in Sibley et al.[8]	1985	—	133	50/133 (38)	71/133 (53)	30/122 (25)	34/116 (29)	
Kroll & Toker[20]	1982	1 yr	23	7 (30)	10 (43)	6 (26)	5 (22)	

* Average F/U, average follow-up period; Dmet, distant metastasis; Local Rec, local recurrences; RLNM, regional lymph node metastasis.

multiple local recurrences. Several studies have shown that local and regional recurrences are not necessarily predictive of a fatal outcome.[8, 28] The most common cause of death from the disease is distant metastasis. Distant metastasis usually is preceded by nodal metastasis.[8, 15, 19, 28, 64] In a review of 309 cases reported between 1972 and 1989, 63% of the female and 85% of the male patients who developed distant metastases died of the disease, with a median time to death of 23 and 16 months, respectively.[28] In contrast, in cases without distant metastases, only 4% died of the disease by the end of the follow-up.[28] The mortality rate varied widely among the different studies. In a review of the literature by Haag and coworkers[15] in 1995, the reported survival rate ranged from 30% to 64%. A publication showed that the differential expression of thyroid transcription factor (TTF-1) in small cell lung carcinoma and Merkel's cell carcinoma may be useful in separating these two lesions.[65]

References

1. Toker C: Trabecular carcinoma of the skin. Arch Dermatol 1972; 105:107.
2. Tang C-K, Toker C: Trabecular carcinoma of the skin: An ultrastrutural study. Cancer 1978; 42:2311.
3. Skelton HG, Smith KJ, Hitchcock CL, et al.: Merkel cell carcinoma: Analysis of clinical, histologic, and immunohistologic features of 132 cases with relation to survival. J Am Acad Dermatol 1997; 37:734.
4. Chan JK, Suster S, Wenig BM, et al.: Cytokeratin 20 immunoreactivity distinguishes Merkel cell (primary cutaneous neuroendocrine) carcinomas and salivary gland small cell carcinomas from small cell carcinomas of various sites. Am J Surg Pathol 1997; 21:226.
5. Parrado C, Bjornhagen V, Eusebi V, et al.: Prognosticating tools in primary neuroendocrine (Merkel-cell) carcinomas of the skin: Histopathological subdivision, DNA cytometry, cell proliferation analyses (Ki-67-immunoreactivity) and NCAM immunohistochemistry. A clinicopathological study in 25 patients. Pathol Res Prac 1998; 194:11.
6. Smith DE, Bielamowicz S, Kagan AR, et al.: Cutaneous neuroendocrine (Merkel cell) carcinoma: A report of 35 cases. Am J Clin Oncol 1995; 18:199.
7. Visscher D, Cooper PH, Zarbo RJ, et al.: Cutaneous neuroendocrine (Merkel cell) carcinoma: An immunophenotypic, clinicopathologic, and flow cytometric study. Mod Pathol 1989; 2:331.
8. Sibley R, Dehner L, Rosai J: Primary neuroendocrine (Merkel cell?) carcinoma of the skin. I. A clinicopathologic and ultrastructural study of 43 cases. Am J Surg Pathol 1985; 9:95.
9. Sibley R, Dahl D: Primary neuroendocrine (Merkel cell?) carcinoma of the skin. II. An immunohistochemical study of 21 cases. Am J Surg Pathol 1985; 9:109.
10. Frigerio B, Capella C, Eusebi V, et al.: Merkel cell carcinoma of the skin: The structure and origin of normal Merkel cells. Histopathology 1982; 7:229.
11. Camisa C, Weissmann A: Friedrich Sigmund Merkel. Part II. The cell. Am J Dermatopathol 1982; 4:527.
12. Murphy G: Histology of the skin. In Elder D, ed.: Lever's Histopathology of the Skin. Lippincott-Raven, Philadelphia, 1997, pp. 5–50.
13. Gruber S, Wilson L: Merkel cell carcinoma. In Miller S, Maloney M, eds.: Cutaneous Oncology. Blackwell Science, Malden, MA, 1998, pp. 710–721.
14. Gould V, Moll R, Moll I, et al.: Biology of disease: Neuroendocrine (Merkel) cells of the skin: Hyperplasia, dysplasia, and neoplasms. Lab Invest 1985; 52:334.
15. Haag ML, Glass LF, Fenske NA: Merkel cell carcinoma. Diagnosis and treatment. Dermatol Surg 1995; 21:669.
16. Shah IA, Netto D, Schlageter MO, et al.: Neurofilament immunoreactivity in Merkel-cell tumors: A differentiating feature from small-cell carcinoma. Mod Pathol 1993; 6:3.
17. Carson HJ, Reddy V, Taxy JB: Proliferation markers and prognosis in Merkel cell carcinoma. J Cutan Pathol 1998; 25:16.
18. Kennedy MM, Blessing K, King G, et al.: Expression of bcl-2 and p53 in Merkel cell carcinoma. An immunohistochemical study. Am J Dermatopathol 1996; 18:273.
19. Krasagakis K, Almond RB, Zouboulis CC, et al.: Merkel cell carcinoma: Report of ten cases with emphasis on clinical course, treatment, and in vitro drug sensitivity. J Am Acad Dermatol 1997; 36:727.
20. Kroll M, Toker C: Trabecular carcinoma of the skin. Arch Pathol Lab Med 1982; 106:404.
21. Cullen K, Subbusswamy S, Lamberty B: Small cell carcinoma of the skin: A report of two cases. Br J Plast Surg 1985; 38:575.
22. Schmidt U, Muller U, Metz KA, et al.: Cytokeratin and neurofilament protein staining in Merkel cell carcinoma of the small cell type and small cell carcinoma of the lung. Am J Dermatopathol 1998; 20:346.
23. Brinkschmidt C, Stolze P, Fahrenkamp A, et al.: Immunohistochemical demonstration of chromogranin A, chromogranin B, and secretoneurin in Merkel cell carcinoma of the skin. Appl Immunohistochem 1995; 3:37.
24. Al-Ghazal S, Arora DS, Simpson RH, et al.: Merkel cell carcinoma of the skin. Br J Plast Surg 1996; 49:491.
25. Goldenhersh MA, Prus D, Ron N, et al.: Merkel cell tumor masquerading as granulation tissue on a teenager's toe. Am J Dermatopathol 1992; 14:560.
26. Schmid C, Beham A, Feichtinger J, et al.: Recurrent and subsequently metastasizing Merkel cell carcinoma in a 7-year-old girl. Histopathology 1992; 20:437.
27. Anderson LL, Phipps TJ, McCollough ML: Neuroendocrine carcinoma of the skin (Merkel cell carcinoma) in a black. J Dermatol Surg Oncol 1992; 18:375.
28. Pitale M, Sessions RB, Husain S: An analysis of prognostic factors in cutaneous neuroendocrine carcinoma. Laryngoscope 1992; 102:244.
29. Li S, Brownstein S, Addison DJ, et al.: Merkel cell carcinoma of the eyelid. Can J Ophthalmol 1997; 32:455.
30. Straka JA, Straka MB: A review of Merkel cell carcinoma with emphasis on lymph node disease in the absence of a primary site [review]. Am J Otolaryngol 1997; 18:55.
31. Pilotti S, Rilke F, Lombardi L: Neuroendocrine (Merkel cell) carcinoma of the skin. Am J Surg Pathol 1982; 6:243.
32. Gil-Moreno A, Garcia JA, Gonzalez BJ, et al.: Merkel cell carcinoma of the vulva. Gynecol Oncol 1997; 64:526.
33. Kokoska ER, Kokoska MS, Collins BT, et al.: Early aggressive treatment for Merkel cell carcinoma improves outcome. Am J Surg 1997; 174:688.
34. Formica M, Basolo B, Funaro L, et al.: Merkel cell carcinoma in renal transplant recipient. Nephron 1994; 68:399.
35. Gooptu C, Woollons A, Ross J, et al.: Merkel cell carcinoma arising after therapeutic immunosuppression. Br J Dermatol 1997; 137:637.
36. Lunder EJ, Stern RS: Merkel-cell carcinomas in patients treated with methoxsalen and ultraviolet A radiation [letter]. N Engl J Med 1998; 339:1247.
37. Williams RH, Morgan MB, Mathieson IM, et al.: Merkel cell carcinoma in a renal transplant patient: Increased incidence? Transplantation 1998; 65:1396.
38. LeBoit PE, Crutcher WA, Shapiro PE: Pagetoid intraepidermal spread in Merkel cell (primary neuroendocrine) carcinoma of the skin. Am J Surg Pathol 1992; 16:584.
39. Rocamora A, Badia N, Vives R, et al.: Epidermotropic primary neuroendocrine (Merkel cell) carcinoma of the skin with Pautrier-like microabscesses. Report of three cases and review of the literature. J Am Acad Dermatol 1987; 16:1163.
40. Smith KJ, Skelton H, Holland TT, et al.: Neuroendocrine (Merkel cell) carcinoma with an intraepidermal component. Am J Dermatopathol 1993; 15:528.
41. Leong AS-Y, Phillips G, Pieterse A, et al.: Criteria for the diagnosis of primary endocrine carcinoma of the skin (Merkel cell carcinoma). A histological, immunohistochemical and ultrastructural study of 13 cases. Pathology 1986; 18:393.

42. Gottschalk SS, Ne'eman Z, Glick T: Merkel cell carcinoma diagnosed by fine-needle aspiration. Am J Dermatopathol 1996; 18:269.

43. Gould E, Albores-Saavedra J, Dubner B, et al.: Eccrine and squamous differentiation in Merkel cell carcinoma. Am J Surg Pathol 1988; 12:768.

44. Cerroni L, Kerl H: Primary cutaneous neuroendocrine (Merkel cell) carcinoma in association with squamous and basal-cell carcinoma. Am J Dermatopathol 1997; 19:610.

45. Battifora H, Silva E: The use of antikeratin antibodies in the immunohistochemical distinction between neuroendocrine (Merkel cell) carcinoma of the skin, lymphoma, and oat cell carcinoma. Cancer 1986; 58:1040.

46. Miettinen M: Keratin 20: Immunohistochemical marker for gastrointestinal, urothelial, and Merkel cell carcinomas. Mod Pathol 1995; 8:384.

47. Moll R, Franke W: Cytoskeletal differences between human neuroendocrine tumors: A cytoskeletal protein of molecular weight 46,000 distinguishes cutaneous from pulmonary neuroendocrine neoplasms. Differentiation 1985; 30:165.

48. Moll R, Lowe A, Laufer J, et al.: Cytokeratin 20 in human carcinomas. A histodiagnostic marker detected by monoclonal antibodies. Am J Pathol 1992; 140:427.

49. Scott M, Helm K: Cytokeratin 20: A marker for diagnosing Merkel cell carcinoma. Am J Dermatopathol 1999; 21:16.

50. Velasco M, Sabater V, Alzaga A: Cytokeratin 20 expression in primary neuroendocrine carcinoma of the skin [abstract]. J Cutan Pathol 1997; 24:130.

51. Mount SL, Taatjes DJ: Neuroendocrine carcinoma of the skin (Merkel cell carcinoma). An immunoelectron-microscopic case study. Am J Dermatopathol 1994; 16:60.

52. Eusebi V, Capella C, Cossu A, et al.: Neuroendocrine carcinoma within lymph nodes in the absence of a primary tumor, with special reference to Merkel cell carcinoma [see comments]. Am J Surg Pathol 1992; 16:658.

53. Woo HH, Kencian JD: Metastatic Merkel cell tumour to the bladder. Int Urol Nephrol 1995; 27:301.

54. Ro JY, Ayala AG, Tetu B, et al.: Merkel cell carcinoma metastatic to the testis. Am J Clin Pathol 1990; 94:384.

55. Penneys NS, Shapiro S: CD44 expression in Merkel cell carcinoma may correlate with risk of metastasis. J Cutan Pathol 1994; 21:22.

56. Harnett P, Kearsley J, Hayward N, et al.: Loss of allelic heterozygosity on distal chromosome 1p in Merkel cell carcinoma; A marker of neural crest origins? Cancer Genet Cytogenet 1991; 54:109.

57. Koduru P, Dicostanzo D, Jhanwar S: Non random cytogenetic changes characterize Merkel cell carcinoma. Dis Markers 1989; 7:153.

58. Sozzi G, Bertoglio M, Pilotti S, et al.: Cytogenetic studies in primary and metastatic neuroendocrine Merkel cell carcinoma. Cancer Genet Cytogenet 1988; 30:151.

59. Smadja N, de Gramont A, Gonzalez-Canali G: Cytogenetic study in a bone marrow metastatic Merkel cell carcinoma. Cancer Genet Cytogenet 1991; 51:85.

60. Perlman E, Hawkins A, Griffin C: Primary cutaneous neuroendocrine carcinoma (Merkel cell carcinoma): Cytogenetic and MIC2 analysis [abstract]. Cancer Genet Cytogenet 1993; 66:153.

61. Zhang P, Sait S, Aljada I, et al.: Trisomy 6 (Tri 6) in Merkel cell carcinoma (MCC); A fluorescence in-situ hybridization (FISH) study [abstract]. Mod Pathol 1999; 12:65A.

62. Ronan S, Green A, Shilkaitis A: Merkel cell carcinoma: In vitro and in vivo characteristics of a new cell line. J Am Acad Dermatol 1993; 29:715.

63. Larsimont D, Verhest A: Chromosome 6 trisomy as sole anomaly in a primary Merkel cell carcinoma. Virchows Arch 1996; 428:305.

64. Yiengpruksawan A, Coit DG, Thaler HT, et al.: Merkel cell carcinoma. Prognosis and management. Arch Surg 1992; 126:1514.

65. Bryd-Gloster AL, Khoor A, Glass LF, et al.: Differential expression of thyroid transcription factor 1 in small cell lung carcinoma and Merkel cell tumor. Hum Pathol 2000; 31:58.

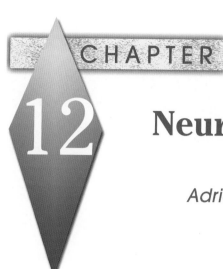

Neuroendocrine Tumors of the Ovary

Adriana Reyes and Maria J. Merino

Ovarian neuroendocrine neoplasms comprise a heterogeneous group of tumor entities with a common characteristic: the potential for endocrine differentiation. The spectrum of ovarian neoplasms with an extensive or partial neuroendocrine component is wide and includes carcinoid tumors of insular, trabecular, and strumal types, and small cell carcinomas of pulmonary type. In addition, it has been clearly demonstrated that neuroendocrine cells can be present in association with other types of ovarian neoplasm, and that tumors often show mixed or "divergent" differentiation. In the ovary, pathologists are describing the admixture of two distinct histologic patterns, such as surface epithelial tumors (benign or malignant) and nonsmall cell neuroendocrine carcinoma. Finally, for completeness, we have also included small cell carcinomas of hypercalcemic type (of unproved neuroendocrine differentiation) and neuroendocrine tumors metastatic to the ovaries.

An important concept in understanding the clinical behavior of neuroendocrine neoplasms is that all of them are at least potentially malignant tumors. Even with regard to classic carcinoid tumor (generally regarded as a tumor at the low end of the spectrum of biologic behavior), there are many documented examples of metastasizing lesions.[1-6]

PRIMARY CARCINOID TUMORS OF THE OVARY

Carcinoid tumors are most frequently localized in different areas of the gastrointestinal tract and less frequently in the pulmonary bronchi, biliary tract, and ovaries. These neoplasms have been divided into three categories according to their site of origin: foregut, midgut, and hindgut. Each type is associated with certain histologic appearances and histochemical reactions, as well as characteristic clinical findings. Primary ovarian carcinoids are rare, accounting for less than 1% of all carcinoid tumors.

Carcinoid tumors of the ovary were first described in 1939 by Stewart and associates,[7] who reported two cases of an insular carcinoid tumor arising in association with an ovarian teratoma. Although these tumors occur predominantly in postmenopausal women, they can affect all age groups. The most common clinical manifestation is that of a pelvic mass. Ovarian carcinoid tumors are invariably unilateral; however, in 15% of cases, cystic teratomas, Brenner's tumors, and mucinous tumors have been reported in the contralateral ovary. The majority occur in association with mature cystic teratomas, but a considerable number of carcinoids present in a pure form. Primary carcinoid tumors of the ovary have been divided into three major histologic types: insular (midgut derivation), trabecular (foregut or hindgut derivation), and strumal (struma ovarii and carcinoid). The insular carcinoid is by far the most common, followed by the strumal type and the rare pure trabecular carcinoid. Mixed patterns (trabecular/insular) and rare cell types of carcinoid (mucinous carcinoid) have been reported.[8, 9] The heterogeneity of morphologic and histochemical features also extends to ultrastructural characteristics, in particular the size and shape of secretory granules. Ovarian carcinoid tumors confined to one ovary should be treated by surgery alone, with a good expected outcome. The possibility of metastatic spread (from a gastrointestinal primary) should be excluded, especially in patients who present with advanced-stage disease.

Ovarian Insular Carcinoid

Considered to be the most common type of ovarian carcinoid, the insular or islet carcinoid tumor (midgut derivation) is frequently a component of a mature cystic teratoma.[1, 2, 10, 11] In rare instances, insular carcinoid can occur in association with mucinous cystadenoma of borderline malignancy, mucinous adenocarcinoma,[12] and Sertoli-Leydig cell tumors.[13]

313

Patients range in age from approximately 30 to 80 years[2] and usually present with signs and symptoms of an enlarging ovarian mass (usually abdominal pain).

Clinical Manifestations of Carcinoid Syndrome

Carcinoid syndrome[1, 4] is found only in association with tumors of the insular type, reflecting their more active secretion of 5-hydroxyindole acetic acid (5-HIAA) and vasoactive kinins. Approximately one-third of reported cases show preoperative clinical evidence of the syndrome, including hot flashes, diarrhea, cardiac murmur, and peripheral edema. The signs and symptoms of the syndrome usually disappear after the removal of the tumor.[1, 5, 10] In the case of ovarian carcinoids, the syndrome occurs in the absence of hepatic or other metastases because the tumor products enter the systemic circulation directly, bypassing the portal venous system and inactivation by the liver. This is in contrast to intestinal carcinoids, which are symptomatic if extensive metastatic (predominantly hepatic) disease is present. Patients with carcinoid syndrome are most commonly over 50 years of age.

It has been documented that the larger the tumor mass, the higher the probability of developing carcinoid syndrome. Prominent morphologic features such as acinar differentiation seem also to correlate with clinical evidence of the syndrome.[1] Urinary 5-HIAA levels can be elevated and usually return to normal after surgical removal of the tumor.

Pathology

Ovarian insular carcinoid tumors are usually unilateral and confined to the ovary. Grossly, these tumors vary in size from incidental microscopic findings to large bulky masses that appear as firm, homogeneous, yellow-to-brown nodules in the wall of cystic teratomas or mucinous tumors[12] (Fig. 12–1). The cut surface of pure insular carcinoids has a solid, gray-to-yellow appearance, with small cystic areas.[5, 10] Mature cystic teratomas or mucinous tumors affect the contralateral ovary in about 16% of the cases.[1]

Histologically, these tumors resemble midgut carcinoids. They are composed of nests and islands of tumor cells forming small acinar structures that are separated by variable amounts of fibrous stroma. Luminal formation is not infrequently found. Tumor cells are uniform, with little or no variation in size. The nucleus is small, round, and centrally located, with stippled chromatin (Fig. 12–2). The cells lining the acini are cuboidal to columnar, with basally located nuclei and finely granular cytoplasm. Acinar structures may contain a small amount of eosinophilic secretion that can become calcified within the lumen of the glands. The peripheral cells

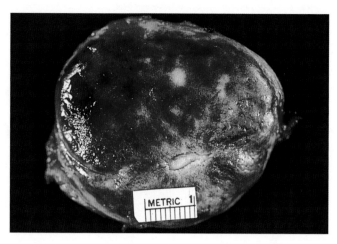

Figure 12–1. Gross appearance of an ovarian carcinoid presenting in a 57-year-old woman with carcinoid syndrome. On cut section, the tumor shows the characteristic yellow-brown color.

of the islands contain coarse granules that appear reddish-brown when stained with hematoxylin and eosin (H&E). They can exhibit argentaffin and argyrophil reactions when stained with the Masson-Fontana, Grimelius, and Pascal stains.[1] Necrosis, hemorrhage, and mitotic figures are rare.

Immunohistochemistry studies demonstrate positivity to neuroendocrine markers such as neuron-specific enolase (NSE), serotonin, synaptophysin (Fig. 12–3) and chromogranin. In 7% of cases, immunoreactivity has been demonstrated for one or more peptide hormones, including somatostatin, glucagon, and pancreatic polypeptide,[14] but this finding is much less frequent than in trabecular (53% of cases) or strumal carcinoids (42% of cases). Ultrastructurally, polymorphic electron-dense core granules, separated from the limiting membrane by a translucent zone, are present.[1, 5, 15] These granules vary greatly in size, ranging from 150 to 400 nm, and often show a reniform dumbbell shape, characteristic of insular carcinoids.

Differential Diagnosis

The differential diagnosis of insular carcinoid, especially in the pure form, includes metastatic insular carcinoid tumors, usually of gastrointestinal origin. Bilateral involvement, multiple tumor nodules, extraovarian metastases, and the presence of an intestinal carcinoid tumor are all helpful in establishing the diagnosis of a metastatic lesion. Overall, if an ovarian carcinoid is unilateral, associated with a teratoma, and without evidence of metastatic disease, it is most probably primary.

Granulosa cell tumors can be confused with the acini of insular carcinoid tumors. However, Call-Exner bodies are frequently not as sharply outlined as the acinar formation of carcinoids, and the granulosa cells around Call-Exner bodies lack the abun-

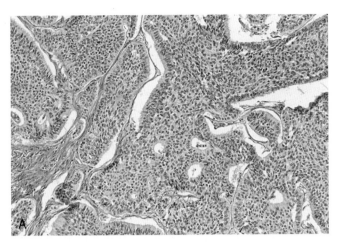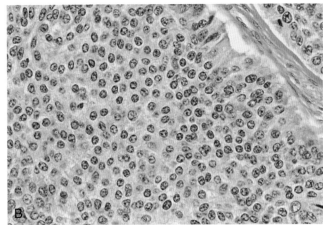

Figure 12-2. A, B, Histologically, carcinoids are composed of nests of cells with round nuclei. Coarse chromatin glands with round small acini are also present. (*A,* H&E ×150; *B,* H&E ×400.)

dant cytoplasm of cells forming the lumen of a carcinoid acinus. Also, the secretions of granulosa cell tumors are frequently watery and eosinophilic. Meanwhile, the acini of insular carcinoid tumors often contain dense eosinophilic secretions that can become calcified. In addition, carcinoids have a characteristic nuclei with coarse chromatin. In difficult cases, immunohistochemistry should assist in and confirm the diagnosis of neuroendocrine origin. Ovarian insular carcinoids can also be misdiagnosed with Brenner's tumors, but the urothelial transitional cell appearance with grooved "coffee bean" nuclei seen in Brenner's tumors is diagnostic of this entity. The absence of argentaffin granules in Brenner's tumors further helps in the differential diagnosis. Additionally, the acini within the Brenner nests are often lined by mucinous cells, unlike those of a carcinoid acinus. Other entities that can be included in the differential diagnosis include Sertoli-Leydig cell tumors and adenocarcinomas. Insular carcinoid tumors have been reported arising within a Sertoli-Leydig tumor and adjacent to Brenner's tumors.[1, 13]

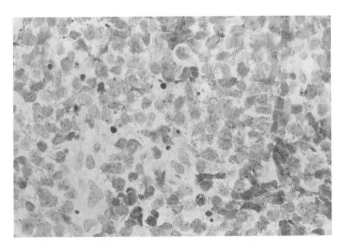

Figure 12-3. Immunohistochemistry shows positive staining for synaptophysin.

Prognosis

Insular carcinoids are slow-growing neoplasms, and few cases of recurrence or metastasis have been documented.[1-3, 5] However, in one particular study,[4] 6 of 17 patients presented with advanced disease, including extensive peritoneal involvement. Three patients developed metastases to the lung or liver. All six patients had insular carcinoid, five of the pure form. Patients with rare cases of right-sided heart disease caused by carcinoid syndrome have died (due to progression of cardiac symptoms) despite complete resection of the neoplasm.[5, 16] Carcinoid heart disease must be ruled out in all patients by means of a clinical examination and two-dimensional echocardiography.[4]

Treatment

Bilateral salpingo-oophorectomy and hysterectomy is the recommended modality of treatment. Younger patients in whom preservation of ovarian function is important should undergo unilateral salpingo-oophorectomy with biopsy of the contralateral ovary. Most insular carcinoids behave in a benign manner, with an excellent overall reported survival rate for patients with disease confined to one ovary. Advanced-stage disease is associated with poor prognosis, a median survival of 1.2 years, and a 33% 5-year survival rate, after treatment with radiotherapy or chemotherapy.[4] Postoperatively, patients can be followed with serial urinary 5-HIAA determinations to monitor recurrences.

Ovarian Trabecular Carcinoid

Carcinoid tumors showing the trabecular pattern are considered to be of foregut or hindgut derivation. These tumors are the least common type of ovarian carcinoids, with fewer than 50 cases reported in the literature.[4, 17-20] Primary trabecular carcinoid tumors share many characteristics with the more common primary insular carcinoids: age distribution, gross appearance, frequent association with mature teratomas, and rare occurrence in a pure form.[19, 20] Clinically, they are slow-growing tumors that, in contrast to insular carcinoids, are not associated with the signs and symptoms of carcinoid syndrome. The age of presentation ranges from 24 to 74 years, with a mean of 46 ± 12 years.[19,20] The most frequent complaints are of abdominal pain and swelling.[19] Rare cases are associated with long-term constipation[4, 18, 21, 22] (a gut hormone called peptide tyrosine is presumed to cause this specific symptom) and elevated levels of serum carcinoembryonic antigen (CEA).[18]

Pathology

The size of the tumor ranges from 4 to 25 cm, with a mean of 11.6 ± 5.8 cm.[17] Macroscopically, when found in association with cystic teratomas, the tumor forms a small mass in an otherwise obvious dermoid cyst. In a pure form, these tumors have a smooth outline and glistening capsule. The cut surface is tan-yellow, firm to hard in consistency, and finely granular. These tumors are usually unilateral and can be found in association with a dermoid cyst in the contralateral ovary.[19]

Histologically, the tumor is composed of long, wavy, ramifying, and anastomosing cords, ribbons, or trabeculae surrounded by connective tissue stroma, which varies from loose and edematous to dense and fibrous[23] (Fig. 12–4). The tumor cells are columnar, arranged with their long axes parallel to each other, and usually forming one or two layers without glandular or insular structures. The cells are uniform, with abundant cytoplasm and oval-to-elongated nuclei with a fine chromatin pattern.

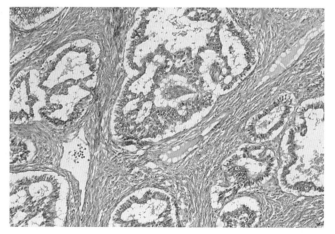

Figure 12–4. Trabecular carcinoids are composed of cords and ribbons of uniform round-to-oval cells with variable amounts of cytoplasm. The tumor cells are surrounded by fibrous stroma. (H&E ×150.)

Mitotic activity is low. Occasional cells may contain small orange-to-red-brown granules in the cytoplasm that stain positive with argyrophilic reactions and are rarely positive for argentaffin reactions, by the Masson-Fontana method.[19, 20] Immunohistochemical studies show positivity for chromogranin[18, 24] neuron-specific enolase,[18, 24] and synaptophysin. In one study by Sporrong and coworkers,[14] 53% of trabecular carcinoids were immunoreactive to neurohormone peptides, including somatostatin, glucagon, pancreatic polypeptide, substance P, calcitonin, and enkephalin. The incidence of these findings is much higher than in insular carcinoids. When examined ultrastructurally, many round-to-oval, membrane-bound, dense neurosecretory granules, with only slight variation in size (ranging from 170 to 290 nm in diameter) and uniform in shape, are typically found.[17, 19, 20]

The differential diagnosis of trabecular carcinoid tumors of the ovary includes metastatic trabecular carcinoid tumors, Sertoli-Leydig cell tumors, and strumal carcinoid. Metastatic trabecular carcinoids are very rare, with few cases reported.[19, 25] The differences between a metastatic carcinoid and a primary ovarian carcinoid are similar to those described for insular carcinoids. Metastatic lesions are usually bilateral and associated with metastasis in other organs. The presence of teratomatous elements helps exclude a metastatic lesion.

Trabecular carcinoids can be misdiagnosed as Sertoli-Leydig cell tumors of the ovary with a pronounced trabecular or cordlike pattern, because of the resemblance of the ribbons to the cords of the latter. However, the ribbons of carcinoids are larger, more uniform, and more numerous than the shorter, thinner, more sparsely distributed cords of a Sertoli-Leydig cell tumor, which is usually associated with other histologic patterns. Carcinoid ribbons are set in a fibrous stroma, and the cells are larger and have abundant cytoplasm with argentaffin granules, whereas the cells of the Sertoli-Leydig cell tumor have little cytoplasm and are often separated by Leydig's cells.[19] In difficult cases, electron microscopy studies can demonstrate the presence of neurosecretory granules within the cytoplasm; these are round, homogeneous, and specific for trabecular carcinoids. Another entity that can cause confusion is the presence of thyroid follicles within a trabecular carcinoid, indicating that the tumor is a strumal carcinoid (struma ovarii and carcinoid) and not a pure trabecular carcinoid. In addition, some cases of primary ovarian carcinoid composed of both trabecular and insular patterns have been described.[1, 19, 24]

Prognosis

The prognosis of these tumors is usually favorable. As mentioned, these are unilateral, slow-growing tumors that behave like tumors of low malignant potential. There is only one report of a patient who died of the disease with metastasis to the lung, 14 years after the initial diagnosis, following a 13-year disease-free interval.[4] Another case of peritoneal recurrence 2 years after removal of the tumor has also been reported.[19] In younger women, the treatment is unilateral salpingo-oophorectomy, whereas in postmenopausal patients bilateral salpingo-oophorectomy and hysterectomy is the treatment of choice.

Ovarian Strumal Carcinoid

Strumal carcinoid was first described by Scully in 1970,[26] and the largest reported group (50 cases) was reviewed by Robboy and Scully 10 years later.[6] Strumal carcinoid is the second most common type of primary ovarian carcinoid tumor, and numerous case reports have been published.[6, 27-44] Overall, it is an uncommon ovarian tumor composed of an intimate mixture of thyroid tissue and a carcinoid that usually has a trabecular arrangement. Trabecular and strumal carcinoids have similar age distributions and biologic behavior, but strumal carcinoids are characterized by the presence of thyroid tissue admixed with the carcinoid component.

Patients range in age from 21 to 77 years (median, 53 years).[6] Patients usually present with an enlarging unilateral mass, or with no symptoms, the tumors being an incidental finding detected during routine gynecologic or urologic examination.[6, 28, 32] There are reported cases in the literature of strumal carcinoids associated with chronic constipation or pain with defecation,[4, 21] hyperinsulinemic hypoglycemia and cutaneous melanosis,[38] multiple endocrine neoplasia type IIA,[34] virilization and hirsutism,[6] and symptoms related to function of the thyroid component.[2, 6] In contrast to insular carcinoids, only once has a strumal carcinoid occurred in association with carcinoid syndrome.[36]

Pathology

Ovarian strumal carcinoid tumors are frequently found as the predominant component of a mature solid teratoma.[6] Grossly, the tumors vary in size from 5.0 to 22.0 cm in diameter, with a median of 7.0 cm[32] (Fig. 12–5). When the tumor is part of a teratoma, it appears as a yellow-tan solid nodule in the cavity of the cyst. In a pure form, it forms characteristic solid yellow-brown masses. Often, the carcinoid and thyroid components can be recognized grossly, with both areas sharply demarcated in color. These tumors occasionally can be associated with mucinous tumor of the ovary.[6, 27, 33, 35]

Histologically, the two components, thyroid follicles and the carcinoid cells, are usually mixed (Fig. 12–6), and other teratomatous elements are also present frequently in skin and respiratory epithelium (Fig. 12–7A). Either component may predominate. Most frequently, the carcinoid is of the trabecular type (columnar or cuboidal cells forming cords and ribbons), or of the mixed trabecular-insu-

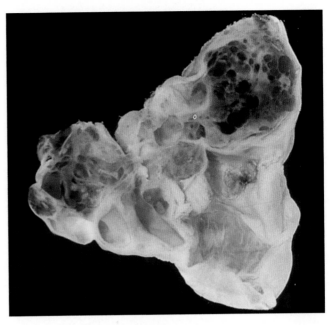

Figure 12–5. Strumal carcinoid, gross appearance. Brown nodules of variable sizes are identified in association with simple ovarian cysts.

lar pattern (with the trabecular pattern usually predominating); in rare instances the tumor may exhibit only the insular pattern.[6, 28] The thyroidal portion of the mass is composed of follicular structures of various sizes, containing eosinophilic dense colloid that resembles normal thyroid, colloid goiter, or a follicular adenoma.[6, 32] The cells lining the follicles range from flat to columnar, and the nuclei range from flat to round with evenly distributed chromatin.[6] Occasionally, the presence of thyroid follicles has been described covering the ovarian surfaces (see Fig. 12–7B). In more than 50% of cases, birefringent calcium oxalate monohydrate crystals are present in the colloid material.[2,6] The areas of follicle formation usually blend into areas of trabecular carcinoid, and

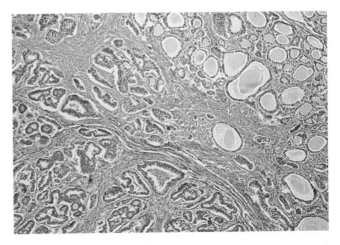

Figure 12–6. Histologically, the areas of normal thyroid follicles merge with the cords and trabeculae of the strumal carcinoid. (H&E ×150.)

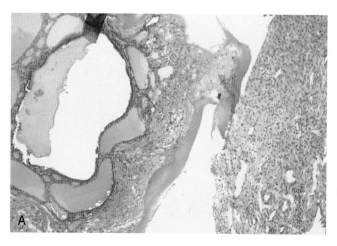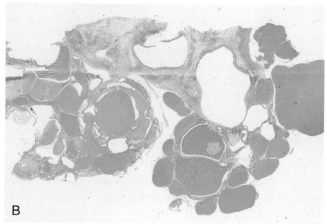

Figure 12–7. A, Struma ovarii. Benign thyroid follicles are distributed throughout the ovarian surface. *B,* Peritoneal implants composed primarily of thyroid follicles. (*A,* H&E ×100; *B,* H&E ×50.)

the intermediate zone between the two tissue elements shows mixed characteristics. The mass is set in a dense fibrous stroma and typically exhibits low mitotic activity. Rare cases have contained amyloid[30, 45, 46] and a variable number of mucus-secreting glands in the carcinoid component.[6, 33, 37, 43]

As in other carcinoids, ovarian strumal carcinoids contain argyrophil and argentaffin granules. However, the granules are in the carcinoid portion, as well as in those areas that merged into or are next to thyroid follicles and (in some cases) in cells lining the thyroid follicles.[6, 31, 32] Immunohistochemical reactions and electron microscopy findings have been contradictory in several reported studies. Immunohistochemically, the tumor cells are reactive for neuron-specific enolase, chromogranin, serotonin, and synaptophysin. Sporrong and coworkers[14] demonstrated immunoreactivity in the carcinoid component (42% of cases) for different neurohormonal peptides, including pancreatic polypeptide, glucagon, enkephalin, calcitonin, somatostatin, vasoactive intestinal polypeptide (VIP), substance P, and endorphin. In another series of cases studied by Stagno and colleagues,[33] somatostatin, serotonin, glucagon, insulin, and gastrin were detected, in that order of frequency. Thyroglobulin has been reported in the strumal component and, in several cases, in the carcinoid portion of the tumor.[30, 32, 36, 39, 43, 47] The presence of calcitonin has been demonstrated,[6, 30, 36, 43] as well as that of CEA.[27, 35] Motoyama and associates[21] reported the presence of the peptide YY in association with clinical symptoms of chronic constipation.

Electron microscopic examination has demonstrated the presence of thyroidal follicular epithelial cells,[31, 33, 36, 39, 43, 48] as well as round, uniform, electron-dense secretory granules in the cytoplasm of the carcinoid, and some cells forming the follicles of the thyroid component. These granules are similar to those observed in trabecular carcinoids.[32, 33, 37, 40, 43]

Carcinoma of the thyroid has been reported in association with struma ovarii (teratoma in which the thyroid tissue is the predominant component). Carcinoma can be follicular or papillary in type and is similar to malignant tumors primary in the thyroid gland. The cells do not contain argentaffin or argyrophil granules, and carcinoid elements are absent.[11] Strumal carcinoids, with few exceptions, have a benign behavior, and their accurate recognition is greatly enhanced by histology, electron microscopy, and particularly immunohistochemistry studies.

Prognosis

The prognosis of patients with strumal carcinoid is excellent following excision of the tumor. The treatment is that of a tumor of low malignant potential, similar to that described earlier for other types of carcinoid tumors. Strumal carcinoid tumor has been associated with metastases in only two reported cases. In one case, the metastatic tumor consisted only of well-differentiated thyroid follicular epithelium.[44] In the other patient, the metastatic lesions were composed only of the carcinoid component. This patient died from the disease 2.5 years postoperatively.[6]

The peculiar combination of thyroid tissue and carcinoid tumor has prompted investigation and debate regarding the histogenesis of this tumor. All evidence supports the germ cell origin of the various tissue elements. Yet it remains unknown whether the neuroendocrine cells of strumal carcinoids originate from C cells of struma ovarii, neuroendocrine cells of teratomatous epithelium that secondarily infiltrate the thyroid follicles, or pluripotential teratomatous endodermal cells capable of differentiation into both thyroid follicles and carcinoid cells.[33] However, even the existence of strumal carcinoids has been questioned by several investigators who concluded that these tumors were pure carcinoid neoplasms.[40–42, 46] There is no longer any doubt as to the identity of thyroid follicles within strumal carcinoids. Their presence has been demonstrated by multiple studies that used immunohistochemical and ultrastructural analyses.[6, 32, 36, 43, 48] Furthermore, many investigators[26, 32, 49, 50] have found similarities between strumal carcinoids and medullary thyroid carcinoma, including the presence of amyloid, calcitonin, CEA reactivity, and dense core granules observed by electron microscopy. The proliferation of neuroendocrine carcinoid cells within follicles, with progressive displacement of thyroid epithelial cells, is similar to the development of C-cell hyperplasia and medullary carcinoma of the thyroid gland. At this time, the theory by Robboy and Scully[6] of both thyroid and carcinoid components originating from the same endodermal germ cell primordium seems most appropriate.

SMALL CELL CARCINOMA, PULMONARY TYPE

This tumor has microscopic features and the neuroendocrine profile of primary small cell carcinoma of the lung. In contrast to small cell carcinomas of the hypercalcemic type, the neuroendocrine differentiation of these tumors has been demonstrated by the histologic growth pattern, the presence of argyrophilic granules, ultrastructural characteristics, and the expression of neuroendocrine markers. However, their histogenesis remains uncertain. Only a few series of cases have been published. Eichhorn and colleagues[51] studied 11 cases. Three more case reports of primary neoplasms of this type have been published: Fukunaga and associates[52] reported a case of a small cell carcinoma of the pulmonary type mixed with carcinoid tumor, and there were two other cases arising in mature cystic teratomas.[53, 54]

This unusual tumor affects predominantly elderly women, but it may occur in younger women as well. The clinical presentation is nonspecific. At the initial time of presentation, 5 of 11 tumors (45%) were bilateral, and most had spread outside the ovary.

Pathology

On gross examination, these tumors appear as large, solid masses, ranging in size from 4.5 to 26 cm with a mean diameter of 13.5 cm. These masses often show areas of cystic degeneration, necrosis, and hemorrhage. Histologically, the tumor typically grows as sheets of closely packed cells forming islands or arranged in a trabecular pattern. The tumor cells are round to oval to spindle-shaped, with little cytoplasm. The nuclei are hyperchromatic, with stippled chromatin and inconspicuous nucleoli. The large nests and sheets of tumor often show central coagulative necrosis. Numerous mitotic figures are present. The stroma can be fibrous with focal edema and hyalinization. Other epithelial elements such as endometrioid carcinoma, squamous differentiation, mucin-producing cells, and Brenner's tumors can be identified in association with the small cell component.[51, 52]

Grimelius stain has been used to show many tumor cells with argyrophil granules. Immunohistochemistry shows variable reactivity for keratin, S-100, *Leu-7,* synaptophysin, epithelial membrane antigen, neuron-specific enolase, chromogranin, and carcinoembryonic antigen.[51, 52, 54] Tumor cells have been negative for vimentin, neurofilament, calcitonin, ACTH, somatostatin, glucagon, and gastrin.[52] In addition, p53 protein accumulation has been reported as strongly positive in one case.[54] Electron microscopy examination demonstrated electron-dense neurosecretory granules.[52, 54] Prominent rough endoplasmic reticulum, a consistent finding in small cell carcinomas with hypercalcemia, has not been found in small cell carcinomas of pulmonary type.[55] In addition, flow cytometry studies have shown the majority of cases to be aneuploid[51, 52] and rare cases to be diploid.[51, 54]

Ovarian small cell tumors are not very common and, when encountered, may pose a problem in diagnosis. The differential diagnosis of small cell carcinoma of the pulmonary type includes mainly small cell carcinoma of the hypercalcemic type and metastatic small cell tumors from the lung, cervix, or gastrointestinal tract. Obtaining adequate clinical information is essential to establish the primary or metastatic nature of the tumor. When a pulmonary small cell carcinoma is found in the presence of a similar tumor in an ovary, the probability is that the pulmonary tumor is primary. This is because pulmonary tumors of this type are more common than primary ovarian small cell carcinomas of the same type.

The presence of other histologic elements will favor an ovarian primary. Primary ovarian small cell carcinomas of the pulmonary type can be misdiagnosed as small cell carcinomas of the hypercalcemic type. Most small cell carcinomas of the pulmonary type are found predominantly in elderly postmenopausal patients, in contrast to small cell carcinomas of the hypercalcemic type. Small cell carcinomas of the hypercalcemic type are usually unilateral, whereas the pulmonary type has been reported as bilateral in 45% of the cases.[51] The hypercalcemic type shows follicles with eosinophilic fluid and foci of larger cells, with prominent nucleoli in about half of the cases. In addition, the trabecular and solid nesting growth patterns that are seen frequently in the hypercalcemic type are not seen in the pulmonary type. Overall, even though the features of these two neoplasms can overlap in some cases, they differ histologically and ultrastructurally (the hypercalcemic type has cells with dilated rough endoplasmic reticulum and lacks the dense core granules seen in the pulmonary type), and in their DNA flow cytometric features (usually aneuploid in the pulmonary type and diploid in the hypercalcemic type).[56, 57] Immunohistochemistry is not always useful due to overlapping in staining patterns.

These tumors behave aggressively. The prognosis of these patients is poor. In the largest published series of cases, most patients with follow-up died of the disease or had recurrences.[51]

SMALL CELL CARCINOMA, HYPERCALCEMIC TYPE

Ovarian small cell carcinoma, which is associated with paraneoplastic hypercalcemia in two-thirds of cases, is a rare and distinctive type of undifferentiated carcinoma. First described by Dickersin and coworkers[58] in 1982, the largest series of cases was published by Young and coworkers in 1994.[59] Numerous case reports can be found in the literature.[60-69] The histogenesis of these tumors remains uncertain. The nature of the substance secreted by the ovarian small cell carcinoma that results in hypercalcemia is also unclear. Some publications have reported reactivity to parathyroid hormone or parathyroid hormone–related protein.[59, 70, 71] Nevertheless, in most instances, attempts to recover these substances have been unsuccessful. Presently, the neuroendocrine differentiation of these tumors has not been proved. For completeness, we have included these tumors in this review.

These are rare and often lethal neoplasms that occur in young women. The age of the patients has ranged from 9 to 45 years of age (average, 24).[58, 59, 67, 70, 72] These tumors are the most frequently encountered forms of undifferentiated ovarian carcinoma in women under 40 years of age. The familial occurrence of small cell carcinoma of the hypercalcemic type appears to be a rare phenomenon; few such cases have been reported.[59, 62, 63, 72] Most patients have presented with nonspecific symptoms, including abdominal pain or swelling, nausea, vomiting, anorexia, and weight loss;[59, 61, 63] symptoms have rarely been related to hypercalcemia.[61] These tumors are unilateral in 99% of cases.[59] By the time of discovery at laparotomy, extraovarian spread is already present in about 50% of patients.[59]

The tumors range in size from 6 to 26 cm (average, 15.3).[59] On gross examination, the neoplasms are usually large and solid, often with cystic degeneration. The cut surface of the ovary reveals a lobu-

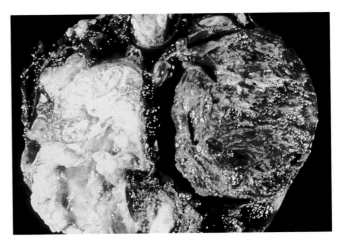

Figure 12-8. Large small cell carcinoma of the ovary. Extensive areas of hemorrhage and necrosis are present.

lated, white-cream-to-gray, fleshy, or friable surface with large or focal areas of necrosis and hemorrhage (Fig. 12–8). Cystic degeneration can be seen, and one tumor was described in the literature as a unilocular cyst.[67]

On light microscopy, different histologic patterns have been described. The most common appearance is a diffuse, solid sheet of generally small and rounded, closely packed epithelial cells. These cells can also grow in nests, cords, trabeculae, and irregular groups. Individual cells have little cytoplasm and small round-ovoid, hyperchromatic nuclei with single small nucleoli (Fig. 12–9). Focal areas with a spindle cell pattern have also been noted.[59] Follicle-like structures of varying sizes lined with neoplastic cells are present in 80% of the tumors. These spaces can be either empty or can contain an eosinophilic or basophilic material.[59] Mitotic figures are numerous and often atypical. Mucin-rich cells ranging from benign-appearing and atypical to scattered signet-ring cells are seen in about 12% of cases.[59] The

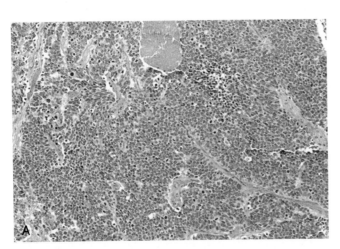

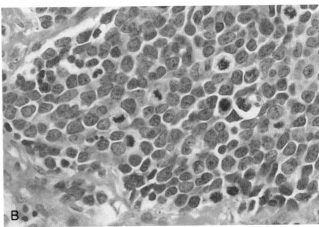

Figure 12-9. A, B, Histologically, small cell carcinomas are identical to their lung counterpart. The cells are oval to round, with small amounts of cytoplasm. Numerous mitotic figures are present.

scant stromal matrix can be dense, myxoid, or edematous.

In approximately 50% of the tumors, there are focal areas composed of large cells with copious, pale to slightly eosinophilic cytoplasm, central and often vesicular nuclei, and prominent nucleoli. Large, pale intracytoplasmic hyaline globules have been described within these large cells.[59, 60] However, these cells rarely predominate. Young and associates[59] designated small cell carcinomas of the hypercalcemic type with a predominance of large cells as the large cell variant of small cell carcinoma, hypercalcemic type. A case report of this variant has been recently published.[60] The clinicopathology, immunohistochemistry, and range of histologic patterns are similar to those of the conventional small cell carcinomas of the hypercalcemic type. The presence of large cells does not appear to predict a worse outcome.[56]

Special staining and ultrastructural examination have not revealed any features that identify the cell of origin of this tumor. Tumor cells have been reported variably positive for vimentin, cytokeratin, neuron-specific enolase, chromogranin, synaptophysin (Figs. 12–10 and 12–11), parathyroid hormone–related protein, and epithelial membrane antigen.[59, 60, 70, 71] Seidman[63] reported that 80% of tumors exhibit p53 protein accumulation in immunohistochemistry studies. Electron microscopy discloses that large amounts of dilated and filled cisternae of rough endoplasmic reticulum have been their most constant feature; in addition, the epithelial nature of the tumor cells has been demonstrated.[55, 57, 73] A prominent ultrastructural finding in cases of large cell variant is the presence of numerous paranuclear whorls of microfilaments, which corresponds with the dense globular appearance of the cytoplasm under light microscopy.[57, 72, 74] The presence of convincing neurosecretory granules has not yet been confirmed in ovarian small cell carcinomas,[55] although there is one report of scattered structures that were interpreted as dense core granules of the neuroendocrine type.[70] Flow cytometry analysis reveals that

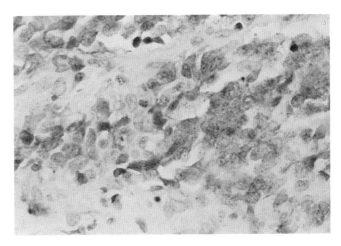

Figure 12–11. Small cell ovarian cancer showing positive immunohistochemical staining for synaptophysin.

the tumor cells show a diploid DNA pattern,[56, 62] a surprising characteristic in view of the high degree of malignancy of this tumor. However, one case of the large cell variant of small cell carcinoma with hypercalcemia was reported as aneuploid.[60] Overall, DNA ploidy and the proliferative activity of this neoplasm do not correlate with stage and outcome.[56]

Small cell carcinomas of the hypercalcemic type can be confused with ovarian small cell carcinomas of the pulmonary type, granulosa cell tumors (adult or juvenile), malignant lymphomas, primitive neuroectodermal tumors, primary or metastatic malignant melanoma, metastatic alveolar rhabdomyosarcoma, and desmoplastic small round cell tumors.

Differentiation of small cell carcinomas of the hypercalcemic type from the pulmonary type has already been discussed. The cells of small cell carcinoma do not have the characteristic pale and often grooved nuclei of adult granulosa cell tumors. The much higher mitotic rate in small cell carcinomas and the formation of Call-Exner bodies in adult granulosa cell tumors also aid in the distinction between these two entities. The morphologic appearance of the tumor with the follicle-like spaces and the young age of most patients results in misinterpretation of some cases as juvenile granulosa cell tumors (JGCT) (Figs. 12–12 and 12–13). Typical small cell carcinomas are composed of small cells with little cytoplasm in contrast to JGCT cells that have abundant amounts of cytoplasm. More difficulty exists with the large cell variant of small cell carcinoma; however, these tumors tend to have at least focal areas of typical small cell carcinoma with scant cytoplasm, which are not features of JGCTs. JGCTs have mitotic figures but usually much less than small cell carcinomas. A thecal cell component, which is usually present in JGCTs, is not observed in small cell carcinomas. In addition, clinical evidence of estrogen production, which is associated with most granulosa cell tumors, has not been found in cases of small cell carcinoma, nor has hypercalcemia been seen in

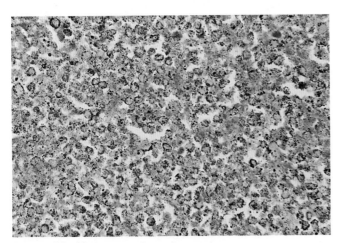

Figure 12–10. Positive Grimelius stain.

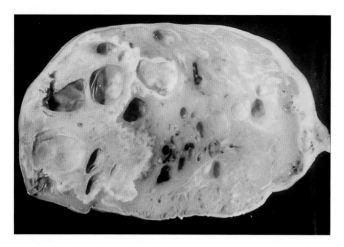

Figure 12–12. Juvenile granulosa cell tumor. Cut section shows solid and cystic areas. Foci of hemorrhage and necrosis are also present.

cases of granulosa cell tumors. Finally, small cell carcinomas are negative for inhibin-α and can be positive for epithelial membrane antigen, in contrast to JGCTs.[47]

Small cell carcinomas can be differentiated from diffuse malignant lymphomas by determining the epithelial nature of the tumors with immunohistochemistry stains, which show reactivity to various cytokeratins, vimentin, and epithelial membrane antigen. However, in most cases the clinical and cytologic features of the two tumors permit their distinction. Confusion with metastatic malignant melanoma has occurred in cases of melanoma with small cells and follicle-like structures. The clinical history and special studies are important in making the correct diagnosis in these cases. The differential diagnosis of small cell carcinoma also includes other small cell malignant tumors of the ovary, such as primitive neuroectodermal tumors and various small cell sarcomas. All these tumors have distinctive clini-

cal, light microscopic, immunohistochemical, and electron microscopic features that differ from those of the small cell carcinoma of hypercalcemic type. As in any case, thorough sampling of the tumor is very important.

Small cell carcinoma of the hypercalcemic type is a very aggressive tumor with poor prognosis. In the largest series of these cases in the literature, by Young and coworkers,[59] almost all the patients with stages higher than IA died of disease. Of 42 patients with stage IA tumors (with follow-up information), 14 had disease-free follow-up, which ranged from 1 to 13 years (average, 5.7) postsurgery; 23 died of the disease within 2 years, and 5 were alive with recurrences. Apparently, there is no significant difference in prognosis between the large cell variant and the classic small cell carcinoma of hypercalcemic type.[59] Tumors that occur in women older than 30 years of age, lack hypercalcemia, and are less than 10 cm are associated with a more favorable prognosis. There appears to be no place for conservative surgery regardless of an early stage of disease, or the young age of the patient. The role of adjuvant therapy is unclear. Combination chemotherapy and radiation therapy for high-stage tumors have been generally unsuccessful.[59] Serum calcium levels can be used as a marker in monitoring treatment response and recurrence, since levels usually fall to normal for those cases in which the tumor has been completely removed.[75]

EPITHELIAL TUMORS WITH NEUROENDOCRINE DIFFERENTIATION

Neuroendocrine cells have been identified in a variety of ovarian surface epithelial neoplasms, including endometrioid adenocarcinoma,[76, 77] mucinous tumors (benign, borderline, and malignant),[77–80] serous tumors,[81] and Brenner's tumors.[82] However, the presence of such cells has not affected progno-

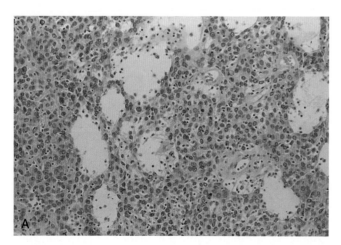
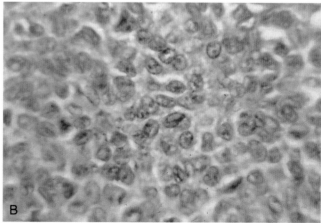

Figure 12–13. A, B, Juvenile granulosa cell tumor, showing oval follicles, and lined by round to oval cells with variable amounts of cytoplasm. The nuclei may show the characteristic groove or exhibit variable degrees of anaplasia and pleomorphism.

sis. Carcinomas with neuroendocrine differentiation accompanied by surface epithelial neoplasia are neoplasms in which the neuroendocrine component lacks the small cell phenotype but are of a higher grade than carcinoid tumors. These are rare tumors that probably belong in the category of surface epithelial neoplasms, which express endocrine pathways of differentiation.

To date, to the best of our knowledge, eight ovarian neuroendocrine carcinomas have been described: seven admixed with a mucinous tumor[83-86] and one with an endometrioid carcinoma[84] (Fig. 12–14A). Patient age ranged from 22 to 77 years old. They presented with abdominal distention, a palpable mass, or abdominal pain.[83-86] Six of the patients presented with stage I disease; one was stage II, and another patient was stage III. The tumors are typically unilateral, and the gross features are similar to those of other ovarian surface epithelial neoplasms. Most of the tumors have cystic and solid components. The solid (neuroendocrine) components of the tumors range in size from 2 to 9 cm.[84]

On microscopic examination, tumors mixed with mucinous neoplasms usually have separate glandular and solid neuroendocrine components (see Fig. 12–14B). The neuroendocrine component is characterized by the presence of islands, irregular sheets, and trabeculae, with little intervening stroma. The stroma ranges from loose to densely fibrous. The tumor cells are of medium-to-large size, with moderate amounts of eosinophilic cytoplasm and large, ovoid vesicular nuclei with coarse, clumped chromatin. Focal areas of necrosis are usually seen, as well as a high mitotic rate.[84] The mucinous glandular component of the tumor was mucinous adenocarcinoma in two cases,[84] mucinous borderline tumor with small foci of mucinous carcinoma in four cases,[83, 84, 86] and mucinous cystadenoma in one case.[85] Only in one case, the glandular component was an endometrioid carcinoma grade 1 of 3.[84]

The neuroendocrine and glandular components of these tumors show a variable number of cells that stain positively for argyrophil and/or argentaffin granules[83, 84, 86] (see Fig. 12–14C) and mucin (Fig. 12–14D). Immunohistochemistry shows positive reactivity (of variable intensity) to chromogranin, neuron-specific enolase, serotonin, synaptophysin, and cytokeratin. In addition, hormone neuropeptides were

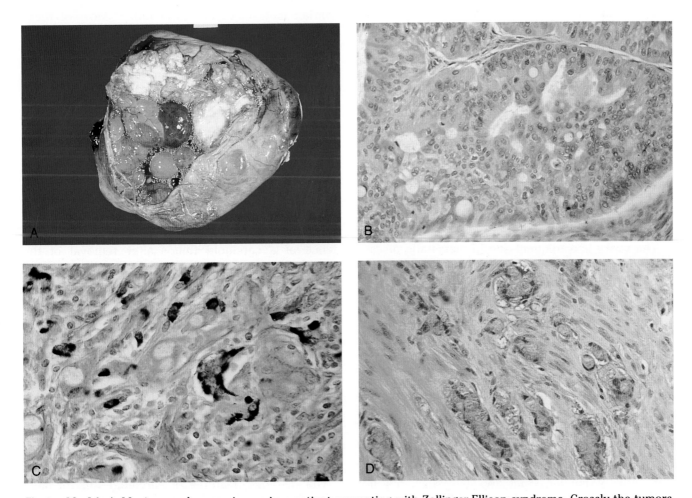

Figure 12–14. A, Mucinous adenocarcinoma in a patient presenting with Zollinger-Ellison syndrome. Grossly the tumors resemble other types of mucinous adenocarcinoma. *B,* Histologically, a moderately differentiated adenocarcinoma with prominent neuroendocrine cells. *C,* Numerous neuroendocrine cells stain positive for Grimelius. *D,* Mucicarmine positivity in tumor cells.

detected in some cases, including vasoactive intestinal peptide, somatostatin, gastrin, and glucagon.[84] When electron microscopy examination was performed, dense core granules were detected.[83, 85, 86]

The differential diagnosis includes the less malignant carcinoid tumor, small cell carcinoma, undifferentiated carcinomas, and metastatic lesions. Unlike carcinoid tumors, these tumors show a predominantly solid growth pattern, extensive necrosis, and high mitotic rate. Overall, the greater atypia of these tumors (in contrast to that of carcinoids) helps in the differential diagnosis. Epithelial tumors with neuroendocrine differentiation can also be confused with undifferentiated growth of the associated surface epithelial tumor, but the trabecular and insular patterns and the uniform nuclei should suggest the neuroendocrine differentiation of the tumor. In these cases, special stains further help in the recognition of the neuroendocrine origin. The differential diagnosis with small cell carcinomas, which is based on nuclear size, has academic but no prognostic significance. The association of these tumors with surface epithelial tumors and the clinical history help exclude the possibility of a metastatic neuroendocrine neoplasm.

Initial observations suggest that, unlike primary carcinoid tumors of the ovary, which are considered to have low malignant potential, neuroendocrine carcinomas of the ovary associated with epithelial tumors behave in an extremely aggressive manner. The prognosis was poor in all the cases with follow-up information.[83–86] It would be expected that the responses to therapy and behavior of these mixed lesions would also be a hybrid of each component in pure form. Optimal therapeutic approaches for these tumors have yet to be delineated.

SECONDARY (METASTATIC) NEUROENDOCRINE TUMORS

The ovary is a frequent site of metastatic disease from numerous sites, the most common being the gastrointestinal tract, breast, hematopoietic system, and other organs in the genital tract (endometrium and cervix).[2, 87] As many as 5% to 10% of malignant tumors involving the ovary that are encountered as surgical pathology specimens are metastatic.[88] Recognition of the metastatic nature of an ovarian tumor depends on an adequate clinical history, thorough search for a primary tumor elsewhere, and a detailed evaluation of the gross and microscopic features of the neoplasms. In some instances, special stains and electron microscopy can be helpful. Malignant tumors spread to the ovary by contiguity, surface implantation, and hematogenous and lymphatic routes. Gross features of metastatic tumors vary greatly. Findings that are suggestive, but not pathognomonic, of metastases are the presence of multiple discrete nodules within the ovary, the location of tumor deposits on its surface, and the presence of bilateral tumors.

Most secondary ovarian tumors (70%) are bilateral. The possibility of metastases should be seriously considered when evaluating bilateral cancers. However, although metastatic tumors as a group are bilateral more often than primary tumors, many metastatic tumors are unilateral. Accordingly, unilaterality should not dissuade the pathologist from considering the possibility of metastases if the histologic features suggest it.[88] Under microscopic examination, the presence of focal implants on the surface or superficial cortex of the ovary, growth in the form of multiple nodules, and lymphatic or blood vessel invasion strongly suggest metastasis.[47] In addition, certain tumors, such as primary carcinoid tumors (which are usually benign) should be diagnosed with caution in cases where there is also extraovarian disease. The most common metastatic neuroendocrine tumors to the ovary are carcinoid tumors, small cell carcinomas of pulmonary origin, and other (nonpulmonary) small cell malignant tumors.

Metastatic Carcinoid Tumors

A review of the literature shows that about 2% of ovarian metastases are carcinoids.[25] Most of these tumors are from the small intestine and rarely originate from colon, stomach, pancreas, or lung.[25, 36, 88–91] In the small intestine, the primary site is usually the ileum, but the cecum, jejunum, and vermiform appendix are also sources in some cases.[25] In contrast to primary ovarian carcinoids, they are usually bilateral. When bilateral ovarian carcinoid tumors are encountered, a search for an extraovarian primary site is mandatory.

In the largest series of carcinoids metastatic to the ovaries published by Robboy and colleagues,[25] the age of the patients ranged from 21 to 82 years, with a median of 57 years. Carcinoid syndrome was present in approximately 50% of cases.[25] Persistence of the carcinoid syndrome or laboratory evidence of a carcinoid tumor after removal of the mass is more consistent with a metastatic carcinoid tumor than a primary neoplasm. In this series, extraovarian metastases were found in 90% of cases. Goblet cell carcinoids of the appendix spread to the ovary in one-third of cases and in 50% of cases the patient presented with an ovarian mass. These tumors may also have foci resembling Krukenberg's tumors.[47] Grossly, as mentioned, most metastatic carcinoids are bilateral and not associated with teratomatous elements. They form large, nodular masses that are predominantly solid and firm, but they may contain small cystic areas.[91] These tumors may resemble thecomas or fibromas. Cysts are occasionally present and can grossly mimic a cystadenofibroma.

The cytologic features of carcinoid tumors have been already discussed: metastatic carcinoid tumors are similar microscopically to primary ovarian tumors of the same type, except that teratomatous elements are not present. The insular pattern is the most common, followed by the trabecular, mixed, and rarely the solid tubular pattern.[91] The tumor is usually multifocal and may show diffuse involvement of the ovary. The prognosis of patients with metastatic carcinoid tumors depends on the extent of the disease, the presence of carcinoid syndrome, and its severity. In a study of 35 patients with carcinoid tumor metastatic to the ovary, the prognosis was poor, with one-third of patients dying within 1 year, and two-thirds dying within 4 years after the diagnosis of ovarian involvement.[25] As in primary ovarian carcinoid tumors, levels of 5-HIAA can be used to monitor disease activity.

Metastatic carcinoid tumors of the ovary must be differentiated mainly from primary ovarian carcinoid. In the absence of teratomatous elements, primary carcinoids may be difficult to distinguish from metastatic carcinoids. Evidence favoring or establishing the diagnosis of metastatic disease includes the presence of a definite or probable carcinoid in the small bowel or elsewhere, extraovarian metastases, bilateral involvement, and persistence of carcinoid syndrome after removal of the ovarian tumor. Overall, in the absence of a demonstrable intestinal primary tumor, a unilateral ovarian carcinoid is most likely primary even if teratomatous elements are not demonstrable, whereas bilateral carcinoid tumors are considered metastatic until proved otherwise.[25] Metastatic carcinoids may be confused with a number of tumors other than primary ovarian carcinoids, including granulosa cell tumors, Sertoli-Leydig cell tumors, and Brenner's tumors.[25] The differential diagnosis with these entities has already been discussed.

Carcinoid tumors metastatic to the ovaries can elicit an extensive stromal proliferation that may resemble an ovarian fibroma or adenofibroma. Nevertheless, the carcinoid tumor shows a more uniform cellular and nuclear appearance compared with an adenofibroma. In difficult cases, special stains for argentaffin and argyrophil granules; immunohistochemical stains for chromogranin, neuron-specific enolase, peptide hormones, and serotonin; and electron microscopy to demonstrate electron-dense core granules can further confirm the diagnosis of a carcinoid. Metastatic insular carcinoids must be differentiated from primary well-differentiated adenocarcinomas of the ovary. The carcinoid has smaller cells and acini when compared with adenocarcinomas, as well as a more uniform appearance. Finally, metastatic mucinous carcinoids should be differentiated from primary mucinous ovarian carcinoids and from Krukenberg's tumors. In these cases, the possibility of a primary gastric or intestinal neoplasm must be carefully excluded (Fig. 12–15).

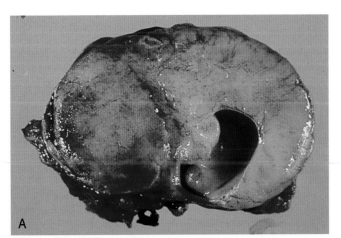

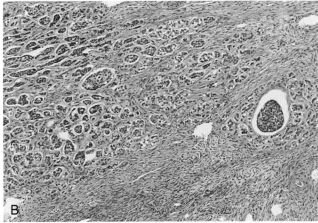

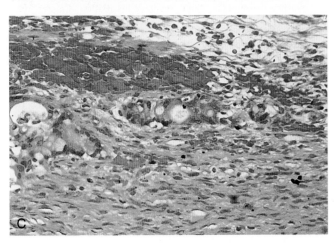

Figure 12–15. A, Metastatic mucinous carcinoid from the appendix to the ovary. *B, C,* Clusters of cells infiltrate diffusely through the ovarian parenchyma, forming glandular structures. The cells are cuboidal and rich in mucins.

Metastatic Pulmonary Neuroendocrine Tumors

Approximately 5% of women with lung cancer have ovarian metastases at autopsy. In a series of ovarian metastases from lung tumors published by Young and Scully,[90] three of the tumors were small cell carcinomas. In two of these cases, the ovarian tumor was recognized before the existence of a lung tumor was known. The majority of the ovarian lesions were unilateral. When reviewing metastatic neuroendocrine tumors, small cell carcinomas of the lung are the primary consideration. Small cell carcinomas account for most metastatic tumors from the lung. Small cell carcinomas of pulmonary type (as we already discussed) can be primary in the ovary; however, these tumors are generally unassociated with pulmonary metastases. The presence of a surface epithelial component in the ovarian tumor provides strong evidence for a small cell carcinoma (pulmonary type) of ovarian origin.

Metastatic Nonpulmonary Small Cell Malignant Tumors

Four cases have been reported in which small cell carcinomas, mixed tumors of the cervix (with components of adenocarcinoma and small cell carcinoma), and poorly differentiated carcinoid have been associated with ovarian metastases.[92] Two patients have been reported to have mediastinal small cell carcinoma, apparently of thymic origin, and ovarian metastases at the time of presentation.[93] Three patients had small cell carcinomas of the small intestine metastatic to the ovary.[93] There is one case report of a primary Merkel cell tumor in the skin of the groin metastatic to the ovary.[93] Approximately 25% to 50% of women with adrenal neuroblastoma have ovarian involvement at autopsy.[89] The fibrillary background of neuroblastoma and the presence of Wright's pseudorosettes help in the distinction of neuroblastoma from other small, round cell tumors. Immunohistochemical and ultrastructural examination may be necessary to establish the diagnosis in some cases. Finally, desmoplastic small round cell tumors should be in the differential diagnosis when dealing with a small cell tumor in the ovary, particularly in young women.[94]

All these neoplasms have the common feature of being small cell carcinomas. Small cell carcinomas metastatic to the ovary differ both clinically and pathologically from the distinctive form of primary small cell carcinoma with hypercalcemia. As already discussed, the latter occurs in a much younger age group, and the histologic, immunohistochemical, and electron microscopic features are quite different. They should also be distinguished from the primary ovarian small cell carcinoma, of the pulmonary type: in these cases, consideration of clinical and pathologic features should enable the pathologist to make the appropriate diagnosis.

References

1. Robboy SJ, Norris HJ, Scully RE: Insular carcinoid primary in the ovary. A clinicopathologic analysis of 48 cases. Cancer 1975; 36:404.
2. Scully RE: Tumors of the Ovary and Maldeveloped Gonads. Fascicle 16, 2nd series. Armed Forces Institute of Pathology, Washington, D.C., 1979.
3. Sens MA, Levenson TB, Metcalf JS: A case of metastatic carcinoid arising in an ovarian teratoma. Cancer 1982; 49:2541.
4. Davis KP, Hartmann LK, Keeney GL, et al.: Primary ovarian carcinoid tumors. Gynecol Oncol 1996; 61:259.
5. Qizilbash AH, Trebilcock RG, Patterson MC, et al.: Functioning primary carcinoid tumor of the ovary. A light and electron microscopic study with review of the literature. Am J Clin Pathol 1974; 62:629.
6. Robboy SJ, Scully RE: Strumal carcinoid of the ovary: An analysis of 50 cases of a distinctive tumor composed of thyroid tissue and carcinoid. Cancer 1980; 46:2019.
7. Stewart MJ, Willis RA, deSaram GS: Argentaffin carcinoma (carcinoid tumor) arising in an ovarian teratoma. A report of two cases. J Pathol Bacteriol 1939; 49:207.
8. Wolpert HR, Fuller AF, Bell DA: Primary mucinous carcinoid tumor of the ovary. A case report. Int J Gynecol Pathol 1989; 8:156.
9. Alenghat E, Okagaki T, Talerman A: Primary mucinous carcinoid tumor of the ovary. Cancer 1986; 58:777.
10. Holtz G, Tucker E, Holtz F: Primary pure insular ovarian carcinoids. Obstet Gynecol 1979; 53:85S.
11. Talerman A: Carcinoid tumors of the ovary. J Cancer Res Clin Oncol 1984; 107:125.
12. Robboy SJ: Insular carcinoid of ovary associated with malignant mucinous tumors. Cancer 1984; 54:2273.
13. Young RH, Prat J, Scully RE: Ovarian Sertoli-Leydig cell tumors with heterologous elements: Gastrointestinal epithelium and carcinoid components. A clinicopathologic analysis of 36 cases. Cancer 1982; 50:2448.
14. Sporrong B, Falkmer S, Robboy SJ, et al.: Neurohormonal peptides in ovarian carcinoids: An immunohistochemical study of 81 primary carcinoids and of intraovarian metastases from six mid-gut carcinoids. Cancer 1982; 49:68.
15. Hilton P, Tweddell A, Wright A: Primary insular argentaffin carcinoma of ovary. Case report and literature review. Br J Obstet Gynaecol 1988; 95:1324.
16. Trell E, Ransing A, Ripa J: Carcinoid heart disease. Clinicopathologic findings and follow-up in 11 cases. Am J Med 1973; 54:433.
17. Hayashi M, Yabuki Y, Asamoto A, et al.: Primary trabecular carcinoid of the ovary. Acta Pathol Jpn 1987; 37:837.
18. Ren JH, Chang DY, Huang SC: Primary trabecular carcinoid tumor of the ovary [letter]. Int J Gynecol Obstet 1996; 52:195.
19. Robboy SJ, Scully RE, Norris HJ: Primary trabecular carcinoid of the ovary. Obstet Gynecol 1977; 49:202.
20. Talerman A, Evans MI: Primary trabecular carcinoid tumor of the ovary. Cancer 1982; 50:1403.
21. Motoyama T, Katayama Y, Watanabe H, et al.: Functioning ovarian carcinoids induce severe constipation. Cancer 1992; 70:513.
22. Yaegashi N, Tsuiki A, Shimizu T, et al.: Ovarian carcinoid with severe constipation due to peptide production. Gynecol Oncol 1995; 56:302.
23. Talerman A, Okagaki T: Ultrastructural features of primary trabecular carcinoid tumor of the ovary. Int J Gynecol Pathol 1985; 4:153.
24. Mungen E, Ertekin AA, Yergok YZ, et al.: Primary mixed trabecular and insular carcinoid tumor of the ovary: A case report. Acta Obstet Gynecol Scand 1997; 76:279.
25. Robboy SJ, Scully RE, Norris HJ: Carcinoid metastatic to the ovary. A clinicopathologic analysis of 35 cases. Cancer 1974; 33:798.
26. Scully RE: Recent progress in ovarian cancer. Hum Pathol 1970; 1:73.
27. Takemori M, Nishimura R, Sugimura K, et al.: Ovarian strumal carcinoid with markedly high serum levels of tumor markers. Gynecol Oncol 1995; 58:266.

28. De Wilde R, Raas P, Zubke W, et al.: A strumal carcinoid primary in the ovary. Eur J Obstet Gynecol Reprod Biol 1986; 21:237.

29. Kimura N, Sasano N, Namiki T: Evidence of hybrid cell of thyroid follicular cell and carcinoid cell in strumal carcinoid. Int J Gynecol Pathol 1986; 5:269.

30. Morgan K, Wells M, Scott JS: Ovarian strumal carcinoid tumor with amyloid stroma—report of a case with 20-year follow-up. Gynecol Oncol 1985; 22:121.

31. Senterman MK, Cassidy PN, Fenoglio CM, et al.: Histology, ultrastructure, and immunohistochemistry of strumal carcinoid: A case report. Int J Gynecol Pathol 1984; 3:232.

32. Snyder RR, Tavassoli FA: Ovarian strumal carcinoid: Immunohistochemical, ultrastructural, and clinicopathologic observations. Int J Gynecol Pathol 1986; 5:187.

33. Stagno PA, Petras RE, Hart WR: Strumal carcinoids of the ovary. An immunohistologic and ultrastructural study. Arch Pathol Lab Med 1987; 111:440.

34. Tamsen A, Mazur MT: Ovarian strumal carcinoid in association with multiple endocrine neoplasia, type IIA. Arch Pathol Lab Med 1992; 116:200.

35. Tsubura A, Sasaki M: Strumal carcinoid of the ovary. Ultrastructural and immunohistochemical study. Acta Pathol Jpn 1986; 36:1383.

36. Ulbright TM, Roth LM, Ehrlich CE: Ovarian strumal carcinoid. An immunocytochemical and ultrastructural study of two cases. Am J Clin Pathol 1982; 77:622.

37. Takubo K, Yasui H, Toi K: Strumal carcinoid of the ovary. A case report. Acta Pathol Jpn 1986; 36:765.

38. Ashton MA: Strumal carcinoid of the ovary associated with hyperinsulinemic hypoglycemia and cutaneous melanosis. Histopathology 1995; 27:463.

39. De Maurizi M, Bondi A, Betts CM, et al.: Strumal carcinoid of the ovary: An immunohistochemical and electron microscopic study. Tumori 1983; 69:261.

40. Hart WR, Regezi JA: Strumal carcinoid of the ovary: Ultrastructural observations and long-term follow-up study. Am J Clin Pathol 1978; 69:356.

41. Livnat EJ, Scommegna A, Recant W, et al.: Ultrastructural observations of the so-called strumal carcinoid of the ovary. Arch Pathol Lab Med 1977; 101:585.

42. Ranchod M, Kempson RL, Dorgeloh JR: Strumal carcinoid of the ovary. Cancer 1976; 37:1913.

43. Greco MA, LiVolsi VA, Pertschuk LP, et al.: Strumal carcinoid of the ovary: An analysis of its components. Cancer 1979; 43:1380.

44. Armes JE, Ostor AG: A case of malignant strumal carcinoid. Gynecol Oncol 1993; 51:419.

45. Arhelger RB, Kelly B: Strumal carcinoid. Report of a case with electron microscopical observations. Arch Pathol 1974; 97:323.

46. Dayal Y, Tashjian AH, Wolfe HJ: Immunocytochemical localization of calcitonin-producing cells in a strumal carcinoid with amyloid stroma. Cancer 1979; 43:1331.

47. Scully RE, Young RH, Clement PB: Tumors of the ovary, maldeveloped gonads, fallopian tube, and broad ligaments. Fascicle 22, 3rd series. Armed Forces Institute of Pathology, Washington, D.C., 1998.

48. Ueda G, Sato Y, Yamasaki M, et al.: Strumal carcinoid of the ovary: Histological, ultrastructural, and immunohistological studies with anti-human thyroglobulin. Gynecol Oncol 1978; 6:411.

49. Horvath E, Kovacs K, Ross RC: Medullary cancer of the thyroid gland and its possible relations to carcinoids: An ultrastructural study. Virchows Arch 1972; 356:281.

50. Serratoni FT, Robboy SJ: Ultrastructure of primary and metastatic ovarian carcinoids: Analysis of 11 cases. Cancer 1975; 36:157.

51. Eichhorn JH, Young RH, Scully RE: Primary ovarian small cell carcinoma of pulmonary type. A clinicopathologic, immunohistologic, and flow cytometric analysis of 11 cases. Am J Surg Pathol 1992; 16:926.

52. Fukunaga M, Endo Y, Miyazawa Y, et al.: Small cell neuroendocrine carcinoma of the ovary. Virchows Arch 1997; 430:343.

53. Chang DH, Hsueh S, Soong YK: Small cell carcinoma with neurosecretory granules arising in an ovarian dermoid cyst. Gynecol Oncol 1992; 46:246.

54. Lim SC, Choi SJ, Suh CH: A case of small cell carcinoma arising in a mature cystic teratoma of the ovary. Pathol Int 1998; 48:834.

55. Dickersin GR, Scully RE: Ovarian small cell tumors: An electron microscopic review. Ultrastruct Pathol 1998; 22:199.

56. Eichhorn JH, Bell DA, Young RH, et al.: DNA content and proliferative activity in ovarian small cell carcinomas of the hypercalcemic type. Implications for diagnosis, prognosis, and histogenesis. Am J Clin Pathol 1992; 98:579.

57. Dickersin GR, Scully RE: An update on the electron microscopy of small cell carcinoma of the ovary with hypercalcemia. Ultrastruct Pathol 1993; 17:411.

58. Dickersin GR, Kline IW, Scully RE: Small cell carcinoma of the ovary with hypercalcemia: A report of eleven cases. Cancer 1982; 49:188.

59. Young RH, Oliva E, Scully RE: Small cell carcinoma of the ovary, hypercalcemic type. A clinicopathological analysis of 150 cases. Am J Surg Pathol 1994; 18:1102.

60. Fukunaga M, Endo Y, Nomura K, et al.: Small cell carcinoma of the ovary: A case report of large cell variant. Pathol Int 1997; 47:250.

61. Reed WC: Small cell carcinoma of the ovary with hypercalcemia: Report of a case of survival without recurrence 5 years after surgery and chemotherapy. Gynecol Oncol 1995; 56:452.

62. Lamovec J, Bracko M, Cerar O: Familial occurrence of small-cell carcinoma of the ovary. Arch Pathol Lab Med 1995; 119:523.

63. Seidman JD: Small cell carcinoma of the ovary of the hypercalcemic type: p53 protein accumulation and clinicopathologic features. Gynecol Oncol 1995; 59:283.

64. Chan LC, Cheung A, Cheng D: Small cell carcinoma of the ovary associated with ins(10;5)(p13;q31q13). Cancer Genet Cytogenet 1994; 77:89.

65. Holtz G, Johnson TR, Schrock ME: Paraneoplastic hypercalcemia in ovarian tumors. Obstet Gynecol 1979; 54:483.

66. Pruett KM, Gordon AN, Estrada R, et al.: Small-cell carcinoma of the ovary: An aggressive epithelial cancer occurring in young patients. Gynecol Oncol 1988; 29:365.

67. Jensen ML, Rasmussen KL, Jacobsen M: Ovarian small cell carcinoma. A case report with histologic, immunohistochemical and ultrastructural findings. APMIS 1991; 23:126.

68. Peccatori F, Bonazzi C, Lucchini V, et al.: Primary ovarian small cell carcinoma: four more cases. Gynecol Oncol 1993; 49:95.

69. Taraszewski R, Rosman PM, Knight CA, et al.: Small cell carcinoma of the ovary. Gynecol Oncol 1991; 41:149.

70. Abeler V, Kjorstad KE, Nesland JM: Small cell carcinoma of the ovary. A report of six cases. Int J Gynecol Pathol 1988; 7:315.

71. Aguirre P, Thor AD, Scully RE: Ovarian small cell carcinoma. Histogenetic considerations based on immunohistochemical and other findings. Am J Clin Pathol 1989; 92:140.

72. Ulbright TM, Roth LM, Stehman FB, et al.: Poorly differentiated (small cell) carcinoma of the ovary in young women: Evidence supporting a germ cell origin. Hum Pathol 1987; 18:175.

73. McMahon JT, Hart WR: Ultrastructural analysis of small cell carcinomas of the ovary. Am J Clin Pathol 1988; 90:523.

74. Lifschitz-Mercer B, David R, Dharan M, et al.: Small cell carcinoma of the ovary: An immunohistochemical and ultrastructural study with a review of the literature. Virchows Arch A 1992; 421:263.

75. Scully R: Small cell carcinoma of hypercalcemic type. Int J Gynecol Pathol 1993; 12:148.

76. Ueda G, Yamasaki M, Inoue M: Argyrophil cells in the endometrioid carcinoma of the ovary. Cancer 1984; 54:1569.

77. Ueda G, Shimizu C, Saito J, et al.: An immunohistochemical study of neuroendocrine cells in gynecologic tumors. Int J Gynecol Obstet 1989; 29:165.

78. Scully RE, Aguirre P, DeLellis R: Argyrophilia, serotonin, and peptide hormones in the female genital tract and its tumors. Int J Gynecol Pathol 1984; 3:51.

79. Aguirre P, Scully RE, Dayal Y, et al.: Mucinous tumors of the ovary with argyrophil cells. An immunohistochemical analysis. Am J Surg Pathol 1984; 8:345.

80. Sasaki E, Sasano N, Kimura N, et al.: Demonstration of neuroendocrine cells in ovarian mucinous tumors. Int J Gynecol Pathol 1989; 8:189.

81. Lin M, Hanai J, Wada A, et al.: Argyrophilia in ovarian serous tumors. A comparative study in 127 epithelial ovarian tumors. Histol Histopathol 1991; 6:477.

82. Aguirre P, Scully RE, Wolfe HF, et al.: Argyrophil cells in Brenner tumors: Histochemical and immunohistochemical analysis. Int J Gynecol Pathol 1986; 5:223.

83. Collins RJ, Cheung A, Ngan HY, et al.: Primary mixed neuroendocrine and mucinous carcinoma of the ovary. Arch Gynecol Obstet 1991; 248:139.

84. Eichhorn JH, Lawrence WD, Young RH, et al.: Ovarian neuroendocrine carcinomas of non-small-cell type associated with surface epithelial adenocarcinomas. Int J Gynecol Pathol 1996; 15:303.

85. Jones K, Diaz JA, Donner LR: Neuroendocrine carcinoma arising in an ovarian mucinous cystadenoma. Int J Gynecol Pathol 1996; 15:167.

86. Khurana KK, Tornos C, Silva EG: Ovarian neuroendocrine carcinoma associated with a mucinous neoplasm. Arch Pathol Lab Med 1994; 118:1032.

87. Mazur MT, Hsueh S, Gersell DJ: Metastases to the female genital tract. Analysis of 325 cases. Cancer 1984; 53:1978.

88. Young RH, Scully RE: Metastatic tumors in the ovary: A problem-oriented approach and review of the recent literature. Semin Diagn Pathol 1991; 8:250.

89. Young RH, Kozakewich HP, Scully RE: Metastatic ovarian tumors in children: A report of 14 cases and review of the literature. Int J Gynecol Pathol 1993; 12:8.

90. Young RH, Scully RE: Ovarian metastases from cancer of the lung: Problems in interpretation. A report of seven cases. Gynecol Oncol 1985; 21:337.

91. Ulbright TM, Roth LM, Stehman FB: Secondary ovarian neoplasia. A clinicopathologic study of 35 cases. Cancer 1984; 53:1164.

92. Young RH, Gersell DJ, Roth LM, et al.: Ovarian metastases from cervical carcinomas other than pure adenocarcinomas: A report of 12 cases. Cancer 1993; 71:407.

93. Eichhorn JH, Young RH, Scully RE: Nonpulmonary small cell carcinomas of extragenital origin metastatic to the ovary. Cancer 1993; 71:177.

94. Young RH, Eichhorn JH, Dickersin GR, et al.: Ovarian involvement by the intra-abdominal desmoplastic small round cell tumor with divergent differentiation: A report of three cases. Hum Pathol 1992; 23:454.

CHAPTER 13

Testis

C.S. Foster

INTRODUCTION

In contrast to more common testicular tumors of germ cell origin (Table 13–1), a separate group of testicular neoplasms is characterized by the frequent common feature of ectopic endocrine activity. This group, the gonadal stromal tumors, comprises a histogenetically heterogeneous collection of neoplasms that originate within the stromal compartment of the testes (Table 13–2). Gonadal stromal tumors represent about 4% of all testicular neoplasms[1] but account for approximately 8% of those in prepubertal males,[2] the majority being in men between the ages of 20 and 60 years.

Interstitial cell tumors, the most common gonadal stromal neoplasm, makes up from 1%–3% of all testis tumors. In well-differentiated tumors, the cells resemble non-neoplastic Sertoli's cells, Leydig's cells,[3] or other histologic types that arise among the nonspecific stromal cells of the testes. Leydig's cell tumor is the most common pure sex cord–stromal tumor, followed by Sertoli's cell tumors, granulosa cell tumors, and pure stromal tumors. All other neoplasms frequently contain elements of two or more of these types or cannot be specifically placed into any clear category. Semantic and histogenic uncertainties have contributed to difficulties in classifying these lesions. Lack of objective criteria with which to distinguish between hyperplasia and neoplasms of benign or malignant types has added to the problems of classification.[4, 5]

SERTOLI'S CELL TUMORS

Origins

Otherwise known as androblastoma or gonadal stromal tumor, true Sertoli's cell tumors may occur at any age but account for less than 1% of testicular neoplasms.[2, 6-9] In addition to the common type of Sertoli's cell tumor, there are also the large-cell calcifying and sclerosing variants. Insufficient examples of a pure "lipid-rich" variant of Sertoli's cell tumor have been described to warrant a separate subtype. While the cause of these tumors remains uncertain, the majority have been reported in morphologically normal intrascrotal testes, although occurrence in maldescended or cryptorchid testes has been reported. Their histogenic origin is unconfirmed, although derivation from the primitive gonadal mesenchyme is suspected.

Approximately 30% of Sertoli's cell tumors are reported in children younger than 12 years of age, many younger than 1 year.[10] Unfortunately, different criteria have been applied to the diagnosis of these tumors. Many of the cases had features of juvenile granulosa cell tumor, with reports antedating the description of that entity. One series of pediatric neoplasms did not report any Sertoli's cell tumors, although they contained four juvenile granulosa cell tumors.[11] In contrast, the problem of distinguishing juvenile granulosa cell tumor from Sertoli's cell tumor, particularly in the pediatric age group, is highlighted by a report that included 18 Sertoli's cell tumors and 11 juvenile granulosa cell tumors.[12] In the largest series (60 Sertoli's cell tumors) yet reported, only 2 occurred in patients younger than 20 years of age, the mean age being 46 years.[13] When strict contemporary diagnostic criteria are applied, only rarely do confirmed cases occur in children younger than 10 years.[14-16]

Occasional tumors develop in patients with androgen insensitivity syndrome.[17] The large-cell calcifying variant is associated with unclassified Carney's syndrome[18] when the clinical features cause the patient to be presented. Seven Sertoli's cell tumors have occurred in boys from 1 to 8 years of age with Peutz-Jeghers syndrome.[9, 19-23] All these boys had gynecomastia and elevated estradiol levels, and many tumors had unusual microscopic features. Despite these associations, the majority of Sertoli's cell tumors appear to be incidental, lacking any recognized predisposing condition and presenting as a testicular mass.

Table 13–1. Histologic Classification of Testicular Tumors

Category	Histologic Type	Cytologic Entity
Primary		
Germinal Neoplasms	Seminoma	Classical (typical) seminoma
		Anaplastic seminoma
		Spermatocytic seminoma
	Embryonal carcinoma	Embryonal carcinoma
	Teratoma	Mature
		Immature
	Choriocarcinoma	Choriocarcinoma
	Yolk sac tumor	Endodermal sinus tumor
		Embryonal adenocarcinoma of prepubertal testis
Sex Cord–Stromal Tumors	Specialized gonadal stromal neoplasms	Leydig's cell tumor
		Sertoli's cell tumor (androblastoma)
		Other gonadal stromal tumors
	Tumors of dysgenic gonads	Gonadoblastoma
	Miscellaneous neoplasms	Adenocarcinoma of the rete testis
		Mesenchymal neoplasms
		Carcinoid
		Adrenal rest tumor
Secondary		
	Reticuloendothelial malignancies	Lymphoma
		Leukemia
	Metastases	
Paratesticular		
	Adenomatoid	
	Cystadenoma of epididymis	
	Mesenchymal neoplasms	
	Mesothelioma	
	Metastases	

Gross Appearances

Tumors vary in size from 1 cm to more than 20 cm in diameter. The tumors peculiar to patients with Peutz-Jeghers syndrome are frequently smaller. On sectioning, the surface is uniformly gray-white to creamy yellow but almost always contains focal cystic change that is increasingly evident with increasing tumor size. Benign lesions are well-circumscribed, whereas malignant lesions are larger and less demarcated. In these lesions, focal hemorrhage may be present (Fig. 13–1). Features suggesting malignancy include large size, poor tumor demarcation, invasion of adjacent paratesticular structures, vascular and lymphatic invasion, and increased mitotic activity. Unfortunately, confirmation of malignancy is made only following development of metastasis.

Table 13–2. Classification of Histologic Tumors of the Testis

Category	Histologic Type	Subtype
Sex cord–stromal tumors	Sertoli's cell tumors	Sertoli cell tumor
		Large-cell calcifying variant
		Sclerosing variant
		Lipid-rich variant
	Leydig's cell tumor	Leydig's cell tumor
	Sertoli-Leydig cell tumor	Sertoli-Leydig cell tumor
	Granulosa cell tumor	Juvenile type
		Adult type
	Fibroma-thecoma-cell tumors	
	Mixed cell types	

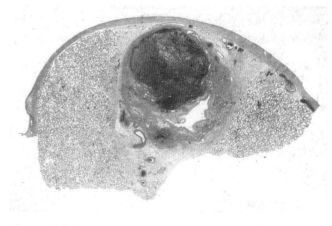

Figure 13–1. Cross-section of enlarged testis containing Sertoli's cell tumor, 1.5-cm diameter, that is well demarcated, partly cystic, partly hemorrhagic, and extending to the tunica albuginea (magnification ×3).

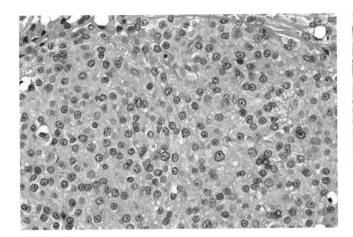

Figure 13-2. Sertoli's cell tumor comprising solid sheets of bland eosinophilic cells in which no tubular differentiation is seen and in which mitoses are not present. Nuclei contain characteristic pinpoint nucleoli (magnification ×250).

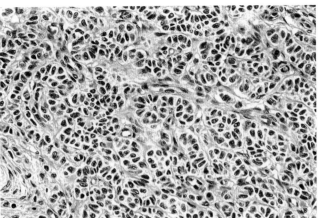

Figure 13-4. Sertoli's tumor in which cells are ranged into distinct tubules as well as discrete but rudimentary rosettes that may contain Call-Exner bodies (magnification ×250).

Microscopic Appearances

Sertoli's tumor cells usually have moderate-to-abundant eosinophilic cytoplasm (Fig. 13–2) but may appear pale due to lipid accumulation (Fig. 13–3). This accumulation may take the form of fine droplets or large vacuoles. The stroma may be scanty or composed of prominent hyalinized fibrous tissue that contains vascular structured vessels. The majority of Sertoli's cell tumors have bland cytologic features and little mitotic activity, although occasional tumors exhibit prominent pleomorphism with conspicuous mitotic figures. The hallmark of this tumor is tubular differentiation; however, the extent of this feature is very variable and may require a detailed search. Tubules may be hollow and round, or solid and elongated (Fig. 13–4). Rarely do they exhibit marked

irregularity in size and shape or have a retiform pattern. In some tumors, cords are prominent. Many Sertoli's cell tumors include foci of solid growth, but tubular differentiation elsewhere facilitates the diagnosis. Rare neoplasms that have an entirely solid growth pattern can be diagnosed as Sertoli's cell tumor, following exclusion of any alternative diagnosis and supported by immunohistochemical findings. Other appearances include peripheral compression of surrounding tissue with the formation of a dense pseudocapsule (Fig. 13–5), foci of hemorrhage (Fig. 13–6), and intracellular lipid accumulation (Fig. 13–7).

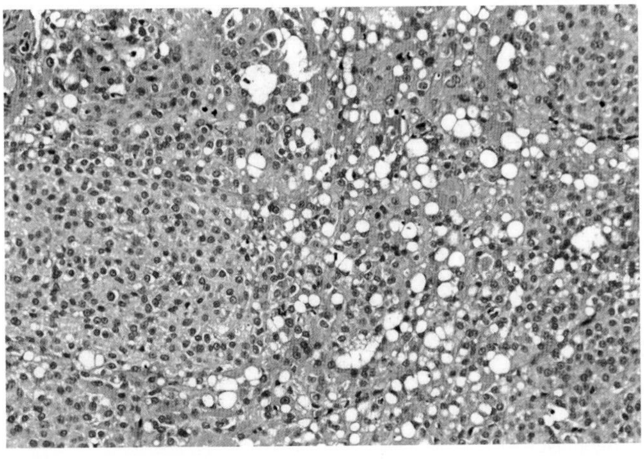

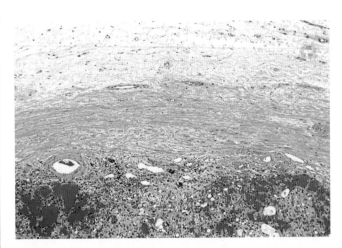

Figure 13-5. Microscopic appearance of periphery of Sertoli's cell tumor similar to that in Fig. 13–1. There is a pseudocapsule formed by compression of stromal connective tissues. The underlying tumor is cystic and hemorrhagic. Vascular invasion was not present, no spread beyond the pseudocapsule was identified, and no metastases developed during a long postdiagnostic period (magnification ×60).

Figure 13-3. Sertoli's cell tumor containing foci of lipid accumulation. Cells are bland, and mitoses are absent. These features are insufficient to warrant diagnosis of "lipid-rich" tumor, unlike that in Fig. 13–7 (magnification ×120).

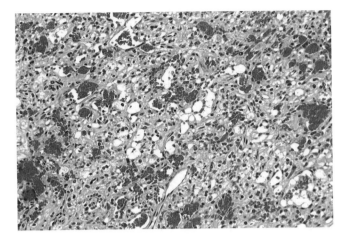

Figure 13-6. Sertoli's cell tumor in which multiple foci of hemorrhage are associated with small cysts and intracellular lipid accumulation. A few rudimentary tubules are scattered between the otherwise diffuse tumor (magnification ×120).

In cryptorchid testes and in 25% of patients with testicular feminization, nodules of immature seminiferous tubules containing lumina lined by undifferentiated cells are commonly found. A wide heterogeneity of microscopic appearances is evident not only among these tumors but also among different areas within the same tumor. Pathognomonic diagnostic features include epithelial elements resembling Sertoli's cells and varying amounts of stroma. Foci of hemorrhage may be present, although necrosis is rare. With the exception of tumors in Peutz-Jeghers patients or some of the large-cell calcifying variants, Sertoli's cell tumors are almost invariably unilateral. There is only one confirmed case of bilateral Sertoli's cell tumor of otherwise conventional type.[14] Secretory material forming

Call-Exner–like bodies is occasionally seen within the neoplastic tubules, and their morphologic appearance resembles that of granulosa cell tumors. The stromal elements may be sufficiently differentiated to be recognizable as Leydig's cells.

Ultrastructural Appearances

Sertoli's cell tumors typically have a well-developed Golgi apparatus, variably prominent smooth endoplasmic reticulum, lipid droplets, lateral desmosomes, and a peripheral surrounding basement membrane.[24] Cisternae of rough endoplasmic reticulum may be prominent, although convincing Charcot-Böttcher filaments have not been identified in the few cases in the Sertoli cell tumor category that have been reported ultrastructurally, unlike the large-cell calcifying variant.[24, 25]

Immunohistochemistry

Sertoli's cell tumors are usually positive for cytokeratin and vimentin and negative for epithelial membrane antigen.[14, 26, 27] Inhibin is usually positive, although often focal. Such positivity favors Sertoli's cell tumor over germ-cell tumor or metastatic carcinoma. It may also help to identify the Sertoli nature of peculiar biphasic neoplasms in which the epithelial component is of uncertain type.[28] Seminoma cells stain strongly for glycogen and placental alkaline phosphatase (in contrast to neoplastic Sertoli's cells), whereas Sertoli's cells stain for lipid, cytokeratins, and inhibin (Table 13–3).

Differential Diagnosis

Sertoli's cell tumors may be misdiagnosed as seminoma because of the common occurrence of seminoma and its frequently diffuse pattern. Although Sertoli's cell tumors may have a focal, nonspecific, chronic, and inflammatory cell infiltrate (Fig. 13–8), they generally lack a consistent sprinkling of lymphocytes throughout their stroma. Rare seminomas have well-developed solid-tubular patterns that suggest Sertoli's cell tumor. In contrast, tubular seminomas have the typical lymphocytes

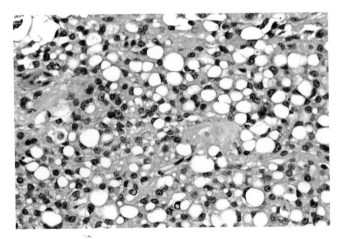

Figure 13-7. Sertoli's cell tumor in which there is prominent intracellular lipid accumulation throughout the tumor; thus the term "lipid-rich." As these tumors mature, so features of chronic inflammation and foci of sclerosis supervene (magnification ×250).

Table 13-3. Features Distinguishing Sertoli's Cell Tumors from Seminoma

Feature	Sertoli's Cell Tumor	Seminoma
Lymphocytic infiltrate	+/−	+++
Intratubular germ cell neoplasia	−	+/−
Glycogen	−	+++
Alkaline phosphatase	−	+++
Lipid	+/++	−
Cytokeratins	+/++	−
Inhibin	+/++	−

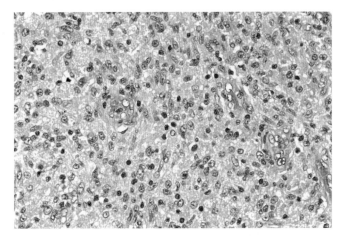

Figure 13-8. Sertoli's cell tumor solid pattern in which there is a focal scattering of lymphocytes. Despite the tumor being composed of sheets of bland pale cells with vesicular nuclei and pinpoint nucleoli, these appearances should not be confused with seminoma (magnification ×120).

and cytologic features of seminoma in addition to foci of typical seminoma usually being apparent in other areas. The presence of adjacent intratubular germ cell neoplasia provides additional evidence that a tubular tumor is a seminoma.

Clinical Features

The majority of Sertoli's cell tumors are benign, although approximately 10% have proved malignant following subsequent development of metastases. There are no definitive diagnostic criteria of malignancy. The typical signs and symptoms at presentation are those of testicular mass with or without pain and with or without gynecomastia. About one-third of patients have gynecomastia. In the presence of a testis tumor in the prepubertal age group, gynecomastia is an important finding in the differential diagnosis, because feminization in boys with Leydig's cell tumors is always superimposed on virilism.

To date, no sclerosing Sertoli's cell neoplasm or tumor in a patient with Peutz-Jeghers syndrome has proved clinically malignant. A study of 60 Sertoli's cell tumors confirmed 7 to be clinically malignant.[9] Four had evidence of spread beyond the testis at presentation and all four had lymph node involvement. One patient also had lung and bone metastases. Three additional patients developed metastases at different times up to 12 years postoperatively. When the features of the malignant tumors were compared with those having an uneventful follow-up of 5 years or more, the pathologic features identified to correlate with a likely malignant course are listed in Table 13-4. Only 1 of 9 benign tumors with follow-up data of 5 years or longer had more than 1 of these features, whereas 5 of the 7 malignant tumors exhibited at least 3. The course of the disease, even in patients with metastases, may be protracted when compared

Table 13-4. Features Correlating with Malignant Progression of Sertoli's Cell Tumors

- Diameter >5 cm
- Necrosis
- Moderate to severe nuclear atypia
- Vascular invasion
- Mitotic rate >5 per 10 high-power fields

with that of patients with metastatic germ-cell tumors. Lung and bone metastases may occur and warrant the inclusion of chest films and bone scans during staging evaluation.

Based on a critical analysis of true Sertoli's cell tumors in the literature, with the exclusion of Sertoli-Leydig cell tumors or unclassified sex cord–stromal tumors, only rare patients without Peutz-Jeghers syndrome have endocrine manifestations such as gynecomastia. The latter is more common in patients with Leydig's cell tumors, Sertoli-Leydig cell tumors, or tumors in the mixed and unclassified sex cord–stromal categories. Although approximately 10%–20% of all patients with sex cord–stromal tumors have gynecomastia. This manifestation is seen more often when the tumors are malignant. Despite the association of some types of Sertoli's cell tumor with endocrinologic abnormalities, studies of the hormonal production by these tumors are rare.[29] Gabrilove and colleagues[10] reviewed 72 cases of Sertoli's cell tumor and identified occasional patients with elevated serum testosterone, plasma estradiol, urinary estrogen, and urinary 17-ketosteroids levels. It is assumed but not confirmed that gynecomastia is a consequence of estrogen production, but whether it is the Sertoli cells or the stromal elements that are responsible remains uncertain. Elevated plasma testosterone has been reported in association with virilizing features in one patient with Sertoli's cell tumor.[10] Although hormone production is a potential marker for follow-up in patients with apparently malignant tumors, evidence as to the clinical value of this feature is currently lacking.

Sertoli's Cell Tumour: Large-Cell Calcifying Variant

Origins

Large-cell calcifying Sertoli's cell tumors have been reported in patients 2–51 years of age.[25, 30–35] One-third of these cases arise in unusual clinical situations, particularly endocrine abnormalities that include acromegaly, pituitary gigantism, hypercortisolemia, sexual precocity, sudden death, spotty mucocutaneous pigmentation, and Peutz-Jeghers syndrome. Infrequently associated pathologic conditions include pituitary adenomas, bilateral primary adrenocortical hyperplasia, testicular Leydig's cell tumors, cardiac myxomas, and lentigines.[18]

Gross Appearances

Tumors are usually 4 cm or less in diameter. Frequently multifocal, about 20% are bilateral. Multifocal and bilateral tumors are almost exclusively seen in patients with Carney's syndrome. Cut section reveals well-circumscribed, firm, yellow-tan to white tissue, often with granular, calcific foci. Necrosis is occasionally present.

Microscopic Appearances

Tumor cells are arranged in sheets, nests, trabeculae, cords, small clusters, or solid tubules. Foci of intratubular tumor are found in approximately half of cases, supporting their Sertoli's cell origin. The stroma varies from loose and myxoid to densely collagenous. Some tumors exhibit a prominent neutrophilic infiltrate. The characteristic calcification is frequently prominent, occasionally massive, with large, wavy, laminated nodules. Small psammoma bodies and ossification are occasionally seen. The neoplastic cells are large and round but occasionally cuboidal or columnar. Rarely, they may be spindle-shaped. Cytoplasm is usually abundant, eosinophilic, and finely granular, but occasionally amphophilic and slightly vacuolated. Nuclei are round or oval, with one or two small to moderate nucleoli. Mitotic figures are rare. Sertoli's cell tumors arising in males with Peutz-Jeghers syndrome often exhibit some features of the large-cell calcifying Sertoli's cell tumor, but they frequently lack calcification. Cysts may be present.

Ultrastructural Appearances

Ultrastructural studies support Sertoli's cell origin of the tumor, with identification of Charcot-Böttcher filament bundles, the specific cytoplasmic inclusions of Sertoli's cells, in occasional cases.[25, 30, 35]

Differential Diagnosis

Sertoli's cell tumors are distinguished from Sertoli's cell nodules by focal clusters of benign tubules. These are of microscopic size but occasionally visible as white nodules up to a few millimeters in diameter. Microscopic examination reveals collections of tubules with interspersed Leydig's cells. Tubules within these nodules are lined by small, immature Sertoli's cells and may contain scattered spermatogonia. Some lesions have a radial arrangement of Sertoli's cells around small hyaline bodies that resemble Call-Exner bodies. Intratubular laminated calcified bodies may also be present. Pure Sertoli's cell tumors are distinguished from mixed sex cord–stromal tumors by the prominent, cellular, stromal component of the latter. This contrasts with the fibrotic to hyalinized non-neoplastic appearance of the stroma in pure Sertoli's cell tumor.

Adult granulosa cell tumor is a rare neoplasm in the testis. The cells generally contain conspicuous eosinophilic cytoplasm together with other typical architectural features lacking from pure Sertoli's cell tumors. Juvenile granulosa cell tumor typically occurs in the first few months of life whereas, in the largest series of Sertoli's cell tumors, no patient was younger than 15 years.[9] In contrast to the tubular differentiation of Sertoli's cell tumors, juvenile granulosa cell tumors exhibit prominent follicle differentiation; the follicles are usually irregular in size and shape. Some juvenile granulosa cell tumors have little or no follicular differentiation; in such cases, intercellular basophilic fluid may impart a chondroid appearance suggestive of the diagnosis. Juvenile granulosa cell tumors typically include more immature-appearing nuclei and more conspicuous mitotic activity than the majority of Sertoli's cell tumors.

Despite superficial similarity, many features distinguish Leyding's cell tumours from Sertoli's cell tumours in which there is a diffuse growth of cells with prominent eosinophilic cytoplasm. Leydig's cell tumors are more often yellow or brown on cut sectioned surface. The pathognomonic difference is the presence of tubular differentiation in most Sertoli's cell tumors, a finding that excludes the diagnosis of Leydig's cell tumor, although focal pseudotubules may be found in occasional Leydig's cell tumors. Additionally, 30%–40% of testicular Leydig's cell tumors contain intracytoplasmic Reinke's crystalloids, which are absent from all Sertoli's cell tumors. Immunostaining for cytokeratin may assist, with typically stronger and more diffuse reactivity in Sertoli's cell tumors and focal, weak, or absent reactivity in Leydig's cell tumors. Inhibin immunoreactivity is typically more intense and diffuse in Leydig's cell tumors than in Sertoli's cell tumors. Nevertheless, individual case variation limits the diagnostic utility of these markers. Confusion between Sertoli's cell tumors of the large-cell calcifying variety and Leydig's cell tumors has been particularly problematic. Before the former tumor was recognized, it was often misdiagnosed as Leydig's cell tumor. Large-cell calcifying Sertoli's cell tumors often show intratubular growth and common bilaterality or multifocality, in contrast to Leydig's cell tumors. Although ossification has rarely been described in Leydig's cell tumor, the presence of calcification strongly favors large-cell calcifying Sertoli's cell tumor.

The rare endometrioid adenocarcinoma of the testis may enter into the differential diagnosis because the tubular glands of this tumor may simulate the hollow tubules seen in occasional Sertoli's cell tumors. However, in other areas, the growth patterns of the two neoplasms are so distinctive that this should not be a problem. Lack of staining of Sertoli's cell tubules for epithelial membrane antigen[14, 27] may be helpful. Inhibin positivity in Sertoli's cell tumors may support the diagnosis.[14, 26, 27, 36]

Adenomatoid tumor and the Sertoli cell tumor may contain cells with conspicuous eosinophilic cytoplasm. However, the latter usually lacks the characteristic vacuolated cells typically seen in the adenomatoid tumor. Although adenomatoid tumors may involve the testis, they are primarily paratesticular, in contrast to the intratesticular Sertoli cell tumors.

A rare neoplasm that might pose diagnostic confusion is the sertoliform rete cystadenoma, but its usual confinement to the rete should make distinction easy in most instances. However, a rare tumor of this type of rete origin that extensively involves the parenchyma may be impossible to distinguish from a Sertoli cell tumor of parenchymal origin on microscopic evaluation alone. Metastatic adenocarcinoma with relatively regular tubular glands, such as from the stomach, might mimic a Sertoli cell tumor. However, such a neoplasm would tend to have a more variegated microscopic appearance than that of a Sertoli cell tumor, including a prominent intertubular growth pattern. A study has shown that the large-cell calcifying variant of Sertoli's cell tumor often stains for S-100 protein,[31] as do some Sertoli's cell tumors.[14, 26, 27]

Sertoli's Cell Tumor: Sclerosing Variant

Sertoli's cell tumors that are predominantly sclerotic are classified as sclerosing Sertoli's cell variant.[37] In these cases, tubules are small and solid (Fig. 13–9). The intensely sclerotic stroma (Fig. 13–10) is not as vascular as in Sertoli's cell tumors. With rare exceptions, these tumor cells have bland cytologic features, and mitotic figures are infrequent. A common finding is entrapped, non-neoplastic tubules reminiscent of the immature tubules of the Sertoli cell nodules in cryptorchid testes (Figs. 13–11 and 13–12). Sertoli's cell tumours in which

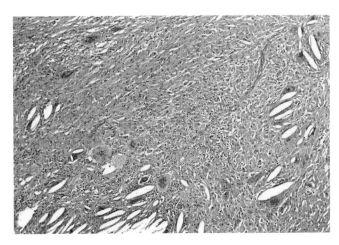

Figure 13–10. Sertoli's cell tumor (sclerosing variant) similar to that in Fig. 13–9 but in which tumor cells with prominent intracellular lipid droplets are replaced by dense sclerotic stroma containing cholesterol clefts (magnification ×30).

the sclerotic stroma contains a prominent infiltration by lymphocytes, in addition to a relatively few residual tumor cells, should cause little confusion with seminoma or lymphoma, including Hodgkin's disease, despite the prominence of the lymphoid infiltration. Sertoli's cell tumor is composed of eosinophilic cells together with (in this field) foci of ossification. Elsewhere, the presence of tubular differentiation confirms the diagnosis of Sertoli's cell tumor. Sertoli's cell tumors (sclerosing variant), in which the entire tumor is composed of isolated tumor cells, either singly or in groups, are dispersed through sclerotic and hyalinized connective tissue. The most significant differential diagnosis is with Leydig's cell tumor.

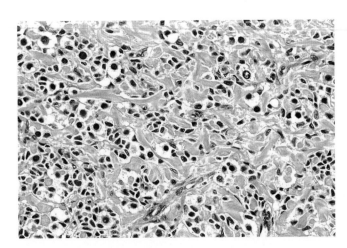

Figure 13–9. Sertoli's cell tumor (sclerosing variant) in which there is diffuse proliferation of background stromal connective tissue cells with concomitant attrition of tumor cells. The pattern of tumor cells may be as effete tubules or cords, but the pattern eventually appears as scattered and apparently discontinuous clusters or individual cells (magnification ×250).

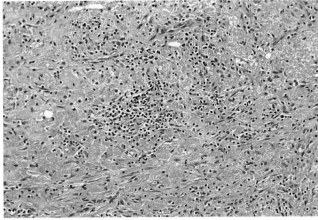

Figure 13–11. Sertoli's cell tumor (sclerosing variant) in which the sclerotic stroma contains a prominent infiltration by lymphocytes in addition to relatively few residual tumor cells. There should be little confusion of this appearance with seminoma or lymphoma, including Hodgkin's disease, despite the prominence of the lymphoid infiltration (magnification ×45).

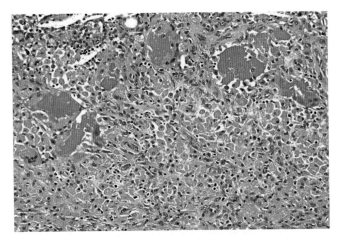

Figure 13-12. Sertoli's cell tumor composed of eosinophilic cells together with foci of ossification. Elsewhere, the presence of tubular differentiation confirms the diagnosis of Sertoli's cell tumor. Sertoli's cell tumor (sclerosing variant), in which the entire tumor is composed of isolated tumor cells, either singly or in groups, dispersed through sclerotic and hyalinized connective tissue. The most significant differential diagnosis is with Leydig's cell tumor (magnification ×60).

LEYDIG'S CELL TUMORS

Origins

Leydig's cell tumors account for about 2% of testicular neoplasms.[38, 39] In contrast to germ cell tumors, there is no demonstrable association with cryptorchidism. Although their exact cause is unknown, experimental development of Leydig's cell tumors in mice following long-term estrogen administration is consistent with a hormonal origin. Approximately 20% of these tumors are detected in the first decade of life, 25% between 10 and 30 years, 30% between 30 and 50 years, and 25% beyond that age. Bilateral occurrence is rare. The presence of an undescended testis or a history of it in 5%–10% of cases[40] suggests that cryptorchidism may predispose to the development of Leydig's cell tumors. Rare examples have occurred in patients with Klinefelter's syndrome, but they should be distinguished from the Leydig cell hyperplasia that is common in that disorder (Fig. 13–13). One malignant "Leydig's cell" tumor has been reported associated with the adrenogenital syndrome despite Reinke's crystals being absent from the tumor cells.[41]

The common histogenic origin of interstitial cells and adrenocortical cells as well as the occurrence of adrenal rests in the testis complicates interpretation. The paradox of the tumor's arising in the interstitial cells of a prepubertal testis and behaving metabolically like its adult counterpart, in conjunction with cells in the normal prepubertal testis containing enzymes capable of producing testosterone, explains the occurrence of spermatogenesis in the seminiferous tubules more remote from the tumor.

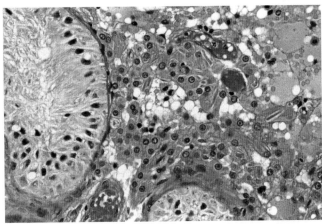

Figure 13-13. Leydig's cell hyperplasia in which large foci of the interstitium are replaced by an overgrowth of Leydig's cells of unremarkable structure. Reinke's crystalloids may be identified. The adjacent seminiferous tubules appear atrophic (magnification ×250).

Gross Appearances

Leydig's tumors are sharply circumscribed, 3–5 cm in diameter, and may be lobulated by fibrous septa. On sectioning, they are usually uniformly solid and yellow or yellow-tan through green-brown to gray-white. Foci of hemorrhage or necrosis may be present.

Microscopic Appearances

Tumors consist of relatively uniform, polyhedral, closely packed cells (Figs. 13–14, 13–15, and 13–16) with round and slightly eccentric nuclei and eosinophilic granular cytoplasm with lipoid vacuoles,

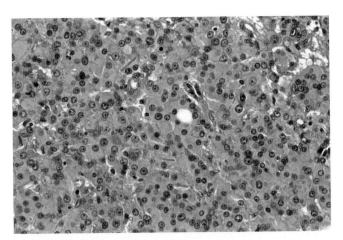

Figure 13-14. Leydig's cell tumor composed of relatively uniform and closely packed polyhedral cells with round and slightly eccentric nuclei and eosinophilic granular cytoplasm. Sometimes these cells contain lipoid vacuoles, brownish pigmentation, and occasional crystalline inclusions (magnification ×250).

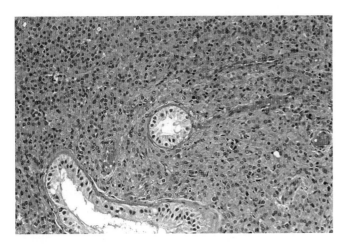

Figure 13-15. Leydig's cell tumor composed of solid sheets of bland eosinophilic tumor cells effacing normal testicular architecture. Residual atrophic tubular elements are identified (magnification ×120).

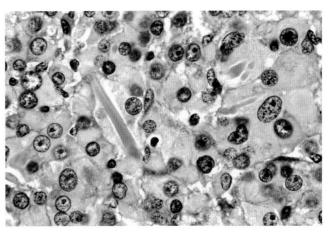

Figure 13-17. Reinke's crystalloids, both intracellular and extracellular, are a characteristic feature (magnification ×625). See Fig. 13-13.

brownish pigmentation, and occasional characteristic inclusions known as Reinke's crystals (Fig. 13-17). Pleomorphism with large and bizarre cell forms may occur, and mitotic figures may or may not be identified. None of these features appear to be consistently related to malignant potential. The two most common microscopic patterns are diffuse and nodular. In the diffuse, the stroma is inconspicuous and of a nondescript fibrous type. When the stroma is prominent, and occasionally extensively hyalinized, broad bands subdivide the tumor into isolated nodules. The stroma may be focally or conspicuously edematous or myxoid. Tumor cells may be dispersed as relatively regular nests, irregular clusters, trabeculae, or cords. Rarely, a pseudotubular pattern is seen.

Approximately 10% of interstitial cell tumors are malignant, although there are no pathognomonic histologic criteria of malignancy. Large size, exten-

sive necrosis, gross or microscopic evidence of infiltration, invasion of blood vessels, and excessive mitotic activity are all features that suggest likely aggressive behavior, although metastasis is the only reliable criterion of malignancy. Two studies confirmed the predictive value of these features for malignant behavior and found that aneuploid DNA content and high proliferative fraction as assessed by the MIB-1 antibody also correlated with malignant behavior.[42, 43] In common with testicular tumors, metastases may involve retroperitoneal lymph nodes, lung, and bone. Occasionally, cytoplasm is extensively vacuolated or spongy because of abundant lipid and appears pale to clear. Focal, well-defined cytoplasmic vacuoles may impart a partial microcystic appearance in unusual cases. Rarely, the cells are small with scanty cytoplasm and have nuclei-containing grooves; exceptionally, the tumor cells are spindle-shaped.[44] These two cell types are usually associated with the characteristic polygonal cell type. Reinke's crystals are identified in the cytoplasm in approximately one-third of cases,[45] and lipochrome pigment is identified in 10%–15% of cases. The nuclei are typically round and contain a single prominent nucleolus. Nuclear atypicality is usually absent or slight but is marked in approximately 30% of cases. The mitotic rate varies greatly: it is usually low, in accord with the bland cytology of most tumors, but it is typically appreciable in cases with striking nuclear atypia.

Ultrastructural Appearances

There are features of steroid-secreting cells, including prominent vesicles of smooth endoplasmic reticulum that are sometimes arranged in concentric whorls around lipid droplets,[46] mitochondria with either tubular or lamellar cristae, and lipid droplets. In some cases, Reinke's crystals, showing the distinctive periodicity, are identified. Limited

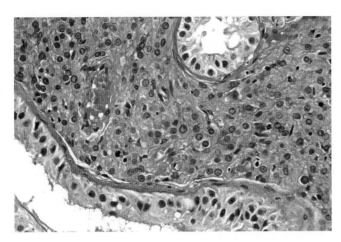

Figure 13-16. Leydig's cell tumor in Fig. 13-15 but at higher magnification. Residual germ cells are identified within the tubules. Mitotic figures are prominent within the tumor (magnification ×250).

observations suggest that ultrastructural features do not categorically distinguish between normal and neoplastic Leydig's cells, whether benign or malignant.

Immunohistochemistry

Important findings that assist in diagnosis of Leydig's cell tumors include positivity for inhibin, negativity for epithelial membrane antigen and HMB-45, and usually negative or weak and focal staining for cytokeratin. The tumors are strongly vimentin-positive, which, in conjunction with inhibin-positivity, negative staining for epithelial membrane antigen, and variable cytokeratin immunoreactivity, supports their differential diagnosis from metastatic carcinoma. Some Leydig's cell tumors are S-100 protein–positive, so this stain has limited value when considering melanoma,[26, 27, 47, 48] although a negative result favors Leydig's cell tumor. An antibody to melan-A has stained a small number of Leydig's cell tumors and has proved to be a diagnostic aid.[49]

Differential Diagnosis

Leydig's cell tumors require differentiation from three non-neoplastic lesions.

Leydig's Cell Hyperplasia

Leydig's cell hyperplasia may be florid, particularly in cryptorchid testes. However, the lack of a discrete mass on gross inspection and the presence of atrophic tubules in the midst of the Leydig's cells should suggest the correct diagnosis. When macroscopically apparent, Leydig's cell hyperplasia is generally multifocal, and nodules are small (see Fig. 13–13).

Malakoplakia

Malakoplakia is a more common problem because it may result in formation of a single, homogeneous, yellow or brown mass macroscopically indistinguishable from a Leydig cell tumor, although the presence of an abscess is a major clue to the diagnosis of malakoplakia. On microscopic examination the eosinophilic histiocytes (von Hansemann's cells) of malakoplakia may be mistaken for Leydig's cells, although they usually involve tubules as well as the interstitium and are admixed with other inflammatory cells. The presence of Michaelis-Gutmann bodies is pathognomonic of malakoplakia.

Adrenogenital Syndrome Tumors

Testicular "tumors" developing in patients with adrenogenital syndrome resemble Leydig's cell tumors but differ in their bilaterality, multifocality, and characteristic dark brown color. Leydig's cell tumors may be brown but are more often yellow or yellow-tan. Seminiferous tubules may be present within these non-neoplastic lesions but are found only rarely within Leydig's cell tumor. The cells of the adrenogenital tumor are larger, with more abundant cytoplasm, and contain lipochrome pigment more frequently and in greater amounts than do cells of Leydig's cell tumors. Reinke's crystalloids have not been identified within cells of the adrenogenital syndrome. Similar morphologic criteria assist in differentiating Leydig's cell tumors from hyperplastic nodules of steroid cells found in patients with Nelson's syndrome.

Leydig's cell tumors are relatively easily distinguished from Sertoli's cell tumors and other tumors in the sex cord–stromal category because the resemblance of the neoplastic cells to Leydig's cells is sufficiently striking to suggest the correct diagnosis. The rare Leydig's cell tumor that contains cells with nuclear grooves and focally resembles a granulosa cell tumor has other areas characteristic of Leydig's cell tumor that are easily found. Leydig's cell tumors may be confused with malignant lymphomas, particularly when their cells have scant cytoplasm and atypical nuclei. Lymphomas are usually bilateral and commonly involve the epididymis and spermatic cord. The characteristic intertubular infiltration of the tumor cells, with invasion of tubules in one third of cases, and the distinctive cytologic features of the neoplastic cells are present.

Occasional Leydig's cell tumors contain foci with small cytoplasmic vacuoles. Rare cases have prominent large vacuoles that may be confused with the microcystic pattern of yolk sac tumor.[50] The presence of areas of typical Leydig's cell tumor—low mitotic rate, cells with foamy cytoplasm, and absence of other patterns reminiscent of yolk sac tumor—are helpful distinguishing features in these cases. Additional support can be obtained with immunostains: inhibin is positive in Leydig's cell tumor, alpha-fetoprotein (AFP) is negative, and cytokeratins (AE1/AE3) are weak or negative.[26, 43] Converse patterns of reactivity are expected in yolk sac tumors.

Clinical Feature

Adults usually complain of testicular swelling, but gynecomastia causes the patient to seek medical attention in 15% of cases and is present in an additional 15% of patients on clinical evaluation.[40] Impalpable tumors may be detected by ultrasound examination of an adult.[51] Decreased libido or potency may be an accompaniment in some cases. Children almost always present with isosexual pseudoprecocity, at between 5 and 9 years of age.[52] Frequently, there are small tumors requiring special studies for detection. Approximately 10% of patients are asymptomatic and have tumors discovered on physical examination. Approximately 3% of Leydig's cell tumors are bilateral, and the tumor has extended beyond the testis at the time of presentation in up to 15% of cases.[40]

Testosterone is the major androgen produced by Leydig's cell tumors, but secretion of androstenedione and dehydroepiandrosterone has also been reported.[52, 53] Urinary 17-ketosteroids may be normal or raised. In patients with and without gynecomastia, elevated estrogen levels were recorded, and estradiol was present in high concentrations in spermatic vein blood in several cases.[10] Testosterone levels and values for gonadotropins, particularly follicle-stimulating hormone, are reported as low in patients with gynecomastia and elevated estradiol levels.[54, 55] In other cases, plasma progesterone or urinary pregnanediol values were elevated.[56, 57] Abnormal hormonal levels may return to normal or may persist after resection of the tumor.[58]

In prepubertal cases, presenting manifestations are of isosexual precocity with prominent external genitalia, mature masculine voice, and pubic hair growth. Unfortunately, in these patients, hormonal assays have been few, generally incomplete, and noncontributory to understanding the diseases. Increased testosterone production is usually demonstrable, and urinary 17-ketosteroid output may or may not be elevated. Virilizing types of congenital adrenocortical hyperplasia may also produce the endocrine signs and symptoms of interstitial cell tumors; differential tests must be performed to clarify the diagnosis. Such tests include estimation of urinary 17-hydroxy and 17-ketosteroid levels as well as plasma cortisol levels before and after corticotropin stimulation and dexamethasone suppression. Interstitial cell tumors may possess some of the same functional activities as adrenocortical tissue; interstitial cell carcinomas have been shown to possess 21-hydroxylase activity and are capable of producing cortisol and hydroxylating steroids at the 11 β position.

Elevation of urinary and plasma estrogen values in association with this tumor is relatively common. In adults, the majority of reported cases have shown inappropriate endocrine release. Such manifestations may precede the palpable testis mass, the most common presenting feature. In the remaining adult cases, impotence, decreased libido, and gynecomastia may occur for a long time before the testicular mass becomes apparent. Such a time lag ranges from 6 months to 10 years and averages more than 3 years. Measurement of AFP and β-hCG may be helpful in the differential diagnosis, which includes feminizing adrenocortical disorders, Klinefelter's syndrome, and other feminizing testicular disorders.

Prognosis for Leydig's cell tumors is good because of its generally benign nature. In the largest series of Leydig's cell tumors,[40] 5 of 30 patients with follow-up developed metastases. There is one report of bilateral malignant Leydig's cell tumor.[59] A number of features viewed in aggregate are helpful in assessing the likelihood of a malignant course. The average age of

patients is 63 years, in contrast to 40 years for Leydig's cell tumors in general.[40] Only an occasional patient with a malignant tumor has presented with endocrine manifestations,[60, 61] despite frequently elevated levels of various hormones or their metabolites. A malignant course in a prepubertal patient with Leydig's cell tumor is exceptional.[29] Tumors that metastasize are typically larger than those with a benign course. In one series, benign tumors had an average diameter of 2.7 cm compared with 6.9 cm for malignant ones.[40] The latter have characteristic infiltrative margins, invade lymphatics or blood vessels, and contain foci of necrosis. They also have a high mitotic rate (more than 3 per 10 high-power fields) and significant nuclear pleomorphism. Persistence of virilizing and feminizing features following orchiectomy is not necessarily an indication of malignancy, because these effects are not entirely reversible. The average survival time from surgery for patients with a malignant Leydig cell tumor is approximately 3 years. Of importance is the observation that malignancy is nonexistent in the prepubertal age group. Malignant Leydig's cell tumors spread most commonly to regional lymph nodes, lung, liver, and bone.[62] About one fifth of patients with clinically malignant tumors have metastases at the time of diagnosis.[62] Treatment of metastatic Leydig's cell tumor has been generally unsatisfactory.[62-64] Most patients with a clinically malignant Leydig's cell tumor die within 5 years, but occasionally there is a prolonged course.

SERTOLI-LEYDIG CELL TUMOR

Origins

Testicular tumors similar to the Sertoli-Leydig cell tumor of the ovary are rare. Six published cases had an unequivocal tubular component and/or patterns consistent with Sertoli-Leydig cell tumor of the ovary, with a stromal component containing at least focal Leydig's cells.[65-69] One patient was 3.5 months of age; the others were 4, 53, 54, 63, and 66 years of age. Two patients had gynecomastia. One tumor with an unusual structure (areas resembling osteosarcoma and malignant giant cell tumor) metastasized to the groin and lung 7 months after presentation.[67] Another tumor with areas of osteosarcoma is perhaps best placed in the Sertoli-Leydig cell category because of the neoplastic stromal component, although Leydig's cells were not identified.[28]

Gross Appearances

Testicular Sertoli-Leydig cell tumors have been reported from 1.8 cm to 12 cm in diameter. They are predominantly solid and usually yellow and commonly have a lobulated surface on cut section. The single known malignant tumor contained regions of hemorrhage and necrosis.[67]

Microscopic Appearances

Most of the tumors are composed of tubules, cords, and trabeculae in haphazard arrangements in a background stroma that usually contains focal Leydig's cells. However, a Sertoli-stromal cell tumor is placed in the Sertoli-Leydig group, even if Leydig's cells are absent, provided the stroma has a cellular, neoplastic appearance. The majority are of intermediate differentiation, according to the classification of ovarian cases, but some are poorly differentiated; there is only one report of a well-differentiated tumor.[70] Retiform differentiation, with slitlike glands and cysts, is unusual.[71] One tumor had areas of osteosarcoma and foci that resembled a malignant giant cell tumor.[67] The metastases in that case were composed predominantly of osteosarcoma, but one lung lesion had the features of a malignant Leydig cell tumor with typical Reinke's crystals.

Clinical Features

Eight of the 47 reported cases of large cell calcifying Sertoli's cell tumor have been clinically malignant.[31] The mean age of patients with malignant tumors is 39 years, compared with 17 years for those with benign tumors. Only one patient with a malignant tumor had any of the unusual clinical findings of Carney's syndrome. In contrast to the benign tumors, a significant number of which are bilateral and multifocal, all the malignant tumors were unilateral and unifocal. Pathologic features that suggest a malignant course include large size and other features generally similar to those useful in determining prognosis in cases of Sertoli's cell tumors. Lymphatic involvement is likely to become associated with clinical evidence of tumor elsewhere.

Immunohistochemistry

Epithelial membrane antigen positivity in most adenocarcinomas provides additional diagnostic aid in difficult cases because this antigen is not expressed in Sertoli's cell tumors.[14] Positivity for inhibin provides additional support for Sertoli's cell tumor, because inhibin is negative in metastatic adenocarcinoma.[36] The distinction of Sertoli's cell tumor from carcinoid may be made by the latter's reactivity with antibodies for S-100, chromogranin A, or NSE.

Differential Diagnosis

Differential diagnosis for tumors with a prominent tubular pattern is similar to that for pure Sertoli's cell tumors. In general, the resemblance of these tumors to the rare but well-known ovarian Sertoli-Leydig cell tumor should facilitate their recognition. The presence of a cellular, neoplastic stroma, sometimes with a Leydig cell component, separates these tumors from pure Sertoli's cell tumors and, in contrast to unclassified tumors in the sex cord–stromal category, they have a less conspicuous fibrothecomatous stroma and lack areas of granulosa cell differentiation.

GRANULOSA–STROMAL CELL TUMORS

Granulosa cell tumors are subdivided into two categories: adult and juvenile. It is impossible to make any conclusive statement concerning the relative frequency of the two because the juvenile type has been recognized only recently, and criteria for distinguishing the adult type from unclassified sex cord–stromal tumors are subjective and inconsistent between reports.

Adult-Type Granulosa Cell Tumor

Origins

Few adult granulosa cell tumors are well documented.[7, 72–76] The tumors generally occur in adults who are an average age of 42 years. Twenty percent of the reported cases were associated with gynecomastia. Some patients had a history of testicular enlargement of several years' duration. These tumors present as a testicular mass but without evidence of endocrine disorder, although some individual cases are reported to be associated with gynecomastia.

Gross Appearances

Tumors measure up to 13 cm in diameter and are homogeneous, yellow-gray through white, firm, and lobulated. Cysts may be present (Fig. 13–18). Tumors associated with metastases at presentation contained areas of hemorrhage or necrosis.

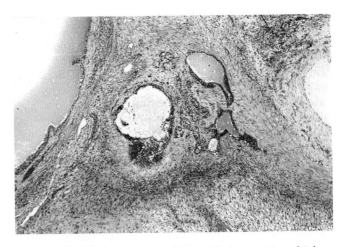

Figure 13–18. Cystic granulosa cell tumor in which a prominent fibrous stroma contains cysts lined by small tumor cells with scanty cytoplasm and pale nuclei (magnification ×30). (See Figs. 13–21 and 13–22).

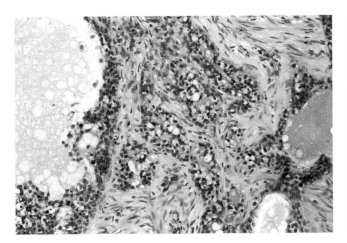

Figure 13-19. Microfollicular appearance of granulosa cell tumor cells (magnification ×120).

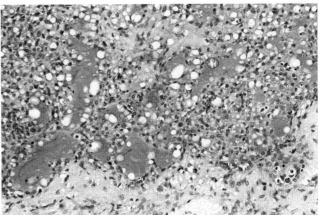

Figure 13-21. Solid and cystic variant of granulosa cell tumor in which the tumor is predominantly solid and diffuse with little stroma. Tumor cells appear variably degenerative and apoptotic with identifiable lipid droplets (magnification ×120).

Microscopic Appearances

The patterns are usually either microfollicular (Fig. 13-19) or diffuse, although other patterns, sometimes with Call-Exner bodies, may occur. Cytoplasm is typically scanty, and nuclei are pale with variably prominent grooves. If architectural features are typical, a paucity of nuclear grooves remains consistent with the diagnosis. The mitotic rate is generally low, although a high rate has been reported.[73] These tumors may have a prominent fibrous-to-thecomatous stroma, often undergoing myxoid change (Figs. 13-20 and 13-21). In occasional cases, the stromal cells have abundant pale-to-eosinophilic cytoplasm.

Clinical Features

Common presenting symptoms are either a painless, slowly-growing testicular mass that has been present for up to 10 years or the tumors are found incidentally on clinical examination. Retroperitoneal lymph node metastases are present or have developed during the prolonged course of the tumors.

Immunohistochemistry

Immunohistochemistry has been performed in only occasional cases. Staining for cytokeratin or epithelial membrane antigen is usually either absent or only focally positive, whereas vimentin (Fig. 13-22) is usually strongly positive.[73] S-100 protein and smooth muscle actin (SMA) may be demonstrated in both the juvenile and adult types,[48, 77] and desmin has also been demonstrated in the juvenile variant.[48] The spindle cell areas of granulosa cell tumors may stain for desmin, whereas these areas in unclassified tumors may be immunoreactive for S-100 protein

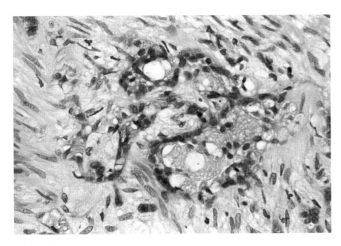

Figure 13-20. Tumor cells are small and pale-looking with scant cytoplasm. The cysts contain granular basophilic secretory material (magnification ×250).

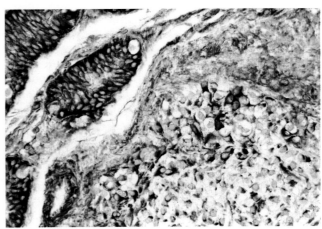

Figure 13-22. Granulosa cell tumor expressing vimentin. This marker is strongly expressed by the adjacent residual non-neoplastic tubular cells (magnification ×250).

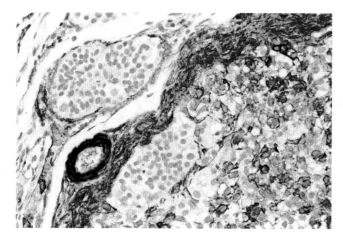

Figure 13–23. Tissue section adjacent to that in Fig. 13–22. Granulosa tumor cells express SMA, distinguishing them from adjacent residual non-neoplastic tubular cells (magnification ×250).

and smooth muscle actin and focally positive for cytokeratin and vimentin, in keeping with the myoepithelial or myofibroblastic differentiation of some of the cells (Fig. 13–23).

Differential Diagnosis

Unclassified tumors in the sex cord–stromal category often have a focal appearance compatible with that of a granulosa cell tumor, but a specific diagnosis of granulosa cell tumor should be made only when most of the neoplasm has granulosa cell features. Rare Leydig's cell tumors also contain cells with nuclear grooves; in these cases other features of Leydig's cell tumor are also present. Abundant pale cytoplasm in the stromal component of an adult granulosa cell tumor may simulate the germ cell component of the rare mixed germ cell–sex cord–stromal tumor. However, the nuclei in the sex cord–stromal tumors are typically smaller and may be irregular, unlike the larger, round nuclei of germ cells. The neoplastic germ cell nature of cells in possible mixed germ cell–sex cord–stromal tumors should be confirmed by periodic acid–Schiff and placental alkaline phosphatase staining. It is likely that many other of these supposed "mixed" tumors actually represent a sex cord–stromal tumor with entrapped, non-neoplastic germ cells. Each reported example contained foci of non-neoplastic germ cells that were crucial in establishing their nature[44] which, if not present, may result in the erroneous diagnosis of sarcoma. Such cases may also be misinterpreted as mixed sex cord–stromal tumors if the spindled cells are not recognized as Leydig's cell variants.

Clinical Features

In the literature, four patients with granulosa cell tumor had metastases. In two, there was retroperitoneal lymph node spread at presentation.[73, 74] One

patient was alive 14 months later and the other 14 years later. One of the other two patients with malignant tumors died of disease at 5 months[7] and the other at just over 11 years.[73] Size greater than 7 cm, vascular or lymphatic invasion, and hemorrhage or necrosis are features of malignant tumors.[73]

Juvenile-Type Granulosa Cell Tumor

Origins

In the first 6 months of life, this is the most common neoplasm of the testis.[12, 78–86] The tumor is occasionally seen in older children but is rare in adults. Occasional juvenile granulosa cell tumors occur in undescended testes of infants with intersexual disorders,[83, 86] and one developed in a patient with Drash's syndrome.[87]

Gross Appearances

Tumors measure up to 6 cm in diameter and may be partly solid and partly cystic. The solid component is nodular and yellow-orange or tan-white. Cysts are thin-walled and contain viscid or gelatinous fluid or altered blood.

Microscopic Appearances

The architectural patterns of growth are variably solid but contain follicles that vary from large and round to oval to small and irregular. They contain basophilic or eosinophilic fluid. In solid, nonfollicular areas, cells grow in sheets, nodules, and irregular clusters. Hyalinization can be extensive. Intercellular basophilic mucinous fluid may be so prominent that the consequence is a chondroid appearance (Fig. 13–24). In some cases tumor cells are dispersed

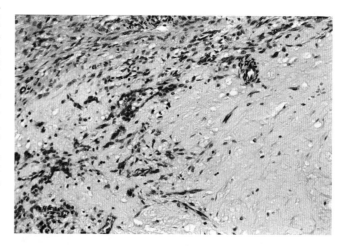

Figure 13–24. Juvenile-type granulosa cell tumor composed of rudimentary tubules within a predominantly myxoid stroma, giving a chondroid appearance (magnification ×120).

throughout the stroma, simulating the reticular pattern of yolk sac tumor. Tumor cells contain moderate to large amounts of pale eosinophilic cytoplasm and hyperchromatic with round to oval nuclei, some of which contain nucleoli. Mitoses are usually frequent and conspicuous.

Clinical Features

A testicular mass is the invariable presenting feature. All reported cases have had a benign outcome.

Differential Diagnosis

Potentially, four tumors may be confused with juvenile granulosa cell tumors (Table 13–5). Yolk sac tumors normally occur later than 6 months of age but may be confused with juvenile granulosa cell tumors if the latter are arranged in a "reticular" pattern with prominent mitotic activity. The presence of follicles, absence of characteristic patterns of yolk sac tumor, and lack of strong and diffuse immunohistochemical staining for cytokeratin and for AFP support the diagnosis of juvenile granulosa cell tumor rather than yolk sac tumor.

Juvenile granulosa cell tumors are usually found in the first year of life and are distinguished from the adult form by their more abundant cytoplasm, immature nuclear appearance, prominent mitotic activity, greater irregularity in size and shape of the follicles, and presence of intraluminal basophilic fluid.

Sertoli's tumor cells usually have moderate-to-abundant eosinophilic cytoplasm, but they may appear pale due to lipid accumulation. The majority of Sertoli's cell tumors have bland cytologic features and little mitotic activity, although occasional tumors exhibit prominent pleomorphism with conspicuous mitotic figures. The characteristic feature of this tumor is tubular differentatiation, which does not occur in juvenile granulosa cell tumors.

Embryonal rhabdomyosarcoma with scattered rhabdomyoblastic cells may be suggested by primitive appearances of nuclei, raised mitotic activity, and eosinophilic cytoplasm of a juvenile granulosa cell tumor. However, embryonal rhabdomyosarcoma almost always occurs as a paratesticular tumor in older children. Rare testicular cases do occur, possibly as sarcomatous overgrowth in teratomas, but have not been reported in infants. Although cystic degeneration may occur, the fluid-filled follicles

Table 13–5. Differential Diagnosis of Juvenile Granulosa Cell Tumors

- Yolk sac tumor
- Adult-type granulosa cell tumor
- Sertoli's cell tumor
- Embryonal rhabdomyosarcoma

characteristic of juvenile granulosa cell tumor do not occur in embryonal rhabdomyosarcoma. Immunostains, including protein kinase C (PKC)-δ and PKC-μ for smooth muscle and skeletal muscle differentiation, respectively, may confirm skeletal muscle differentiation.

FIBROMA-THECOMA TUMORS

Origins

These tumors are uncommon and resemble either the typical ovarian fibroma or its cellular variant.[88] Four tumors of the testicular parenchyma have been reported as resembling ovarian fibroma.[6] It is likely that some cases are not of testicular stromal origin but arise from nonspecific soft-tissue fibroblasts.

Gross Appearances

Tumors range from 0.5 to 7.0 cm in diameter and are circumscribed, firm, and yellow to tan-white. Hemorrhage and necrosis are absent, even in the largest reported tumors.

Microscopic Appearances

These tumors are characterized by spindle-shaped fibroblasts associated with variable amounts of collagen and often grow in storiform patterns, sometimes associated with edema and modest vascularity. Occasional cellular tumors contain up to 2 mitotic figures per 10 high-power fields.

Clinical Features

The age incidence of these tumors has ranged from 5 to 52 years of age. Typically, the tumors presented with a testicular mass.[6, 89–95] Follow-up has been unremarkable although limited.

Ultrastructural Appearances

Electron microscopic studies reveal fibroblastic or myofibroblastic differentiation, with the tumor cells containing filaments, subplasmalemmal electron-dense bodies, pinocytotic vesicles, discontinuous basal lamina, and intercellular desmosomes.

Immunohistochemistry

Immunohistochemical staining of fibromatous tumors is rarely indicated. However, their negativity for desmin provides evidence against a smooth muscle tumor. Weak desmin staining and actin staining have to be interpreted in the context of the overall microscopic findings. Absence of PKC-δ or PKC-μ staining excludes myogenic smooth-muscle or skeletal-muscle types. Although experience is limited, unclassified sex cord–stromal tumors with a predominance of spindle cells are frequently positive for both S-100 protein and SMA, whereas fibromas are positive for SMA but negative for S-100 protein.[77]

Differential Diagnosis

Noncellular fibromas are similar to fibromatous tumors of the testicular tunica and are distinguished by their macroscopic characteristics. Cellular fibromas may require differentiation from the rare fibrosarcoma of the testis. No established criteria distinguish these two tumors in the testis.[88] The tumors are distinguished from leiomyomas of both typical and cellular type according to criteria applicable in the ovary and soft tissues. Unclassified sex cord–stromal tumors may have prominent fibromatous areas but have at least some focal epithelial differentiation that permits distinction from pure fibromas. Because occasional tumors in the sex cord–stromal (unclassified) category are malignant, this distinction is clinically important because of the benign course of all reported fibromas.

MIXED AND UNCLASSIFIED TUMORS

Origins

Some testicular sex cord–stromal tumors have patterns of two or more of the previously discussed subtypes. Unclassified sex cord–stromal tumors occur at all ages and frequently lack specific differentiation or contain patterns and cells resembling degrees of both testicular and ovarian elements.[7, 96] Approximately one third of the reported tumors have been from children. The most common clinical symptom is painless testicular enlargement. Gynecomastia is present in about 10% of patients.

Gross Appearances

Tumors vary in size, with many replacing most or all of the affected testis. These tumors are well circumscribed and are composed of white-to-yellow, often lobulated, tissue, sometimes traversed by gray-white fibrous septa. Cysts may be present. Hemorrhage and necrosis are uncommon.

Microscopic Appearances

The spectrum of these patterns ranges from predominantly epithelial to predominantly stromal. The better-differentiated tumors typically contain solid-to-hollow tubules or cords composed of or lined by cells resembling Sertoli's cells. Islands and masses of cells resembling granulosa cells and containing

Call-Exner–like bodies may be present, but usually the nuclei lack grooves. Despite appearances suggestive of granulosa cell tumor, the overall architectural and cytologic features are usually not typical of that tumor. The cytoplasm of cells lining sertoliform tubules varies from scanty to abundant, and may be eosinophilic, amphophilic, or vacuolated and lipid-laden. Nuclei are round to oval and often vesicular, sometimes containing single small nucleoli. Mitotic figures are variably prominent. The stromal component may be from densely cellular to fibromatous, possibly containing Leydig's cells (Fig. 13–25). Some stromal cells may have abundant vacuolated or eosinophilic cytoplasm. Less differentiated tumors exhibit varying degrees of nuclear pleomorphism and mitotic activity. Diffuse and sarcomatoid patterns are frequent, and in some areas it may be difficult or impossible to distinguish the epithelial and stromal components on routine staining. Spindle cell–predominant cases are often reactive for S-100 protein and SMA, similar to granulosa cell tumors.[77]

Differential Diagnosis

The greatest problem is in distinguishing tumors of the "unclassified and mixed" category from pure tumors of the various subtypes already defined. Analysis of the morphologic features should enable the pure tumors to be separated from those in the mixed and unclassified categories, particularly the prominent cellular stromal component of many unclassified tumors and the typical presence of both granulosa-like and Sertoli-like areas. When the epithelial component is small, areas of the tumor may resemble one or another form of pure sarcoma of the testis. This diagnosis should be made only after

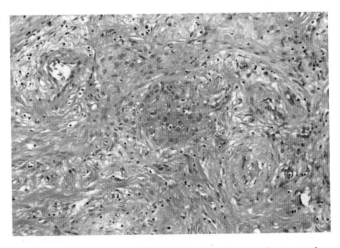

Figure 13–25. Unclassified testicular tumor of mesenchymal origin in which there is proliferation of tumor cells in a densely fibromatous stroma with formation of endothelial-lined slitlike spaces and thick-walled blood vessels. Foci of benign Leydig's cells without Reinke's crystalloids are scattered throughout the tumor (magnification ×250).

extensive sampling, together with appropriate immunohistochemistry, to exclude epithelial elements consistent with a sex cord–stromal neoplasm.

Clinical Features

An important characteristic of these tumors is the rarity of malignant behavior in children when compared with 25% malignancy in adults. Features that generally correlate with aggressive behavior include large size, extratesticular spread, necrosis, vascular invasion, marked nuclear pleomorphism, and brisk mitotic activity. The patterns of spread are predominantly to inguinal and retroperitoneal lymph nodes, but visceral metastases are not rare. In cases with overt malignant features on microscopic examination, a staging lymph node dissection is indicated.

OTHER TESTIS NEOPLASMS

These comprise a heterogeneous group of tumors of relatively infrequent occurrence but constituting 5%–10% of all testis tumors.

Gonadoblastoma

Origins

Otherwise known as tumor of dysgenetic gonads, mixed germ cell tumor, or gonadocytoma, these rare tumors occur in patients with some form of gonadal dysgenesis and comprise 0.5% of all testis neoplasms. They occur in all age groups from infancy to beyond 70 years, although the majority have been reported below 30 years of age. Although gonadoblastomas are currently regarded as neoplasms, the possibility that they represent hamartomas or nodular hyperplasia in response to pituitary gonadotrophins has been suggested.

Gross Appearances

These lesions may be unilateral or bilateral and may vary in size from microscopic to greater than 20 cm in diameter. Tumors weighing more than 1000 g have been reported. Aggressive growth may efface the testis from which the tumor arises. Tumors generally are round, with a smooth and slightly lobulated surface, and vary in consistency from soft and fleshy to firm or hard. Calcified areas are frequent and may reflect the extensive spontaneous retrogressive changes common with these lesions. The cut surface is grayish-white to yellow but can vary considerably.

Microscopic Appearances

Tumors comprise the three elements of Sertoli's cells, interstitial tissue, and germ cells, although the proportions in individual neoplasms vary widely.[97] In half of these tumors, germ cell overgrowth, with the appearance of seminoma, or germ cell elements exhibiting histologic features of embryonal carcinoma, teratoma, choriocarcinoma, or yolk sac tumor may occur. Throughout the tubules, characteristic Call-Exner bodies may be identified, consisting of PAS-positive material similar to that seen in tubular basement membranes. The germ cells of gonadoblastoma are similar to those of seminoma. If germ cell proliferation occurs, gonadoblastoma may progress from an in situ stage to invasive germinoma (seminoma), defined as gonadoblastoma with germinoma (seminoma).

Clinical Features

Clinical manifestations are the consequence of the usual concurrence of gonadal dysgenesis with resultant abnormalities in the external genitalia and gonads, presence of germ cells with malignant potential, and endocrine function of the gonadal stromal components of the tumor (usually production of androgen). Although interstitial cells may not be evident on light microscopy, a steroidogenic potential of the tumor may exist. Furthermore, demonstration of Leydig's cells in the tumor does not necessarily dictate virilism, either because the resultant steroids may be biologically inactive or because the end organs may be defective. The usual appearance is of solid tubules of varying size containing germ cells in close association with Sertoli's cells and of mature interstitial cells evident between the tubules.

The majority of patients with gonadoblastomas are phenotypic females, usually presenting with primary amenorrhea but occasionally with lower abdominal masses. The remainder are phenotypic males, almost always presenting with cryptorchidism, hypospadias, and some female internal genitalia. However, gonadoblastoma has been described in an anatomically normal male.[98] In phenotypic females, breasts are small, the internal genitalia are hypoplastic, and the gonads are usually of the streak type. Sex chromatin assessment is negative, and chromosome analysis usually shows XY, XO, or XO/XY patterns. In the phenotypic male, gynecomastia may be present, and there is often hypospadias, some female internal genitalia, and dysgenetic testes usually located in the abdomen or inguinal region. Sex chromatin assessment is negative, and the chromosome pattern is XY or XO/XY.

Miscellaneous Neoplasms of Mesenchymal Origin

Occurring as painless masses, these lesions raise the possibility of malignant tumors. A variety of neoplasms derived from mesenchymal elements may arise on the tunica albuginea within the testes. These include benign fibroma, angioma, neurofibroma, and leiomyoma. Differential diagnosis includes abnormalities of the testicular appendages, fibrous pseudotumors, adenomatoid tumors, and non-neoplastic cystic lesions.

Epidermal Cyst

Occuring as 1% of testis tumors,[99] approximately half occur in the 3rd decade, and most of the remainder occur between the 2nd and 4th decades. Their histogenesis remains uncertain but is widely accepted to represent a monophasic teratoma. Such an origin is supported by the age and racial incidences of these tumors as well as by the occasional association with cryptorchidism. These lesions appear as round, sharply circumscribed, firm, and encapsulated intratesticular nodules (Fig. 13–26). Cut surface reveals a grayish-white to yellowish, cheesy, amorphous mass. Microscopically, the wall is composed of dense fibrous tissue lined by stratified, squamous, and keratinized epithelium, desquamations from which, with degeneration and microcalcification, make up the amorphous interior. The clinical behavior of these tumors has been consistently benign: apparently, no instance of associated, clinically unrecognized but microscopically confirmed germ cell tumor has been reported. Rare instances of bilaterality have been reported, as with germ cell tumors.[100] Testicular ultrasonography may demonstrate a well-circumscribed lesion with a solid central core and may aid in the distinction from a germ cell tumor.

Adenocarcinoma of the Rete Testis

These rare but highly malignant tumors occur in adults in the age range of 20–80 years. The clinical presentation is of a painless scrotal mass, commonly with an associated hydrocele (Fig. 13–27). Microscopic examination reveals a multicystic papillary adenocarcinoma composed of small cuboidal

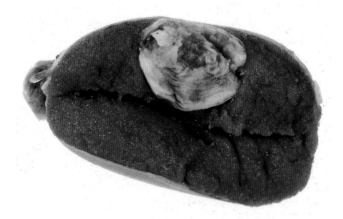

Figure 13–26. Epidermal cyst appearing as a round, sharply circumscribed, firm, and encapsulated intratesticular nodule 1 cm in diameter. Cut surface reveals a grayish-white to yellowish, cheesy, amorphous mass.

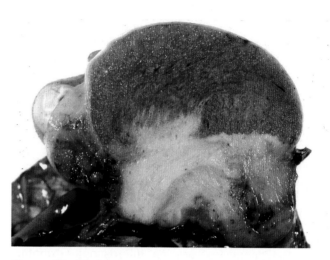

Figure 13–27. Adenocarcinoma of the rete testis. Macroscopically, there is invasion into the substance of the testis together with development of a small hydrocele (left). Focal hemorrhage indicates the likely sinister nature of this small malignancy.

cells with elongated nuclei and scanty cytoplasm, presumably arising from the rete tubules of the testicular mediastinum. Despite radical orchiectomy, half of the patients die within a year from the time of diagnosis. Metastasis has occurred in inguinal and retroperitoneal lymph nodes, lungs, bone, and liver. The observation that retroperitoneal deposits may represent the sole site of metastasis supports the rationale of retroperitoneal lymphadenectomy in the absence of distant metastasis.

Adrenal Rest Tumors

These bilateral testis tumors are defined by their association with congenital adrenal hyperplasia, and the remission of endocrine manifestations and tumors following cortcosteroid treatment denotes these unusual lesions. Whether they represent neoplasms or hyperplasia and whether they derive from "normal" adrenal rests or from abnormal interstitial cells remain uncertain in some cases. Luteinizing hormone may contribute to the growth of these tumors; high serum LH levels are found in association with incomplete suppression of adrenal steroid secretion, and there is evidence of gonadotropin secretion with testicular tumors in some patients with congenital adrenal hyperplasia.[101]

Adenomatoid Tumors

These lesions are characteristically small benign tumors peculiar to the genital tract of males and females. Occuring primarily in the epididymis in the male (Fig. 13–28), occasional instances of tumor confined to the testis have been reported. They consist of a fibrous stroma in which disoriented spaces of epithelial cells occur, resembling endothelium,

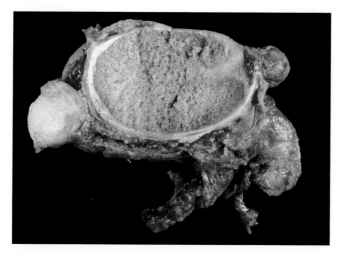

Figure 13–28. Adenomatoid tumor comprising a 0.8-cm–diameter solid nodule arising in the epididymis of the testis.

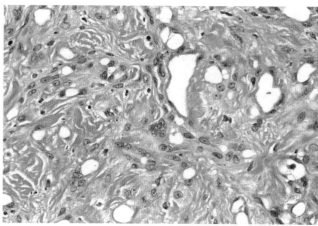

Figure 13–30. Adenomatoid tumor in which individual neoplastic cells are scattered throughout the lesion and form the lining of the various spaces (magnification ×250).

epithelium, or mesothelium (Figs. 13–29 and 13–30). Histogenesis remains debatable. Immunophenotyping usually confirms the simultaneous expression of a spectrum of divergent phenotypes (Figs. 13–31 to 13–33). Microscopically, despite florid proliferation of slitlike vascular spaces, these tumors should not be mistaken for hemangiopericytoma (Fig. 13–34).

Carcinoid

Carcinoid is uncommon outside the gastrointestinal tract. In the testis, the histogenesis of these tumors remains uncertain, but monophasic development of a teratoma or origin from argentaffin or enterochromaffin cells within the testis is an alternative. A slow, progressive, painless testicular enlargement is the most frequent presentation. On macroscopic examination, the tumors are circumscribed and limited to the

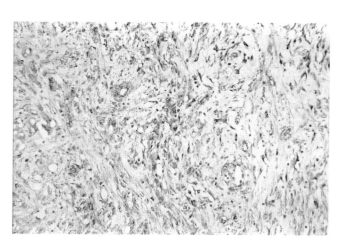

Figure 13–31. Adenomatoid tumor: diffusely vimentin-positive (magnification ×60).

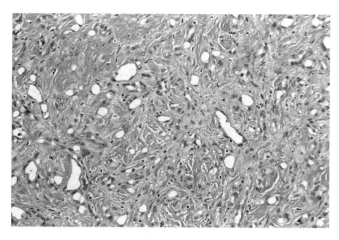

Figure 13–29. Adenomatoid tumor composed of a fibrous stroma containing disoriented spaces lined by tumor cells resembling endothelium, epithelium, or mesothelium (magnification ×120).

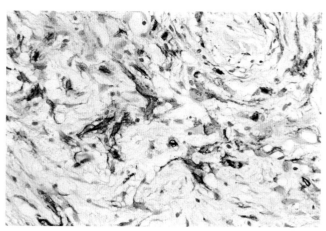

Figure 13–32. Adenomatoid tumor: individual tumor cells strongly CD-34–positive, confirming their endothelial phenotype (magnification ×250).

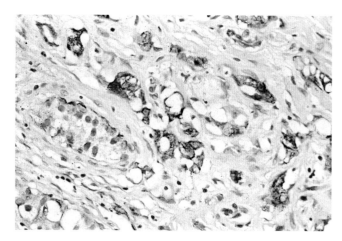

Figure 13-33. Adenomatoid tumor: individual tumor cells strongly cytokeratin-positive, confirming their epithelial phenotype (magnification ×250).

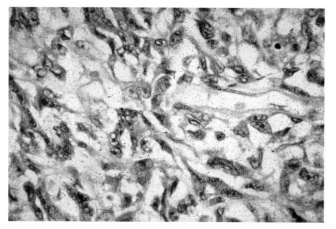

Figure 13-34. Hemangiopericytoma of testis comprising characteristic large neoplastic cells forming slitlike channels but without the fibroblastic background of the adenomatoid tumor (magnification ×625).

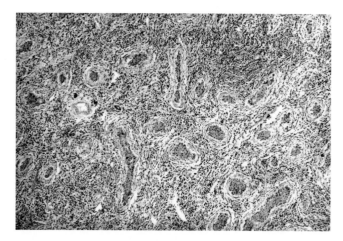

Figure 13-35. Non-Hodgkin's malignant lymphoma involving testis. Normal architecture is effaced, leaving a few residual but effete tubules in a sea of neoplastic lymphoma cells (magnification ×60).

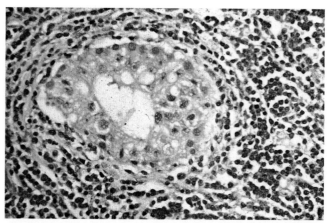

Figure 13-36. Chronic lymphatic leukemia obliterating normal architecture. Residual tubules are not directly involved but appear atrophic with maturation-arrest. This appearance is likely to be attributed to the effects of cytotoxic chemotherapy rather than to the leukemia (magnification ×625).

testis, with diameters ranging up to 8 cm. Microscopically, the tumors comprise islands, nests, or discrete masses of round, oval, or polygonal cells separated by fibrous strands and exhibit a solid acinar structure. Although most reported cases have been pure carcinoids, a few have arisen in association with teratoma. Detailed serum serotonin and 5-hydroxyindoleacetic acid estimations have not been performed despite minimal symptoms suggesting carcinoid syndrome in one patient.

Mesothelioma

Malignant mesothelioma may arise from any site on the mesothelial membrane-pleura, peritoneum, pericardium, or tunica vaginalis. Fewer than 20 cases involving the tunica vaginalis have been reported. The lesion occurs in patients 21–78 years of age, and the usual presentation is with a hydrocele. Although not reported, these tumors can be, potentially, endocrineactive, in common with their more frequent pleural counterparts.

SECONDARY NEOPLASMS

Reticuloendothelial Malignancies

The two most common malignancies to involve the testes are malignant lymphoma (Fig. 13-35) and leukemia (Fig. 13-36). Although endocrine manifestations of these malignancies are extremely rare, other secondary systemic effects are not infrequent.

References

1. Scully RE: Testicular tumors with endocrine manifestations. In De Groot U, ed.: Endocrinology. WB Saunders, Philadelphia, 1995, p. 2442.

2. Kaplan GW, Cromie WJ, Kelalis PP, et al.: Gonadal stromal tumors: A report of the prepubertal testicular tumor registry. J Urol 1986; 136:300.

3. Ober WB, Sciagura C: Leydig, Sertoli, Reinke: Three anatomists who were on the ball. Pathol Annu 1981; 16:1.

4. Teilum O: Arrhenoblastoma-androblastoma: Homologous ovarian and testicular tumors. Acta Pathol Microbiol Scand 1946; 23:252.

5. Teilum O: Special tumors of ovary and testis and related extragonadal lesions. Lippincott, Philadelphia, 1971.

6. Collins DII, Symington T: Sertoli-cell tumor. Br J Urol 1964; 36:52.

7. Mostofi FK, Theiss EA, Ashley DJ: Tumors of specialized gonadal stroma in human male subjects. Cancer 1959; 12:944.

8. Talerman A: Malignant Sertoli cell tumor of the testis. Cancer 1971; 28:446.

9. Wilson DM, Pitts WC, Hintz RL, et al.: Testicular tumors with Peutz-Jeghers syndrome. Cancer 1986; 57:2238.

10. Gabrilove JL, Freiberg EK, Leiter E, et al.: Feminizing and non-feminizing Sertoli cell tumors. J Urol 1980; 124:757.

11. Goswitz JJ, Pettinato G, Manivel JC: Testicular sex cord stromal tumors in children: Clinicopathologic study of sixteen children with review of literature. Pediatr Pathol Lab Med 1996; 16:451.

12. Harms D, Kock LR: Testicular juvenile granulosa cell and Sertoli cell tumours: A clinicopathologic study of 29 cases from the Kiel Paediatric Tumor Registry. Virch Arch 1997; 430:301.

13. Young RH, Koelliker DD, Scully RE: Sertoli cell tumors of the testis, not otherwise specified: A clinicopathologic analysis of 60 cases. Am J Surg Pathol 1998; 22:709.

14. Amin MB, Young RH, Scully RE: Immunohistochemical profile of Sertoli and Leydig cell tumors of the testis. Mod Pathol 1998; 11:76A.

15. Rosvoll RV, Woodard JR: Malignant Sertoli cell tumor of the testis. Cancer 1968; 22:8.

16. Sharma S, Seam RK, Kapoor HE: Malignant Sertoli cell tumour of the testis in a child. J Surg Oncol 1990; 44:129.

17. Rutgers JL, Scully RE: The androgen insensitivity syndrome (testicular feminization): A clinicopathologic study of 43 cases. Gynecol Pathol 1991; 10:126.

18. Carney JA, Gordon H, Carpenter PC: The complex of myxomas, spotty pigmentation, and endocrine overactivity. Medicine 1985; 64:270.

19. Caccamea A, Cozzi F, Farragiana T, et al.: Feminizing Sertoli cell tumor associated with Peutz-Jeghers syndrome. Tumori 1985; 7:379.

20. Cantu JM, Rivera H, Ocampo-Campos R: Peutz-Jeghers syndrome with feminizing Sertoli cell tumor. Cancer 1980; 46:223.

21. Coen P, Kuhn H, Ballantine T: An aromatase-producing sex-cord tumor resulting in prepubertal gynecomastia. New Engl J Med 1991; 324:317.

22. Dubois RS, Hoffman WH, Krishnan TH: Feminizing sex cord tumor with annular tubules in a boy with Peutz-Jeghers syndrome. J Pediatr 1982; 101:568.

23. Young S, Gooneratne S, Straus FH, et al.: Feminizing Sertoli cell tumors in boys with Peutz-Jegher syndrome. Am J Surg Pathol 1995; 19:50.

24. Erlandson RA: Diagnostic transmission electron microscopy of tumors with clinicopathological, immunohistochemical and cytogenetic correlations. Raven Press, New York, 1994.

25. Tetu B, Roy JY, Ayala AG: Large cell calcifying Sertoli cell tumor of the testis: A clinicopathologic, immunohistochemical and ultrastructural study of two cases. Am J Clin Pathol 1991; 96:717.

26. Iczkowskj KA, Bostwick DG, Cheville JC: Inhibin is a sensitive and specific marker for testicular sex cord stromal tumors. Mod Pathol 1998; 11:774.

27. McCluggage WG, Shanks JH, Whiteside C, et al.: Immunohistochemical study of testicular sex cord–stromal tumors, including staining with anti-inhibin antibody. Am J Surg Pathol 1998; 22:615.

28. Gilcrease MZ, Delgado R, Albores-Saavedra J: Testicular Sertoli cell tumor with a heterologous sarcomatous component: Immunohistochemical assessment of Sertoli cell differentiation. Arch Pathol Lab Med 1996; 122:907.

29. Freeman DA: Steroid hormone-producing tumors in man. Endocr Rev 1986; 7:203.

30. Horn T, Jao W, Keh PC: Large cell calcifying Sertoli cell tumor of the testis: A case report with ultrastructural study. Ultrastruct Pathol 1983; 4:359.

31. Kratzer SS, Ulbright TM, Talerman A: Large cell calcifying Sertoli cell tumor of the testis: Contrasting features of six malignant and six benign tumors and a review of the literature. Am J Surg Pathol 1997; 21:1271.

32. Plata C, Algaba F, Anjudar M: Large cell calcifying Sertoli cell tumor of the testis. Histopathology 1995; 26:255.

33. Proppe KH, Scully RE: Large cell calcifying Sertoli cell tumor of the testis. Am J Clin Pathol 1980; 74:607.

34. Rosenzweig JL, Lawrence DA, Vogel DL: Adrenocorticotropin-independent hypercortisolemia and testicular tumors in a patient with a pituitary tumor and gigantism. J Clin Endocrinol Metab 1982; 55:421.

35. Waxman M, Damjanov I, Khapra A, et al.: Large cell calcifying Sertoli tumor of testis: Light microscopic and ultrastructural study. Cancer 1984; 54:1574.

36. Rishi M, Howard LN, Bratthauer GL, et al.: Use of monoclonal antibody against human inhibin as a marker of sex cord stromal tumors of the ovary. Am J Surg Pathol 1997; 21:583.

37. Zukerberg LR, Young RH, Scully RE: Sclerosing Sertoli cell tumor of the testis: A report of 10 cases. Am J Surg Pathol 1991; 15:829.

38. Dilworth JP, Farrow GM, Oesterling JE: Non-germ cell tumors of testis. Urology 1991; 37:399.

39. Kay R: Prepubertal testicular tumor registry. J Urol 1993; 150:671.

40. Kim I, Young RH, Scully RE: Leydig cell tumors of the testis: A clinicopathological analysis of 40 cases and review of the literature. Am J Surg Pathol 1985; 9:177.

41. Davis JM, Woodroff J, Sadasivan R, et al.: Case report: Congenital adrenal hyperplasia and malignant Leydig cell tumor. Am J Med Sci 1995; 309:63.

42. Cheville JC, Sebo TJ, Lager DJ, et al.: Leydig cell tumor of the testis: A clinicopathologic DNA content and MIB-1 comparison of non-metastasizing and metastasizing tumors. Am J Surg Pathol 1998; 22:1261.

43. McCluggage WG, Shanks JH, Arthur K, et al.: Cellular proliferation and nuclear ploidy assessments augment prognostic factors in predicting malignancy in testicular Leydig cell tumours. Histopathology 1998; 33:361.

44. Richmond I, Banerjee SS, Eyden BP, et al.: Sarcomatoid Leydig cell tumor of testis. Histopathology 1995; 27:578.

45. Reinke F: Beiträge zur Histologie des Menschen. Arch Mikr Anat 1896; 47:34.

46. Dickersin GR: Diagnostic electron microscopy: A text/atlas. Igaku-Shoir, New York, 1988.

47. McClaren K, Thomson D: Localization of S-100 protein in a Leydig and Sertoli cell tumor of testis. Histopathology 1989; 15:1271.

48. Perez-Atayde AR, Joste N, Mulhern H: Juvenile granulosa cell tumor of the infantile testis: Evidence of a dual epithelial–smooth muscle differentiation. Am J Surg Pathol 1996; 20:72.

49. Busam KJ, Iversen K, Coplan KA, et al.: Immunoreactivity for A103, an antibody to Melan-A (Mart-i) in adrenocortical and other steroid tumors. Am J Surg Pathol 1998; 22:57.

50. Billings SD, Roth LM, Ulbright TM: Microcystic Leydig cell tumors mimicking yolk sac tumor: A report of four cases. Am J Surg Pathol 1999; 23:546.

51. Haas GP, Pittbiga S, Gomella L: Clinically occult Leydig cell tumor presenting with gynecomastia. J Urol 1989; 142:1325.

52. Wilson BE, Netzloff ML: Primary testicular abnormalities causing precocious puberty: Leydig cell tumor, Leydig cell hyperplasia and adrenal rest tumor. Ann Clin Lab Sci 1983; 13:315.

53. Boulanger P, Somma M, Chevalier S, et al.: Elevated secretion of androstenedione in a patient with a Leydig cell tumour. Acta Endocrinol 1984; 107:104.

54. Bercovici P, Nahoul K, Tater D: Hormonal profile of Leydig cell tumors with gynecomastia. J Clin Endocrinol Metab 1984; 59:625.

55. Mineur P, DeCooman S, Hustin J, et al.: Feminizing testicular Leydig cell tumor: Hormonal profile before and after unilateral orchidectomy. J Clin Endocrinol Metab 1987; 64:686.

56. Czernobilsky H, Czernobilsky B, Schneider HG: Characterization of a feminizing testicular Leydig cell tumor by hormone profile, immunocytochemistry, and tissue culture. Cancer 1985; 56:1667.

57. Perez C, Novoa J, Alcaniz J, et al.: Leydig cell tumour of the testis with gynaecomastia and elevated oestrogen, progesterone and prolactin levels: Case report. Clin Endocrinol 1980; 13:409.

58. Bercovici P, Nahoul L, Ducasse M: Leydig cell tumor with gynecomastia: Further studies—the recovery after unilateral orchidectomy. J Clin Endocrinol Metab 1985; 61:957.

59. Sugimura J, Suzuki Y, Tamura C, et al.: Metachronous development of malignant Leydig cell tumor. Hum Pathol 1997; 28:1318.

60. Balsitis M, Sokol M: Ossifying malignant Leydig (interstitial) cell tumour of the testis. Histopathology 1990; 16:597.

61. Shapiro CM, Sankovitch A, Yoon WJ: Malignant feminizing Leydig cell tumor. J Surg Oncol 1984; 27:73.

62. Grem JL, Robins I, Wilson KS, et al.: Metastatic Leydig cell tumor of the testis: Report of three cases and review of the literature. Cancer 1986; 58:2116.

63. Bertrem KJ, Bratloff B, Hodges GF, et al.: Treatment of malignant Leydig cell tumor. Cancer 1991; 68:4.

64. Bokemeyer C, Harstrick A, Gonnermann O: Metastatic Leydig cell tumours of the testis: Report of four cases and review of the literature. Int J Oncol 1993; 2:241.

65. Fain A, Ishak KG: Androblastoma of the testicle: Report of a case in an infant three months old. J Urol 1958; 79:859.

66. Fugisang F, Ohlse NS: Androblastoma predominantly feminizing: With report of a case. Acta Chir Scand 1957; 112:405.

67. Oosterhuis JW, Castedo SM, de Jong B: A malignant mixed gonadal stromal tumor of the testis with heterologous components and i(12p) in one of its metastases. Cancer Genet Cytogen 1989; 41:105.

68. Teilum G: Arrhenoblastoma-androblatoma: Homologous ovarian and testicular tumors. II. Including the so-called luteomas and adrenal tumors of the ovary and the interstitial cell tumors of the testis. Acta Pathol Microbiol Scand 1943; 23:252.

69. Teilum G: Homologous tumours in the ovary and testis: Contributions to classification of the gonadial tumors. Acta Obstetticia Gynecologica Scand 1944; 24:480.

70. Perito PE, Ciancio G, Civantos F, et al.: Sertoli Leydig cell testicular tumor: Case report and review of sex cord/gonadal stromal tumor histogenesis. J Urol 1992; 148:883.

71. Young RH, Scully RE: Ovarian Sertoli Leydig cell tumours with a retiform pattern: A problem in histopathologic diagnosis: A report of 25 cases. Am J Surg Pathol 1983; 7:775.

72. Gaylis FD, August C, Yeldandi A, et al.: Granulosa cell tumor of the adult testis: Ultrastructural and ultrasonographic characteristics. J Urol 1989; 141:126.

73. Jimenez-Quintero UP, Ro JY, Zavala-Pompa A: Granulosa cell tumor of the adult testis: A clinicopathologic study of seven cases and a review of the literature. Hum Pathol 1993; 24:1120.

74. Matoska J, Ondrus D, Talerman A: Malignant granulosa cell tumor of the testis associated with gynecomastia and long survival. Cancer 1992; 69:1769.

75. Nistal M, Lazaro R, Garcia J, et al.: Testicular granulosa cell tumor of the adult type. Arch Pathol Lab Med 1992; 116:284.

76. Talerman A: Pure granulosa cell tumor of the testis: Report of a case and review of the literature. Appl Pathol 1985; 138:117.

77. Renshaw AA, Gordon M, Corless CL: Immunohistochemistry of unclassified sex cord stromal tumors of the testis with a predominance of spindle cells. Mod Pathol 1997; 10:693.

78. Chan JK, Chan VS, Mak KL: Congenital juvenile granulosa cell tumour of the testis: Report of a case showing extensive degenerative changes. Histopathology 1990; 17:75.

79. Crump WD: Juvenile granulosa cell (sex cord stromal) tumor of fetal testis. Urology 1983; 129:1057.

80. Lawrence WD, Young RH, Scully RE: Juvenile granulosa cell tumor of the infantile testis: A report of 14 cases. Am J Surg Pathol 1985; 9:87.

81. Nistal M, Redondo E, Paniagua R: Juvenile granulosa cell tumor of the testis. Arch Pathol Lab Med 1988; 112:1129.

82. Pinto MM: Juvenile granulosa cell tumor of the infant testis: Case report with ultrastructural observations. Pediatr Pathol 1985; 4:277.

83. Raju U, Fine G, Warner R, et al.: Congenital testicular juvenile granulosa cell tumor in a neonate with X/XY mosaicism. Am J Surg Pathol 1986; 10:577.

84. Uehling DT, Smith JE, Logan R, et al.: Newborn granulosa cell tumor of the testis. J Urol 1987; 138:385.

85. White JM, McCarthy MP: Testicular gonadal stromal tumors in newborns. Urology 1982; 20:121.

86. Young RH, Lawrence WD, Scully RE: Juvenile granulosa cell tumor: Another neoplasm associated with abnormal chromosomes and ambiguous genitalia: A report of three cases. Am J Surg Pathol 1985; 9:737.

87. Manivel JC, Sibley RK, Dehner LP: Complete and incomplete Drash syndrome: A clinicopathologic study of five cases of a dysontogenetic neoplastic complex. Hum Pathol 1987; 18:80.

88. Prat J, Scully RE: Cellular fibromas and fibrosarcomas of the ovary: A comparative clinicopathological analysis of seventeen cases. Cancer 1981; 47:2663.

89. Allen PR, King AR, Sage MD, et al.: A benign gonadal stromal tumor of the testis of spindle fibroblastic type. Pathology 1990; 22:227.

90. Greco MA, Feiner HD, Theil KS, et al.: Testicular stromal tumor with myofilaments: Ultrastructural comparison with normal gonadal stroma. Hum Pathol 1984; 15:228.

91. Jones MA, Young RH, Scully RE: Benign fibromatous tumors of the testis and paratesticular region: A report of 9 cases with a proposed classification of fibromatous tumors and tumor-like lesions. Am J Surg Pathol 1997; 7:47.

92. Miettinen M, Salo J, Virtanen I: Testicular stromal tumor: Ultrastructural, immunohistochemical and gel electrophoretic evidence of epithelial differentiation. Ultrastruct Pathol 1986; 10:515.

93. Nistal M, Puras A, Perna C, et al.: Fusocellular gonadal stromal tumour of the testis with epithelial and myoid differentiation. Histopathology 1996; 29:259.

94. Schenkman NS, Moul JW, Nicely ER, et al.: Synchronous bilateral testis tumor: Mixed germ cell and theca cell tumors. Urology 1993; 42:593.

95. Weidner N: Myoid gonadal stromal tumor with epithelial differentiation: Testicular myoepithelioma. Ultrastruct Pathol 1991; 15:409.

96. Eble JN, Hull MT, Warfel KA, et al.: Malignant sex cord–stromal tumor of testis. J Urol 1984; 131:546.

97. Scully RE: Gonadoblastoma: A gonadal tumor related to the dysgerminoma (seminoma) and capable of sex-hormone production. Cancer 1953; 6:455.

98. Talerman A: A distinctive gonadal neoplasm related to gonadoblastoma. Cancer 1972; 30:1219.

99. Shah KH, Maxted WC, Chun B: Epidermoid cysts of the testis. Cancer 1981; 47:577.

100. Forrest JB, Whitmore WFJ: Bilateral synchronous epidermoid cysts. World J Urol 1984; 2:76.

101. Kirkland RT, Kirkland JL, Keenan BS, et al.: Bilateral testicular tumors in congenital adrenal hyperplasia. J Clin Endocrinol Metab 1977; 44:367.

Placenta

Ana-Maria Bamberger and Christoph Bamberger

The human placenta is a multifunctional organ that apart from supplying nutrients and oxygen to the fetus and eliminating CO_2 from its circulation,[1] contains entire immune and endocrine networks of considerable complexity.[1-3] The latter resemble those in the hypothalamus and the pituitary, and most of the hormones originally described there have been found to be expressed in the placenta.[4] Furthermore, the placenta is an important site of steroid hormone production and, thus, fulfills the criteria of a peripheral endocrine organ. Depite our extensive knowledge of placental hormone expression and regulation, their function and physiologic significance remain largely obscure in most cases. This chapter gives an overview of placental endocrine physiology and pathophysiology and relates them to histologic and histopathologic findings, respectively.

MACROSCOPIC AND MICROSCOPIC STRUCTURE OF THE HUMAN PLACENTA

Macroscopically, the human placenta is a flat (average thickness: 2.5 cm) and disk-like (average diameter 22 cm) organ with an average weight of 470 g. However, shape and weight may vary considerably, depending on mode of birth and postnatal treatment of the tissue. The fetal surface has a glossy appearance because it is covered by amniotic epithelium. The cord is usually inserted in or near the center of the disk, with chorionic veins and arteries branching in a centrifugal pattern to cover the entire surface.

The maternal (uterine) surface of the placenta appears more opaque. It is composed of maternal (decidual) and fetal (trophoblast) tissue as well as of debris, fibrinoid, and blood clots. It is characterized by several grooves forming 10–40 placental lobes. The grooves correspond to septae, i.e., incomplete separations between the lobes that originate from the basal plate (see next paragraph). Each placental lobe may contain one or several villous trees, which, in situ, are bathed in maternal blood flowing from the spiral arteries into the intervillous space. As does the fetus, the placental villi depend entirely on maternal blood for nutrition and oxygenation. Because maternal blood and villous trophoblast cells come into direct contact, the human placenta belongs to the *villous hemochorial*–type placentas.

At the microscopic level, using low magnification, the following structural elements can be distinguished. The *villous tree* originates from the *chorionic plate* (fetal side). The most proximal villi are stem villi, which branch to give rise to intermediate villi, which in turn form terminal villi. The villous tree is surrounded by the *intervillous space*. The *basal plate* forms the maternal side of the placenta. It is penetrated by the spiral arteries, from which oxygenated maternal blood flows directly into the intervillous space. As mentioned, incomplete septae protrude from the basal plate into the intervillous space to form the placental lobes. In routine paraffin sections, these structures are hardly ever seen at once. Instead, one sees an array of villous and extravillous islands lacking any apparent order. It is, thus, very helpful to keep in mind this overall architecture when dealing with placental histology and histopathology.

Higher magnification of the placental villus reveals the following structural elements. The *villous core* contains fetal vessels and mesenchymal tissue. A thin *basement membrane* separates the core from the trophoblast. The villous trophoblast consists of two layers, the inner *cytotrophoblast* (Langhans' cells) and the outer *syncytiotrophoblast*. The cytotrophoblast is a discontinuous layer of mitotically active (Ki-67–positive) stem cells that differentiate into the postmitotic syncytiotrophoblast, a true syncytium covering the surface of all placental villi as well as of the chorionic and basal plate, thus forming a continuous line out of the intervillous space. Cytotrophoblast cells stain positive for proteins that promote the cell cycle, such as cyclin E, and negative for cell-cycle inhibitors, such as p27 (Fig. 14–1A). In contrast, the postmitotic

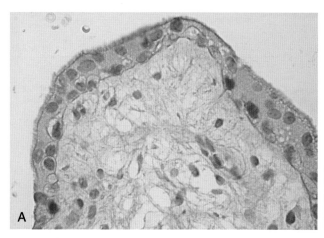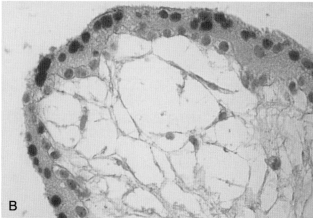

Figure 14–1. A, Expression of the cell-cycle promoter cyclin E in the mitotically active cytotrophoblast but not in the postmitotic syncytiotrophoblast (×400). *B,* Complementary staining pattern for the cell-cycle inhibitor p27 (×400).

syncytiotrophoblast is cyclin E–negative and p27-positive[5] (see Fig. 14–1B).

Specialized placental structures, *anchoring villi,* have evolved at those loci where direct contact is established between trophoblast (fetal) and decidual (maternal) cells. The cells infiltrating the decidua share morphologic and functional features of both cytotrophoblast and syncytiotrophoblast. Hence, they are termed *intermediate trophoblast* cells.[6–8] These cells are also found outside the implantation site, i.e. in the chorion laeve (chorionic-type intermediate trophoblast). Scientists have not been able to agree on a unified terminology for the different trophoblast cell types. Whereas the term intermediate trophoblast is generally used by pathologists and clinicians, the generally synonymous term *extravillous trophoblast* is largely preferred by cell biologists.[9] The extravillous trophoblast can be further divided into proximal extravillous trophoblast of the anchoring villi, deep interstitial extravillous trophoblast invading the endometrial stroma and the myometrium, and endovascular trophoblast, which invades the spiral arteries and assumes endothelial-like characteristics.[9]

Several immunohistochemical markers have been introduced to distinguish trophoblast cells from decidual structures and from one another. Because trophoblast cells are of epithelial origin, they stain positive for cytokeratin, which is negative for decidual cells. Therefore, cytokeratin staining is especially useful for distinguishing intermediate/extravillous trophoblast and decidual cells.[8, 9] A complementary staining pattern occurs with antivimentin antibodies, because vimentin is expressed by mesenchymal cells only. The antibodies Ki-67, MIB-1, and anti-PCNA are useful for distinguishing proliferating cells, e.g., cytotrophoblast, from mitotically inactive cells, e.g., syncytiotrophoblast. The cell adhesion molecule CEACAM-1 is specifically expressed by the intermediate/extravillous trophoblast[10] (Fig. 14–2). Similar results have been published for Mel-CAM[11] and pregnancy-associated major basic protein.[12]

Even though the function of these molecules in this context remains to be shown, they seem to be suitable markers for this particular cell type.

PLACENTAL HORMONES: EXPRESSION, REGULATION, AND FUNCTION

Most hormones that have been found in the hypothalamus and the pituitary are also expressed in the placenta.[4] In addition, numerous steroid hormones are produced by this endocrine organ. Whether so-called pregnancy-associated placental proteins, such as pregnancy-associated placental protein A, Schwangerschaftsprotein 1, and placental protein 12, can bind to and activate specific receptors in distant tissues, i.e., act as hormones, has not been determined.[3] As opposed to the hypothalamus and the pituitary and their dependent glands, no feedback mechanism controlling placental hor-

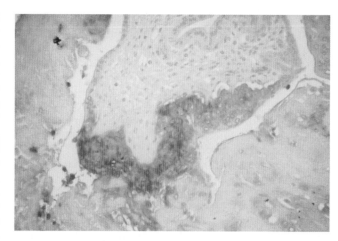

Figure 14–2. Expression of CEACAM-1 in intermediate/extravillous trophoblast cells (×160).

mone synthesis has been described. It appears that the rate of secretion of the respective hormones is directly proportional to placental mass. Human chorionic gonadotropin (hCG) represents one important exception to this rule (see the following section).

Hormones Produced by the Villous Cytotrophoblast and the Syncytiotrophoblast

The majority of peptide hormones released by the placenta are produced by the villous syncytiotrophoblast. They include hCG, human placental lactogen (hPL), prolactin, thyrotropin, adrenocorticotropin (ACTH), gonadotropin-releasing hormone (GRH), corticotropin-releasing hormone (CRH), and α-inhibin.[3, 13–20] Accordingly, electron microscopic analysis reveals abundant secretory granules in syncytiotrophoblast cells, whereas cytotrophoblast cells display only very few such granules. Again, hCG synthesis seems to be more complex, because it is also observed in the cytotrophoblast (see later). Placental steroid hormone synthesis is also very much restricted to the syncytiotrophoblast. Consistent with these findings, the presence of steroidogenic enzymes has been demonstrated in syncytiotrophoblast cells, using immunohistochemistry.[3, 21]

hCG is a 38,000-kDa glycoprotein composed of two subunits termed α-subunit and β-subunit. The α-subunit is encoded by a single gene, and the β-subunit is encoded by seven genes.[3, 22] The α-subunit is virtually identical to that of follicle-stimulating hormone, luteinizing hormone (LH), and thyroid-stimulating hormone (TSH). The β-subunit of hCG is highly homologous to that of LH.[23]

Whereas the expression of the β-subunit is confined to the syncytium, α-subunit mRNA and protein expression have been demonstrated both in the villous cytotrophoblast and syncytiotrophoblast.[16, 24] It appears that β-subunit expression is a sign of maturation of the cytotrophoblast toward the syncytial trophoblast.[25]

hCG levels can be detected in the maternal circulation from day 8 onward (pregnancy test) to reach a maximum between the 8th and the 10th week of gestation and then rapidly falls by about 90%. Thereafter, hCG levels remain low yet detectable until the end of pregnancy.[26] hCG production therefore rather reflects trophoblast maturation than pure trophoblast mass.[25, 27] In vitro, hCG expression has been shown to be stimulated by placental GRH[28–31] and inhibited by prolactin.[32, 33] Whether this plays a role in vivo remains to be shown. At the cellular and molecular levels both hCG α- and β-subunit expression is stimulated via the cyclic adenosine monophosphate pathway leading to activation of ets-2 and AP-2 transcription factors, for which specific binding sites have been demonstrated in the hCG promoter.[34, 35]

The main function of hCG is to maintain the corpus luteum of pregnancy and, thus, sufficient progesterone production until placental progesterone production takes over.[36, 37] Additional functions of hCG have been postulated but not proven in vivo, including stimulation of fetal testosterone synthesis and placental estrogen production.[3] Because of its weak thyrotropic activity, hCG-induced hyperthyroidism can be observed in some women in the first trimester of pregnancy.[38] hCG-mediated antitumoral and immunosuppressive effects have been demonstrated in vitro, which may be due to inhibition of intracellular NF-kB activity.[39, 40]

Human placental lactogen (hPL), also known as chorionic somatomammotropin, is a 22,000-kDa protein, which is 85% homologous to hypophyseal growth hormone (GH) and also shares a high degree of homology with prolactin. hPL is encoded by four different genes (*CS-A, CS-B, CS-L,* and *GH-V*) located close to each other and to the *GH* gene on the short arm of chromosome 17.[41–46] Finally, transcription and translation of the *CS* genes give rise to one single hPL protein. Interestingly, hPL expression is not restricted to the syncytiotrophoblast; it is also present in intermediate/extravillous trophoblast cells (see later).[8] However, cytotrophoblast cells are clearly hPL-negative.

hPL levels rise later in pregnancy than do hCG levels and continue to do so until 37 weeks of gestation. Little information is available about how hPL expression is regulated. Lipoproteins may participate in hPL regulation; it has been shown that pre-β–high density lipoprotein (HDL) particles can stimulate hPL release from cultured trophoblast cells.[47] Furthermore the concentration of pre-β-HDL constantly rises after the 10th week of gestation.[47] It appears that apolipoprotein-A1 is the HDL constituent stimulating hPL expression by means of MAP kinase activation.[48] Further downstream, transcription factors belonging to the AP-2 family play a crucial role in transcriptional activation of the different hPL genes.[49] It can be demonstrated that the transaction factor Pit-1, which was originally thought to be restricted to the anterior pituitary, is expressed in the human placenta as well.[50] Binding sites for Pit-1 are present in all hPL gene promoters.[51, 52] Furthermore, gene transfer experiments in pituitary cells revealed that the CS-A and GH-V promoters can be activated by Pit-1.[53]

What is the physiologic function of hPL? Successful pregnancies in women expressing low or even undetectable levels of hPL suggest that this hormone does not play an essential functional role.[54, 55] hPL has been shown to stimulate fatty acid mobilization from maternal depots,[56] thus allowing the mother to spare glucose needed by the fetus. Consistent with these findings, hPL is suppressed in diabetic women in the first and third trimesters.[57] hPL also clearly binds to prolactin receptors and stimulates milk production in mammals.[58] It may exert these functions as part of a redundant hormonal network, with other hormones taking over when hPL is absent.[59]

The primate placenta is a major source of CRH. Placental CRH is a 34,000-kDa protein that is encoded by the same gene as and is identical to hypothalamic CRH.[60] It has paracrine effects within the uteroplacental unit as well as endocrine effects on mother and fetus.[60] Placental CRH is expressed almost exclusively in the syncytiotrophoblast. As opposed to hypothalamic CRH, placental CRH is upregulated by glucocorticoids establishing a positive feedback loop, leading to CRH concentrations up to 100 times higher than in nonpregnant women.[61]

Placental CRH is thought to regulate placental blood flow; to stimulate placental, pituitary, and fetal pituitary ACTH expression and, thus, fetal adrenal dehydroeplandrosterone (DHEA) release (see later); and to stimulate uterine contractility.[62, 63] The latter effect may participate in the onset of labor; free CRH reaches a maximum at term because of the decrease in placental CRH binding protein.[61, 62, 64–66] Higher CRH levels and lower CRH binding protein levels are found in women with preterm labor.[63, 67]

Steroid hormones are considered the real pregnancy hormones that play essential roles for the maintenance of pregnancy and the proper development of the fetus.[68] They are synthesized in multistep pattern by enzymatic modification of precursor molecules. Steroidogenic enzymes and the transcription factors required for their expression, e.g., steroidogenic factor–1, are expressed by the syncytiotrophoblast cells and, to a lesser extent, by the cytotrophoblast.[69] In the second and third trimesters, when ovarian steroid production subsides, the placenta is the predominant source of female reproductive hormones.

Progesterone is synthesized from cholesterol, which is made available by maternal low-density lipoprotein.[70, 71] Progesterone levels rise continuously until the end of pregnancy, thus increasing with growing trophoblast mass and maturation. Because precursors are abundant in maternal blood, they are not rate-limiting. The same is probably true for regulatory mechanisms shown in vitro, e.g., ACTH or GRH stimulating placental steroidogenesis.[72] Many different functions have been proposed for progesterone, including a suppressive role on the immune system to prevent rejection of the fetal allograft and preventing premature labor.[62, 73–75] However, successful pregnancies at much lower levels of progesterone have been observed, e.g., in familial hypobetalipoproteinemia.[68, 76]

The placenta does not posses the enzymatic equipment to synthesize estrogens from cholesterol. It thus depends on precursor molecules made by the fetal adrenal, most importantly DHEA.[3] As with progesterone, estrogen concentrations rise continuously throughout pregnancy. Estrogen production rates mirror trophoblast mass and maturation but also depend on sufficient fetal adrenal DHEA production.[77] Vice versa, estriol levels in maternal blood (grossly) reflect fetal growth and well-being. Estrogens enhance uteroplacental blood flow to provide optimal oxygen and nutrient supply. In turn, estrogens have stimulatory effects on the receptor-mediated uptake of low-density lipoprotein by syncytiotrophoblast cells, thus promoting the biosynthesis of progesterone.[68] Partial or complete lack of placental estriol synthesis is nevertheless compatible with a normal outcome of pregnancy,[78] again indicating the high level of redundancy established to maintain pregnancy and fetal growth.

Hormones Produced by the Intermediate/Extravillous Trophoblast

Not all hormones produced by the uteroplacental unit are expressed by villous trophoblast cells. In fact, hPL expression is more abundant in the intermediate/extravillous trophoblast and is used as a marker to differentiate these cells from decidual structures.[7, 8] The decidua itself is another important source of various hormones, the most important examples being prolactin and relaxin.[79, 80]

ENDOCRINE PATHOLOGY OF THE HUMAN PLACENTA

Endocrine Pathology of Gestational Trophoblastic Disease

The terms gestational trophoblastic disease and gestational trophoblastic neoplasia refer to a heterogeneous group of diseases that originate from the trophoblast but are by no means all true neoplasms. Originally, this group included only hydatidiform moles (complete and incomplete) and choriocarcinoma. Exaggerated placental site, placental site trophoblastic tumor, placental site nodule, and epithelioid trophoblastic tumor have been added to this category.[8]

Hydatidiform Moles and Choriocarcinoma

Hydatidiform moles are immature placentas that appear excessively edematous because of massive fluid accumulation within the villous parenchyma.[81] They occur in about 1:1000 pregnancies, with certain ethnic groups, e.g., the Japanese, having a much higher incidence.

In *complete hydatidiform moles,* all villi have that edematous appearance. Except for very few cases, no embryo is present in this condition. The villi are fluid-filled cavities lacking blood vessels and being connected to each other by thin strands of connective tissue. Various degrees of anaplasia and cellular pleomorphism are observed, which do not strictly correlate with the clinical behavior of the lesion. Genetically, complete hydatidiform moles have only paternal chromosomes (androgenetic moles) and are, thus, thought to originate from fertilized "empty eggs."[82] The molar tissue may invade the uterus and even metastasize to distant organs, such as the lung. In this case, the lesion is termed *invasive mole*. The most important differential diagnosis is choriocarcinoma, which can be distinguished from invasive moles by the absence of villi.

In partial moles, only a portion of villi is hydropic, whereas the others appear normal. An embryo or remnants thereof may be present. Partial moles do not fulfill the criteria of true neoplasms. As opposed to complete moles, they are characterized by a triploid karyotype.[83, 84]

Complete moles and (less so) partial moles can produce excessive amounts of hCG, which tends to rise after the 10th week of gestation when hCG levels begin to fall in normal pregnancies. As a consequence, ovarian cysts are frequently found. They usually regress after delivery. Attempts to differentiate moles from choriocarcinoma by hCG levels have not been successful. However, after removal of the lesion, determination of hCG levels is used to detect recurrent disease. hPL levels are low or undetectable in molar disease, as are estriol levels. This is not due to an incapacity of the molar tissue to synthesize estrogens but by the lack of fetal tissue providing the required precursor molecules.

Choriocarcinoma is a malignant tumor composed of cytotrophoblast and syncytiotrophoblast.[85] Its incidence is about 1:40,000. It may be preceded by complete moles or normal pregancy. Histopathologic analysis shows solid sheets of trophoblast cells invading vessels and, thus, causing considerable hemorrhage. A few intermediate/extravillous trophoblast cells may also be present. The most frequent target organs for metastasis are lung and brain. hCG production is excessive and resembles that in complete moles. In rare cases, androgen production by a choriocarcinoma has been described. The majority of choriocarcinoma cells are mitotically active as indicated by strong staining for Ki-67 (Fig. 14–3).

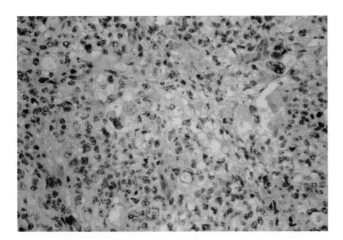

Figure 14–3. Example of a choriocarcinoma staining strongly positive for the mitotic marker Ki-67 (×200).

Lesions Originating from the Intermediate/Extravillous Trophoblast

Exaggerated placental site, placental site trophoblastic tumor, placental site nodule, and epithelioid trophoblast tumor are lesions considered to have arisen from the intermediate/extravillous trophoblast.[8] Kurman[8] has further categorized these lesions into those originating from the implantation site intermediate/extravillous trophoblast (exaggerated placental site, placental site trophoblastic tumor) and those arising from chorionic-type intermediate/extravillous trophoblast (placental site nodule, epithelioid trophoblastic tumor).[8]

The *exaggerated placental site* represents the extreme end of normal myometrial infiltration by the intermediate/extravillous trophoblast. Thus, no cutoff as to the degree of infiltration has been defined to separate this entity from the normal implantation process. The cells infiltrating the endometrium and myometrium do not differ from normal intermediate/extravillous trophoblastic cells, neither as to form nor to immunostaining patterns (positive for Mel-CAM and hPL). They are not proliferating and, thus, are Ki67–negative.

Placental site trophoblastic tumor is a rare neoplasm that occurs following normal pregnancy or nonmolar abortion. The tumor is usually confined to the uterine wall and/or cavity, but extension into neighboring structures has been described. Histologically, it is composed of monomorphic cells bearing the features of intermediate/extravillous trophoblast cells. Hence, immunostaining is positive for cytokeratin, hPL, Mel-CAM, and CEACAM-1[86] (Fig. 14–4A and B) but weakly positive or negative for hCG (reflected by slightly elevated serum hCG levels). Necrosis of the invaded structures may be present and is considered a sign of a more aggressive behavior. Chorionic villi are usually absent. Ki-67 staining is elevated and can serve to differentiate this tumor from exaggerated placental site lesions (see Fig. 14–4C).

Placental site nodule is a benign lesion that is most often found incidentally in curettage material or hysterectomy specimens. It is not clear whether it is derived from tissue remaining from previous pregnancies or whether it represents a new gestation. It is composed of trophoblastic cells resembling those of the chorionic-type intermediate/extravillous trophoblast, embedded in abundant hyalinized or fibrinoid matrix, and surrounded by a slim border of lymphocytes and decidual cells. Trophoblast cells stain positive for hPL, albeit less extensively than in the preceding lesions, as well as for cytokeratin and CEACAM-1[86] and Mel-CAM.[8] The Ki-67 index is equal to or less than 5%, indicating weak proliferative activity.

The *epithelioid trophoblast tumor* has been recognized as a separate entity by Kurman and coworkers.[8] Tumor cells are of the mononucleate trophoblast type. Typically, they are arranged in nests and cords surrounded by hyalin-like material and necrotic debris. As do the chorionic-type intermedi-

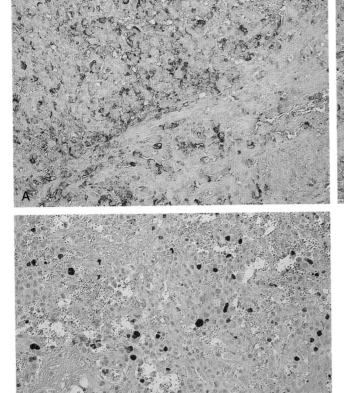

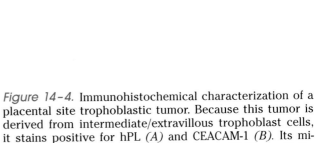

Figure 14-4. Immunohistochemical characterization of a placental site trophoblastic tumor. Because this tumor is derived from intermediate/extravillous trophoblast cells, it stains positive for hPL *(A)* and CEACAM-1 *(B)*. Its mitotic activity is indicated by moderate Ki-67 positivity *(C)* (×100).

ate/extravillous trophoblast cells they are thought to originate from, epithelioid trophoblast tumor cells stain (focally) positive for hPL and hCG.

Endocrine Placental Pathology in Complicated Pregnancy

Ectopic Pregnancy

The placenta in ectopic (tubal) pregnancy is abnormal in most cases, because it is at least a placenta accreta, if not percreta.[9] In ruptured tubal pregnancies, a placenta percreta is the most common finding. Moreover, numerous infarcts are usually found on closer examination. hCG levels are generally low in women with tubal pregnancies.[87] In addition, there is a tendency toward lower estradiol and progesterone levels. However, there is a significant overlap with normal pregnancies in both hCG and steroid concentrations. Hormone levels are, thus, not suitable screening parameters in suspected ectopic pregnancies.

Spontaneous Abortion

In the placenta of spontaneous abortion, hydropic villi are the most frequent finding. This may sometimes render it difficult to differentiate them from moles and partial moles. Very low hCG levels are indicative of threatened abortion if the fetus is no longer alive.[3] For this reason, examination of fetal heart movements by ultrasonography is a much more reliable method for predicting abortion. hCG levels in pregnancies that eventually undergo spontaneous abortion of a *living* fetus do not differ significantly from those in normal pregnancies.[88]

Twin Pregnancy

There are two types of placentation in twin pregnancies: monochorionic and dichorionic.[89-93] As a general rule, monochorionic placentas belong to monozygotic twins. There are hardly any exceptions to this rule. Dichorionic placentas belong to dizygotic twins in the majority of cases (90%). Monochorionic placentas can be further categorized as either monoamniotic (the twins are in one amniotic sac, quite rare) or diamniotic. The experienced placental pathologist makes the correct diagnosis of the chorionic status macroscopically. Histologically, analysis of a cross-section of the dividing membranes or of a so-called T section, i.e., the site where the membranes insert, will allow the diagnosis. In multiple pregnancies, hCG levels tend to be higher than in single pregnancies, even though a cut-off value that would separate both entities with sufficient sensitivity and specificity does not exist.

hPL levels are much higher in twin/multiple pregnancies as well, whereas estriol levels are only marginally elevated.

Intrauterine Fetal Growth Retardation

The macroscopic and microscopic appearance of the placenta in pregnancies complicated by fetal growth retardation is as diverse as the causes leading to this condition.[94-101] The variety of pathologic findings include, for instance, small placentas, a high degree of placental infarctions, fetoplacental vasculopathy, villous hypermaturity, and deficiency of the terminal villus. If maternal (preplacental) or uteroplacental hypoxia is the underlying cause of growth retardation, there are signs of increased trophoblastic proliferation and villous capillary branching, a compensatory reaction to the hypoxic state. Histologically, syncytial knotting, also known as Tenney-Parker change, is a typical finding in this condition. If umbilical blood flow is diminished (postplacental hypoxia), a characteristic deficiency of terminal villi is observed. In all these conditions, hPL and estriol levels tend to be in the low-normal range or slightly below. The considerable overlap between uncomplicated pregnancies and those complicated by fetal growth retardation makes hPL and estriol levels poor prognostic parameters.

Pregnancy-Induced Hypertension

The term pregnancy-induced hypertension (PIH) refers to a condition of unknown cause that is characterized by maternal arterial hypertension occurring in the second or third trimester of pregnancy.[102] When it is accompanied by edema and proteinuria, the term preeclampsia is used.[103] PIH depends on the presence of trophoblast but not of fetal tissue. Hence, it also occurs in molar pregnancies. After delivery, blood pressure values usually return to normal quickly. The return is significantly accelerated by postpartum curettage. As mentioned, the cause and pathogenesis of PIH and preeclampsia are poorly understood. It has been shown that the endovascular trophoblast, i.e., the part of the intermediate/extravillous trophoblast invading the maternal vessels, is not properly established in PIH/preeclampsia.[104] There is no pathognomonic histopathologic sign of preeclampsia. Typical findings include decidual arteriolopathy ("arthetosis"), infarction in the central portion of the placenta, placental abruption, and syncytial knotting (Tenney-Parker change) as a sign of uteroplacental hypoxia. Earlier observations of low hPL and estriol levels in PIH have been confirmed only in those cases in which fetal growth retardation was present.

Premature Onset of Labor

Despite intense efforts to determine hormone levels that would predict premature onset of labor, no such parameter has been found. This is especially true for hPL, which has the same range in women proceeding to term and going into premature labor.[3] Recent observations point to corticotropin-releasing hormone (CRH) as a central player governing the "placental clock." Accordingly, higher CRH levels and lower CRH-binding protein levels (i.e., even higher free CRH levels) have been reported in patients with premature onset of labor.[60, 62, 66, 74] However, as long as standard methods for measuring CRH in human plasma are not readily available, routine predictions of imminent premature labor based on this parameter cannot be made.

Placental Pathology in Maternal Endocrine Disease

Diabetes Mellitus

Diabetes mellitus is the most frequent endocrine disorder in nonpregnant and in pregnant women.[105-107] Preexisting diabetes mellitus type I and type II can exert their adverse effects throughout the whole course of pregnancy. In contrast, gestational diabetes mellitus usually occurs by the end of the second trimester. Most known complications of pregnancy are more frequent in diabetic than in nondiabetic women. These include abortion, prematurity, congenital anomalies, preeclampsia/eclampsia, and macrosomia. The latter is caused by elevated maternal glucose crossing the placenta and stimulating fetal pancreatic insulin secretion (maternal insulin does not cross the placental barrier).

The pregnancy outcome in diabetic women largely depends on blood glucose control. Placental changes observed in diabetic patients are by no means specific and correlate with metabolic control as well.[108] Earlier reports of excessive placental calcifications in diabetic women, for instance, probably reflect very poor glucose control, which is rarely observed today. In poorly controlled diabetic women, the placenta appears enlarged and somewhat plethoric and edematous. Microscopically, there is an increased number of villous trophoblast cells, probably caused by an increased proliferative index.[109-113] Another finding is the higher frequency of fetal and placental thrombosis.

Placental hormone expression may also be altered in diabetic women, although reports on this issue are sometimes contradictory. hCG levels tend to be lower,[114, 115] even though placental hCG immunostaining appears to be more intense.[116] The reason for this discrepancy is not known. Both elevated and reduced levels of hPL have been reported in pregnant women with diabetes mellitus.[117, 118] It appears that first-trimester hPL levels are low in insulin-dependent diabetic women, leading to an increased risk of abortion and fetal growth retardation.[57] Later in pregnancy, increased hPL levels may participate in causing fetal macrosomia. Schonfelder et al.[119] reported that nitric oxide synthase is preferentially expressed in diabetic as compared to nondiabetic placentas.[119] The authors speculated that nitric oxide could cause vasodilation of placental vessels, leading to increased placental blood flow and, thus, nutrient supply.

Thyroid Disease

Thyroid hormone physiology undergoes major changes in pregnancy.[120, 121] The marked increase in serum thyroxine–binding globulin levels has to be met by an increase in thyroid hormone synthesis in order to maintain normal free thyroxin levels. This and the iodine demand of the fetal thyroid gland make sufficient iodine intake by the mother (200 μg/day) essential to adequate nutrition during pregnancy. In recent years, it has become clear that even subclinical hypothyroidism in pregnant women is associated with impaired neuropsychologic development of the child and has to be treated.[122]

Overt hypothyroidism is rare in pregnant women, because it is a frequent cause of infertility. Nevertheless, several cases have been published, in many of which pregnancy was complicated by either placental abruption, preeclampsia, postpartum hemorrhage, fetal growth retardation, or even fetal death.[123]

Hyperthyroidism is more frequently encountered in pregnant women. Transient hyperthyroidism often occurs by the end of the first trimester and is caused by the thyrotropic activity of hCG (see earlier). It rarely needs treatment. However, persistent hyperthyroidism, e.g., in Graves' disease, is associated with a higher risk of abortion, preterm labor, preeclampsia, fetal growth retardation, and fetal death. Therefore, is treated with thyrostatic drugs, which cross the placenta[124] and may induce goitrogenesis in the fetus. In maternal Graves' disease, TSH receptor auto-antibodies may be transferred to the fetus as well and cause fetal hyperthyroidism. Thyroid dysfunction does not cause specific morphologic changes in the placenta. However, as it is associated with preeclampsia, placental infarction and abruption are more frequently observed.

References

1. Battaglia FC, Regnault TR: Placental transport and metabolism of amino acids. Placenta 2001; 22:145.
2. Saito S: Cytokine network at the feto-maternal interface. J Reprod Immunol 2000; 47:87.
3. Fox H: The placenta. In Kovacs K, Asa S, eds.: Functional Endocrine Pathology. Blackwell Science Inc., Nalden, MA, 1998, p. 733.
4. Waddell BJ: The placenta as hypothalamus and pituitary: Possible impact on maternal and fetal adrenal function. Reprod Fertil Dev 1993; 5:479.
5. Bamberger A, Sudahl S, Bamberger CM, et al.: Expression patterns of the cell-cycle inhibitor p27 and the cell-cycle promoter cyclin E in the human placenta throughout gestation: Implications for the control of proliferation. Placenta 1999; 20:401.
6. Kurman RJ, Main CS, Chen HC: Intermediate trophoblast: A distinctive form of trophoblast with specific morphological, biochemical and functional features. Placenta 1984; 5:349.
7. Kurman RJ, Young RH, Norris HJ, et al.: Immunocytochemical localization of placental lactogen and chorionic gonadotropin in the normal placenta and trophoblastic tumors, with emphasis on intermediate trophoblast and the placental site trophoblastic tumor. Int J Gynecol Pathol 1984; 3:101.
8. Shih IM, Kurman RJ: The pathology of intermediate trophoblastic tumors and tumor-like lesions. Int J Gynecol Pathol 2001; 20:31.
9. Frank HG, Kaufmann P: Nonvillous parts and trophoblast invasion. In Benirschke K, Kaufmann P, eds.: Pathology of the Human Placenta. Springer, New York, Berlin, Heidelberg, 2000, p. 171.
10. Bamberger AM, Sudahl S, Löning T, et al.: The adhesion molecule CEACAM1 (CD66a, C-CAM, BGP) is specifically expressed by the extravillous intermediate trophoblast. Am J Pathol 2000; 156:1165.
11. Shih IM, Kurman RJ: Expression of melanoma cell adhesion molecule in intermediate trophoblast. Lab Invest 1996; 75:377.
12. Rhoton-Vlasak A, Wagner JM, Rutgers JL, et al.: Placental site trophoblastic tumor: Human placental lactogen and pregnancy-associated major basic protein as immunohistologic markers. Hum Pathol 1998; 29:280.
13. Watkins WB: Use of immunocytochemical techniques for the localization of human placental lactogen. J Histochem Cytochem 1978; 26:288.
14. de Ikonicoff LK, Cedard L: Localization of human chorionic gonadotropic and somatomammotropic hormones by the peroxidase immunohistoenzymologic method in villi and amniotic epithelium of human placentas (from six weeks to term). Am J Obstet Gynecol 1973; 116:1124.
15. Al-Timimi A, Fox H: Immunohistochemical localization of follicle-stimulating hormone, luteinizing hormone, growth hormone, adrenocorticotrophic hormone and prolactin in the human placenta. Placenta 1986; 7:163.
16. Gaspard UJ, Hustin J, Reuter AM, et al.: Immunofluorescent localization of placental lactogen, chorionic gonadotrophin and its alpha and beta subunits in organ cultures of human placenta. Placenta 1980; 1:135.
17. Perkins AV, Linton EA: Identification and isolation of corticotrophin-releasing hormone-positive cells from the human placenta. Placenta 1995; 16:233.
18. Petraglia F, Garuti GC, Calza L, et al.: Inhibin subunits in human placenta: Localization and messenger ribonucleic acid levels during pregnancy. Am J Obstet Gynecol 1991; 165:750.
19. Cheng KW, Chow BK, Leung PC: Functional mapping of a placenta-specific upstream promoter for human gonadotropin-releasing hormone receptor gene. Endocrinology 2001; 142:1506.
20. Cheng KW, Nathwani PS, Leung PC: Regulation of human gonadotropin-releasing hormone receptor gene expression in placental cells. Endocrinology 2000; 141:2340.
21. Dobashi K, Ajika K, Kambegawa A, et al.: Localization and distribution of unconjugated steroid hormones in normal placenta at term. Placenta 1985; 6:445.
22. Boorstein WR, Vamvakopoulos NC, Fiddes JC: Human chorionic gonadotropin beta-subunit is encoded by at least eight genes arranged in tandem and inverted pairs. Nature 1982; 300:419.
23. Fiddes JC, Talmadge K: Structure, expression, and evolution of the genes for the human glycoprotein hormones. Recent Prog Horm Res 1984; 40:43.
24. Muyan M, Boime I: Secretion of chorionic gonadotropin from human trophoblasts. Placenta 1997; 18:237.
25. Castellucci M, Kaufmann P: Basic structure of the villous trees. In Benirschke K, Kaufmann P, eds.: Pathology of the Human Placenta. Springer, New York, Berlin, Heidelberg, 2000, p. 50.
26. Braunstein GD, Grodin JM, Vaitukaitis J, et al.: Secretory rates of human chorionic gonadotropin by normal trophoblast. Am J Obstet Gynecol 1973; 115:447.
27. Hoshina M, Boothby M, Hussa R, et al.: Linkage of human chorionic gonadotrophin and placental lactogen biosynthesis to trophoblast differentiation and tumorigenesis. Placenta 1985; 6:163.

28. Siler-Khodr TM, Khodr GS: Content of luteinizing hormone-releasing factor in the human placenta. Am J Obstet Gynecol 1978; 130:216.
29. Siler-Khodr TM, Khodr GS, Rhode J, et al.: Gestational age-related inhibition of placental hCG, alpha hCG and steroid hormone release in vitro by a GnRH antagonist. Placenta 1987; 8:1.
30. Siler-Khodr TM, Grayson M: Action of chicken II GnRH on the human placenta. J Clin Endocrinol Metab 2001; 86:804.
31. Islami D, Chardonnens D, Campana A, et al.: Comparison of the effects of GnRH-I and GnRH-II on HCG synthesis and secretion by first trimester trophoblast. Mol Hum Reprod 2001; 7:3.
32. Yuen BH, Moon YS, Shin DH: Inhibition of human chorionic gonadotropin production by prolactin from term human trophoblast. Am J Obstet Gynecol 1986; 154:336.
33. Wurfel W, Beckmann MW, Austin R, et al.: Effects of prolactin on secretion and synthesis of human chorionic gonadotropin in human term placentas in vitro: Short-term increase in secretion, followed by medium-term suppression of synthesis and secretion. Gynecol Obstet Invest 1992; 33:129.
34. Johnson W, Jameson JL: Role of Ets2 in cyclic AMP regulation of the human chorionic gonadotropin beta promoter. Mol Cell Endocrinol 2000; 165:17–24.
35. LiCalsi C, Christophe S, Steger DJ, et al.: AP-2 family members regulate basal and cAMP-induced expression of human chorionic gonadotropin. Nucleic Acids Res 2000; 28:1036.
36. Rodway MR, Rao CV: A novel perspective on the role of human chorionic gonadotropin during pregnancy and in gestational trophoblast disease. Early Pregnancy 1995; 1:176.
37. Rao CV: Potential novel roles of luteinizing hormone and human chorionic gonadotropin during early pregnancy in women. Early Pregnancy 1997; 3:1.
38. Yoshimura M, Hershman JM: Thyrotropic action of human chorionic gonadotropin. Thyroid 1995; 5:425.
39. Manna SK, Mukhopadhyay A, Aggarwal BB: Human chorionic gonadotropin suppresses activation of nuclear transcription factor-kappa B and activator protein-1 induced by tumor necrosis factor. J Biol Chem 2000; 275:13307.
40. Song XY, Zeng L, Jin W, et al.: Suppression of streptococcal cell wall–induced arthritis by human chorionic gonadotropin. Arthritis Rheum 2000; 43:2064.
41. Chen EY, Liao Y, Smith DH, et al.: The growth hormone locus: Nucleotide sequence, biology, and evolution. Genomics 1989; 4:479.
42. Cooke NE, Ray J, Emery JG, et al.: Two distinct species of human growth hormone variant mRNA in the human placenta predict the expression of novel growth hormone proteins. J Biol Chem 1988; 263:9001.
43. Liebhaber SA, Urbanek M, Ray J, et al.: Characterization and histologic localization of human growth hormone-variant gene expression in the placenta. J Clin Invest 1989; 83:1985.
44. Frankenne F, Closset J, Scippo ML, et al.: The physiology of growth hormones (GHs) in pregnant women and partial characterization of the placental GH variant. J Clin Endocrinol Metab 1988; 66:1171.
45. Miller WL, Eberhardt NL: Structure and evolution of the growth hormone gene family. Endocr Rev 1983; 4:97.
46. Alsat E, Guibourdenche J, Couturier A, et al.: Physiological role of human placental growth hormone. Mol Cell Endocrinol 1998; 140:121.
47. Handwerger S, Datta G, Richardson B, et al.: Pre-beta-HDL stimulates placental lactogen release from human trophoblast cells. Am J Physiol 1999; 276:E384.
48. Kanda Y, Richards RG, Handwerger S: Apolipoprotein A-I stimulates human placental lactogen release by activation of MAP kinase. Mol Cell Endocrinol 1998; 143:125.
49. Richardson BD, Langland RA, Bachurski CJ, et al.: Activator protein-2 regulates human placental lactogen gene expression. Mol Cell Endocrinol 2000; 160:183.
50. Bamberger AM, Bamberger CM, Pu LP, et al.: Expression of pit-1 messenger ribonucleic acid and protein in the human placenta. J Clin Endocrinol Metab 1995; 80:2021.
51. Nachtigal MW, Nickel BE, Cattini PA: Pituitary-specific repression of placental members of the human growth hormone gene family. J Biol Chem 1993; 268:8473.
52. Nickel BE, Nachtigal MW, Bock ME, et al.: Differential binding of rat pituitary-specific nuclear factors to the 5′-flanking region of pituitary and placental members of the human growth hormone family. Mol Cell Biochem 1991; 106:181.
53. Cattini PA, Eberhardt NL: Regulated expression of chimaeric genes containing the 5′-flanking regions of human growth hormone related genes in transiently transfected rat pituitary tumor cells. Nucl Acids Res 1987; 15:1297.
54. Hubert C, Descombey D, Mondon F, et al.: Plasma human chorionic somatomammotropin deficiency in a normal pregnancy is the consequence of low concentration of messenger RNA coding for human chorionic somatomammotropin. Am J Obstet Gynecol 1983; 147:676.
55. Rygaard K, Revol A, Esquivel-Escobedo D, et al.: Absence of human placental lactogen and placental growth hormone (HGH-V) during pregnancy: PCR analysis of the deletion. Hum Genet 1998; 102:87.
56. Gaspard UJ, Luyckx AS, George AN, et al.: Relationship between plasma-free fatty acid levels and human placental lactogen secretion in late pregnancy. J Clin Endocrinol Metab 1977; 45:246.
57. Pedersen JF, Sorensen S, Molsted-Pedersen L: Serum levels of human placental lactogen, pregnancy-associated plasma protein A and endometrial secretory protein PP14 in first trimester of diabetic pregnancy. Acta Obstet Gynecol Scand 1998; 77:155.
58. Akers RM: Lactogenic hormones: Binding sites, mammary growth, secretory cell differentiation, and milk biosynthesis in ruminants. J Dairy Sci 1985; 68:501.
59. Handwerger S, Freemark M: The roles of placental growth hormone and placental lactogen in the regulation of human fetal growth and development. J Pediatr Endocrinol Metab 2000; 13:343.
60. Fadalti M, Pezzani I, Cobellis L, et al.: Placental corticotropin-releasing factor: An update. Ann N Y Acad Sci 2000; 900:89.
61. Majzoub JA, Karalis KP: Placental corticotropin-releasing hormone: Function and regulation. Am J Obstet Gynecol 1999; 180:S242.
62. Challis JRG, Matthews SG, Gibb W, et al.: Endocrine and paracrine regulation of birth at term and preterm. Endocr Rev 2000; 21:514.
63. Majzoub JA, McGregor JA, Lockwood CJ, et al.: A central theory of preterm and term labor: Putative role for corticotropin-releasing hormone. Am J Obstet Gynecol 1999; 180:S232.
64. Behan DP, De Souza EB, Lowry PJ, et al.: Corticotropin-releasing factor (CRF) binding protein: A novel regulator of CRF and related peptides. Front Neuroendocrinol 1995; 16:362.
65. Challis JR, Matthews SG, Van Meir C, et al.: Current topic: The placental corticotropin-releasing hormone–adrenocorticotrophin axis. Placenta 1995; 16:481.
66. McLean M, Smith R: Corticotropin-releasing hormone and human parturition. Reproduction 2001; 121:493.
67. Lockwood CJ: Stress-associated preterm delivery: The role of corticotropin-releasing hormone. Am J Obstet Gynecol 1999; 180:264.
68. Pepe GJ, Albrecht ED: Actions of placental and fetal adrenal steroid hormones in primate pregnancy. Endocr Rev 1995; 16:608.
69. Bamberger AM, Ezzat S, Cao B, et al.: Expression of steroidogenic factor-1 (SF-1) mRNA and protein in the human placenta. Mol Hum Reprod 1996; 2:457.
70. Grimes RW, Pepe GJ, Albrecht ED: Regulation of human placental trophoblast low-density lipoprotein uptake in vitro by estrogen. J Clin Endocrinol Metab 1996; 81:2675.
71. Albrecht ED, Pepe GJ: Placental steroid hormone biosynthesis in primate pregnancy. Endocr Rev 1990; 11:124.
72. Petraglia F, de Micheroux AA, Florio P, et al.: Steroid-protein interaction in human placenta. J Steroid Biochem Mol Biol 1995; 53:227.
73. Szekeres-Bartho J, Faust Z, Varga P: The expression of a progesterone-induced immunomodulatory protein in pregnancy lymphocytes. Am J Reprod Immunol 1995; 34:342.

74. Keelan JA, Coleman M, Mitchell MD: The molecular mechanisms of term and preterm labor: Recent progress and clinical implications. Clin Obstet Gynecol 1997; 40:460.

75. How H, Huang ZH, Zuo J, et al.: Myometrial estradiol and progesterone receptor changes in preterm and term pregnancies. Obstet Gynecol 1995; 86:936.

76. Parker CR Jr, Illingworth DR, Bissonnette J, et al.: Endocrine changes during pregnancy in a patient with homozygous familial hypobetalipoproteinemia. N Engl J Med 1986; 314:557.

77. Tulchinsky D, Osathanondh R, Belisle S, et al.: Plasma estrone, estradiol, estriol and their precursors in pregnancies with anencephalic fetuses. J Clin Endocrinol Metab 1977; 45:1100.

78. Bradley LA, Canick JA, Palomaki GE, et al.: Undetectable maternal serum unconjugated estriol levels in the second trimester: Risk of perinatal complications associated with placental sulfatase deficiency. Am J Obstet Gynecol 1997; 176:531.

79. Goldsmith LT, Weiss G, Steinetz BG: Relaxin and its role in pregnancy. Endocrinol Metab Clin North Am 1995; 24:171.

80. Telgmann R, Gellersen B: Marker genes of decidualization: Activation of the decidual prolactin gene. Hum Reprod Update 1998; 4:472.

81. Benirschke K, Kaufmann P. Molar pregnancies. In Benirschke K, Kaufmann P, eds.: Pathology of the Human Placenta. Springer, New York, Berlin, Heidelberg, 2000, p. 718.

82. Lawler SD: Genetic studies on hydatidiform moles. Adv Exp Med Biol 1984; 176:147.

83. Szulman AE, Philippe E, Boue JG, et al.: Human triploidy: Association with partial hydatidiform moles and nonmolar conceptuses. Hum Pathol 1981; 12:1016.

84. Seckl MJ, Fisher RA, Salerno G, et al.: Choriocarcinoma and partial hydatidiform moles. Lancet 2000; 356:36.

85. Benirschke K, Kaufmann P: Trophoblastic neoplasms. In Benirschke K, Kaufmann P, eds.: Pathology of the Human Placenta. Springer, New York, Berlin, Heidelberg, 2000, p. 754.

86. Bamberger AM, Sudahl S, Wagener C, et al.: Expression pattern of the adhesion molecule CEACAM1 (C-CAM, CD66a, BGP) in gestational trophoblastic lesions. Int J Gynecol Pathol 2001; 20:160.

87. Lehner R, Kucera E, Jirecek S, et al.: Ectopic pregnancy. Arch Gynecol Obstet 2000; 263:87.

88. Westergaard JG, Teisner B, Sinosich MJ, et al.: Does ultrasound examination render biochemical tests obsolete in the prediction of early pregnancy failure? Br J Obstet Gynaecol 1985; 92:77.

89. Benirschke K, Kim CK: Multiple pregnancy: 1. N Engl J Med 1973; 288:1276.

90. Benirschke K, Kim CK: Multiple pregnancy: 2. N Engl J Med 1973; 288:1329.

91. Bardawil WA, Reddy RL, Bardawil LW: Placental considerations in multiple pregnancy. Clin Perinatol 1988; 15:13.

92. Lantz ME, Johnson TR: Multiple pregnancy. Curr Opin Obstet Gynecol 1993; 5:657.

93. ESHRE: Multiple gestation pregnancy. The ESHRE Capri Workshop Group. Hum Reprod 2000; 15:1856.

94. Gluckman PD, Harding JE: The physiology and pathophysiology of intrauterine growth retardation. Horm Res 1997; 48:11.

95. Garnica AD, Chan WY: The role of the placenta in fetal nutrition and growth. J Am Coll Nutr 1996; 15:206.

96. Altshuler G: Role of the placenta in perinatal pathology (revisited). Pediatr Pathol Lab Med 1996; 16:207.

97. Kingdom J, Huppertz B, Seaward G, et al.: Development of the placental villous tree and its consequences for fetal growth. Eur J Obstet Gynecol Reprod Biol 2000; 92:35.

98. Robinson JS, Moore VM, Owens JA, et al.: Origins of fetal growth restriction. Eur J Obstet Gynecol Reprod Biol 2000; 92:13.

99. Gaziano EP, De Lia JE, Kuhlmann RS: Diamnionic monochorionic twin gestations: An overview. J Matern Fetal Med 2000; 9:89.

100. Bell AW, Hay WW Jr, Ehrhardt RA: Placental transport of nutrients and its implications for fetal growth. J Reprod Fertil Suppl 1999; 54:401.

101. Salafia CM: Placental pathology of fetal growth restriction. Clin Obstet Gynecol 1997; 40:740.

102. Sosa ME: Pregnancy-induced hypertension, preeclampsia, and eclampsia. J Perinat Neonatal Nurs 1997; 10:8.

103. Roberts JM: Preeclampsia: Not simply pregnancy-induced hypertension. Hosp Pract (Off Ed) 1995; 30:25.

104. Bolte AC, van Geijn HP, Dekker GA: Pathophysiology of preeclampsia and the role of serotonin. Eur J Obstet Gynecol Reprod Biol 2001; 95:12.

105. Ryan EA: Pregnancy in diabetes. Med Clin North Am 1998; 82:823.

106. Linn T, Bretzel RG: Diabetes in pregnancy. Eur J Obstet Gynecol Reprod Biol 1997; 75:37.

107. Garner P: Type I diabetes mellitus and pregnancy. Lancet 1995; 346:157.

108. Singer DB: The placenta in pregnancies complicated by diabetes mellitus. Perspect Pediatr Pathol 1984; 8:199.

109. Jacomo KH, Benedetti WL, Sala MA, et al.: Pathology of the trophoblast and fetal vessels of the placenta in maternal diabetes mellitus. Acta Diabetol Lat 1976; 13:216.

110. Teasdale F: Histomorphometry of the placenta of the diabetic women: Class A diabetes mellitus. Placenta 1981; 2:241.

111. Teasdale F: Histomorphometry of the human placenta in class B diabetes mellitus. Placenta 1983; 4:1.

112. Teasdale F: Histomorphometry of the human placenta in class C diabetes mellitus. Placenta 1985; 6:69.

113. Teasdale F, Jean-Jacques G: Morphometry of the microvillous membrane of the human placenta in maternal diabetes mellitus. Placenta 1986; 7:81.

114. Wald NJ, Densem JW, Cheng R, et al.: Maternal serum free alpha- and free beta-human chorionic gonadotropin in pregnancies with insulin-dependent diabetes mellitus: Implications for screening for Down's syndrome. Prenat Diagn 1994; 14:835.

115. Crossley JA, Berry E, Aitken DA, et al.: Insulin-dependent diabetes mellitus and prenatal screening results: Current experience from a regional screening programme. Prenat Diagn 1996; 16:1039.

116. Greco MA, Kamat BR, Demopoulos RI: Placental protein distribution in maternal diabetes mellitus: An immunocytochemical study. Pediatr Pathol 1989; 9:679.

117. Lopez-Espinoza I, Smith RF, Gillmer M, et al.: High levels of growth hormone and human placental lactogen in pregnancy complicated by diabetes. Diabetes Res 1986; 3:119.

118. Botta RM, Donatelli M, Bucalo ML, et al.: Placental lactogen, progesterone, total estriol and prolactin plasma levels in pregnant women with insulin-dependent diabetes mellitus. Eur J Obstet Gynecol Reprod Biol 1984; 16:393.

119. Schonfelder G, John M, Hopp H, et al.: Expression of inducible nitric oxide synthase in placenta of women with gestational diabetes. Faseb J 1996; 10:777.

120. Glinoer D: What happens to the normal thyroid during pregnancy? Thyroid 1999; 9:631.

121. Fantz CR, Dagogo-Jack S, Ladenson JH, et al.: Thyroid function during pregnancy. Clin Chem 1999; 45:2250.

122. Fukushi M, Honma K, Fujita K: Maternal thyroid deficiency during pregnancy and subsequent neuropsychological development of the child. N Engl J Med 1999; 341:201.

123. Davis LE, Leveno KJ, Cunningham FG: Hypothyroidism complicating pregnancy. Obstet Gynecol 1988; 72:108.

124. Mortimer RH, Cannell GR, Addison RS, et al.: Methimazole and propylthiouracil equally cross the perfused human term placental lobule. J Clin Endocrinol Metab 1997; 82:3099.

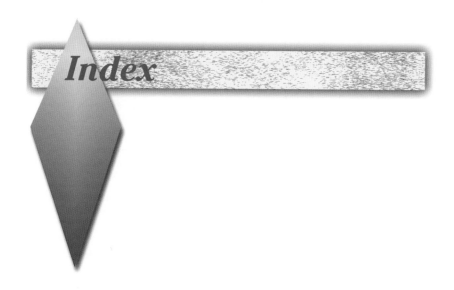

Index

Note: Page numbers followed by the letter f refer to figures and those followed by t refer to tables.

A

Acetylcholine, 1
Acquired immunodeficiency syndrome
    (AIDS)
    adrenal insufficiency and, 193
    mesenchymal adrenocortical tumors and,
        190
    secondary hypophysitis and, 38
    thyroiditis and, 65
Acromegaly, 41
    mammosomatotroph adenoma and, 43
    neuronal tumors and, 51
    pancreatic endocrine tumors and, 209t
Addison's disease, 191–193
    adrenoleukodystrophy and, 177
    autoimmune, 191–192, 192f
    corticotroph hyperplasia in, 39
    from histoplasmosis, 193
    from tuberculosis, 192, 192f
Addison-Schilder disease, 177
Adenocarcinoid, 250–253, 251f–252f, 251t.
        See also Carcinoid(s).
    treatment of, 252–253
Adenocarcinoma, 19
    inflammatory bowel disease and, 255
    mucinous, ovarian, 323, 323f
    neuroendocrine differentiation and, 253f,
        279
    of rete testis, 346, 346f
    poorly differentiated, with neuroendocrine
        features, 253, 253f
    vs. bowel carcinoids, 243
    with poorly differentiated neuroendocrine
        carcinoma of lung, small cell type, 287,
        291f
Adenohypophysis, 31–32, 32f, 33–34
    ectopic, 34
    Sheehan's syndrome and, 38, 38f
Adenoma(s)
    acidophil stem cell, 42t, 44, 45–46, 45f
        treatment of, 46
    adrenal, 181, 181f–182f, 185f, 186, 189. *See
        also* Conn's syndrome.
        magnetic resonance imaging of, 185f
        pathogenesis of, 189
    corticotroph, 42t, 46–47
        Cushing's disease and, 47, 180
        densely granulated, 42t, 47, 47f
        sparsely granulated, 42t, 47, 48f
        type I silent, 49
        type II silent, 49
    Crooke's cell, 47–48, 48f
    follicular, 67–68
        signet-ring cell, 69
        vs. papillary carcinoma, 68

Adenoma(s) *(Continued)*
    gonadotroph, 42t, 48–49, 49f
        female type, 50
        silent, 49
        treatment of, 48
    Hürthle cell, 68, 79
    hyalinizing trabecular, 68–69, 69f
        papillary carcinoma and, 69
    lactotroph, 42t, 44
        densely granulated, 42t, 45, 45f
        silent, 49
        sparsely granulated, 42t, 44–45, 44f–45f
        treatment of, 44, 46, 46f
    mammosomatotroph, 42t, 43–44
        treatment of, 44
    null cell, 49
    parathyroid, 110f, 118–121, 119f–121f
        cytoplasmic fat and, 110, 110f
        differential diagnosis of, 124
        genomic alterations and, 112, 113
        hyperplasia and, 113, 118, 121–123, 131,
            132
        immunohistochemistry of, 122–123
        incidence of, 113
        large clear cell, 120f, 124
        lipoadenoma as, 123–124
        oncocytic, 120f, 121f, 123, 123f
        parathyroid hormone messenger RNA
            and, 107
        parathyroid hormone secretion by, 111
        treatment of, 115
        tumor cell mean diameter in, 126
        vs. medullary thyroid carcinoma, 124
        vs. papillary thyroid carcinoma, 119, 124
        vs. parathyroid carcinoma, 122, 128–129
        vs. thyroid tissue, 124
        water–clear cell, 121f, 124
        with stromal components, 123–124
    pituitary, 40–50, 40f
        classification of, 40–41, 40f–41f, 42t
        ectopic, 41
        multiple endocrine neoplasia type I with,
            40, 231
        nonfunctioning, 49
        plurihormonal, 50
        vs. metastatic tumors, 54
    secondary hypophysitis and, 37
    silent, subtype III, 50
    somatotroph, 41–42, 42t
        densely granulated, 42–43, 42t, 43f
        silent, 49
        sparsely granulated, 42t, 43, 43f
            pleomorphism and, 43f, 54
        treatment of, 41, 44
    thyroid, paraganglioma-like, 68–69, 69f

Adenoma(s) *(Continued)*
    thyrotroph, 42t, 46, 46f
        silent, 49
        thyrotoxicosis and, 62–63
        treatment of, 46
    vs. granulomatous hypophysitis, 37
Adenomatous polyposis coli *(APC)* gene, and
    neoplastic progression, 241–242, 254
Adrenal cortex, 171–172, 172f. *See also*
    Tumor(s), adrenocortical.
    capsular extrusions and, 175, 176f
    cysts and, 191, 191f
    drug effects on, 194
    fetal cytomegaly in, 176
    growth regulation in, 173
    innervation of, 173
    insufficiency of, 193
        chronic, 191–193. *See also* Addison's
            disease.
    stress response and, 178–179, 179f
    vasculature of, 173, 173f
    zona fasciculata of, 172–173, 172f
    zona glomerulosa of, 172, 172f
        aldosterone from, 174
    zona reticularis of, 172, 172f, 173
        dehydroepiandrosterone and, 174
Adrenal hyperplasia
    congenital, 177–178, 178f
        adrenal rest tumors and, 346
    macronodular, 181
Adrenal hypoplasia, congenital, 176
Adrenal medulla, 149, 150f
    cortex boundary and, 171
    epinephrine from, 152
    hyperplasia of, 153, 153f, 156f. *See also*
        Adrenal hyperplasia, macronodular.
        vs. pheochromocytoma, 153–154
    maturation of, 150
    medullary weight of, 153
    paraganglioma of, 152. *See also*
        Paraganglioma.
Adrenalectomy, and Cushing's disease, 47,
    180
Adrenalitis, autoimmune, 191–192, 192f
Adrenocorticotropic hormone (ACTH)
    adrenal cortex growth and, 173
    big, 6
    dexamethasone and, 180, 181
    ectopic secretion of, 181, 214
        malignancy and, 209t, 211
    from foregut gastrointestinal carcinoid, 242
    in hypothalamic-pituitary-adrenal axis, 174,
        175f
    in neuroendocrine carcinoma of prostate,
        25f, 26f

Adrenocorticotropic hormone (ACTH)
  (Continued)
  pancreatic endocrine tumors and, 209t,
    214
    malignancy of, 209t, 211
  pituitary adenomas and, 42t
  terminal illness and, 171
  tumor secretion of, 6, 19t
  vs. big ACTH, 6
Adrenocytomegaly, 176
Adrenogenital syndrome, 184, 338
Adrenoleukodystrophy, 177
Alcohol
  for secondary hyperparathyroidism, 116
  parathyroid ablation by, 116
Aldosterone, 174f, 174t
  action of, 175
  production of, 174, 174f, 175
Alfacalcidol, for secondary
    hyperparathyroidism, 116
Alpha-fetoprotein. *See* α-Fetoprotein (AFP).
Algorithm, for neuroendocrine lung tumor
    diagnosis, 278t
Alkaline phosphatase, and germinoma, 53
Aminoglutethimide
  cortisol synthesis and, 194
  for Cushing's disease, 47
Amyloid
  in medullary thyroid carcinoma, 13, 15f, 82,
    83
  in pancreatic endocrine tumors, 17f, 221,
    221f
  parathyroid glands and, 105
Amyloidosis
  adrenal insufficiency and, 193
  hypophysial, 39
Androblastoma. *See* Sertoli cell tumor.
Androgen insensitivity syndrome, and Sertoli
    cell tumors, 329
Androgens, 174f, 174t
  production of, 174, 174f
Androstenedione, 174f, 174t, 175
Angiography, carotid, pituitary apoplexy and,
    38
Angiosarcoma, thyroid, 88
Anorexia, and germ cell tumors, 53
Antibodies, heterophilic, 6
Antigens, in differential diagnosis, 158t. *See
    also specific antigens.*
Antiserotoninergic agents, for Cushing's
    disease, 47
Aorticopulmonary paraganglia, 150, 151f
  central nervous system and, 152
Appendectomy, for appendiceal carcinoid
    tumors, 250, 252
Arachnoid cysts, 35
Argyrophil cells, 238f
  bronchial distribution of, 264f
Argyrophilia, in parathyroid carcinoma, 128
Arteriography, pancreatic endocrine tumors
    by, 219, 219f
Arteritis, temporal, pituitary apoplexy and, 38
Astrocytomas, 51
Atherosclerosis, and pituitary apoplexy, 38
Autocrine hormonal systems, 1
Autoimmune polyendocrinopathy–
    candidiasis–ectodermal dystrophy
    (APECED), 191–192, 192f
Azzopardi effect, 285, 287f, 289f, 290f

B
Barbiturates, and steroid metabolism, 194
Basedow's disease, 61. *See also* Graves'
    disease (GD).
Beckwith-Wiedemann syndrome, 176
  adrenal medullary hyperplasia in, 153
  familial tumors in, 189
  islet hyperplasia in, 227, 227f

Benign prostatic hyperplasia (BPH), and
    prostate-specific antigen concentration, 7
BETA2 protein, in secretin cell differentiation,
    238–239
Biopsy. *See also* Fine-needle aspiration (FNA).
  parathyroid glands and, 104, 108–109
Birbeck's granules, and Langerhan's cell
    histiocytosis, 53
Blastoma, adrenocortical, 190
Bombesin-like peptides (BLPs), 266t, 268
  in fetal lung development, 262f
Bromocriptine
  for lactotroph adenomas, 44, 46
  gonadotroph adenomas and, 48
Bronchopulmonary dysplasia (BPD), 271
Bulimia, and germ cell tumors, 53

C
C (calcitonin) cells, 62, 81
  hyperplasia of, 81, 83
  pulmonary neuroendocrine cells and, 262
CA 125, 7, 8
Calcitonin (CT), 266t, 268
  as tumor marker, 8, 19t
  C cells and, 62, 81
  fetal pulmonary expression of, 261, 262f
  hypercalcemia medical management and,
    116
  in large cell neuroendocrine carcinoma of
    lung, 21f
  in non-neoplastic lung disease, 268
  medullary thyroid carcinoma and, 13, 15f,
    82–83
  pancreatic endocrine tumors and, 214,
    215
Calcitonin gene–related peptide (CGRP), 266t,
    268
  in fetal lung development, 262f
  lung hypoplasia and, 271
Calcium
  for hypoparathyroidism, 134
  for secondary hyperparathyroidism, 116
  parathyroid hormone and, 107
Calcium oxalate, and thyroid colloid, 62
Carcinoembryogenic antigen (CEA), 247
  in medullary carcinoma of thyroid, 13, 15f
Carcinoid(s), 17–18, 241f, 313. *See also*
    Tumor(s).
  appendiceal, 23, 23f–24f, 245–246, 245f,
    250
    gender predominance and, 250
    ovarian metastases of, 324, 325f
    patient age and, 243
    serotonin in, 24f
  bronchial, 21, 272, 273, 279–280, 280f,
    281–282
    atypical, versus typical carcinoids, 19t,
      21–22, 273, 277
    classification of, 19t, 276t, 277, 279
    peripheral, 280–281, 280f–282f
    pulmonary neuroendocrine cells and,
      263–264
    vs. pulmonary tumorlets, 271, 273f
    vs. well-differentiated neuroendocrine
      carcinoma, 19t, 277, 278t, 282,
      283f
  cytokeratin and, 280, 304t
  detection of, 256–257
  diffuse, 18, 19f–20f
  formation of, transgenic models in, 255
  gallbladder, 22f
  gastric, 23, 24, 247–249, 248f
    multiple endocrine neoplasia type I and,
      214f, 215–216, 247–248
    pernicious anemia and, 249
    REG1A gene in, 255
    Zollinger-Ellison syndrome and, 213, 214f,
      215, 216, 247–248

Carcinoid(s) *(Continued)*
  gastrointestinal, 23–24, 241, 241f–244f,
    242–243, 244t
    immunohistochemistry of, 244–247,
      246f
    metastatic, 23–24, 243, 245f
    patient survival and, 245f
    presentation of, 247, 247t
    serotonin from, 24, 242, 247
  goblet cell, 250–253, 251f–252f, 251t
    ovarian metastases of, 324
    treatment of, 252–253
  ileal, 23, 24
    carcinoid syndrome and, 26
    serotonin production in, 24
    vs. Crohn's disease, 256
  insular, 313–315, 314f–315f
    heart disease and, 315
    in ovarian strumal carcinoid, 317
    vs. adenocarcinomas, 325
    vs. Brenner's tumors, 315
    vs. granulosa cell tumors, 314–315
  metastatic, 23–24, 26, 243, 245f, 316,
    324–325, 325f
  middle ear, 26
  ovarian, 26, 313, 314f
    metastatic, 316, 324–325, 325f
    strumal, 317–319, 317f–318f
      immunohistochemistry and, 318
      insular carcinoid in, 317
      thyroid follicles in, 317, 317f–318f,
        318–319
      trabecular carcinoid in, 317–318
    trabecular, 315–317, 316f
      in ovarian strumal carcinoid, 317–318
      metastases and, 316
      treatment of, 317
      vs. Sertoli-Leydig cell tumors, 316
  rectal, 23, 24, 257
  renal, 26
  testicular, 347–348
  thymic, 26
  treatment of, 257
Carcinoid syndrome, 24, 26, 242, 256–257
  heart disease and, 256, 257, 315
  hepatic artery embolization and, 256,
    257
  liver transplantation and, 257
  octreotide for, 231, 256
  ovarian carcinoids and, 314
    metastatic, 324, 325
  pancreatic endocrine tumors and, 209t,
    214
  serotonin in, 21, 209t, 242, 256
  substance P and, 214
  valvular lesions and, 256, 257
Carcinoma. *See also* Adenocarcinoma;
    Choriocarcinomas; Tumor(s).
  adrenal cortical, 186–187, 186f–187f
    immunocytochemistry and, 188–189,
      188f
    pathogenesis of, 189
    staging of, 188, 188t
    vs. hepatocellular carcinoma, 188
    vs. pheochromocytoma, 189
    vs. renal carcinoma, 188
  columnar cell, 75–76
  crypt cell, 250–253, 251f–252f, 251t
    treatment of, 252–253
  ectopic adrenocorticotropic hormone
    secretion and, 181
  embryonal, 52
    α-fetoprotein and, 53
  follicular, 77–79, 78f
    vs. papillary thyroid carcinoma, 74, 78
  Hürthle cell, 75, 79–80
    aneuploidy and, 80
  insular, 80–81, 80f
  large cell neuroendocrine, 19–20, 19t, 21f,
    22–23, 272, 273

Carcinoma *(Continued)*
lung, 275. *See also* Carcinoma, small cell lung.
neuroendocrine, 282, 282f–283f, 283–284
moderately differentiated, 283, 284, 284f
ovarian metastases of, 326
poorly differentiated. *See* Poorly differentiated neuroendocrine carcinoma of lung.
prognosis of, 284, 284t
vs. poorly differentiated tumor, 283, 283f, 286–287
non–small cell, neuroendocrine differentiation in, 291, 291f
medullary thyroid, 13, 15f, 81–83, 82f
cytology of, 15f, 82f, 83
ectopic adrenocorticotropic hormone secretion and, 181
mixed tumor with, 83
vs. Hürthle cell tumors, 83
vs. papillary carcinoma, 83
vs. parathyroid adenoma, 124
with pheochromocytoma, 13
Merkel cell. *See* Merkel cell carcinoma (MCC).
mucoepidermoid thyroid, 86–87, 86f
neuroendocrine, 18–19. *See also* Carcinoma, lung, neuroendocrine; Carcinoma, small cell.
adenomatous component with, 253, 253f. *See also* Poorly differentiated neuroendocrine carcinoma *entries.*
breast tumors as, 26, 27f
cutaneous. *See* Merkel cell carcinoma (MCC).
ovarian, 323–324, 323f
prostatic, 25f–26f, 26
ovarian. *See* Carcinoma, small cell ovarian.
pancreatic endocrine, 210
poorly differentiated, 226–227, 226f
papillary thyroid, 67, 70–72, 71f
composite tumor as, 83
cribriform, 75
cytokeratin 19 marker for, 68
cytology of, 71f, 77
diffuse sclerosing variant, 76–77
follicular variant, 71f, 73–74, 77
hyalinizing trabecular adenoma and, 69
lymphatic thyroid tissue and, 62
nodular fasciitis–like stroma variant, 75
oncocytic variant, 74–75
prognostic indicators for, 72
radiation and, 73, 76
tall cell variant, 71f, 74
vs. Hürthle cell tumors, 77
treatment for, 73
vs. follicular adenoma, 68, 74
vs. follicular carcinoma, 74, 78
vs. Graves' disease hyperplasia, 64
vs. Hashimoto's thyroiditis, 66, 66f, 75
vs. medullary carcinoma, 83
vs. parathyroid adenoma, 119
vs. Reidel's disease, 75
Warthin's-like, 71f, 75
cytology of, 77
parathyroid, 124–128, 125f, 127f
aneuploidy in, 111
argyrophilia in, 128
cardiac calcinosis from, 129f
differential diagnosis of, 129
genetic mutations and, 112, 113
immunohistochemical stains and, 128
incidence of, 113–114, 124
prognosis of, 129–130
S-phase fractions in, 128
surgery for, 116
vs. parathyroid adenoma, 122, 128–129
vs. thyroid tumors, 129

Carcinoma *(Continued)*
pituitary, 50
pulmonary. *See* Carcinoma, lung; Carcinoma, small cell lung.
renal, versus adrenal tumors, 158t, 188
small cell, 19, 23
ovarian metastases of, 326
surgical pathology and, 12, 13
small cell lung, 19t, 272, 273. *See also* Carcinoma, small cell ovarian.
autocrine growth factors in, 274
chromogranin A expression in, 267f
classification schemes and, 276t, 277–278
human achaete-scute homologue-1 and, 275
myc oncogenes in, 272
ovarian metastases of, 326
pulmonary neuroendocrine cells and, 263
tumorigenesis in, 273
vs. Merkel cell carcinoma, 302–303, 304t, 306, 310
vs. pulmonary tumorlets, 271, 273f
small cell ovarian, 319
hypercalcemic type, 320–322, 320f–321f
large cell variant of, 321
treatment of, 322
vs. granulosa cell tumors, 321–322
vs. lymphoma, 322
vs. metastatic small cell carcinoma, 326
small cell pancreatic, 226–227, 226f
thyroid, 69–70. *See also* Carcinoma, medullary thyroid; Carcinoma, papillary thyroid.
anaplastic, 84
mortality of, 67, 70
vs. nodular fasciitis–like stroma variant carcinoma, 75
vs. Reidel's thyroiditis, 84
lymphoepithelioma-like, 85–86, 85f
mixed, 83
mucoepidermoid, 86–87, 86f
vs. Hodgkin's disease, 87
oncogenes in, 72–73
poorly differentiated, 80
squamous cell, 84–85
struma ovarii with, 318
vs. parathyroid carcinoma, 129
Cardiac dysfunction, and carcinoid syndrome, 256, 257, 315
Carney complex, 182
Carotid bodies, 149, 150, 151f
central nervous system and, 152
chronic hypoxemia and, 154, 161
hyperplasia of, 154
innervation of, 149
paraganglioma of, 161, 161f
malignancy of, 161
size of, 151
CASTLE (carcinoma showing thymus-like differentiation), 85–86, 85f
Catecholamines
adrenal medullary hyperplasia and, 153
paraganglion tumors and, 152
neuroblastic, 165
CD57 (Leu-7), 223, 266t
in neuroendocrine differentiation, 276
Chief cells. *See* Neuroendocrine cells.
Cholesteatomas, 35–36
Cholesterol, 174f
craniopharyngioma and, 52
human placental lactogen and, 353
in steroidogenesis, 174, 354
Chordomas, 51
Choriocarcinomas, 52–53, 355, 355f
Chorionic somatomammotropin, 353
Chromogranin A (CGA, ChrA), 8, 11, 152, 222, 246, 266t, 267f
gastrin and, 241
in adrenal medulla, 12f

Chromogranin A (CGA, ChrA) *(Continued)*
in differential diagnosis, 19t, 158t
in gallbladder carcinoid, 22f
in large cell neuroendocrine carcinoma of lung, 21f
in liver carcinoids, 28f
in neuroendocrine breast carcinoma, 27f
in neuroendocrine differentiation, 276
in pheochromocytoma, 16f
in rectal carcinoid, 24f
in type A gastritis, 20f
pancreatic endocrine tumors and, 211, 222–223, 222f
Chronic obstructive pulmonary disease. *See also* Pulmonary neuroendocrine cells (PNECs), in non-neoplastic lung disease.
carotid bodies and, 154
Chvostek's sign, 133
Cigarette smoke, and tumorigenesis, 274–275
Cisplatin, for pancreatic poorly differentiated (small cell) endocrine carcinoma, 227
Clinical pathology laboratory, 1
analytic test assessments by, 1–2
neuroendocrine tumors and, 11–13
Clinical pathology tests
competitive-binding assays in, 3–5
efficiency of, 3
precision and, 1
predictive value of, 2–3
reference range for, 2
sensitivity of, 2, 2f
specificity of, 2, 2f
Coagulopathy
adrenal insufficiency and, 193
pituitary apoplexy and, 38
Colitis, ulcerative, neoplastic progression and, 255–256
Computed tomography (CT)
of pancreatic endocrine tumors, 219, 219f
of Rathke's cleft cysts, 35
Congenital adrenal hyperplasia (CAH), 177–178, 178f
adrenal rest tumors and, 346
Congenital lipoid hyperplasia, 178
Conn's syndrome, 182–184, 183f
spironolactone and, 183–184, 184f
Corticotroph(s), 33, 33f
adenoma. *See* Adenoma(s), corticotroph.
hyperplasia of, 39
Corticotropin-releasing hormone (CRH), 353–354
pancreatic endocrine tumors and, 209t
premature labor and, 357
Cortisol, 174f, 174t
Cushing's disease and, 47
Cushing's syndrome and, 180
dexamethasone and, 180
production of, 174, 174f–175f
Cranial nerve palsy
from pituitary apoplexy, 38
granulomatous hypophysitis and, 37
Craniopharyngioma, 52
Cretinism, 64–65
Crohn's disease, 256
neoplastic progression and, 255–256
Crooke's cell adenoma, 47–48, 48f
Crooke's hyaline change, 33, 33f
Cushing's disease, 47, 180, 180f
corticotroph hyperplasia and, 39, 180
ectopic pituitary adenomas and, 41
neuronal tumors and, 51
Cushing's syndrome, 179–182, 179f. *See also* Tumorlets.
adrenal cortical carcinoma and, 186
big ACTH and, 6
ectopic adrenocorticotropic hormone secretion and, 181, 214
central carcinoids and, 280
from adrenal tumor, 181, 181f–182f, 186
from exogenous steroids, 180

Cushing's syndrome (Continued)
  hypophysectomy for, 39
  mixed, 180
  pancreatic endocrine tumors and, 209t, 214
  renal carcinoids and, 26
  Zollinger-Ellison syndrome and, 214
Cyproheptadine, for Cushing's disease, 47
Cystic fibrosis
  adrenal medullary hyperplasia with, 153
  carotid bodies and, 154
Cytochrome P-450 enzymes, in
    steroidogenesis, 174, 174f
Cytokeratin
  as papillary thyroid carcinoma marker, 68
  carcinoids and, 280, 304t
    gastrointestinal, 245, 246f
  fetal trophoblasts and, 352
  in Merkel cell carcinoma, 29f, 297, 301–303,
    303f, 304t, 305t, 306
  pancreatic endocrine tumors and, 222f

D

De Quervain's disease, 65
Dehydroepiandrosterone (DHEA), 174t. See
    also Adrenogenital syndrome.
  in pregnancy, 354
  in steroidogenesis, 174, 174f
Depression, and Cushing's syndrome, 180
Dermoid cysts, 35–36
Dexamethasone
  adrenocorticotropic hormone and, 180
  ectopic adrenocorticotropic hormone
    secretion and, 181
Dexamethasone suppression testing, 47
Diabetes insipidus
  from arachnoid cysts, 35
  from pituitary apoplexy, 38
  from Rathke's cleft cysts, 35
  germ cell tumors and, 53
  intracranial hematologic tumors and, 53
  lymphocytic hypophysitis and, 36
Diabetes mellitus
  adrenal cortical nodules and, 184
  autoimmune adrenalitis and, 192
  familial benign hypercalcemia and, 117
  from glucagonomas, 14
  in Cushing's syndrome, 180
  pituitary apoplexy and, 38
  pregnancy and, 357–358
  somatostatinoma syndrome and, 212, 249
Diazoxide, for insulinoma, 231
DiGeorge's syndrome, 103, 134
5-Dimethyltriazeno-4-carboxamide, for
    pancreatic endocrine tumor metastases,
    231
Diplopia, from pituitary apoplexy, 38
Dopamine, 266t
  from hindgut gastrointestinal carcinoid, 242
  parathyroid hormone and, 107
  pheochromocytoma and, 154
Dopaminergic agonists
  for lactotroph adenomas, 46, 46f
  for lactotroph hyperplasia, 39
Doxorubicin, for pancreatic endocrine tumor
    metastases, 231
Drugs
  adrenal cortex and, 194
  parathyroid hormone and, 107

E

Echovirus, and adrenal insufficiency, 193
Ectopic ACTH (adrenocorticotropic hormone)
    syndrome, 181
Embolization, hepatic artery
  carcinoid syndrome and, 256, 257
  for pancreatic endocrine tumor metastases,
    231

Empty sella syndrome, 35, 35f
Endocrine feedback loops, 1
Enterochromaffin cells, 237, 238, 238f, 240,
    241, 241f
  hyperplasia of, gastrinoma and, 213, 214f,
    247–248
Enteroendocrine cells, 237, 238, 238f, 240,
    241, 241f
Enzyme-multiplied immunoassay technique, 5
Enzyme-linked immunosorbent assays, 5
Epidermoid cysts, 35–36
Epinephrine
  adrenal medullary hyperplasia and, 153
  from adrenal medulla, 152
  from sympathetic paraganglia tumors,
    152
  parathyroid hormone and, 107
  pheochromocytoma and, 154
Epithelioid trophoblast tumor, 355–356
Estradiol, 174t
  ectopic pregnancy and, 356
  Leydig cell tumors and, 339
Estriol
  in pregnancy, 354
  multiple pregnancy and, 357
Estrogen(s), 174f, 174t
  hypercalcemia medical management and,
    116
  Leydig cell tumors and, 339
  parathyroid hormone and, 107
  pregnancy and, 354
Ethanol
  for secondary hyperparathyroidism, 116
  parathyroid ablation by, 116
Etomidate, and cortisol synthesis, 194
Etoposide, for pancreatic poorly
    differentiated (small cell) endocrine
    carcinoma, 227

F

Familial benign (hypocalciuric)
    hypercalcemia (FBH), 117
  incidence of, 115, 117
Feedback loops, 1
Ferritin, serum, neuroblastoma prognosis
    and, 165
α-Fetoprotein (AFP), 8
  intracranial germ cell tumors and, 53
  liver carcinoids and, 26
Fibromas, testicular, 343–344
Fine-needle aspiration (FNA), 63
  anaplastic carcinoma and, 84
  Hürthle cell tumors and, 79
  of medullary thyroid carcinoma, 82f, 83,
    109
  of pancreatic endocrine tumors, 219–220,
    219f
  of papillary thyroid carcinoma, 71f, 77
  of parathyroid cysts, 109
  of spindle epithelial tumor with thymus-like
    differentiation, 85
  parathyroid glands and, 104, 108–109, 119,
    131
Fluorescent polarization immunoassay, 5
5-Fluorouracil, for pancreatic endocrine
    tumor metastases, 231
Folliculostellate cells, 33, 34f
Furosemide, and hypercalcemia medical
    management, 116

G

G protein, adrenal tumor, 190
Gangliocytomas, 50–51
Ganglioneuroblastomas, 163, 164, 164f
Ganglioneuromas, 163, 164, 164f–165f
  from neuroblastoma, 166

Gastrin, 6, 240
  chromogranin A and, 241
  in gastric acid secretion, 240–241, 240f
  pancreatic endocrine tumors and, 209t, 212
    malignancy of, 209t, 211
  parietal cell hypertrophy and, 242
Gastrinoma, 14–16, 212, 213, 213f
  distribution of, 15, 220
  enterochromaffin-like cell hyperplasia and,
    213, 214f, 247–248
  frequency of, 209
  malignancy and, 16, 211
  multiple endocrine neoplasia type I and,
    15–16, 212, 213f, 215, 248–249
  p16INK4a gene methylation and, 229–230
  parietal cell hypertrophy and, 213, 214f,
    242
  peptide production in, 6
  Zollinger-Ellison syndrome and, 212, 213f,
    214f, 248–249
Gastrin-producing tumors. See Gastrinoma.
Gastrin-releasing peptide (GRP), 19t, 266t,
    268–269
  small cell lung carcinoma and, 274
Gastritis
  atrophic
    gastric carcinoid tumors and, 247, 248f
    lymphocytic hypophysitis and, 36
  type A, 18, 19f–20f
Genetic mutation
  adrenocortical tumors and, 189–190
  in congenital adrenal hyperplasia, 177–178
  in gastrointestinal tract, 254
  in hyperparathyroidism, 112–113
  in MEN1 gene, 229, 242, 255
  in multiple endocrine neoplasia type I, 242,
    255
  neuroblastic tumors and, 165–166
  parasympathetic paragangliomas and, 163
  pheochromocytoma and, 158–159
  pulmonary neuroendocrine tumorigenesis
    and, 272–274
  thyroid tumors and, 72–73, 75, 81
Germinoma, 52, 53
  gonadoblastoma with, 345
Gestational trophoblastic disease, 354
Gliomas, 51
Glucagon
  from islets of Langerhans, 14f, 207, 207t,
    208f
  pancreatic endocrine tumors and, 209t, 212
    malignancy of, 209t, 211
Glucagon-like peptide-1 (GLP-1), 255
Glucagonoma, 212, 212f, 225f
  frequency of, 209
Glucagonoma syndrome, 209t, 212
Glucocorticoid(s), 174f
  action of, 175
  corticotropin-releasing hormone and, 354
  for pituitary apoplexy, 38
  parathyroid hormone and, 107
  synthesis of, 174f–175f
Glucocorticoid deficiency, familial, 176
P-Glycoprotein, 172
  adrenal cortical carcinoma and, 186
  neuroblastoma prognosis and, 165
Goiter, 62–64
  dyshormonogenetic, 64–65
  lymphadenoid. See Hashimoto's thyroiditis.
  papillary hyperplasia in, 63f
  toxic, 61, 63, 64, 64f, 66
Gonadoblastoma, 345
Gonadotroph(s), 33
  hyperplasia of, 39
Gonadotroph adenomas, 48
Gonadotropin, and pituitary adenomas, 42t
Gonadotropin-releasing hormone, and
    gonadotroph adenomas, 48
Graft-versus-host disease, 256
Granular cell tumors, in neurohypophysis, 51

Granuloma. *See also* De Quervain's disease.
  eosinophilic, 53
Granulosa cell tumors, 340–342, 340f–342f
  juvenile-type, 322f, 342–343, 342f, 343t
    vs. embryonal rhabdomyosarcoma, 343
    vs. ovarian small cell carcinoma,
      321–322
    vs. Sertoli cell tumors, 343
    vs. yolk sac tumors, 343
  malignancy and, 342
  vs. insular carcinoids, 314–315
  vs. ovarian small cell carcinoma, 321–322
  vs. Sertoli cell tumor, 334, 343
Graves' disease (GD), 61, 63, 64
  hyperparathyroidism following, 111
  lymphocytic thyroiditis and, 64, 66
  papillary hyperplasia in, 64f
  pregnancy and, 358
  vs. papillary carcinoma, 64
Grimelius stain, 11, 21f, 27f, 238f, 321f, 323f
Growth hormone (GH)
  acromegaly and, 41, 209t
  pancreatic endocrine tumors and, 209t
  pituitary adenomas and, 42t
Gynecomastia
  Leydig cell tumors and, 338, 339
  Sertoli cell tumors and, 333

H
H₂ antagonists
  for hyperchlorhydria, 213
  for Zollinger-Ellison syndrome, 213, 231
³H (tritium), 4
Hand-Schüller-Christian disease, 53
Hashimoto's thyroiditis, 66–67, 66f
  familial benign hypercalcemia and, 117
  fibrous variant, 66–67, 75
  Graves' disease and, 64, 66
  Hürthle cells in, 66, 79
  hyperparathyroidism and, 111
  RET/PTC oncogene and, 73
  sclerosing mucoepidermoid carcinoma and,
    86, 86f, 87
  vs. papillary carcinoma, 66, 66f, 75
  vs. Reidel's disease, 67
  vs. thyroid lymphoma, 66
  Warthin's-like carcinoma and, 75
hCG. *See* Human chorionic gonadotropin
  (hCG).
Heart disease
  carcinoid syndrome and, 256, 257
    insular carcinoid in, 315
  cyanotic congenital, carotid bodies and,
    154
Hemangiopericytoma, of testis, 348f
Hemicolectomy
  appendiceal adenocarcinoids and,
    252–253
  for appendiceal carcinoid tumors, 250
Hemochromatosis, and adrenal cortex, 193,
  194f
Hemorrhage
  chronic prolactinoma therapy and, 46
  pheochromocytoma and, 154, 157
Hemosiderin, and chronic prolactinoma
  therapy, 46
Hemosiderosis
  adrenal cortex and, 193
  hypophysial, 39
Herpesviruses, and adrenal insufficiency,
  193
HISL-19, 223
Histamine
  in carcinoid syndrome, 242, 256
  in gastric acid secretion, 240f
Histamine H₂ antagonists. *See* H₂ antagonists.
Histoplasmosis, adrenal insufficiency from,
  193

Hormones, 1
  analytic test assessments for, 1–2
  identification methods for, 11
  peptide, 11
Human achaete-scute homologue-1 (hASH1)
  in pulmonary neuroendocrine cell
    differentiation, 263, 263f
  lung carcinoma and, 275
Human autoimmune polyendocrinopathy, 134
Human chorionic gonadotropin (hCG), 8, 353
  diabetic pregnancy and, 357
  ectopic pregnancy and, 356
  from foregut gastrointestinal carcinoids,
    242
  from intracranial germ cell tumors, 53
  hydatidiform moles and, 355
  multiple pregnancy and, 356
  pancreatic endocrine tumors and, 226
  spontaneous abortion and, 356
Human immunodeficiency virus (HIV). *See
  also* Acquired immunodeficiency
    syndrome (AIDS).
  hypothalamic-pituitary-adrenal axis and,
    193
Human placental lactogen (hPL), 353, 354
  diabetic pregnancy and, 357
  multiple pregnancy and, 357
  Pit-1 and, 353
Humoral hypercalcemia of malignancy
  (HHM), 108, 136
Hürthle cell(s), 79
  in Hashimoto's thyroiditis, 66, 79
  in thyroid lesions, 63, 64, 79
Hürthle cell tumors, 75, 79–80. *See also*
  Adenoma(s), Hürthle cell.
  aneuploidy and, 80
  vs. medullary thyroid carcinoma, 83
  vs. tall cell variant papillary thyroid
    carcinoma, 77
Hyaline membrane disease (HMD), 271
Hybridomas, 3
Hydatidiform moles, 354–355
  pregnancy-induced hypertension and, 357
Hydrocephalus
  craniopharyngioma and, 52
  germ cell tumors and, 53
1α-Hydroxycholecalciferol, for secondary
  hyperparathyroidism, 116
5-Hydroxyindoleacetic acid (5-HIAA), and
  insular carcinoids, 314
21-Hydroxylase
  in congenital adrenal hyperplasia, 177
  in steroidogenesis, 174f
3β-Hydroxysteroid dehydrogenase
  in congenital adrenal hyperplasia, 177–178
  in steroidogenesis, 174f
5-Hydroxytryptamine (5-HT). *See* Serotonin
  (5-HT).
Hyperaldosteronism
  Conn's syndrome, 182–184, 183f–184f
  glucocorticoid-suppressible, 184
Hypercalcemia, 136
  familial hypocalciuric, 117
  hyperparathyroidism and, 114, 114t, 115
  in cardiac calcinosis, 129f
  medical management of, 116
  microvillous formation and, 122
  ovarian neuroendocrine carcinoma and,
    320–322
  pancreatic endocrine tumors and, 209t, 214
  parathyroid hormone–related peptides
    and, 8, 108
  water–clear cell hyperplasia and, 133
Hypercapnia, and parasympathetic
  paraganglia, 152
Hypercortisolism. *See* Cushing's syndrome.
Hypergastrinemia
  gastric carcinoid tumors and, 247
  Helicobacter pylori and, 249
  omeprazole and, 249

Hypergastrinemia *(Continued)*
  pernicious anemia and, 249
  Zollinger-Ellison syndrome and, 213,
    247–249
Hyperparathyroidism, 111–116
  chief cell hyperplasia and, 112, 113, 130,
    132
  clinical signs of, 114, 114t
  genetic mutations in, 112–113
  incidence of, 113
  neonatal, 117–118
  radiology and, 114–115, 114f
  recurrence of, 115
    graft-induced, 117, 132
  renal, 116
  secondary, 116–117
  tertiary, 117
    chief cell hyperplasia and, 132
  treatment of, 115–116
Hyperparathyroidism–jaw tumor syndrome,
  113
Hyperprolactinemia
  dermoid cysts and, 36
  empty sellar syndrome and, 35
  gliomas and, 51
  lactotroph adenomas and, 44
  lymphocytic hypophysitis and, 36
  meningiomas and, 51
  neuronal tumors and, 51
  nonfunctioning pituitary adenomas and,
    49
Hypertension
  adrenal cortical nodules and, 184
  adrenal medullary hyperplasia and, 153
  Conn's syndrome with, 182–183
  pheochromocytoma and, 154
  pregnancy-induced, 357
  pulmonary neuroendocrine cells and, 271
Hyperthyroidism
  multiple endocrine neoplasia type I and,
    231
  pregnancy and, 358
Hypogonadism, and gonadotroph
  hyperplasia, 39
Hypokalemia, and ectopic
  adrenocorticotropic hormone secretion,
    181
Hypoparathyroidism, 133–135
Hypophysitis
  granulomatous, 37, 37f
    treatment of, 37
  lymphocytic, 36, 36f
    treatment of, 36
  secondary, 37–38
  xanthomatous, 37, 37f
Hypopituitarism, 34–35
  arachnoid cysts and, 35
  chordomas and, 51
  craniopharyngioma and, 52
  dermoid cysts and, 36
  Rathke's cleft cysts and, 35
Hypothalamic-pituitary-adrenal (HPA) axis,
  174, 175f, 193
Hypothyroidism
  hypopituitarism and, 35
  pregnancy and, 358
  thyrotroph hyperplasia in, 39
Hypoxemia, chronic, paraganglia and, 154
Hypoxia, and parasympathetic paraganglia,
  152

I
Id transcription factor, 31
Idiopathic diffuse hyperplasia of PNECs
  (pulmonary neuroendocrine cells), 270,
    270f
Immunohistopathology, advances in, 152
Immunoradiometric assays (IRMAs), 4, 5f

Indium 111, in somatostatinoma detection, 218, 249–250
Infection
  autoimmune adrenalitis and, 191, 192–193, 192f
  secondary hypophysitis and, 37–38
  thyroiditis from, 65
Insulin, 1
  from islets of Langerhans, 14f, 207–208, 207t, 208f
  pancreatic endocrine tumors and, 209t, 211
    malignancy of, 209t, 211
Insulin-like growth factor I (IGF-I)
  acromegaly and, 41
  small cell lung carcinoma and, 274
Insulinoma, 14, 17f, 211, 212f, 225f
  frequency of, 209
  multiple endocrine neoplasia type I and, 215
α-Interferon, for pancreatic endocrine tumor metastases, 231
International Association for the Study of Lung Cancer (IASLC), pulmonary neuroendocrine tumor classification of, 276t, 277, 278
Intestinal transcription factors, 238–240
Iodine 123, in somatostatin scintigraphy, 218
Iodine 125, 4
Iodine 131
  for papillary thyroid carcinoma, 73
  hypoparathyroidism and, 134
  pheochromocytoma and, 154
Islets of Langerhans, 206–209, 206f, 207f–208f, 207t
  hyperplasia of, 227, 227f
  prohormone convertases in, 14f

K
Ketoconazole
  cortisol synthesis and, 194
  for Cushing's disease, 47
Ki-67 antigen
  pancreatic endocrine tumors and, 226
  pancreatic poorly differentiated (small cell) endocrine carcinoma and, 227
  parathyroid malignancy and, 128
Kidney. See also Renal entries.
  adrenal-renal heterotopia and, 176

L
Lactotrophs, 32
  hyperplasia of, 39
Langerhans' cell histiocytosis, 53
Large cell neuroendocrine carcinoma of lung (LCNCL), 19–20, 19t, 21f, 22–23, 272, 273
  prognosis of, 19t, 23
Leiomyoma, thyroid, 87
Leiomyosarcoma, thyroid, 87
Letterer-Siwe disease, 53
Leu-7 (CD57), 223, 266t
  in neuroendocrine differentiation, 276
Leukemia, in testis, 348f
Leukotrienes, 1
Leydig cell hyperplasia, 336f, 338
Leydig cell tumor, 329, 336–339, 336f–337f
  gynecomastia and, 338, 339
  hormonal anomalies with, 339
  malignancy and, 337, 339
  vs. adrenogenital tumor, 338
  vs. Leydig cell hyperplasia, 338
  vs. lymphoma, 338
  vs. malakoplakia, 338
  vs. Sertoli cell tumor, 334, 338
  vs. yolk sac tumor, 338

Li-Fraumeni syndrome, 189
Ligand competition-binding assays, 3–6
  automated, 6
  enzyme labels in, 5
  fluorescent labels in, 5
  radioactive labels for, 4
Lipoadenoma
  parathyroid, 123–124
  thyroid, 124
Lipohyperplasia, parathyroid, 131
Lipoid hyperplasia, congenital adrenal, 178
Lipothymoadenoma, of parathyroid, 123–124
Lipoxins, 1
Liver
  adrenal-hepatic heterotopia and, 176
  carcinoids of, 26, 28f
Lung. See also Carcinoma, lung.
  inflammatory disease in, 268–269, 270, 270f
Lymph nodes, cervical, thyroid tissue within, 61
Lymphoma
  non-Hodgkin's
    intracranial, 53
    testicular, 348f
  testicular, 348
  thyroid, 88
    vs. lymphocytic thyroiditis, 66
    vs. Leydig cell tumor, 338
    vs. Merkel cell carcinoma, 301
    vs. ovarian small cell carcinoma, 322

M
Magnetic resonance imaging (MRI)
  of adrenal adenoma, 185f
  of craniopharyngioma, 52
  of intracranial hematologic tumors, 53
  of pheochromocytoma, 154
  of pituitary adenoma, 41
Malakoplakia, 338
Mammosomatotrophs, 32–33
  hyperplasia of, 39
McCune-Albright syndrome
  adrenal tumor G protein in, 190
  mammosomatotroph hyperplasia in, 39
MCT. See Carcinoma, medullary thyroid.
MEN. See Multiple endocrine neoplasia entries.
MEN1 gene, in tumorigenesis, 229, 242, 255
MEN1 tumor suppressor mouse knockout model, and pancreatic endocrine tumors, 229
Menin, 229, 255
Meningiomas, 51
Meningitis
  dermoid cysts and, 36
  granulomatous hypophysitis and, 37
  Rathke's cleft cysts and, 35
  secondary hypophysitis and, 37
Merkel cell carcinoma (MCC), 26, 29f–30f, 297–299, 298t, 299f–302f, 301, 306
  cytogenetics of, 309
  cytokeratin in, 29f, 297, 301–303, 303f, 304t, 305t, 306
    neurofilament and, 29f, 303f, 304t, 305t, 306
  immunohistochemical features of, 26, 304t, 305t
  lymph nodes and, 306–307, 307f, 309t
  metastases of, 307–308, 308f, 309, 309t, 310
  patient survival and, 309t, 310
  prognosis of, 308–310, 309t
  treatment of, 309
  vs. lymphoma, 301
  vs. small cell lung carcinoma, 302–303, 304t, 306, 310
Mesothelioma, 348
Metergoline, for Cushing's disease, 47

Metyrapone
  cortisol synthesis and, 194
  for Cushing's disease, 47
MIB-1, and parathyroid malignancy, 122, 128
Microcarcinoma, 70
  papillary thyroid, 76
Mithramycin, and hypercalcemia medical management, 116
Mitochondria, in oxyphil cell adenomas, 123, 123f
Mitosis, and parathyroid carcinoma, 126
Mitotane
  for adrenal cortical carcinoma, 186
  for Cushing's disease, 47
Monoclonal homogeneous antibody–forming cell lines, 3
Mucosa-associated lymphoid tissue (MALT), of thyroid, 88
Mucosal neuroma syndrome. See Multiple endocrine neoplasia type II (MEN-II).
Multiple endocrine neoplasia (MEN), 40
  chief cell hyperplasia and, 112, 130
Multiple endocrine neoplasia type I (MEN-I), 40, 112, 215, 231, 254–255
  gastric carcinoid tumors and, 214f, 215–216, 247–248
  genetic mutation and, 242, 255
  menin and, 229, 255
  pancreatic disease in, 205, 216f
  pancreatic endocrine tumorigenesis in, 229
  pancreatic somatostatinomas with, 249
  pancreatic tumors with, 14, 210, 210t, 213f, 215, 216f, 220, 249. See also *MEN1* tumor suppressor mouse knockout model.
  parathyroid and, 15–16, 115, 215
  parathyroidectomy and, 115
  pituitary adenoma with, 40, 231
  treatment of, 231
  vs. von Hippel–Lindau disease, 217–218
  Zollinger-Ellison syndrome with, 212, 213f, 215, 216, 247–249
Multiple endocrine neoplasia type II (MEN-II), 112–113
  adrenal medullary hyperplasia with, 153, 153f, 156f
  medullary thyroid carcinoma in, 13, 81–82, 113
  ovarian strumal carcinoid and, 317
  pheochromocytoma in, 13, 155, 156f
Myelolipoma, adrenal, 190–191, 191f

N
Nebenkern formations, 45
Nelson's syndrome, 47
  vs. Leydig cell tumors, 338
Neoplasia. See also Multiple endocrine neoplasia (MEN) entries; Tumor(s); Tumorigenesis, neuroendocrine; Von Hippel–Lindau (VHL) disease.
  neuroendocrine, 272–273
  nitrosamines and, 274–275
  paraganglia and, 152
Nesidioblastosis, 227–228, 228f
  multiple endocrine neoplasia type I and, 215, 216f
Neural cell adhesion molecule (NCAM), 11, 247
  in differential diagnosis, 19t, 158t
  in infantile pulmonary neuroendocrine cells, 263
  in neuroendocrine differentiation, 276
Neuroblastoma, 163–165, 164f
  catecholamines and, 165
  classification of, 165
  disorders associated with, 166
  ganglioneuroma from, 166
  incidence of, 166

Neuroblastoma *(Continued)*
  molecular pathogenesis and, 165–166
  ovarian metastases of, 326
  prognostic indicators for, 165
  regression of, 166
Neuroendocrine cells, 11, 151
  bronchiolitis obliterans and, 270
  differentiation
    clinical behavior and, 279
    tumor diagnosis and, 275–276
  gut. *See* Enterochromaffin cells.
  histochemistry and, 11
  pulmonary, 261–262, 262f, 264. *See also*
    Pulmonary neuroendocrine cells
    (PNECs).
  secretory expression by, 151–152
Neuroendocrine markers, 11, 19t, 265–266,
  266t. *See also* Tumor markers.
  in pulmonary localization, 265, 266t, 267f
  in tumor diagnosis, 275–276
Neuroepithelial bodies (NEBs), 261, 264–266,
  265f, 267f, 268f. *See also* Pulmonary
    neuroendocrine cells (PNECs).
  chemoreception by, 266–267
  ultrastructure of, 265, 265f–266f
Neuroepithelial tumors, peripheral, 26. *See
  also* Tumor(s), ovarian epithelial, with
    neuroendocrine differentiation.
Neurofibromatosis. *See* Von Recklinghausen's
  disease.
Neurohypophysis, 34
Neurohypophysitis, infundibular, 36
Neurolemmomas, 51–52
Neuron-specific enolase (NSE), 11, 222
  carcinoids and, 314, 316
  developmental pulmonary neuroendocrine
    cells and, 261
  in differential diagnosis, 19t, 158t
  in neuroendocrine differentiation, 261, 266t,
    276
  in pancreatic endocrine tumors, 222, 222f
Neurotensin, pancreatic endocrine tumors
  and, 215
  malignancy and, 211
Neurotransmitters, 1
Neutral endopeptidase (NEP), 269
NH (neonatal hyperparathyroidism), 117–118
Nicotine, and tumorigenesis, 274–275
Nitric oxide synthase, and diabetic placentas,
  357–358
Nitrosamines, and neoplasia, 274–275
N-*myc* oncogene, and neuroblastoma
  prognosis, 165, 166
Non-Hodgkin's lymphoma
  intracranial, 53
  testicular, 348f
Norepinephrine, 1
  adrenal medullary hyperplasia and, 153
  neuroblastoma prognosis and, 165
  pancreatic endocrine tumors and, 214
  parasympathetic paraganglia and, 152
  pheochromocytoma and, 154

O

Octreotide, 230–231, 256
  cholelithiasis and, 256
  for carcinoid syndrome, 231, 256
  for pancreatic endocrine tumors, 230–231
  for somatostatinoma detection, 218–219,
    219f, 249–250
  gonadotroph adenomas and, 48
Oil red O fat stain, 110, 110f
Omeprazole
  for hyperchlorhydria, 213
  for Zollinger-Ellison syndrome, 213, 231
  hypergastrinemia and, 249
Oncocytoma, 49, 49f
  adrenal, 190, 190f

Organs of Zuckerkandl, 150, 150f
  size of, 151
Osteosarcoma, and Sertoli-Leydig cell tumor,
  339, 340
Ovarian cancer. *See also* Carcinoid(s), insular;
  Carcinoid(s), ovarian; Carcinoma, small
  cell ovarian.
  CA 125 and, 7, 8
  β-human chorionic gonadotropin and, 8
  urinary gonadotropin peptide and, 9
Ovarian thecal metaplasia, 191
Oxytocin, 34

P

p53 protein, 254
  goblet cell carcinoid tumors and, 253
  ovarian small cell carcinoma and, 321
  parathyroid adenomas and, 122
  parathyroid carcinoma and, 122, 128
Pancreas, 205, 206–207, 206f
  developmental, 205–206
  histologic sampling of, 219–220
Pancreatic endocrine tumor(s), 14, 209–211,
  209t, 210f, 210t, 220, 223f, 225f. *See also*
    Vasoactive intestinal peptide *entries;*
    Zollinger-Ellison syndrome (ZE, ZES).
  animal models of, 228–229
  chromogranin A and, 211
  classification of, 209t, 211
  differential diagnosis of, 226
  distribution of, 220
  ectopic hormone secretion and, 14, 209t,
    214
  gastrinoma as, 14–16, 212, 213, 213f. *See
    also* Gastrinoma.
  genetic alteration and, 229–230
  glucagonoma as, 14–15, 212, 212f, 225f
    diabetes mellitus from, 14
  histology of, 220–222, 221f
  immunohistochemistry of, 222–224,
    222f–223f
  insulinoma as, 14, 17f, 211, 212f, 225f
    frequency of, 209
    multiple endocrine neoplasia type I and,
      215
  malignancy of, 14, 210, 211, 214, 224, 225f,
    226
  medical treatment of, 230–231
  multiple endocrine neoplasia type I and,
    14, 205, 210, 210t, 213f, 215, 220
  nonfunctioning, 214–215
  radiology and, 218–219, 219f
  somatostatinoma as, 16, 18f, 212, 225f. *See
    also* Somatostatinoma(s).
  surgery and, 230, 230f, 231
  ultrastructural analysis of, 224, 225f
  von Hippel–Lindau disease and, 210, 210t,
    215, 216–218, 217f, 220
Pancreatic islet cell tumors. *See* Pancreatic
  endocrine tumor(s).
Pancreatic polypeptide (PP), 19t
  from islets of Langerhans, 207t, 208–209,
    208f
  pancreatic endocrine tumors and, 209t,
    215
  malignancy of, 209t, 211
Paracrine hormonal systems, 1
Paraganglia, 149
  cytologic maturation of, 150
  glossopharyngeal, 150, 151f
  histology of, 151
  hyperplasia and, 152, 154. *See also* Adrenal
    medulla, hyperplasia of.
  neoplasia and, 152
  parasympathetic, 150–151, 151f, 152
  physiology of, 151–152
  sympathetic, 149, 150, 150f, 152
  vagal, 150, 151f

Paraganglioma, 152
  aorticopulmonary, 162
  carotid body, 161, 161f
    malignancy of, 161
  cauda equina, 152, 160–161
  cytoskeletal proteins and, 152
  jugulotympanic, 161–162
  laryngeal, 162
  of neck, 162
  orbital, 162
  parasympathetic, 161, 163f
    cytology of, 162–163
  paravertebral, 160
  pulmonary, 162
  sympathetic, 159–160, 160f, 160t
    hyperplasia in, incidence of, 154
    malignancy and, 160, 161
  thyroid, 83–84
  urinary bladder, 160
  vagal, 162
Paraganglioma-like adenoma of thyroid
  (PLAT), 68–69, 69f
Paraquat poisoning, and adrenal cortex, 194
Parathyroid, 103, 104f–106f. *See also*
  Adenoma(s), parathyroid; Parathyroid
  hyperplasia.
  amyloid and, 105
  anatomy of, 104–105, 106–107
  cell ratios of, 104
  density gradients of, 110–111
  DNA cytometry of, 111
  histochemistry of, 105–106
  histologic sampling of, 108–110, 110f
    chief cells in, 110
  innervation of, 104
  multiple endocrine neoplasia type I and,
    115, 215
  normocalcemic hypercellularity in, 136
  secondary malignancy in, 136
  variable location of, 103–104
  vasculature for, 104
Parathyroid cysts, 135–136
  fine-needle aspiration of, 109
Parathyroid hormone (PTH), 107–108
  bone resorption and, 107
  hypoparathyroidism and, 133
  pancreatic endocrine tumors and, 209t, 214
    malignancy of, 209t, 211
Parathyroid hormone–related peptide (PTH-
  RP, PTHrP), 8, 108
  pancreatic endocrine tumors and, 209t, 214
Parathyroid hyperplasia, 130f, 131f. *See also*
  Parathyroid, normocalcemic
  hypercellularity in.
  adenoma and, 113, 118, 121–123, 131, 132
  adenomatous, 131, 131f
  chief cell, 130–132, 130f, 131f
    hyperparathyroidism and, 112, 113, 130
    tertiary hyperparathyroidism and, 132
  intrathyroidal, 130, 130f
  multiple endocrine neoplasia and, 112, 130
  severity of, glandular size and, 132
  treatment of, 115
Parathyroidectomy
  for hyperparathyroidism, 115
  hypoparathyroidism and, 133
Parathyroiditis, chronic, 134f, 135
Parathyroma, 132
Parathyromatosis, 115, 131–132
Pars distalis, 31, 32f
Pars intermedia, 33–34
Pars tuberalis, 34
PDNEC-SC. *See* Poorly differentiated
  neuroendocrine carcinoma of lung, small
  cell (PDNEC-SC).
Peutz-Jeghers syndrome, and Sertoli cell
  tumors, 329, 330, 332, 333, 3
PGP 9.5 (protein gene product 9.5), 223
  pulmonary neuroendocrine cells and,
    266t

Phenylethanolamine *N*-methyltransferase
    (PNMT), 152
Phenytoin, and steroid metabolism, 194
Pheochromocytoma, 13–14, 16f, 152, 154–155,
    155f
  detection of, 154
  ectopic adrenocorticotropic hormone
      secretion and, 181
  frequency of, 154
  hemorrhage and, 154, 157
  histology of, 156–157, 156f–158f
  hypertension and, 154
  malignancy and, 158, 159f, 159t, 161
  medullary carcinoma of thyroid with, 13
  molecular abnormalities and, 158–159
  secretory activity of, 13, 16f, 154
  vs. adrenal cortical carcinoma, 189
  vs. adrenal cortical oncocytoma, 157, 158t
  vs. adrenal medullary hyperplasia,
      153–154, 156f
Phosphate binders, for secondary
    hyperparathyroidism, 116
PHP (primary hyperparathyroidism),
    111–116, 114f, 114t. *See also*
    Hyperparathyroidism.
Pit-1 deficiency, and pituitary hormone
    deficiency, 31
Pituitary, 31–32, 32f
  arterial supply for, 34
  histologic sampling of, 34
  hyperplasia of, 39, 39f. *See also*
      Adenoma(s), pituitary.
  hypoplasia of, 34–35
  inflammatory processes and, 36–38
  metabolic disorders of, 39
  metastatic tumors of, 54
  multiple endocrine neoplasia type I and,
      40, 215
Pituitary apoplexy, 38, 38f
  treatment of, 38
Pituitary hormone deficiency, Pit-1 deficiency
    in, 31
Pituitary infarction, 38
Placenta, 351–352, 353
  fetal growth retardation and, 357
  thyroid disorders and, 358
  twin pregnancy and, 356
Placental site, exaggerated, 355
Placental site nodule, 355
Placental site trophoblastic tumor, 355, 356f
Pneumocystis carinii
  secondary hypophysitis and, 38
  thyroiditis and, 65
Polyendocrine autoimmune syndrome, 134
Pompe's disease, 137
Poorly differentiated endocrine pancreatic
    carcinoma, small cell type, 226–227,
    226f
Poorly differentiated neuroendocrine
    carcinoma, with adenoma, 253, 253f
Poorly differentiated neuroendocrine
    carcinoma of lung. *See also* Carcinoma,
    small cell lung.
  combined (PDNEC-C), 287, 291f
  large cell (PDNEC-LC), 279, 286–287, 288f,
      289f–290f
    classification algorithm and, 278t
    prognosis of, 287, 291
    vs. moderately differentiated carcinoma,
        286–287
  mixed small cell/large cell (PDNEC-SC/LC),
      279, 285–286, 287, 289f
  small cell (PDNEC-SC), 267f, 284–285,
      285f–288f, 287
    adenocarcinoma with, 287, 291f. *See also*
        Poorly differentiated neuroendocrine
        carcinoma, with adenoma.
    classification and, 276t, 279
    vs. moderately differentiated neoplasm,
        283

Poorly differentiated neuroendocrine
    carcinoma of lung *(Continued)*
  vs. tumorlets, 273f
  vs. well-differentiated neoplasm, 283f
PP. *See* Pancreatic polypeptide (PP).
Preeclampsia, 357
Pregnancy. *See also* Sheehan's syndrome.
  corticotropin-releasing hormone in, 354
  diabetes mellitus and, 357–358
  ectopic, 356
  estrogens and, 354
  human chorionic gonadotropin in, 353
  human placental lactogen in, 353
  lactotroph hyperplasia and, 39
  lymphocytic hypophysitis and, 36
  pituitary mass and, 31
  progesterone in, 354
  thyroid disease and, 358
Pregnancy-associated placental proteins,
    352–353
Pregnancy-induced hypertension (PIH), 357
Primary pigmented nodular adrenocortical
    disease, 181–182, 182f
Progesterone, 174f
  in ectopic pregnancy, 356
  in pregnancy, 354
Prohormone convertases (PCs), 11, 14f
Prolactin (PRL)
  human chorionic gonadotropin and, 353
  lactotroph adenomas and, 44
  parathyroid hormone and, 107
  pituitary adenomas and, 42t
Proliferating cell nuclear antigen (PCNA)
  pancreatic endocrine tumors and, 226
  secretin cells and, 239
Prostaglandins, 1
Prostate-specific antigen (PSA), 7
  in neuroendocrine prostatic carcinoma, 25f
Psammoma bodies, 70, 249f
Pseudocarcinoid syndrome, 257
Pseudohypoparathyroidism, 135
PTC. *See* Carcinoma, papillary thyroid.
Pulmonary neuroendocrine cell hyperplasia.
      See also Pulmonary neuroendocrine cells
      (PNECs).
  diffuse idiopathic, 270, 270f
  hypertension and, 271
Pulmonary neuroendocrine cells (PNECs),
    261–262, 262f, 264, 266, 268f. *See also*
    Tumor(s), neuroendocrine.
  as pulmonary tumorlets, 268, 269f, 271,
      272f–274f
  development of, 262–263, 263f
  differentiation of
    clinical behavior and, 279
    tumor diagnosis and, 275–276
  distribution of, 264, 264f
  ectopic neuropeptide expression and,
      269–270
  fetal differentiation of, 263, 263f
    vs. neoplasia, 263–264
  immunocytochemical markers of, 265–266,
      266t, 267f
  in neoplastic lung disease, 274–275
  in non-neoplastic lung disease, 268–270,
      269f
  inflammatory disease and, 268–269, 270, 270f
  neonatal pulmonary disease and, 271
  paracrine function of, 266, 268
  pulmonary hypertension and, 271
  ultrastructure of, 265, 265f–266f

R

Radiation therapy. *See also* Radiology.
  Cushing's disease and, 47
  for germinoma, 53
  gliomas and, 51
  meningiomas and, 51

Radiation therapy *(Continued)*
  papillary thyroid carcinoma and, 73, 76
  pituitary apoplexy and, 38
  sellar region mesenchymal tumors and, 54
  thyroiditis and, 65
Radioassay, 4
Radioimmunoassay (RIA), 3–4, 3f
Radiology. *See also* Angiography;
    Arteriography; Computed tomography
    (CT); Magnetic resonance imaging (MRI);
    Somatostatin receptor scintigraphy
    (SRS).
  granulomatous hypophysitis and, 37
  hyperparathyroidism and, 114–115, 114f
    neonatal, 118
  lymphocytic hypophysitis and, 36
  pancreatic endocrine tumors and, 218–219,
      219f
Rathke's cleft cysts, 35, 35f
  secondary hypophysitis and, 37
Receiver operating characteristic (ROC)
    curve, 3
Receptor assays, 4
Refsum's disease, 177
REG1A gene, and gastric carcinoids, 255
Reidel's disease, 65, 67
  vs. anaplastic carcinoma of thyroid, 84
  vs. nodular fasciitis–like stroma variant
      thyroid carcinoma, 75
Reinke's crystalloids, 336f, 337, 337f
Renal carcinoma, versus adrenal tumors,
    158t, 188
Renal failure, and secondary
    hyperparathyroidism, 116
Renin-angiotensin system, 175
Reserpine, for Cushing's disease, 47
Retinoblastoma (Rb) protein
  parathyroid adenomas and, 122
  parathyroid carcinoma and, 128
Rifampicin, and steroid metabolism, 194

S

S-100 protein, 246
  appendiceal carcinoids and, 246
  sustentacular cell immunoreactivity and, 152
Schwannomas, 51–52
Sclerosing mucoepidermoid carcinoma with
    eosinophilia (SMECE), 86–87, 86f
  vs. Hodgkin's disease, 87
Secretory protein-1. *See* Chromogranin A
    (CGA, ChrA).
Seminoma, 332–333
  α-fetoprotein and, 8
  gonadoblastoma and, 345
  human chorionic gonadotropin and, 8
  vs. Sertoli cell tumor, 332, 332t
Sensitivity, of laboratory tests, 2, 2f
Septicemia, and adrenal insufficiency, 193,
    193f
Septo-optic dysplasia, and hypopituitarism,
    35
Serotonin (5-HT), 19t, 266t, 268
  from carcinoids of unknown primary, 247
  from midgut gastrointestinal carcinoids, 24,
      242
  in appendiceal carcinoid, 24f
  in carcinoid syndrome, 21, 209t, 242, 256
  in fetal lung development, 261, 262f
  insular carcinoids and, 314
  pancreatic endocrine tumors and, 209t
Sertoli-Leydig cell tumors
  insular carcinoids and, 313, 315
  testicular, 339–340
  vs. trabecular carcinoid, 316
Sertoli cell tumor, 329–332, 330f–332f, 330t,
    333
  cryptorchid testes and, 332
  endocrinologic anomalies and, 333

Sertoli cell tumor *(Continued)*
  gynecomastia and, 333
  large-cell calcifying variant of, 333–335
    bilateral occurrence of, 334
    Carney's syndrome and, 329, 334
    malignancy and, 340
    vs. Leydig cell tumors, 334
  malignancy and, 333, 333t
  pediatric patients and, 329
  sclerosing variant of, 335, 335f–336f
  vs. endometrioid adenocarcinoma of testis, 334–335
  vs. granulosa cell tumors, 334, 343
  vs. Leydig cell tumors, 334, 338
  vs. metastatic adenocarcinoma, 335, 340
  vs. seminoma, 332, 332t
  vs. sertoliform rete cystadenoma, 335
SETTLE (spindle epithelial tumor with thymus-like differentiation), 85
Sheehan's syndrome, 38, 38f
SHP (secondary hyperparathyroidism), 116–117
Simian virus (SV) 40
  pancreatic tumors and, 229, 255
  secretin transcription and, 239
Sipple's syndrome. *See* Multiple endocrine neoplasia type II (MEN-II).
Small cell carcinoma, 19, 23
  lung. *See* Carcinoma, small cell lung.
  ovarian. *See* Carcinoma, small cell ovarian.
  ovarian metastases of, 326
  pancreatic, 226–227, 227f
  surgical pathology and, 12, 13
SNAP-25, 11, 13f, 152
SNP. *See* Synaptophysin (SNP, SY38).
Somatomedin C. *See also* Insulin-like growth factor I (IGF-I).
  acromegaly and, 41
Somatostatin (ST), 19t, 256, 266t
  from hindgut gastrointestinal carcinoid, 242
  from islets of Langerhans, 207t, 208, 208f
  pancreatic endocrine tumors and, 18f, 209t, 212
    malignancy of, 209t, 211
Somatostatin receptor scintigraphy (SRS), 256
  gastric carcinoids and, 249
  pancreatic endocrine tumors by, 218–219, 219f
  pheochromocytoma by, 154
Somatostatinoma(s), 16, 18f, 212, 225f, 249–250, 249f
  distribution of, 220
  octreotide in detection of, 218–219, 219f, 249–250
Somatostatinoma syndrome, 209t, 212
  diabetes mellitus and, 212, 249
  von Recklinghausen's disease and, 218
Somatotrophs, 31
  hyperplasia of, 39
Specificity, of laboratory tests, 2, 2f
Spironolactone, and Conn's syndrome, 183–184, 184f
Steroidogenesis, 173–175, 174f–175f
  in pregnancy, 354
Steroids, 175
  nomenclature of, 174, 174t
Streptozotocin, for pancreatic endocrine tumor metastases, 231
Struma lymphomatosa. *See* Hashimoto's thyroiditis.
Struma ovarii, 318, 318f
Substance P, 266t
  carcinoid syndrome and, 214
  pancreatic endocrine tumors and, 214
Sudan IV fat stain, 110
Sudden death, from pituitary apoplexy, 38
Suramin, and cortisol synthesis, 194
Sustentacular cells, 151
  S-100 protein and, 152

SV40
  pancreatic tumors and, 229, 255
  secretin transcription and, 239
Synaptic vesicle, 12f
Synaptophysin (SNP, SY38), 152, 222, 247, 265–266, 266t
  carcinoids and, 314, 315f, 316
  in differential diagnosis, 158t
  in gallbladder carcinoid, 22f
  in neuroendocrine differentiation, 276
  in neuroendocrine prostatic carcinoma, 25f
  in ovarian small cell carcinoma, 321f
  in pancreatic endocrine tumors, 222, 222f
  in pancreatic islet, 13f
  in pheochromocytoma, 16f
  in secretory granules, 13f
  in type A gastritis, 20f
Syphilis
  adrenal insufficiency from, 192–193
  secondary hypophysitis and, 37
  thyroiditis and, 65

T
Target cells, 1
Tenney-Parker change, 357
Teratomas, 52, 53
  ovarian carcinoids and, 313, 314, 316, 317
Testicular tumor(s), 330t. *See also* specific *tumors.*
  epidermal cyst as, 346, 346f
  α-fetoprotein and, 8
  human chorionic gonadotropin and, 8
  mesenchymal, 345–346
  unclassified sex cord–stromal, 344–345, 344f
Testosterone, 1
THP (tertiary hyperparathyroidism), 117, 132
Thromboxanes, 1
Thymoma, intrathyroidal, 85–86, 85f
Thyroglossal duct, 61
Thyroid, 61, 62
  developmental anomalies of, 61–62
  lingual, 61
  mesenchymal tumors of, 87
  vascular tumors of, 88
Thyroid follicles, and ovarian strumal carcinoid, 317, 317f–318f
Thyroid hormone
  ligand-binding of, 6
  pregnancy and, 358
Thyroid tumorigenesis, 72–73
Thyroiditis, 65
  autoimmune. *See* Hashimoto's thyroiditis.
  chronic, 65–67
  lymphocytic, 66–67, 66f
    familial benign hypercalcemia and, 117
    fibrous variant, 66–67, 75
    Graves' disease and, 64, 66
    Hürthle cells in, 66, 79
    hyperparathyroidism and, 111
    RET/PTC oncogene and, 73
    sclerosing mucoepidermoid carcinoma and, 86, 86f, 87
    vs. papillary carcinoma, 66, 66f
    vs. Reidel's disease, 67
    vs. thyroid lymphoma, 66
    Warthin's-like carcinoma and, 75
  palpation, 65
Thyroid-stimulating hormone (TSH) assays, 6
Thyroid-stimulating hormone (TSH). *See also* Thyroid-stimulating immunoglobulins (TSIs).
  fetal concentration of, 61
  goiter and, 62–63
  pituitary adenomas and, 42t
Thyroid-stimulating immunoglobulins (TSIs), 64

Thyrotrophs, 33
  hyperplasia of, 39
  vs. thyrotroph adenoma, 46
Thyroxine, fetal concentration of, 61
Tissue fixation procedures, and pituitary samples, 34
Tobacco smoke, and tumorigenesis, 274–275
Tolbutamide, in somatostatinoma diagnosis, 212
Transcortin, 1
Transferrin, and small cell lung carcinoma, 274
Transplantation
  liver, carcinoid syndrome and, 257
  parathyroid, 115
    chronic hypoparathyroidism and, 134
    graft-induced hyperparathyroidism and, 117, 132
    secondary hyperparathyroidism and, 116, 117
Trauma
  pituitary apoplexy and, 38
  thyroiditis from, 65
Tritium (^{3}H), 4
Trophoblast cells, 351–352, 352f
Trophoblastic disease, gestational, 354
Trousseau's sign, 133
TSH. *See* Thyroid-stimulating hormone (TSH).
Tuberculosis. *See also* Pulmonary neuroendocrine cells (PNECs), in non-neoplastic lung disease.
  autoimmune adrenalitis and, 192, 192f
Tumor(s). *See also* Adenoma(s); Carcinoid(s); Carcinoma; Pancreatic endocrine tumor(s); *and other specific tumors.*
  adenomatoid, 346–347, 347f–348f
  adrenal medullary, 154
    vs. renal carcinoma, 158t
  adrenal rest, 346
  adrenocortical, 184–186, 185f
    Cushing's syndrome from, 181, 181f–182f
    immunocytochemistry of, 188–189, 188f
    malignancy and, 187–188
    mesenchymal, 190
    metastases and, 190
    ovarian thecal metaplasia as, 191
    pathogenesis of, 189–190
    staging of, 188, 188t
  adrenocorticotropic hormone–secreting biologically active hormone produced by, 6
    ectopic, 181, 214
    pancreatic endocrine tumors and, 209t, 214
  endodermal sinus, 52
    α-fetoprotein from, 53
  epithelioid trophoblast, 355–356
  fibroma-thecoma testicular, 343–344
  gastrin-producing, 212, 213, 213f–214f
    distribution of, 220
    pancreatic endocrine tumors and, 209t, 213f
    peptide production in, 6
  germ cell
    intracranial, 52–53
    testicular, 330t
  gonadal stromal, 329, 330t
    differential diagnosis and, 342
  granulosa cell, 340–342, 340f–342f
    juvenile-type, 342–343, 342f, 343t
    malignancy and, 342
    vs. insular carcinoids, 314–315
    vs. ovarian small cell carcinoma, 321–322
    vs. Sertoli cell tumor, 334, 343
  hematologic, intracranial, 53
  Hürthle, 75, 79–80. *See also* Adenoma(s), Hürthle cell; Hürthle cell tumors.
  Leydig cell, 329, 336–339, 336f–337f. *See also* Leydig cell tumor.

Tumor(s) *(Continued)*
mesenchymal
pituitary, 53–54
testicular, 345–346
mixed exocrine-endocrine pancreatic, 227
neuroblastic, 163–165, 164f–165f
catecholamines and, 165
classification of, 165
prognostic indicators for, 165
neuroendocrine, 12–13, 17, 275. *See also specific tumors.*
metastatic, 324–326, 325f
non-neuroendocrine tumors from, 275
ovarian, 313–326, 314f–318f, 323f
pulmonary, 272–273. *See also* Carcinoma, lung, neuroendocrine; Carcinoma, small cell lung.
classification of, 276–279, 276t
diagnostic algorithm for, 278t
pulmonary neuroendocrine cells and, 263–264. *See also* Pulmonary neuroendocrine cells (PNECs).
surgical pathology and, 11–13
treatment of, 257
vs. Merkel cell carcinoma, 306
neurohypophysial granular cell, 51
neuronal, 50–51, 163–165
from sympathetic paraganglia, 152, 163
of dysgenetic gonads, 345
ovarian epithelial, with neuroendocrine differentiation, 322–324
pancreatic endocrine. *See* Pancreatic endocrine tumor(s).
paraganglion, catecholamines and, 152, 165
pituitary. *See also* Adenoma(s), pituitary.
mesenchymal, 53–54
sellar region, 54
placental site trophoblastic, 355, 356f
recurrence of, circulating tumor markers and, 7
Sertoli cell, 329–332, 330f–332f, 330t, 333. *See also* Sertoli cell tumor.
solitary fibrous, 87
testicular, 330t. *See also specific tumors.*
epidermal cyst as, 346, 346f
α-fetoprotein and, 8
fibroma-thecoma, 343–344
human chorionic gonadotropin and, 8
mesenchymal, 345–346
unclassified sex cord–stromal, 344–345, 344f
thyroid, 67. *See also specific neoplasms.*
mesenchymal, 87
metastatic, 88, 88f

Tumor(s) *(Continued)*
mixed, 83
vascular, 88
vs. parathyroid carcinoma, 129
with small cell ovarian carcinoma, 319
Tumor markers, 7–9. *See also* Neuroendocrine markers.
in differential diagnosis, 158t
level of, 7
specificity and, 7
Tumorigenesis, neuroendocrine, 272–274
apoptosis and, 273
Tumorlets, 19, 20, 268, 269f, 271, 272f–274f
Tyrosine kinase receptors, and papillary thyroid carcinoma, 72–73

U
Urinary gonadotropin peptide (UGP), 8–9

V
Valvular lesions, and carcinoid syndrome, 256, 257
Vanillylmandelic acid, and neuroblastoma prognosis, 165
Vasoactive intestinal peptide (VIP)
neuronal tumor maturation and, 165
pancreatic endocrine tumors and, 16, 209t
malignancy of, 209t, 211
pulmonary inflammatory disease and, 270
pulmonary neuroendocrine cell proliferation and, 269–270
Vasoactive intestinal peptide–secreting tumor (VIPoma), 16, 209, 209t, 213–214
octreotide for, 231
Vasopressin, 34
pancreatic endocrine tumor malignancy and, 211, 214
Verner-Morrison syndrome, 209t, 213–214
VHL gene, in von Hippel–Lindau disease, 229
Vimentin, and granulosa cell tumors, 341, 341f, 342
Vitamin D
for hypoparathyroidism, 134
parathyroid hormone and, 107
secondary hyperparathyroidism and, 116
Vitamin D–binding protein, 1
Von Hippel–Lindau (VHL) disease, 216–218, 217f
adrenal medullary hyperplasia with, 153
pancreatic endocrine tumorigenesis in, 229

Von Hippel–Lindau (VHL) disease *(Continued)*
pancreatic endocrine tumors with, 210, 210t, 216–218, 217f, 220
malignancy of, 217
pheochromocytoma with, 155
treatment of, 231
VHL gene in, 229
vs. multiple endocrine neoplasia type I, 217–218
Von Recklinghausen's disease
adrenal medullary hyperplasia with, 153
duodenal somatostatinomas with, 218, 249
pancreatic endocrine tumors with, 210t, 218
pheochromocytoma with, 155

W
Warthin's-like carcinoma, of thyroid, 71f, 75
Water–clear cell hyperplasia, 105, 133
Waterhouse-Friderichsen syndrome, 193, 193f
WDHA (watery diarrhea, hypokalemia, achlorhydria) syndrome, 209t, 213–214
Wermer's syndrome. *See* Multiple endocrine neoplasia type I (MEN-I).
Wilson-Mikity syndrome, 271
Wolman's disease, 176
World Health Organization (WHO)
pancreatic endocrine tumor classification of, 211
papillary thyroid carcinoma diagnostic recognition by, 70
pulmonary neuroendocrine tumor classification of, 276t, 277, 278–279
thyroid microcarcinoma definition by, 76

Z
Zellweger's syndrome, 177
Zollinger-Ellison syndrome (ZE, ZES), 212–213, 247
Cushing's syndrome and, 214
gastric carcinoid tumors in, 213, 214f, 215, 216, 247–248
gastrinomas and, 212, 213f, 214f, 248, 249
hypergastrinemia and, 213, 247–249
lymph node metastasis in, 214, 248–249
mucinous adenocarcinoma with, 323f
multiple endocrine neoplasia type I with, 212, 213f, 215, 216, 247–249
pancreatic endocrine tumors and, 209t, 212, 213f, 214
peptide production in, 6

ISBN 0-443-06595-0